Peripheral Endovascular Interventions
Third Edition

Thomas J. Fogarty · Rodney A. White
Editors

Peripheral Endovascular Interventions

Third Edition

Springer

Editors
Thomas J. Fogarty, MD
Alpine Road 3270
Menlo Park 94028
USA

Rodney A. White, MD
Harbor-UCLA Medical Center
W. Carson St. 1000
Torrance 90509
USA

ISBN 978-1-4939-5023-2 ISBN 978-1-4419-1387-6 (eBook)
DOI 10.1007/978-1-4419-1387-6
Springer New York Dordrecht Heidelberg London

Printed on acid-free paper

Springer is part of Springer Science+Business Media (www.springer.com)

Preface to the Third Edition

It has been nearly 50 years since the original description of balloon thrombectomy catheters as the initial endovascular intervention to treat thromboembolic vascular occlusion disease. The initial description of this innovative technology by Dr. Thomas Fogarty was viewed with skepticism and rejected by many prestigious journals. The publication of this technological advance (*Surg Gynecol Obstet* 1963;116:241–244) detailed a concept that introduced the potential for endovascular therapy of vascular diseases and initiated a progression of technologic advances that have led to the current accepted role of endovascular therapy replacing many conventional surgical procedures. The adoption of Dr. Fogarty's concept, which was developed at the Good Samaritan Hospital (Cincinnati, OH) and the University of Oregon, led to a collaboration with Dr. Charles Dotter in the initial application of balloon technologies to treat occlusive lesions. The eventual impact of this concept on the evolution of balloon angioplasty for treatment of vascular occlusive disease throughout the vascular system is apparent.

Although the evolution of endovascular technologies required many years from Dr. Fogarty's original concept, the eventual trials of occlusive lesion dilation, laser angioplasty, and the eventual development of intraluminal imaging technologies such as angioscopy and ultrasound substantiated the reality that combined catheter-based therapy and improved imaging technologies could convert many of the existing open operative procedures to catheter-based therapies.

The subsequent evolution of improved noncompliant balloon dilation devices and the addition of intraluminal stents to maintain integrity of the vessel lumen not only provided advanced recannulation techniques for medium-sized vessels but also provided the fixation mechanism for intraluminal graft technologies that have evolved rapidly as a standard of practice for aortoiliac aneurysmal and occlusive disease.

The third edition of *Peripheral Endovascular Interventions* updates the current status of endovascular interventions in the treatment of vascular diseases and outlines the current challenges that remain in future development of these technologies. The text outlines the rapid development of these methods and introduces the concepts proposed by Dr. Fogarty for eventual transcutaneous therapies to enhance the exponential development that has occurred in the treatment of vascular lesions.

Thanks to Paula Callaghan and Margaret Burns of Springer for their work on this book.

Rodney A. White, MD

Preface to the Second Edition

The first edition of *Peripheral Endovascular Interventions* was developed to furnish a comprehensive review of the subject for individuals from different disciplines. It offered a thorough overview of accepted techniques and methods, as well as information needed to adapt endovascular technologies to clinical practice. Additional sections briefly discussed new concepts so that the reader was kept informed of future developments.

Since the publication of the first edition in 1996, the field has rapidly evolved and several new technical advances have occurred. The utility and utilization of imaging techniques, particularly ultrasound and spiral computed tomography, and several new devices, including endovascular prostheses, have matured. Therefore, several new chapters have been added to provide detailed discussions of these advances and provide a overview of their potential for clinical application. An additional group of new chapters addresses specific topics, including disobliteration techniques, inferior vena caval filters, brachocephalic angioplasty, tibioperioneal angioplasty, and endoscopic first rib resection. Other developing areas discussed in detail include laparoscopic aortic procedure, endoluminal radiation therapy, and carotid angioplasty and stenting. Approximately 40% of the material in this edition is new, and the entire text updated to reflect the current status of peripheral endovascular treatments.

As with the first edition, our intention is not to recommend or promote the use of endovascular methods before they are proven by appropriate clinical studies, but rather to provide a detailed assessment of potential advantages. To accomplish this goal, we have made timely production and publication of this book a priority.

Thomas J. Fogarty, MD
Rodney A. White, MD

Preface to the First Edition

Catheter-based diagnosis and treatment of vascular diseases has evolved over the last several decades, with a recent increase occurring in the utility of the therapeutic methods. This development has been stimulated by several factors including miniaturization of interventional devices and imaging technologies, and an emphasis on the utilization of minimally invasive, cost-effective treatments that reduce the economic impact of health-care delivery. As part of this evolution, the development and adaption of new interventional techniques and devices has produced a continual need for updating and training physicians in several subspecialties regarding the use of these methodologies. This requires not only adapting the technologies to current clinical practice but also establishing educational training curriculum in subspecialty fellowship programs.

Because endovascular technologies are of multispecialty interest, a review of the entire scope of fundamental information regarding each aspect of the field is required to furnish a comprehensive review that will provide specific utility for individuals from different disciplines.

For this reason, we have undertaken the development of this text to satisfy two goals. The first is to provide a broad overview of the entire range of topics for clinicians with little or no background relative to the subject matter. Second, those with some familiarity will find definitive informational material to allow adaptation of endovascular technologies to their current clinical practice.

To adequately understand and safely use catheter-based interventional therapies, knowledge of a number of topics beyond the clinical indications and techniques for applying endovascular methods is required. A thorough understanding of the pathophysiology of vascular disease, safety issues regarding interventional devices and imaging methods, and a comprehension of fundamental biomaterial concepts is needed. These topics are addressed in detail and represent relatively mature aspects of this field that are otherwise characterized by continual change in devices and techniques as the field expands.

Additional sections of the book attempt to introduce and briefly discuss new concepts that may be of utility in the future, such as endoluminal prostheses, catheter-based drug delivery systems, and percutaneous vascular sealing devices. The obvious liability in including these topics in the text is that some may not be adopted or practical for broad clinical application. In this regard, it is not our intent to recommend or promote the use of investigational endovascular methods before they are proven by appropriate clinical studies, but rather to provide a detailed assessment of potential advances. To accomplish this goal, we have made timely production and publication of this book a priority so that information presented is as current as possible.

Thomas J. Fogarty, MD
Rodney A. White, MD

Contents

Contributors

David E. Allie, MD Chief, Cardiothoracic and Endovascular Surgery, Cardiovascular Institute of the South, Lafayette, LA, USA.

Frank R. Arko, MD Chief, Endovascular Surgery; Associate Professor, Division of Vascular and Endovascular Surgery, Department of Surgery, University of Texas Southwestern Medical Center, Dallas, TX, USA.

Enrico Ascher, MD Director, Division of Vascular Surgery, Department of Surgery, Maimonides Medical Center, New York, NY, USA.

Martin R. Back, MD Associate Professor, Division of Vascular and Endovascular Surgery, Department of Surgery, University of South Florida Health, Tampa, FL, USA.

John J. Bergan, MD, FACS, FACPh, Hon. FRCS (Eng.) Founder, Vein Institute of La Jolla, La Jolla, CA, USA.

Jean Bismuth, MD Assistant Professor, Cardiovascular Surgery Associates, The Methodist Hospital, Houston, TX, USA.

Amitava Biswas, MD Fellow, Department of Surgery, Stanford University Medical Center, Stanford, CA, USA.

Nisha Bunke, MD Fellow, Vein Institute of La Jolla, La Jolla, CA; Clinical Instructor, Department of Surgery, San Diego School of Medicine, University of California, San Diego, CA, USA.

Allison B. Burkett, MD Attending Physician, Department of Vascular Surgery, Atlanta Medical Center, Atlanta, GA, USA.

Tony Chan, MD Resident, Department of Surgery, Harbor-UCLA Medical Center and UCLA School of Medicine, Torrance, CA, USA.

Rabih A. Chaer, MD Assistant Professor, Division of Vascular Surgery, Department of Surgery, The University of Pittsburgh School of Medicine, Pittsburgh, PA, USA.

Joe P. Chauvapun, MD Staff Surgeon, Department of Surgery, Harbor-UCLA Medical Center, Torrance, CA, USA.

Stephen W.K. Cheng, MBBS, MS, FRCS Professor, Department of Surgery, Chief, Division of Vascular Surgery, Queen Mary Hospital, The University of Hong Kong, Hong Kong, China.

G. Patrick Clagett, MD Chairman, Division of Vascular and Endovascular Surgery, Department of Surgery, University of Texas Southwestern Medical Center, Dallas, TX, USA.

Michael C. Dalsing, MD E. Dale and Susan E. Habegger Professor of Surgery, Director of Vascular Surgery, Section of Vascular Surgery, Department of Surgery, Indiana University School of Medicine, Indianapolis, IN, USA.

Christian de Virgilio, MD, FACS Professor, Department of Vascular Surgery, Harbor-UCLA Medical Center and UCLA School of Medicine, Torrance, CA, USA.

Jean-Paul P.M. de Vries, MD, PhD Vascular Surgeon, Department of Vascular Surgery, St. Antonius Hospital, Nieuwegein, The Netherlands.

Wouter J.M. Derksen, MD Surgical Resident, Experimental Cardiology Laboratory, Department of Vascular Surgery, University Medical Center Utrecht, Utrecht, The Netherlands.

Edward Diethrich, MD Medical Director, Arizona Heart Institute and Arizona Heart Hospital, Phoenix, AZ, USA.

Jacques E. Dion, MD Professor and Director, Interventional Neuroradiology, Department of Radiology, Emory University Hospital, Atlanta, GA, USA.

Yves-Marie Dion, MD, MSc, FRCSC, FACS Professor, Department of Surgery, Hôpital St-François d'Assise and Lavel University, Quebec City, Canada.

Tony D. Fang, MD Attending Physician, Division of Vascular Surgery, Southern California Permanente Medical Group, Irvine, CA, USA.

Thomas J. Fogarty, MD Adjunct Clinical Professor, Department of Surgery, Stanford University Medical Center, Stanford, CA, USA.

Angela M. Gerhardinger, BSN, RN Endovascular Case Manager, Department of Minimally Invasive Vascular Surgery, St. Vincent Mercy Medical Center, Toledo, OH, USA.

Seymour Glagov, MD Professor Emeritus of Pathology and Surgery, Department of Pathology, The University of Chicago, Chicago, IL, USA.

Anil Hingorani, MD Attending Physician, Division of Vascular Surgery, Department of Surgery, Maimonides Medical Center, New York, NY, USA.

Melissa E. Hogg, MD Resident, Department of Surgery, Northwestern University Feinberg School of Medicine, Chicago, IL, USA.

Agostino Ingraldi, MD Cardiologist, Cardiovascular Institute of the South, Lafayette, LA, USA.

Thomas Joseph, MBBS, MS, FRCS(Glasgow), FRCS(Gen. Surg) Attending, Department of General and Vascular Surgery, North Cumbria University Hospitals, Cumberland Infirmary, Carlisle, Cumbria, United Kingdom.

Clinton Z. Kakazu, MD Attending Physician, Department of Anesthesiology, Harbor/UCLA Medical Center, Torrance, CA, USA.

Christof Karmonik, PhD Research Scientist, Department of Radiology, Methodist Hospital Research Institute, Houston, TX, USA.

Arash Keyhani, DO Fellow, Department of Vascular Surgery, Harbour-UCLA Medical Center, Torrance, CA, USA.

Ali Khoynezhad, MD, PhD, FACS Associate Professor, Director of Aortic and Arrhythmia Surgery, Division of Cardiothoracic and Vascular Surgery, Department of Surgery, Creighton University Medical Center, Omaha, NE, USA.

Melina R. Kibbe, MD, RVT, PVI Associate Professor, Division of Vascular Surgery, Department of Surgery, Northwestern University Feinberg School of Medicine, Chicago, IL, USA, E-mail: mkibbe@nmh.org.

Neal Kleiman, MD Director, Cardiac Catheterization Laboratories, The Methodist DeBakey Heart and Vascular Center; Professor, Department of Medicine, Weill Cornell Medical College; Department of Cardiology, The Methodist Hospital, Houston, TX, USA.

Paul V. Kochupura, MD Fellow, Department of Vascular Surgery, Atlanta Medical Center, Atlanta, GA, USA.

George E. Kopchok, BS Director, Vascular Surgery Research Laboratory, Department of Vascular Surgery, Los Angeles Biomedical Research Institute, Harbor-UCLA Medical Center, Torrance, CA, USA.

Christopher J. Kwolek, MD Associate Visiting Professor, Program Director, Division of Vascular and Endovascular Surgery, Department of Surgery, Harvard Medical School, Massachusetts General Hospital, Boston, MA, USA.

Maurice Lippmann, MD Professor, Department of Anesthesiology, Harbor/UCLA Medical Center, Torrance, CA USA.

G. Matthew Longo, MD Assistant Professor, Section of Vascular Surgery, Department of Surgery, University of Nebraska Medical Center, Omaha, NE, USA.

Alan B. Lumsden, MD Chairman and Professor, Cardiovascular Surgery Associates, The Methodist Hospital, Houston, TX, USA.

Lucian M. Maidan, MD Fellow, Department of Radiology, Division of Interventional Neuroradiology, Emory University Hospital, Atlanta, GA, USA.

Natalie Marks, MD, RVT Technical Director, Division of Vascular Surgery, Vascular Laboratory, The Vascular Institute of New York, Maimonides Medical Center, New York, NY, USA.

Bernardo D. Martinez, MD, FACS, HECBC Vascular Surgeon, Department of Vascular Surgery, The Toledo Hospital, Toledo, OH, USA.

Richard N. Messersmith, MD, FACR Section Director, Interventional Radiology, Department of Radiology, Advocate Lutheran General Hospital, Park Ridge, IL, USA.

Arnold Miller, MD Attending Vascular Surgeon, Department of Surgery, MetroWest Medical Center, Natick, MA, USA.

Elena V. Mitran, MD, PhD Research Scientist, Cardiovascular Institute of the South, Lafayette, LA, USA.

Frans L. Moll, MD, PhD Professor, Department of Vascular Surgery, University Medical Center Utrecht, Utrecht, The Netherlands.

Erin H. Murphy, MD Postdoctoral Fellow, Department of Vascular Surgery, Stanford University Medical Center, Dallas, TX, USA.

Gerard Pasterkamp, MD, PhD Professor, Experimental Cardiology Laboratory, University Medical Center Utrecht, Utrecht, The Netherlands.

Rajendra Patel, MD Fellow, Division of Vascular and Endovascular Surgery, Department of Surgery, Harvard Medical School, Massachusetts General Hospital, Boston, MA, USA.

Raghotham R. Patlola, MD Cardiologist, Cardiovascular Institute of the South, Lafayette, LA, USA.

Adrienne L. Rochier, MD Postdoctoral Associate, Department of Vascular Surgery, Yale University School of Medicine, New Haven, CT, USA.

David Rosenthal, MD Chief, Department of Vascular Surgery, Atlanta Medical Center, Atlanta, GA, USA.

Constance Ryjewski, MSN, APRN Manager, Department of Surgery, Cardiovascular Risk Reduction Center, Advocate Lutheran General Hospital, Park Ridge, IL, USA.

Juha P. Salenius, MD, MBA Chief of Vascular Surgery, Department of Surgery, University Hospital, Tampere, Finland.

Alan P. Sawchuk, MD Professor, Section of Vascular Surgery, Department of Surgery, Indiana University School of Medicine, Indianapolis, IN, USA.

Peter A. Schneider, MD Chief, Division of Vascular Therapy, Hawaii Permanante Medical Group, Honolulu, HI, USA.

Shoaib Shafique, MD, FACS, FRCSC Attending Physician, Department of Vascular Surgery, St. Anthony Hospital, Oklahoma City, OK, USA.

Kevin M. Sheridan, MD Fellow, Section of Vascular Surgery, Department of Surgery, Indiana University School of Medicine, Indianapolis, IN, USA.

Gregorio Sicard, MD, FACS Eugene M. Bricker Professor, Surgery; Division Head of General Surgery; Section Head of Vascular Surgery; Vice Chairman, Department of Surgery, Washington University School of Medicine, St. Louis, MO, USA.

Inderjeet Singh Julka, MD, MBBS Associate Professor, Department of Anesthesiology, Harbor/UCLA Medical Center, Torrance, CA, USA.

Stephen T. Smith, MD Assistant Professor, Division of Vascular & Endovascular Surgery, Department of Surgery, University of Texas Southwestern Medical Center, Dallas, TX, USA.

Bauer E. Sumpio, MD, PhD Professor and Chief, Department of Vascular Surgery, Yale University School of Medicine, New Haven, CT, USA.

Bradley Thomas, MD Fellow, Division of Vascular Surgery, Department of Surgery, Washington University in St. Louis, St. Louis, MO, USA.

Miguel Valderrábano, MD, FACC Associate Professor, Department of Medicine, Weill Cornell Medical College; Director, Division of Electrophysiology, Department of Cardiology, The Methodist Hospital, Houston, TX, USA.

Ashley K. Vavra, MD Resident, Department of Surgery, Northwestern University Feinberg School of Medicine, Chicago, IL, USA.

William Veale, MD Fellow, Department of Vascular Surgery, Atlanta Medical Center, Atlanta, GA, USA.

Craig M. Walker, MD Interventionist, Cardiovascular Institute of the South, Lafayette, LA, USA.

Irwin Walot, MD, MS, M. Engr Professor, Department of Radiology, Harbor-UCLA Medical Center, Torrance, CA, USA.

Eric D. Wellons, MD Attending Physician, Department of Vascular Surgery, Atlanta Medical Center, Atlanta, GA, USA.

John V. White, MD, FACS Clinical Professor, Department of Surgery, University of Illinois, Chicago School of Medicine; Chairman, Department of Surgery, Advocate Lutheran General Hospital, Park Ridge, IL, USA.

Rodney A. White, MD Associate Chair; Chief, Vascular Surgery, Los Angeles County Harbor-UCLA Medical Center, Torrance, CA, USA.

Chengpei Xu, MD Senior Research Scientist, Department of Surgery, Stanford University School of Medicine, Stanford, CA, USA.

Christopher K. Zarins, MD Professor, Department of Surgery, Stanford University School of Medicine, Stanford, CA, USA.

Part I

Introduction

1 Evolution of Endovascular Therapy: Diagnostics and Therapeutics

Thomas J. Fogarty and Amitava Biswas

Interest in the workings of the circulation goes back to the ancient Greeks: Hippocrates and Galen both wrote about their findings in the heart and blood vessels. The pulmonary circulation was first described by an Arab physician, Ibn Al-Nafiis, in 1230, and no less a figure than Leonardo da Vinci had a keen interest in the hydrodynamic properties of blood. However, it was Harvey's description of the circulation in 1628 that truly marked the beginnings of our modern understanding of the vasculature. Since then, great strides have been made in our understanding of vascular disease, leading to the development of endovascular methods for both diagnosis and treatment [1].

Although endovascular therapy, the manipulation of pathology by an intraluminal approach, is a relatively recent concept, it has a rich history. The history of endovascular therapy can be divided into two 30-year periods. The first 30 years, from about 1929 to 1959, was an era of diagnostics, during which a number of cardiac and vascular diagnostic procedures were rapidly developed (Table 1.1). The second 30 years, from 1960 to the present, can be considered the era of therapeutics, which saw the development of interventional modalities such as embolectomy, angioplasty, and atherectomy (Table 1.2). Although many investigators were involved in the conception, design, and implementation of various diagnostic and therapeutic innovations, a number of individuals and events stand out as pivotal in significantly advancing the field as a whole and in bringing endovascular therapy to the point at which it is today. It is interesting to note the multidisciplinary nature of the advances that have been made in this evolution; the joint participation of cardiologists, surgeons, and radiologists has been critical to the evolution of the current technology of endovascular therapy. From a developmental standpoint, this is a field to which no one discipline can lay sole claim.

Table 1.1 Partial list of significant developments in endovascular diagnostics

Developer	Year	Instrument	Use
Dos Santos	1929	Needle	Visualization
Forssmann	1929	Coax catheter	Physiologic
Cournand	1941	Coax catheter	Clinical diagnosis
Seldinger	1953	Guide	Percutaneous access
Sones	1959	Coax catheter	Coronary visualization

Table 1.2 Partial list of noteworthy contributions to endovascular therapeutics

Developer	Year	Instrument	Use
Fogarty	1963	Coax balloon	Removal
Dotter	1964	Coax catheter	Dilate
Grüntzig	1974	Coax balloon	Dilate
Palmaz	1984	Stent	Stent
Simpson	1985	Coax cutter	Removal
Parodi	1990	Stent/graft	Graft

First 30 Years: Era of Diagnostics (1929–1959)

Roentgen's discovery of X-ray images of bones in 1895 set off a flurry of medical activity, with physicians seeking ever more ways to use the new

T.J. Fogarty (✉)
Adjunct Clinical Professor, Department of Surgery, Stanford University Medical Center, Stanford, CA, USA

T.J. Fogarty, R.A. White (eds.), *Peripheral Endovascular Interventions*,
DOI 10.1007/978-1-4419-1387-6_1, © Springer Science+Business Media, LLC 1998, 2010

technology. Angiograms of cadavers were taken as early as 1896 and experiments to elucidate the vasculature of live animals were attempted shortly thereafter. In both these cases, as well as in early attempts to visualize the extremities of living patients, the limiting factor proved to be the lack of a suitably nontoxic contrast agent. In 1927 the Portuguese neurologist Egas Moniz finally succeeded in using a 22% sodium iodide solution to visualize the cerebral circulation [2].

Arteriography—Dos Santos

Moniz's colleague and countryman, the surgeon Renaldo Dos Santos (Fig. 1.1), felt that Moniz's technique would be well applied to the extremities. With his associates, Augusto Lamas and Jose Pereira Caldas, Dos Santos seized on Moniz's breakthrough to develop arteriography and aortography [3]. Using these new techniques, they were able not only to demonstrate arterial conditions such as atherosclerosis, aneurysms, and ischemic paralysis but also to look at vessel changes in osteomyelitis and tumors. Dos Santos and his group were able to see atheromatous plaques, obstructions, irregular contours of vessels, and collaterals. In their 1931 book, they published 100 peripheral arteriograms and 300 lumbar aortograms, encompassing pathologic findings in various inflammatory conditions and tumors [1]. This work paved the way for the future development of vascular visualization.

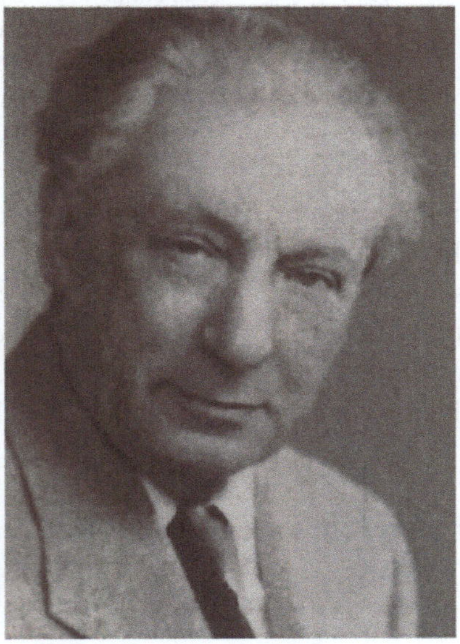

Fig. 1.1 Renaldo Dos Santos, MD, pioneer surgeon and original developer of diagnostic arterial visualization techniques and technologies

Cardiac Catheterization—Forssmann and Cournand

At the same time that Dos Santos was beginning his pioneering work in the peripheral vasculature, Werner Forssmann, a surgical intern in Berlin just out of medical school (Fig. 1.2), was about to conduct another landmark experiment. Until this time, physicians had been very wary of trying to access the heart directly. However, Forssmann felt that it should be possible to insert a catheter into the right side of the heart through a venous channel and thereby monitor cardiac pressures, obtain blood for analysis, and administer therapeutic agents. His superiors flatly refused to allow him to attempt this experiment in any patient, including himself. However, he persisted, and in 1929, working behind a screen where no one

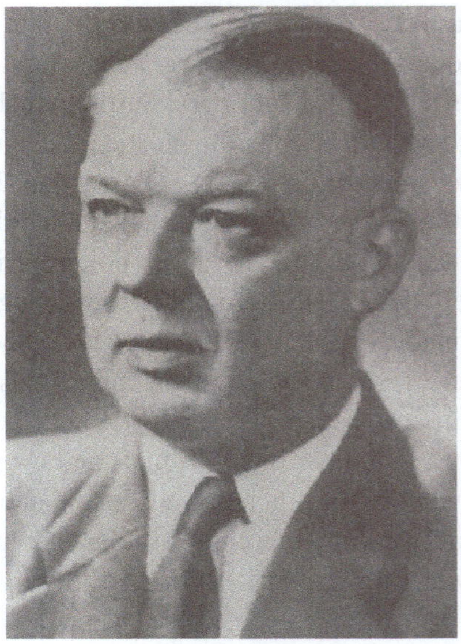

Fig. 1.2 Werner Forssmann, MD, physician credited with developing endovascular diagnostics by courageously demonstrating the potential for cardiac assessment using catheter technology

could see him, he inserted a ureteral catheter into his own basilar vein. After fighting off another physician who wanted to remove the catheter, Forssmann proceeded to advance the catheter into his right ventricle by watching the reflection of his fluoroscopic image in a mirror. This experiment constituted the first use of a cardiac catheter in a living human, and it marked a turning point in the development of endovascular diagnosis.

It was to be another decade before the potential of Forssmann's experiment would be realized. It was not until 1941, when Andre Cournand began his landmark work in cardiopulmonary physiology [4], that the power of cardiac catheterization became apparent. Cournand was able to refine the design of the catheter, adding curved ends to lessen trauma and incorporating double lumens to measure two cavities at once. However, his major contribution was not the instruments he used but what he did with them. He and his colleagues were able to take pressure readings in the right heart, determine blood volumes using dye techniques, catheterize the pulmonary artery, and determine changes in cardiac output in response to physical activity [5]. All of these procedures could now be accomplished without significant harm to the patient, demonstrating the practical utility of a catheter-based technology. For his efforts, Cournand was awarded the 1956 Nobel Prize in physiology or medicine, which he shared with Dickinson Richards and, at Cournand's insistence, Werner Forssmann.

Vascular Access—Seldinger

Vascular access remained a problem at this time. To get an artery for catheter placement or contrast injection, one had to either make a surgical cutdown of the area or insert the catheter percutaneously through a large-bore needle. Both methods left something to be desired. A cutdown was time consuming. Catheterizing through a needle required a hole larger than the catheter, which carried the risk of perivascular bleeding. The problem was solved in 1953 by a Swedish radiologist, Sven Ivar Seldinger. His breakthrough was to insert a flexible guidewire through a relatively small-bore needle and then remove the needle, leaving the wire in place. Subsequently, a larger catheter could be inserted over the guidewire [6]. The Seldinger technique allowed the passage of a catheter through a hole smaller than itself. This method, which continues to be used today for venous and arterial cannulation, was a significant developmental advance in endovascular therapy.

Coronary Angiography—Sones

The next major step in vascular visualization was accomplished by a cardiologist, F. Mason Sones. In 1958, Sones and his colleagues were already performing left heart catheterization through a femoral or brachial access site. Sones was interested in visualizing the coronary arteries, but he found that placement of contrast medium at the ascending aorta—or even into the sinus of Valsalva near the orifice of the coronary arteries—was unsatisfactory. Then one day as he was performing a left ventriculogram, he paused for a cigarette and history was made [7]. The catheter tip slipped into the right coronary artery, giving an excellent picture of the vessel and its branches, and sent the patient into asystole. In the absence of a defibrillator, the patient's forceful cough came in time to avoid disaster. However, the development of direct-current countershock made the procedure more feasible. Sones designed a tapered woven catheter that allowed him direct access to the coronary arteries, and in 1962 he published a landmark collection of coronary arterial images taken in 1,020 patients [8].

Other Diagnostic Modalities

Since the early days of vascular imaging, many new and exciting techniques have emerged, and the field continues to grow. Intravascular ultrasound—the invasive use of ultrasound to generate high-resolution images of vessels, ducts, or organs—began in the 1950 s with research directed toward measuring and recording cardiac motion. The application of ultrasound technology to the peripheral vasculature occurred shortly thereafter. To date, intravascular ultrasound has been used in conjunction with atherectomy and with both balloon and laser angioplasty. At present, research is continuing to find ways to use ultrasound to take advantage of the density differentials in calcified plaques to provide better guidance for therapeutic procedures.

Angioscopy has failed to reach its potential. Clearing the field of blood with saline flush proved difficult, unreliable and time consuming. Volume overload related to the saline flush often resulted in congestive heart failure.

Other diagnostic modalities that have been developed in recent years include radionuclide scanning and the vascular application of computed tomography (CT) and magnetic resonance imaging (MRI). Research continues in this field, and it is probable that we can look forward to even more new and exciting diagnostic options.

Second 30 Years: Era of Therapeutics (1960–1990)

It must of course be remembered that diagnosis is only half the story of the development of endovascular procedures. Ultimately, the goal is not only to describe the vascular pathology but also to manipulate it in the interest of the patient. Manipulation can be done in a number of ways. The pathology can be removed, pulverized, shaved, or disrupted; alternatively, a device can be put in place to mitigate the consequences of pathology. In the three decades since Sones' work, we have seen a flowering of endovascular therapeutic techniques designed to remedy vascular disease. Just as in the development of diagnostic methods, many people were involved in creating and perfecting the therapeutic methods we have today. However, a few events and personalities stand out as pivotal.

Embolectomy—Fogarty

The earliest disease entity to be approached intraluminally was embolic occlusion. Ischemic injury from such events resulted in severe morbidity, and until the early 1960 s there was no resort for the problem other than a major operation requiring large and multiple incisions. These patients all had severe associated cardiac disease; therefore prolonged anesthesia carried a high operative risk. There was no standard technique or instrumentation to manage this difficult patient group. Then in 1961 the balloon embolectomy catheter was introduced, and its results were reported by Thomas Fogarty and colleagues in 1963 [9]. The instrument was comprised of a hollow pliable catheter body with a soft elastomeric balloon situated at the tip. In use, the catheter tip with the deflated latex balloon was passed through and beyond the area of occlusion. Once past the embolus, the balloon was inflated and the catheter withdrawn toward the arteriotomy, the inflated balloon pulling the embolic material as it was retracted. The catheter was passed both antegrade and retrograde from a small femoral cutdown. This approach marked the first conversion of a previously complicated and potentially dangerous open procedure into a safe, relatively easy endovascular procedure, using a much smaller incision and performed under local anesthesia. This was to be the beginning of endovascular therapy and of less invasive interventions.

Balloon Angioplasty—Dotter/Grüntzig

The next major milestone in the evolution of endovascular therapy was the application of catheter-based techniques to the problem of atherosclerotic stenosis. Charles Dotter (Fig. 1.3) was professor and chairman of radiology at the University of Oregon, where Fogarty was a first-year surgical resident. Dotter knew of Fogarty's work, but in 1964 his interest was in treating chronic occlusions percutaneously. That year, he passed an 8F Teflon catheter over a guidewire into an elderly woman with ischemic gangrene who had refused amputation. After the first catheter was in place, he passed a 12F Teflon catheter over it to further dilate the stenotic segment [10].

In Europe, this catheter-based angioplasty was refined by several clinicians using modified catheters, but Dotter and Fogarty made the next advance. In 1965, Dotter used a balloon catheter made by Fogarty with two balloons wrapped over one another to give extra thickness resulting in an almost fixed catheter. Once the tip was in the vicinity of the iliac stenosis, expansion of the balloon caused an increase in the lumen diameter. The balloon was deflated and removed through a very small incision. Fourteen years later, this first balloon angioplasty was still patent [11].

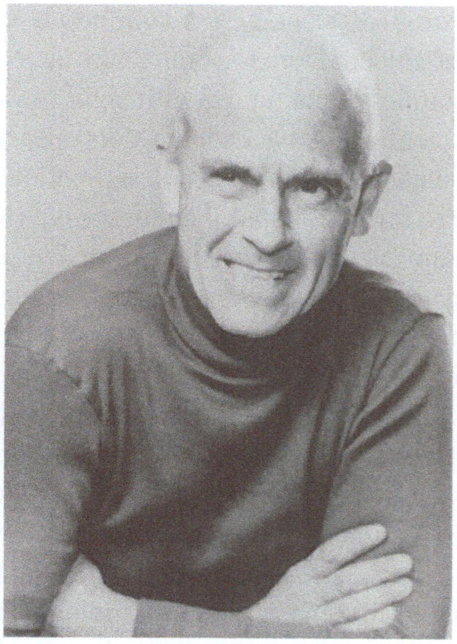

Fig. 1.3 Charles Dotter, MD, "father of interventional radiology," who developed endovascular techniques and demonstrated the utility of catheter-mediated therapies in the radiology setting at the University of Oregon Medical School and Health Sciences Center

In 1974, Andreas Grüntzig made a fundamental improvement in the balloon angioplasty catheter by changing the balloon material from the latex of the embolectomy balloon to polyvinyl chloride [12]. This was a less elastomeric material than the latex balloon and allowed more force to act on the plaque rather than to distend away from the atheroma (as was intended in the design of the embolectomy balloon). Grüntzig began his angioplasty work in the peripheral circulation [12], but his main interest was the heart. He is best remembered for the introduction of coronary angioplasty, which quickly became (and remains) one of the most common endovascular procedures. In 1982, John Simpson developed the movable guidewire concept, which further advanced the ease and versatility of coronary angioplasty [13].

In the 1980 s, some investigators began trying to use laser energy to disrupt atheromatous plaque. These laser methods began with much interest and fanfare. However, the high cost of setting up a workable system coupled with the persistent problem of vessel perforation and the difficulty of the procedure itself all combined to make laser angioplasty less practical than originally hoped. It is possible that better integration of visualization modalities and computer-directed laser systems could make laser angioplasty worthwhile in the future.

Atherectomy—Simpson

About the same time that lasers were being developed, John Simpson (Fig. 1.4) developed the idea of mechanically removing atheroma from diseased vessels. In 1988 he coined the term *atherectomy*, referring to a catheter-based technique to physically remove obstructing atheroma from the vessel lumen. It was felt that this approach would have a number of advantages over balloon angioplasty. In particular, it was intended to reduce restenosis rates because the atherectomy device would selectively cut and remove the atheromatous material from the vessel wall and leave behind a smooth luminal surface. To achieve this aim, Simpson developed the directional atherectomy catheter, which consists of a cylindrical metal housing containing a drum-like cutting element located at the end of a dual-lumen catheter. The cylinder has a cutting window on one side and an inflatable balloon on the opposite side. Inflating the balloon brings the plaque into the cutting window, where it is shaved off with the cutting element and stored in a collecting chamber at the distal end of the catheter for subsequent removal. It is interesting to note that Simpson and Fogarty collaborated on the initial design and clinical application of directional atherectomy [14]. This collaboration occurred at Sequoia Hospital, a small community hospital 6 miles

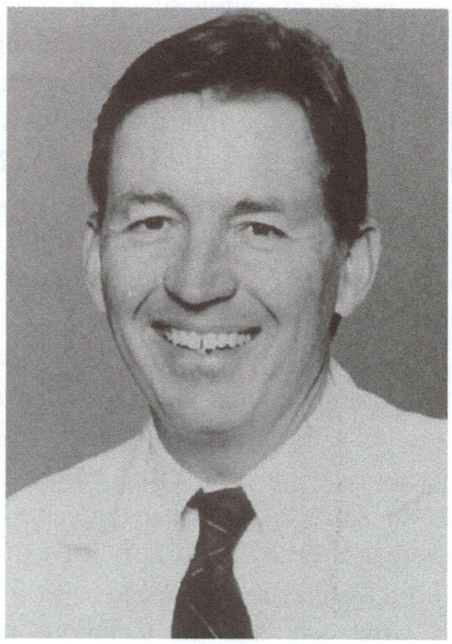

Fig. 1.4 John B. Simpson, MD, cardiologist and innovator of catheter-mediated techniques for treating coronary artery atherosclerosis

north of Stanford University Medical Center where both Simpson and Fogarty had previously worked.

Several other approaches to atherectomy have been developed, including the transluminal extraction catheter (TEC), which contains an open-ended cutter at the distal end of a catheter assembly. This device cuts atheroma located in front of it rather than to the side, as does the Simpson AtheroCath. Thus, it is not "directional." An attached vacuum provides continuous suction to prevent embolization of plaque particles. This design also allows a better approach to total occlusions. Other mechanical plaque disruption catheters that are often called atherectomy devices may be better referred to as atheroablation devices because they do not actually remove atheroma. Instead, they use a high-speed rotational catheter with a spinning tip to pulverize the plaque into particles presumably too small to cause microembolization. Unfortunately, microembolization remains a problem with both of these types of devices, and efforts continue to reduce and eliminate this serious problem.

Stents and Stent–Grafts

Embolectomy and atherectomy were developed to remove the source of arterial occlusion. Angioplasty and atheroablation were intended to disrupt pathology. Another aspect of endovascular therapy was the insertion of a device to circumvent the effects of pathology. The first devices introduced endovascularly were venous filters in the inferior vena cava to prevent pulmonary embolism. In 1958 [15], M.S. De Weese and colleagues passed a grid of silk sutures across the vena cava to trap large embolic material that came up from the pelvis and extremities. Mobin-Uddin, Greenfield, and Roehm applied less invasive endovascular technology to venous implants for venous thromboembolic disease. The idea of introducing a synthetic device endovascularly to manage vascular disease was quickly seized on for use in the arterial system. In fact, Dotter had suggested the idea of a mechanical arterial scaffold in 1964, but it was not until Julio Palmaz's experience with a balloon-expandable wire stent that the technique became a clinical practicality.

Julio Palmaz introduced his first stent in 1985 [16] and then developed a refined version in 1986 [17] Palmaz's original stent was a continuous steel wire with silver-soldered cross-points; his later one was made of stainless steel tubing with eight rows of slots. When the stent was expanded, the slots opened to form diamond-shaped spaces. This design allowed more resistance to radial collapse than mesh-like stents such as the Medinvent, but it was not flexible. Palmaz's stent had application in areas where radial strength was critical and the distances were relatively short, such as the coronary arteries. The stent was delivered to the stenotic site via a catheter and then expanded to its open configuration by balloon inflation. For the first time, a stent was shown to be relatively nonthrombogenic (a significant problem with previous stents). Although clinicians are still concerned about the problem of long-term stenosis, stent technology has rapidly evolved to a state where it has been shown to be highly efficacious in large-bore vessels. Consequently, its utility is now recognized by surgeons who have currently accepted it as a viable method to treat stenotic lesions.

The most recent implantable device to enter the endovascular field is the endograft. Introduced by J.C. Parodi (Fig. 1.5) in 1991, it marks the first significant minimally invasive approach for the treatment of aneurysms. First termed as its name implies, the stent–graft, is a combination of a vascular stent, which

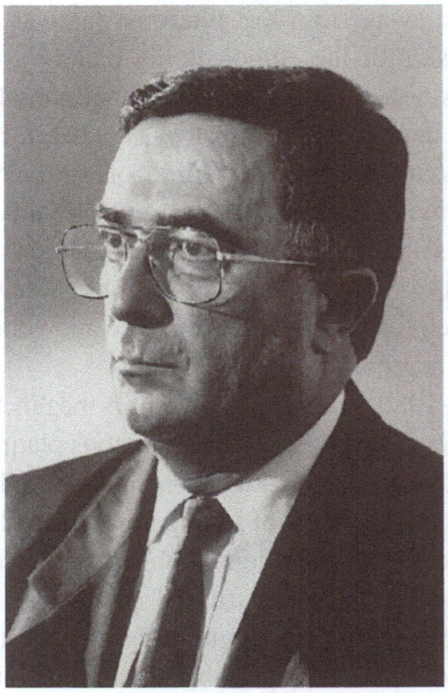

Fig. 1.5 Juan C. Parodi, MD, vascular surgeon and designer who advanced the clinical techniques and applications for the transluminally placed endovascular endograft

provides support, with an enveloping graft material that lines the spaces in the stent. The idea is to introduce the device endovascularly to the affected site and secure it in place by friction or hooks in such a manner that the endograft bridges the aneurysm. Thus, blood flow is diverted through the endograft and never gets to the actual aneurysm. This mechanism is intended to prevent rupture.

Endograft technology is important because it has the potential to replace traditional open aneurysm repair which is a major procedure associated with significant morbidity and mortality. The technology has also been successfully applied to thoracic aortic aneurysms. To date, however, the procedure is still in the investigational stages, and long-term results are currently being obtained.

Future Developments

The concept of predicting what we, as vascular surgeons, will be doing in 5 to 10 years is a daunting task. It is quite possible that all predictions will be wrong. Technology causing major paradigm shifts is innately unpredictable and often spontaneous. Invention and innovation are often fortuitous and occur during the process of trying to solve a problem. The ability to observe a failure and take that failure in different ways or apply it differently often results in innovation or invention. Few things are certain in our lives. It is our prediction that rapid advances in technology will change what all physicians are doing. How one diagnoses, how one treats, who we treat, when we treat, what specialty will do the diagnoses and treatment all are uncertain. Many predict that cell therapy, proteomics, and genomics will be our future. We believe that in 5 years significant progress will be made. However, routine applications of these technologies will not be widespread. The availability of other technologies such as nanotechnology and microtechnology will allow significant miniaturization of current surgical tools and diagnostic approaches. This will be in clinical use in 5 years. The rapid developmental changes bring with it solutions and problems. In the surgical field, a device or procedure begins to be replaced between 5 and 8 years after its initial introduction. Soon it will not be unusual that by the time one finishes medical school and training, being outdated will not be implausible. With the introduction of a new technology an old one is always replaced. The users of the new technology are often shared by multiple specialties. In the cardiovascular field we have cardiologists, cardiac surgeons, vascular surgeons, and interventional radiologists all treating the same diseases and pathology with the same or different techniques and instruments. The relationships and interactions between these specialty groups are inconsistent and vary from poor to good. If technology change occurs so rapidly, the way we teach and train must change. We exist in our own silos. There should be just one silo dedicated to the diagnoses and management of the cardiovascular disease state. If we, as surgeons, plan to survive, we must adapt to change. Other specialties and disciplines have a lot to offer; cooperation and collaboration are essential for innovation.

Patients are continuing to demand less invasive approaches; this includes both diagnoses and therapies. The medical community has responded; catheter technology and port access procedures have already replaced many standard surgical procedures and will continue to do so.

How about transcutaneous procedures, no invasion whatsoever? In diagnosis, most imaging of disease states is done transcutaneously by the use of radiation or other energy forms. Can the same energy source combined with other technologies such as robotics and instantaneous information feedback be used for therapy? The answer is yes; it already is and receiving wide adaptation. Two companies, Accuray and Varian, are using the above combined technology to treat metastatic and benign tumors. The accuracy of the Accuray technology is sub-one millimeter. The implications for cardiac and vascular surgery are significant and enormous. This will be in common practice in the next 10 years. Currently, the application of transcutaneous technology is being applied to cardiac tissue for the purpose of ablating atrial fibrillation. Clinical trials are beginning offshore.

If patients are going to receive the benefit of innovation and new technology, we must encourage those who can implement the above. Currently, the trend is in fact in the opposite direction. Overregulation by institutions, governments, and issues surrounding conflict of interest are impeding those who are capable of making the future happen now. For the benefit of the patients, the physicians, and society in general, those who improve health care should be encouraged and rewarded. Those who say it cannot be done should not get in the way of those who are doing it.

Conclusion

Endovascular therapy is a multidisciplinary field, involving contributions from surgeons, cardiologists, radiologists, physicists, and engineers. It is also a growing field destined to have a fascinating future because it addresses many issues that are of prime importance in medicine and society today. The problems and pathologies that endovascular therapy seeks to remedy are some of today's most common chronic medical problems. Medically, these procedures decrease the risk to the patient and allow a quicker return to normal daily functions. In this era of cost containment and fiscal responsibility, endovascular therapies can decrease operating room time, hospitalization time, and overall time to recovery. In a very real sense, the proven endovascular techniques have actually delivered "more for less." Today, work continues to further refine existing technologies and to develop additional innovations to serve this purpose.

References

1. Doby T: *Development of angiography and cardiac catheterization*, Littleton, Mass, 1976, Publishing Sciences Group.
2. Moniz E: Arterial encephalography: its importance in the location of cerebral tumors, *Revue Neurologique* 48:72, 1927. Reprinted in Viega-Pires J, Grainger R, editors: *Pioneers in angiography: the Portuguese school of angiography*, Boston, 1987, MTP Press.
3. Dos Santos R: Arteriography of the limbs, with the collaboration of Augusto Lamas and J Pereira Caldas, *Medicina Contempanea* 1929. Reprinted in Viega-Pires J, Grainger R, editors: *Pioneers in angiography: the Portuguese school of angiography*, Boston, 1987, MTP Press.
4. Cournand A, Ranges H: Catheterization of the right auricle in man, *Proc Soc Exp Biol Med* 46:462, 1941.
5. Cournand A: Cardiac catheterization: development of the technique, its contributions to experimental medicine and its initial applications in man, *Acta Med Scand* 579(suppl):7, 1975.
6. Seldinger S: Catheter replacement of the needle in percutaneous arteriography, a new technique, *Acta Radiol* 39:368–376, 1953.
7. Loop F: F Mason Sones, Jr, M.D. (1918–1985), *Ann Thor Surg* 43:237–238, 1987.
8. Sones F, Shirey E: Cine coronary arteriography, *Mod Con Cardiovas Dis* 31:735, 1962.
9. Fogarty T, Cranley J, Krause R et al.: A method for extraction of arterial emboli and thrombi, *Surg Gynecol Obstet* 116:241–244, 1963.
10. Dotter C, Judkins M: Transluminal treatment of arteriosclerotic obstruction: description of a new technic and a preliminary report of its application, *Circulation* 30:654–670, 1964.
11. Dotter C: Transluminal angioplasty: a long view, *Radiology* 135:561–564, 1980.
12. Grfintzig A, Hopf H: Perkutane rekanalisation chroischer arterieller verschlusse mit neuen dilatationskatheter: modification der Dotterteknik, *Dtsch Med Wochenschr* 99:2502–2551, 1974.
13. Simpson J, Bairn D, Robert E et al.: A new catheter system for coronary angioplasty, *Am J Cardiol* 49:1216–1222, 1982.
14. Simpson J, Selmon M, Robertson G et al.: Transluminal atherectomy for occlusive peripheral vascular disease, *Am J Cardiol* 61:96G–101G, 1988.
15. DeWeese M, Hunter D: A vena cava filter for the prevention of pulmonary emboli, *Bulletin de la Societe Internationale de Chirurgie* 1:1–9, 1958.
16. Palmaz J, Sibbitt R, Reuter S et al.: Expandable intraluminal graft: preliminary study, *Radiology* 156:72–77, 1985.
17. Palmaz J, Sibbitt R, Tio F et al.: Expandable intraluminal vascular graft: a feasibility study, *Surgery* 99:199–205, 1986.

2 Pathophysiology of Vascular Disease

Christopher K. Zarins, Chengpei Xu, and Seymour Glagov

Vascular disease is the major cause of morbidity and mortality in Western civilization. Its manifestations include heart attacks, strokes, lower extremity occlusive disease, and aneurysmal disease, and its predominant underlying cause is atherosclerosis. Although atherosclerosis is a generalized disorder of the arterial tree associated with well-known risk factors—including hyperlipidemia, hypertension, cigarette smoking, and diabetes mellitus—its clinical expression tends to be focal. Not all individuals with extensive risk factors develop atherosclerotic plaques, and many patients with extensive atherosclerotic plaques have no recognized risk factors. Moreover, morbidity and mortality usually result from localized plaque deposition at certain vulnerable sites in the arterial tree rather than from diffuse disease. For example, the carotid arteries, coronary arteries, and lower extremity arteries are particularly susceptible to plaque formation, whereas the upper extremity arteries are rarely involved. Some arteries with small plaques may become occluded, whereas other arteries with large and extensive plaques may retain a normal lumen caliber. Still others may become aneurysmally enlarged.

The responses of arterial smooth muscle and endothelial cells to physiologic and pathologic stimuli promote the initiation and progression of atherosclerotic plaque. Because there is a close integration between the mechanical and metabolic functions of arteries, an alteration of one type of stimulus affects other aspects of the pathogenetic process. A large body of descriptive clinical and experimental data on the general appearance of human atherosclerotic lesions exist, but the precise initiating and perpetuating pathogenic mechanisms remain obscure. The factors determining lesion composition, rate of enlargement, organization, and disruption still require elucidation. This chapter reviews the pathophysiology of atherosclerosis as it affects the artery wall and considers the factors that affect plaque localization and the mechanisms that are likely to lead to stenoses and aneurysms.

Atherosclerotic Process

Atherosclerosis is not necessarily a continuous process leading inexorably to artery stenosis or other clinically significant complications. Plaque formation involves an interaction among systemic risk factors and local conditions in the lumen and artery wall in the context of a living tissue capable of healing and remodeling. The evolution of atherosclerotic lesions is a combination of initiating and sustaining processes, adaptive responses, and involutional changes. Despite the available experimental data concerning plaque progression and regression, the natural history of atherosclerotic lesions in humans is poorly understood.

Plaque Initiation

Plaque initiation refers to the earliest detectable biochemical and cellular events leading to or preceding the formation of atherosclerotic lesions. Possible mechanisms of plaque initiation have been the subject of extensive study. Principal research foci have

C.K. Zarins (✉)
Professor, Department of Surgery, Stanford University School of Medicine, Stanford, CA, USA

T.J. Fogarty, R.A. White (eds.), *Peripheral Endovascular Interventions*,
DOI 10.1007/978-1-4419-1387-6_2, © Springer Science+Business Media, LLC 1998, 2010

included altered endothelial function or turnover resulting in increased permeability, oxidative alteration of insudated lipids by endothelium, and the subsequent ingress of macrophages [1]. Other possible factors include various stimuli to smooth muscle proliferation, such as circulating mitogens [2], limitations of transmural transfer or egress related to the composition and organization of subendothelial tissues and media [3], and high levels of specific lipoprotein cholesterol fractions [4]. Each of these factors is associated with early lesion development in experimental models, and each may also be related to one or more epidemiologically identified risk factors. Although none has been directly implicated yet in the mural disturbance that leads to plaque formation, some or several of these stimulating mechanisms may well prove to be significant.

Endothelial injury and the response to this injury have been proposed as critical and essential first steps in plaque pathogenesis [1]. According to this response-to-injury hypothesis [5], the endothelial lining of arteries can be damaged or denuded by several factors, including mechanical forces such as shear stress and hypertension, chemical agents such as homocysteine or excessive lipids, immunologic reactions, or hormonal dysfunction. Responses to such injuries include platelet deposition, release of platelet-derived growth factor, leukocyte adhesion and diapedesis, cellular proliferation, and lipid deposition [6–8]. According to this theory, local, repeated endothelial injury, or denudation would determine the location of plaque formation.

There is, however, growing recognition that there is no direct evidence for the response-to-injury hypothesis. There is no in vivo evidence of spontaneous endothelial injury or disruption, with or without platelet adherence, in areas at risk for future lesion development [9, 10]. In animal models, experimentally induced endothelial cell denudation is transient and is restored by rapid regeneration. In addition, there is no direct evidence that experimentally induced endothelial injury or denudation results in eventual sustained lesion formation [11], even in the presence of hyperlipidemia. On the contrary, strong experimental evidence suggests that the formation of intimal plaques requires the presence of a continuous endothelial covering [9, 11–13]. Moreover, the role of platelets in atherogenesis remains unclear and platelet-derived growth factor can be isolated from tissue other than platelets [14].

More recent research has investigated other possible initiating processes. Altered endothelial function may be linked to an inflammatory response to injury, characterized by leukocyte adhesion, diapedesis and cell proliferation, smooth muscle cell migration, and macrophage foam cell formation. This response is accompanied by lipid accumulation—including cholesterol, cholesterol esters, and triglycerides—in both cell types. The pathobiology of this lipid accumulation process may be attributable to increased lipoprotein infiltration, coupled with dysregulation of the cholesterol ester cycle and cholesterol efflux processes. Lipid accumulation may be enhanced by a process in which T cells, macrophages, and smooth muscle cells release specific biologic response modifiers that participate in the dysregulation of lipid metabolism [15, 16].

Very elderly people who have no clinically manifest atherosclerotic disease during life often have substantial and advanced atherosclerotic plaques at autopsy. It is obvious that these people's longevity and good health did not stem from the prevention of plaque initiation or formation; rather, their lack of atherosclerotic disease symptoms must be attributable to the stable nature of the plaque, control of its progression, adequate artery adaptation, and prevention of lesion complications.

Plaque Progression

Plaque progression refers to the continuing increase in intimal plaque volume, which may cause narrowing of the lumen and obstruction of blood flow. Plaque progression may be rapid or slow, continuous, or episodic. Rates of plaque accretion may vary with its stage of development, its composition, and its cell population. Some of these variables may be modulated by clinical risk factors; others may be related to changes in circulation and wall composition that are associated with lesion growth. At the tissue level, plaque progression involves cellular migration, proliferation, and differentiation, intracellular and extracellular lipid accumulation, extracellular matrix accumulation, and degeneration and cell necrosis. Evolution and differentiation of plaque organization and stratification are also characteristics of progression.

Artery Wall Responses

Artery wall responses to intimal plaque accumulation serve to maintain an adequate lumen channel. The formation of a fibrous cap, the sequestration of necrotic and degenerative debris, the persistence of a regular and round lumen cross section, and the adaptive enlargement of the artery are all aspects of an overall adaptive and healing process (Fig. 2.1). If plaque enlargement is accompanied by these responses, plaque progression is well tolerated. Lumen diameter and blood flow can be maintained even with advanced and extensive lesions.

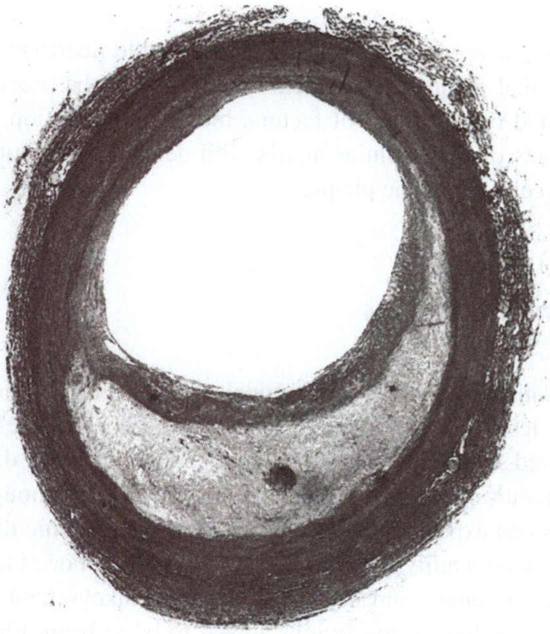

Fig. 2.1 Cross section of a well-adapted atherosclerotic artery. Artery enlargement in response to increasing intimal plaque tends to preserve a normal lumen caliber. Lumen contour remains round and the eccentric lipid-rich necrotic core of the plaque is walled off from the lumen by a fibrous cap containing elastic lamellae that resembles the media

The primary artery wall response to atherosclerotic plaque deposition is arterial enlargement. It is not uncommon to have a twofold enlargement of atherosclerotic arteries, with little or no alteration in the lumen cross-sectional area. The compensatory enlargement of the affected artery segment tends to limit the stenosing effect of the enlarging intimal plaque (Fig. 2.2). Such enlargement of atherosclerotic arteries has been demonstrated in experimental atherosclerosis [17–19], in human coronary [20, 21],

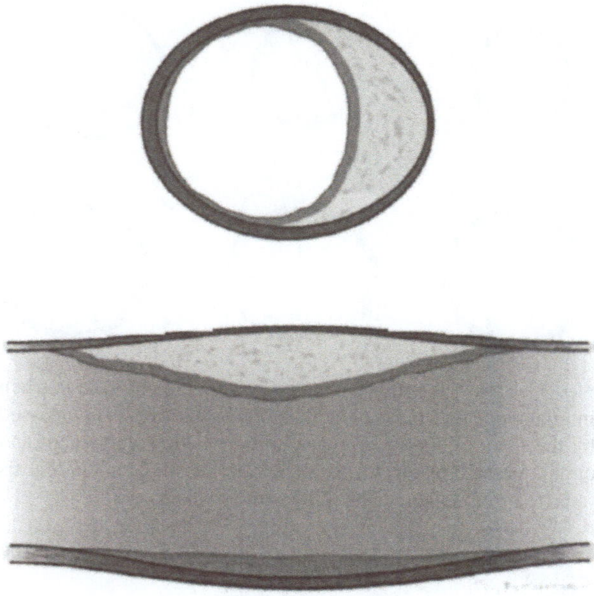

Fig. 2.2 Arterial wall compensatory changes in response to increasing atherosclerotic plaque. The fibrous cap sequesters the plaque contents from the lumen and artery enlargement prevents lumen stenosis

carotid [22, 23], and superficial femoral arteries [24], and in the abdominal aorta. The mechanism by which this enlargement occurs is unclear. Possible explanations include adaptive responses to altered blood flow on the segment of artery wall that is free of plaque formation or direct effects of the plaque on the subjacent artery wall. Focal intimal plaque deposition decreases lumen diameter. The resulting increased local blood flow velocity and wall shear stress induces dilatation of the artery to restore baseline levels of shear stress. In addition, atrophy of the media underlying the plaque could cause outward local bulging of the artery to maintain an adequate lumen caliber (Fig. 2.3). Thus an increase in intimal plaque volume appears to engender an increase in artery size.

In arteries such as the human left main coronary artery, compensatory enlargement keeps pace with increases in intimal plaque. Such enlargement can maintain a normal or near-normal lumen caliber and is effective in preventing lumen stenosis until the cross-sectional area of the plaque occupies approximately 40% of the area encompassed by the internal elastic lamina (Fig. 2.4). Further plaque enlargement or complication appears to exceed the ability of the artery to enlarge. The result is lumen stenosis [21]. Thus

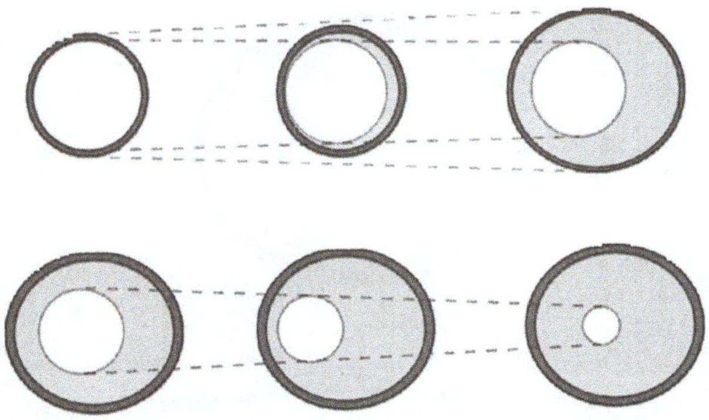

Fig. 2.3 Arterial enlargement can prevent lumen stenosis when intimal plaque occupies more than 40% of the area encompassed by the internal elastic lamina. Further plaque enlargement and circumferential plaque formation usually result in lumen stenosis (adapted from Glagov et al. [20] with permission)

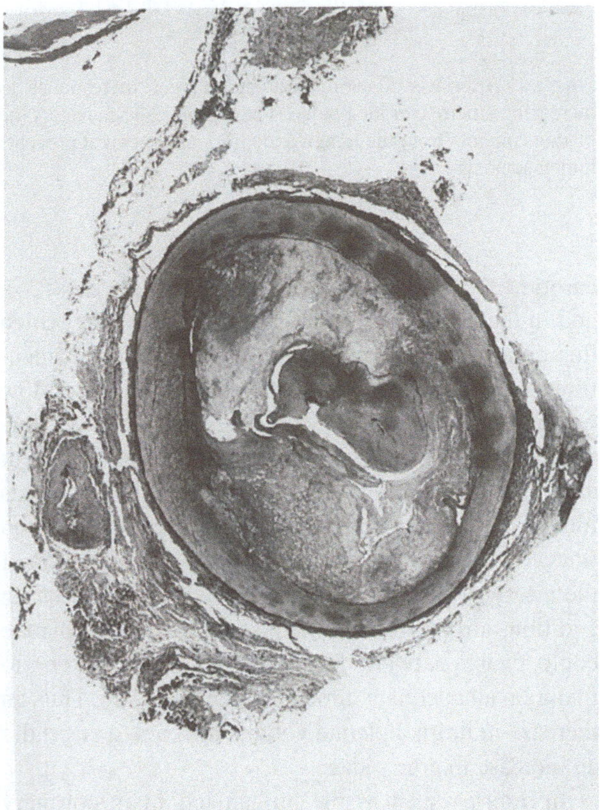

Fig. 2.4 Cross section of occluded atherosclerotic artery. Intimal plaque deposition exceeding the arterial compensatory mechanisms resulted in lumen stenosis. Thrombosis of the stenotic vessel resulted in occlusion of the lumen

atherosclerosis is fundamentally a dilating rather than a constricting disorder of arteries.

Understanding the processes that regulate plaque development, differentiation, and healing is the key to determining why one plaque progression results in unfavorable complications—such as stenosis, ulceration, or thrombosis—while another does not. Rates of cell proliferation, lipid deposition, fibrous cap formation, necrosis and healing, calcification, and inflammation may vary over time. They may also differ with location at the same point in time. Such differences probably account for the wide spectrum of morphologic changes seen in plaques in a given patient at any one time.

Plaque Regression

Plaque regression refers to a discernible decrease in intimal plaque volume. This decrease may be precipitated by a number of factors, including resorption of lipids or extracellular matrix, cell death, or migration of cells out of the plaque.

Animal Studies

In atherosclerotic animal models, significant reduction in lesion volume resulted when experimentally elevated serum lipid levels were markedly reduced by diet alteration or lipid-lowering drugs [25–27]. Although lesions experimentally induced by an atherogenic diet respond readily, the response is not uniform. For example, coronary and aortic lesions in monkeys tend to regress, but carotid lesions appear to be resistant [28]. In swine, severe, longstanding lesions are much more resistant to regression than early foam cell lesions [29]. In most animal studies, induction and regression periods occur over a matter of months. It is unclear whether human lesions, which may have accumulated over decades, would also decrease significantly.

Human Studies

In human trials, apparent regression of atherosclerotic lesions in coronary [30–32] and peripheral arteries has been documented by serial contrast arteriography. In each of these trials, results are based on luminal changes observable by angiography rather than on direct evidence of plaque regression. The fact that each trial has demonstrated simultaneous progression *and* regression of different lesions during the course of treatment indicates the complexity of the process.

Although plaque regression is usually considered to be simply resorption of plaque material, it may proceed by various mechanisms. Changes in plaque metabolism may result in dissolution of the fibrous cap, ulceration and erosion, and embolization of the necrotic core (Fig. 2.5). Also, *apparent regression* may take place when the rate of artery wall enlargement exceeds the rate of plaque deposition. As indicated previously, most human studies performed to date have used angiography, which provides information only on lumen diameter and contour—not on the volume and composition of the atherosclerotic lesion itself. Despite continued plaque progression, arteriography will show no change if intimal plaque deposition and artery wall enlargement keep pace. If arterial enlargement exceeds plaque deposition, the angiographic evidence will indicate regression, even if plaque deposition continues [33]. These phenomena occur at the outset of plaque formation in some vessels and, in some locations, are quite prominent. Direct assessment of the plaque and artery wall, as well as of lumen caliber, is necessary to achieve certainty about reduction in lesion volume or regression of atherosclerosis in humans.

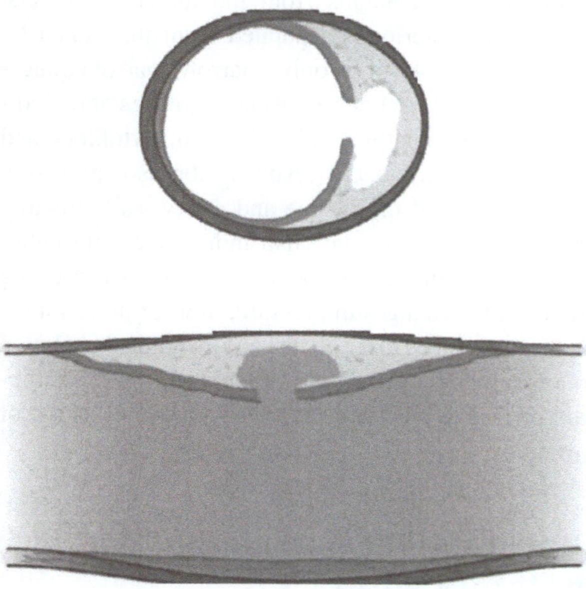

Fig. 2.5 Erosion of the protective fibrous cap exposes the necrotic lipid core of the plaque. This erosion can result in embolization of plaque contents or accumulated platelets and thrombi. It may also promote plaque fissuring, dissection hemorrhage, and thrombosis

Such assessment is now available with newer imaging techniques which allow in vivo imaging of atherosclerotic arteries. Intravascular ultrasound with virtual histology analysis (IVUS-VH) provides cross-sectional image data of arteries and is able to identify atherosclerotic plaques, fibrous caps, and plaque components using radiofrequency backscatter data. The catheter-based technology utilizes ultrasound which is generated from a transducer at the catheter tip. Reflected ultrasound signals from the artery wall produce a color-coded map of the artery lumen, artery wall, and atherosclerotic plaque. Quantitative information on plaque volume and composition can be used to determine plaque progression and regression and help guide treatment strategies (Fig. 2.6) [34–37].

Although the desirability of plaque regression may seem like an a priori assumption, regression regimens could alter plaque composition and organization in unfavorable ways, especially in plaques with soft, semifluid, or pultaceous contents. These alterations could lead to plaque ulceration or disruption, release of plaque debris, and thrombosis or embolism. In certain circumstances, the plaque may provide mechanical support to the artery wall (particularly in cases of well-organized sclerotic plaques). This support may be especially significant when there has been medial atrophy underneath the plaque. Under these circumstances, plaque dissolution could leave a weakened artery wall and the potential for aneurysm formation. Experimental studies have shown that aneurysms form in monkeys undergoing cholesterol-lowering regression regimens [38, 39]. Further studies of the direct effects of regression regimens on plaques and the artery wall are needed, and the specific effects of regression on well-established atherosclerotic plaques must be defined. As alternative therapeutic goals, arrest or control of progression, plaque stabilization, and enhancement of artery wall adaptation might be considered.

Plaque Complication

Clinical sequelae of atherosclerotic lesions are usually caused by plaque complications. Complications such as plaque disruption or ulceration may result in

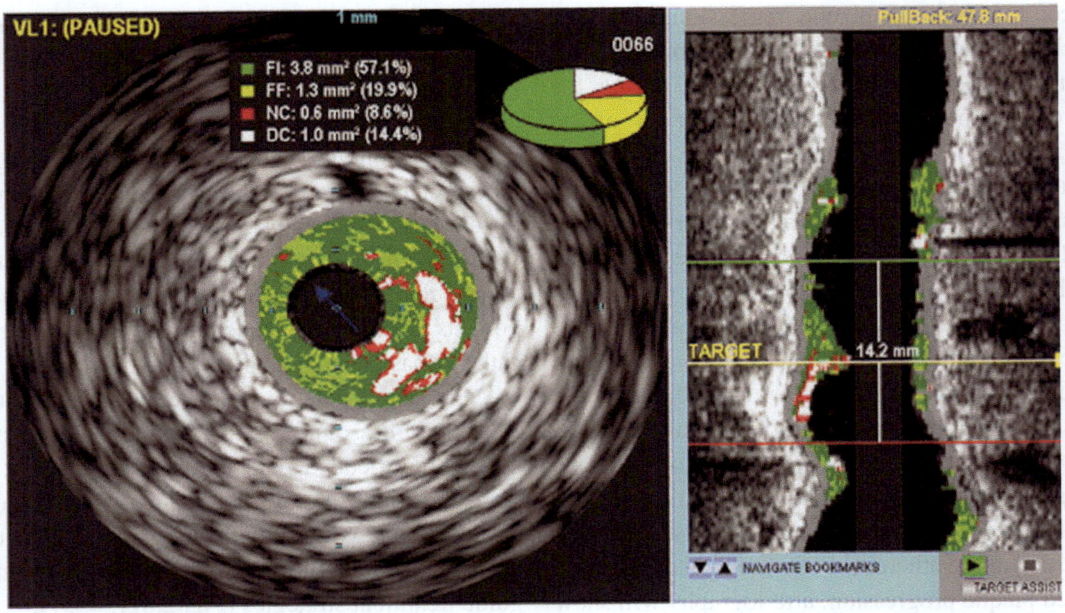

Fig. 2.6 IVUS-virtual histology reconstruction of a coronary artery plaque in vivo. Note the round lumen contour and eccentric plaque contour. Details of plaque composition are visible: fibrous, FI; fibro fatty, FF; necrotic core, NC; and dense calcium, DC are displayed in mm^2 (from Sangiorgi et al. [37] with permission)

the exposure of plaque components to the circulation, resulting in occlusive or embolizing thrombi (Fig. 2.7). The susceptibility of plaques to disruption, fracture, or fissuring probably depends on plaque structure, composition, and consistency. Plaques may be relatively soft and pliable, friable or cohesive, densely sclerotic, or calcific and brittle. Some plaques have well-formed fibrous caps, similar in architecture and thickness to a normal artery wall, that effectively sequester the plaque and its contents from the lumen. In others, the necrotic interior is separated from the lumen by endothelium alone or by only a narrow zone of connective tissue [40]. Activation of macrophages and mediators of inflammation with release of cytokines and proteolytic enzymes can result in fibrous cap erosion and alteration of the plaque and artery wall structure and composition; it may also induce local thrombogenic conditions. Local mechanical stresses resulting from sudden changes in pressure, flow, or pulse rate—or those arising from torsion and bending in relation to organ movements—may then precipitate disruption of friable or brittle plaques with embolization or thrombosis.

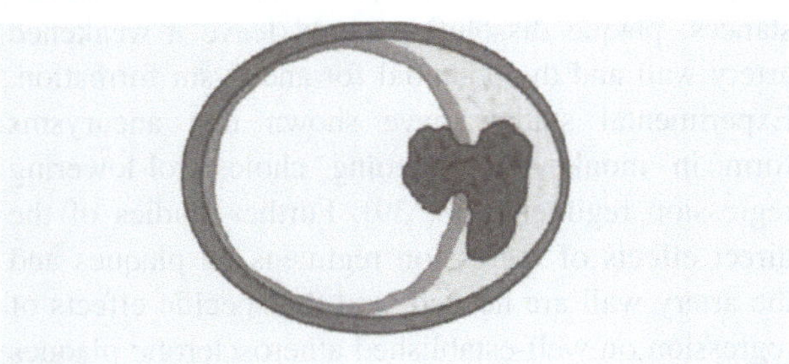

Fig. 2.7 Fibrous cap erosion and plaque fissuring exposes a thrombogenic surface to the lumen, promoting local thrombosis

Hemodynamic Influences in Atherosclerosis

Hemodynamic influences are important determinants of structure and function of both normal and atherosclerotic arteries. Variations in lumen diameters and in vessel curvatures and branchings produce local disturbances in the primary flow field as blood courses through the arterial tree. These disturbances result in regions of varied shear stress and boundary conditions with areas of flow separation, secondary flow patterns, and disordered flow. The complexity of flow conditions at specific sites is exacerbated by the pulsatile nature of blood flow. Branch points are particularly vulnerable to plaque formation and are characterized by wide variations in hemodynamic conditions. Thus it is not surprising that a wide variety of hemodynamic variables have been implicated in plaque pathogenesis. These include high and low wall shear stress, flow separation and stasis, oscillation of flow, turbulence, and hypertension [41].

Wall Shear Stress

Wall shear stress (π_w) in arteries is the tangential drag force produced by blood moving across the endothelial surface. It is described by the Hagen–Poiseuille formula:

$$\pi_w = \frac{4\mu Q}{\pi r^3}$$

where μ is the viscosity of blood, Q the blood flow, and r the radius. Wall shear stress is a function of the velocity gradient of blood near the endothelial surface. Its magnitude is directly proportional to blood flow and blood viscosity and inversely proportional to the cube of the vessel radius. Thus a small change in vessel radius will have a large effect on wall shear stress. Shear stress has an immediate and direct effect on endothelial cells, which respond to increases in shear stress by releasing nitric oxide, producing relaxation of artery wall smooth muscle cells and vasodilation (Fig. 2.8).

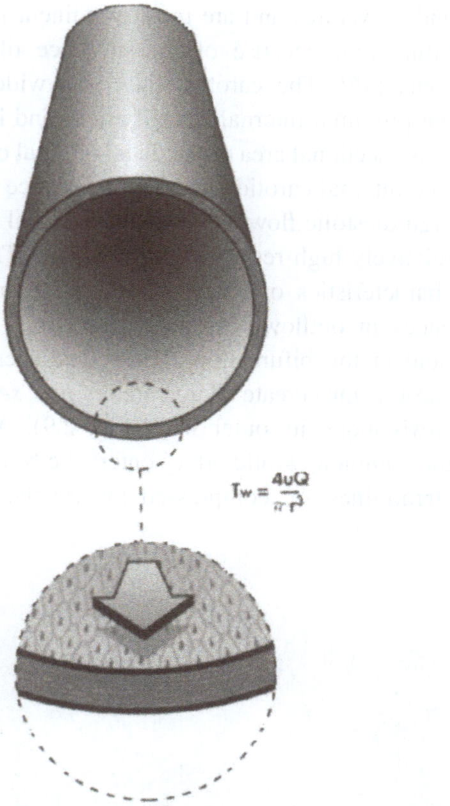

Fig. 2.8 Wall shear stress is the drag force on the endothelial surface and is directly proportional to blood flow and inversely proportional to the cube of the vessel radius. Endothelial cells respond to increased shear by releasing endothelial-derived relaxing factor (EDRF). Small increases in lumen radius will have a large effect on reducing wall shear stress

It was originally thought that high shear stress potentiated plaque formation by producing endothelial injury and disruption, thereby exposing the underlying artery wall to circulating platelets and lipids [1, 4]. It is now recognized that endothelial cells can withstand very high levels of shear and that the reported high shear-induced in vivo endothelial abnormalities were experimental artifacts [42]. Plaques form in areas of low wall shear stress rather than in those of high shear stress. In fact, areas of high shear appear to be relatively spared of plaque formation [43]. This phenomenon may serve to limit the rate of plaque deposition in developing stenoses, which produce local elevations in wall shear stress.

In experimental atherosclerosis, the earliest lesions develop at the upstream rims of aortic ostia, which are regions of low shear stress. Similar plaque localization has been noted in humans. It has been suggested that low wall shear stress rates may retard the mass transport of atherogenic substances away from the vessel wall, resulting in increased accumulation of lipids [44]. Low shear stress may also interfere with turnover of substances at the endothelial surface that are essential for both artery wall nutrition and maintaining optimal endothelial metabolic function [45].

Flow Field Changes

Alterations in the vessel geometry result in local flow field changes. Such changes occur at branch points and curvatures and are most prominent in the carotid bifurcation because of the presence of the carotid sinus [46]. The carotid sinus is a widened area of the proximal internal carotid artery and has twice the cross-sectional area of the distal internal carotid artery. The internal carotid has a low resistance outflow with high diastolic flow, whereas the external carotid has a relatively high resistance outflow bed. The geometric characteristics of the carotid bifurcation and differences in outflow resistance result in a unique flow field at the bifurcation. These characteristics of the carotid sinus create a large area of *flow separation and stasis* along its outer wall (Fig. 2.9). As flow from the common carotid artery enters the bifurcation, flow streamlines are compressed toward the flow divider and inner wall of the internal carotid artery, an area of rapid laminar flow and high shear stress. Plaque formation does not occur in this area. Rather, the earliest intimal plaques develop along the outer wall of the sinus, a region of low flow velocity and shear stress in which a large area of flow separation develops. Late, complicated, stenotic, and ulcerated lesions also tend to develop in this region [47]. In flow separation areas, there is a reversal of axial flow and slow fluid movement upstream. This area is also a zone of complex secondary flow patterns, including counter-rotating helical trajectories. Flow reattaches distally in the sinus. The distal internal carotid, which has relatively rapid axial flow throughout its cross section, is almost always free of plaque (Fig. 2.10).

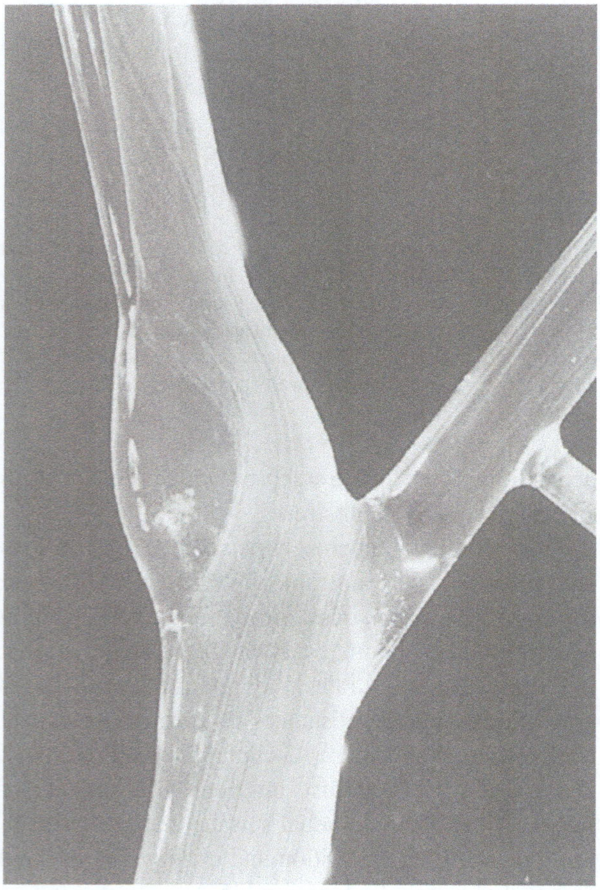

Fig. 2.9 Glass model carotid bifurcation with hydrogen bubble flow visualization, demonstrating large area of flow separation along the outer wall of the internal carotid sinus. This is an area of low flow velocity, low wall shear stress, and increased particle residence time and is the region of the carotid bifurcation most susceptible to plaque deposition

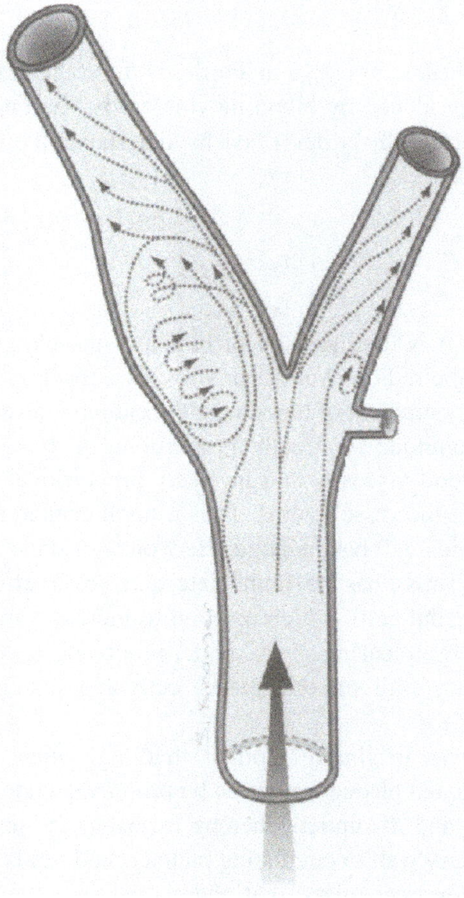

Fig. 2.10 Carotid bifurcation flow field. Flow streamlines are skewed toward the inner wall of the carotid bifurcation, where flow is laminar and velocity and shear stress are high. The outer wall of the carotid sinus is characterized by a region of low and oscillating shear stress with vortex formation, retrograde flow, and irregular flow patterns. This is the region susceptible to plaque formation

Particle Residence Time

Particles are present in the outer region of the carotid sinus, in the area of flow separation and low flow velocity, for a significantly longer period of time than along the inner wall. This is referred to as *increased particle residence time* and is associated with elevated plaque formation. Atherogenic particles would therefore have a greater opportunity to interact with the vessel wall. Time-dependent lipid particle–vessel wall interactions would thus be facilitated in this region, making plaque formation more likely. Increased particle residence time would also increase the probability of the deposition or vessel wall adhesion of blood-borne cellular elements that may play a role in atherogenesis [48]. Flow separation has been shown to favor deposition of platelets in vitro [49], which may stimulate cell proliferation and induce intimal thickening and plaque formation. Radiographic and ultrasound studies in patients have confirmed the presence of flow separation and stasis in this outer wall region of the carotid bifurcation (Fig. 2.10) [50].

Oscillation of Flow

Under conditions of pulsatile flow, dynamic features of the flow field become prominent. The differences between steady flow and pulsatile flow are most prominent along the outer wall of the carotid sinus. Along the inner wall of the carotid sinus, pulsatile flow conditions are similar to those seen under steady flow conditions [51]. Flow remains laminar, with high flow velocity and shear stress. Although there are fluctuations in the magnitude of velocity and shear, there is no change in velocity or shear stress directional vectors.

In contrast, along the outer wall where plaque forms, pulsatile flow produces an *oscillating shear* stress pattern. During early systole, the region of flow separation disappears and there is forward flow throughout the cross-sectional area of the sinus. However, during late systole, the region of separation and flow reversal becomes prominent along the outer wall. There is also a reversal in the shear stress directional vector [51]. During diastole, pulsatile flow conditions are similar to those seen under steady flow conditions. These alternating positive and negative shear stress vectors (oscillations) along the outer wall of the carotid sinus have been shown to correlate strongly with early plaque deposition [52].

Thus, variations in shear stress direction associated with pulsatile flow may lead to increased endothelial permeability, whereas even relatively high shear stresses that remain unidirectional may not be injurious [53]. The oscillating shear stress pattern may cause an increased ingress of plasma constituents through the endothelial monolayer because of its effects on the stability of intercellular junction. Because endothelial cells normally align in the direction of flow in an overlapping arrangement [54], changing shear stress may cause cyclic shifts in the relationship between shear stress direction and the orientation of intercellular overlapping borders. This hypothesis is supported by studies showing increased permeability of cultured, confluent endothelial cells that have been subjected to changes in shear stress [55]. Also, increased Evans blue dye staining has been observed in relation to differences in endothelial organization that may be attributable to changing flow patterns [56]. Oscillation of shear stress direction is a systolic event. Therefore the number of such oscillations is directly related to the number of systoles, or *heart rate,* which has been implicated as an independent risk factor in coronary atherosclerosis.

Turbulence

Turbulence results from the random movement of elements in a flow field. Turbulence in blood flow is dependent on blood flow velocity, artery diameter, and blood viscosity. Causes of focal turbulence include extreme or abrupt changes in geometry resulting from intraluminal projections, severe stenoses, or other obstacles in the flow stream [57]. Although turbulent flow has often been implicated as a factor in plaque pathogenesis [58, 59], neither experimental atherosclerosis studies nor in vitro observations in the model carotid bifurcation support this suggestion.

Various flow field disturbances, such as flow separation, recirculation, and vortex formation, occur in the arterial tree under both normal and abnormal conditions [60]. However, turbulence only develops in the presence of abnormal geometry such as stenoses or shunts. Also, various studies have shown that regions immediately distal to severe stenoses, which are characterized by significant turbulence [61, 62], are free of atherosclerotic lesions [63–65].

In the region where plaques form in the human carotid bifurcation, there is a zone of complex secondary and tertiary flow patterns, including counter-rotating helical trajectories, but there is no turbulence [66]. This lack of turbulence holds true under a wide range of Reynolds' numbers and flow conditions, including both steady and pulsatile flow. Furthermore, in vivo noninvasive studies of carotid arteries in normal human subjects using pulsed Doppler ultrasound have not observed turbulence [67]. In areas of early plaque formation in the normal carotid bifurcation, turbulence may develop late as a result of severe carotid stenosis. Thus turbulence may be a result, rather than a cause, of atherosclerotic plaques.

Hypertension

Postmortem studies have revealed that hypertension is associated with an increase in both the extent and severity of atherosclerosis [68]. Numerous epidemiologic studies have implicated hypertension in the development of serious complications of atherosclerosis in humans, such as myocardial infarction and stroke [69–71]. Nevertheless, recent clinical data revealed no significant difference in the development of myocardial infarction or stroke between patients with and without control of mild to moderate hypertension. These data suggest that a combination of factors interacting with hypertension may be important [72].

The effects of other local hemodynamic variables may influence the effects of hypertension in different portions of the arterial tree. For example, hypertension is known to be a more important factor in cerebrovascular disease and stroke than in coronary artery or peripheral occlusive disease [70, 73]. Severe atherosclerosis can occur in clinically normotensive individuals, and vessels distal to stenoses can be spared, even in the presence of elevated blood pressure. Thus, hypertension may potentiate or enhance atherogenesis but in itself may not be a necessary atherogenic factor.

Experimental studies of hypertension as an important etiologic factor in plaque pathogenesis have produced ambivalent results [74–77]. Inhibition of plaque deposition, despite the presence of hypertension and marked hyperlipidemia, was associated with a decreased pulse pressure [42, 74], decreased wall motion [78], and decreased arterial wall metabolism [79]. Hypertension enhanced experimental plaque formation and plaque progression but inhibited plaque regression [80, 81], despite reduction of hypercholesterolemia. These observations suggest that factors other than blood pressure per se may be of primary importance in atherogenesis.

Plaque Localization

Several major arterial sites are especially prone to plaque formation and the development of advanced atherosclerotic lesions, whereas others are relatively resistant. The coronary arteries, carotid bifurcation, infrarenal abdominal aorta, and iliofemoral vessels are particularly susceptible, whereas the thoracic aorta, common and distal internal carotid, mesenteric, renal, intercostal, mammary, and upper extremity arteries tend to be spared [82]. As discussed previously, the selective localization of plaques that evolve into clinical symptoms has been attributed to differences in local hemodynamic patterns. Although plaques may develop in straight vessels, they are usually located at bifurcations or bends, where hemodynamic variations are especially likely.

Susceptible Regions of the Arterial Vasculature

Carotid Artery Bifurcation

The carotid bifurcation is especially susceptible to plaque formation, with focal plaque deposition occurring principally at the origin of the internal carotid artery (Fig. 2.11). In contrast, plaque does not tend to occur in the proximal common and distal internal carotid arteries. The distribution of lesions at this site is probably associated with the hemodynamic conditions created by the special geometry of the carotid bifurcation, as described previously.

As plaques enlarge at the outer wall of the carotid bifurcation, they modify the geometric configuration of the lumen. These modifications favor subsequent

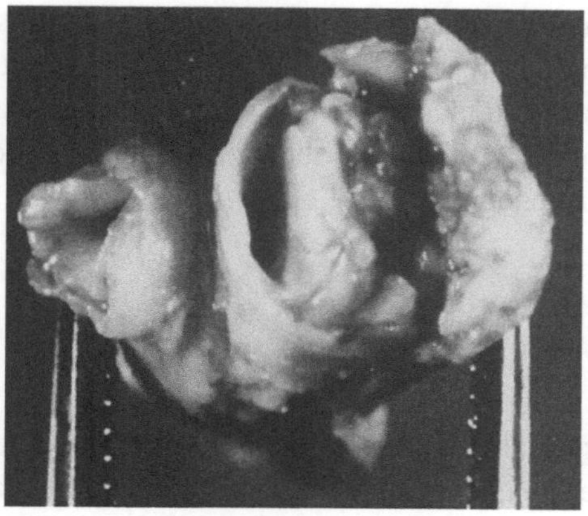

Fig. 2.11 Atherosclerotic plaque removed from carotid bifurcation, viewed on end demonstrating internal and external branches. Plaque is most prominent along outer wall of carotid sinus. Inner wall of internal carotid has minimal intimal thickening

plaque formation on the side and inner walls. In its most advanced and stenotic form, atherosclerotic disease at the carotid bifurcation involves the entire circumference of the sinus, including the region of the flow divider. Nevertheless, plaques in this area remain largest and most complicated at the outer and side walls of the carotid bifurcation. Characteristic hemodynamic conditions at this site, including the turbulence underlying the characteristic bruit, may also compromise the integrity of existing carotid plaques and contribute to their tendency to fissure, ulcerate, and embolize.

Coronary Arteries

The coronary arteries are particularly prone to the development of atherosclerosis [76]. Predisposing factors include the geometric configuration of the vessels and their branches, the mechanical torsion and flexions of the vessels associated with cardiac motion, and the special reactivity of the smooth muscle in these arteries to vasoactive substances and nervous impulses. In addition, the selective localization of plaque in the left coronary artery opposite the flow divider at the bifurcation of the left circumflex indicates the presence of hemodynamic relationships similar to those prevailing at the carotid bifurcation [83]. This is a region characterized by low flow velocity and low and oscillating wall shear stress opposite the flow divider [84].

If oscillation of shear stress direction, which occurs mainly during systole, is a major factor in plaque localization, the coronary arteries may have a higher vulnerability than other systemic arteries. The coronary arteries experience two systolic episodes and one diastolic episode of flow acceleration and deceleration during each cardiac cycle. Coronary arterial flow decreases initially in systole, increases briefly when peak systolic aortic pressure exceeds intracoronary pressure, and decreases again during the remainder of systole [85]. Flow reversal during systole has been demonstrated with tachycardia and in concentric left ventricular hypertrophy.

Because phasic fluctuation in coronary flow is predominantly a systolic occurrence, both the frequency and magnitude of oscillations in shear stress direction should be directly dependent on heart rate. Thus the preferential localization of plaques in the coronary arteries may be related to the fact that the coronary arteries experience at least twice as many oscillations of flow velocity over time as other major arteries. A modest change in heart rate has a remarkable cumulative effect on flow conditions in the coronary arteries.

In experimental studies, sinoatrial node ablation in cynomolgus monkeys resulted in a 20% reduction in mean heart rate. After 6 months on an atherogenic diet, animals with a low heart rate had a 50% reduction in coronary artery atherosclerotic plaque [86]. Heart rate has also been directly implicated as an independent risk factor in human coronary atherosclerosis. A number of major prospective clinical studies have found that high heart rates in men at rest are predictive of future coronary heart disease [87, 88]; conversely, low heart rates appear to protect against coronary atherosclerosis [89]. Although increased resting heart rate seems to correlate significantly with an atherogenic lipid profile in sedentary men [90], both theoretic and experimental evidence suggests that hemodynamic factors associated with cyclic myocardial contraction selectively predispose the coronary arteries to atherosclerosis.

Abdominal Aorta

Although atherosclerotic plaques are regularly found in the adult human thoracic aorta, they are often less abundant, complicated, or calcific than those found in the abdominal aorta. Clinically significant aortic plaque is generally most likely to be found in the abdominal region of the aorta, below the level of the renal arteries. Plaque complications in this region include obstruction, ulceration, thrombus formation, and (potentially) aneurysmal degeneration. The differences in atherogenic susceptibility between the thoracic and abdominal aortas may be related to differences in flow conditions, in mural architecture, or in vasa vasorum distribution and aortic wall nutrition. Suprarenal flow volume is largely independent of skeletal muscular activity. In contrast, infrarenal flow volume is largely dependent on the muscular activity of the lower extremities. Therefore reduced physical activity results in an overall reduction in flow volume and velocity in the infrarenal segment. The long-term effect of reduced flow velocity may be accentuated by the tendency of the aorta to enlarge with age. In addition, the media of the thoracic aorta is well furnished with vasa vasorum, but that of the abdominal aorta is relatively avascular. These differences in medial nutrition may enhance the atherogenic susceptibility of the abdominal aortic segment.

Superficial Femoral Artery

There is no widely accepted explanation for the discrepancy between the incidence of atherosclerotic plaque in the upper and lower extremity arteries. Recognized differences in the two areas include hydrostatic pressure and variations in volume flow depending on the level of physical activity. As in the abdominal aorta, the relative inactivity of a sedentary lifestyle, associated with low flow rates and diminished shear stress, may tend to increase rates of plaque deposition in these arteries [91].

Cigarette smoking and diabetes mellitus are the risk factors most closely associated with atherosclerotic disease of the lower extremities, but their specific mechanisms of action are unknown. Arterial medial density in the lower extremities may be increased because of the chronically heightened smooth muscle tone induced by nicotine use. Such a change could interfere with the transluminal transfer of materials entering the intima, facilitating accumulation of atherogenic materials. Occlusive plaque of the superficial femoral artery tends to be predominantly located at the adductor canal. Possible explanations for this location include repeated mechanical trauma, limitations on vessel compliance, or restrictions on compensatory enlargement because of the closely applied adductor magnus tendon [24].

Aneurysm Formation

Aneurysmal enlargement is the most dramatic degenerative change affecting the human aorta. Most patients with aortic aneurysms have evidence of significant atherosclerosis in the coronary arteries, carotid bifurcation, and/or the lower extremity arteries. Although a causative relationship has not been proven, increasing knowledge of the atherosclerotic process and its effect on the artery wall supports a close pathogenetic relationship between atherosclerosis and aneurysm formation [92].

Arterial Enlargement

As previously noted, arterial enlargement occurs in response to atherosclerosis and tends to compensate for the increase in intimal plaque area. The rate of enlargement in response to atherosclerotic plaque may vary in different segments of the coronary tree under varying conditions. In the human aorta, enlargement is seen both with increasing age and with increasing atherosclerotic plaque. However, whereas the primary determinant of thoracic aortic size is age, the primary determinant of abdominal aortic size is the amount of intimal plaque. This may explain the particular susceptibility of the abdominal aorta to aneurysmal development.

Medical Thinning

In atherosclerosis, the media frequently becomes thin and disappears under large plaques (Fig. 2.12). It is not clear whether this thinning is related to the mechanism of atherosclerotic enlargement or to the erosive effects of plaque components on the artery wall. Cavitary excavations of the media, frequently noted in lipid-rich areas of the plaque, may be associated with

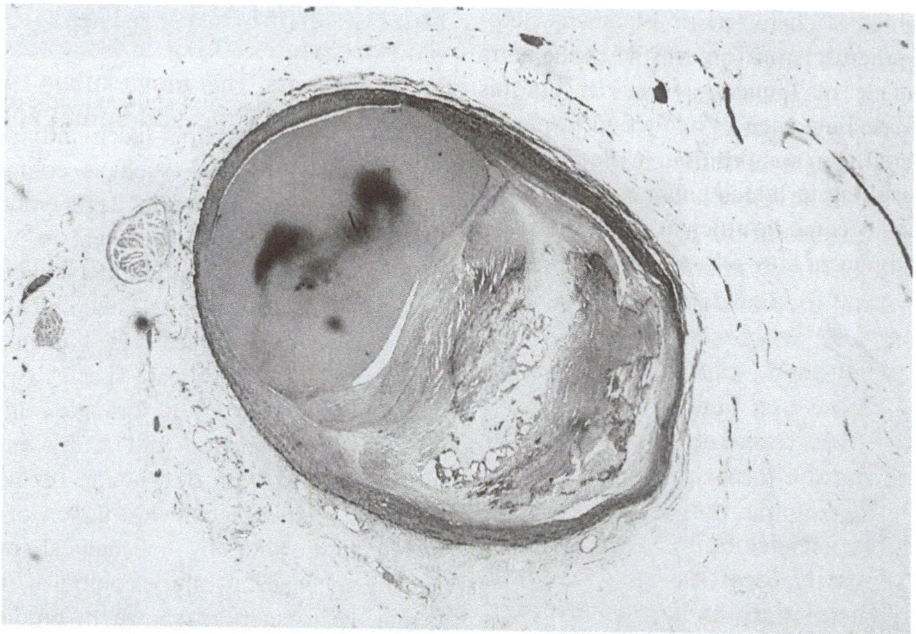

Fig. 2.12 Prominent thinning of the media underneath atherosclerotic plaque. Note the loss of medial lamellar architecture. This may predispose to subsequent aneurysmal degeneration if the plaque ulcerates or regresses

regions of macrophage invasion and inflammation. Under atherosclerotic conditions, collagen and fibrous tissue collect in the adventitia and calcification occurs within the plaque and media. The presence of these materials in the aortic wall may compensate for loss of the media and may even provide structural support. Aortic enlargement can occur in atherosclerosis only if the aortic wall matrix fibers of collagen and elastin are degraded and/or resynthesized in new proportions. Simple passive distention will not permit the aorta to enlarge in excess of its diastolic dimensions without rupture. Thus proteolytic enzymes must be activated for adaptive atherosclerotic arterial enlargement to take place. During active, rapid enlargement, which characterizes aneurysmal development, proteolytic activities would probably be much larger and perhaps less controlled. Indeed, increased collagenase, elastase, and metalloproteinases have been demonstrated in aortic aneurysms, with maximal concentrations noted in those that are rapidly enlarging or ruptured [93–95]. In experimental studies, enzymatic destruction of the medial matrix architecture results in dilatation and rupture of the aorta [96]. Experimental mechanical injury that destroys the medial lamellar architecture can result in aneurysm formation [97]. These observations underscore the importance of the media in maintaining the integrity of the aorta.

Human atherosclerotic aneurysms, particularly those of the abdominal aorta, are characterized by extensive atrophy of the media. The normal lamellar architecture is almost totally effaced, and the aortic wall is replaced by a narrow fibrous band. There are also atrophic changes in the overlying atherosclerotic lesions; plaques may be thinned and left with little residual lipid. Fibrosis and calcification may predominate. Human abdominal aortic aneurysms are rarely found without evidence of atherosclerosis. Atherosclerotic plaques are usually prominent in the neck of the aneurysm and the iliac vessels, and they frequently occur posteriorly along the lumbar ostia.

Mechanism of Aneurysm Formation in Atherosclerosis

Observations of human atherosclerotic arteries suggest a possible mechanism for aneurysm formation. Intimal plaque deposition is accompanied by a compensatory arterial enlargement and by atrophy of the aortic media underlying the plaque. Stable, fibrotic, or calcified atherosclerotic plaques, well nourished by vasa vasorum, may provide structural support to the aortic wall, particularly in association with adventitial fibrogenesis, which is characteristic of atherosclerosis. Late in the atherosclerotic process when the aorta is enlarged, plaque may undergo senescence. This process may be accompanied by reduction in plaque volume and alteration in composition, in ulceration, or in regression resulting in lumen enlargement. Tensile support may thus become insufficient and progressive aneurysmal enlargement may follow (Fig. 2.13).

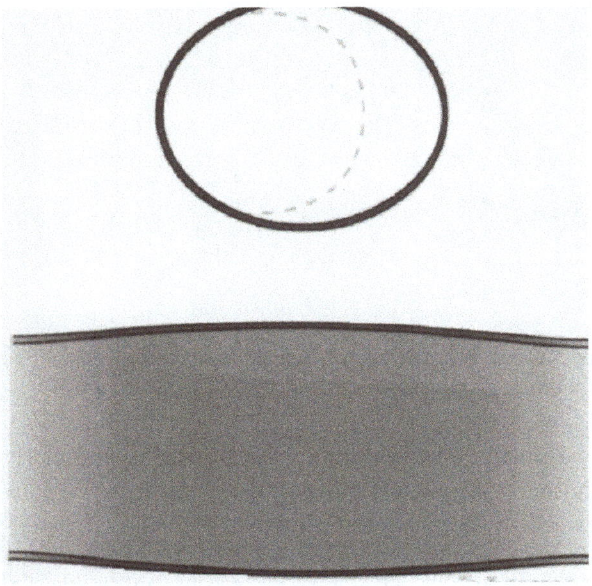

Fig. 2.13 Possible mechanism of atherosclerotic aneurysmal degeneration. Enlargement of the atherosclerotic aorta may be associated with significant medial thinning and loss of elastic architecture beneath atherosclerotic plaques. Under these circumstances, the plaque may provide structural support to the aortic wall. Plaque dissolution resorption and regression would act to enlarge the lumen. The plaque resorptive process may be promoted by macrophage release of proteolytic enzymes, which may weaken the susceptible aortic wall. The enlarged atherosclerotic aorta and thinned aortic wall would result in increased mural tension with progressive aneurysmal dilation

In some atherosclerotic plaques, metabolic alteration in plaque lipid composition may stimulate macrophage activity and inflammation and promote proteolytic activity. The balance between plaque formation, artery wall adaptation, and matrix protein synthesis and degradation probably plays a major role in aneurysmal pathogenesis. Aneurysms appear to occur at a relatively late phase of plaque evolution, when atrophy of the plaque and media is predominant, rather than at an earlier phase of atherosclerosis, when cell proliferation, fibrogenesis, and sequestered lipid accumulation are predominant.

Experimental Observations

In animal models, diet-induced atherosclerosis produces arteries with lipid-laden intimal plaques and artery wall responses—such as compensatory arterial enlargement and medial degeneration—similar to those found in human atherosclerosis. Arterial enlargement in coronary, carotid, and superficial femoral arteries of primates limits lumen stenosis in a manner similar to that seen in human arteries [17–19]. Particularly in primate species (which are more susceptible to aneurysm formation in atherosclerosis), plaque formation and artery enlargement are also associated with destruction of medial architecture [97]. Experimental destruction of aortic medial architecture, both by mechanical methods alone and by mechanical injury combined with hyperlipidemia, has also been shown to produce aneurysms [98].

Our own experience with more than 500 nonhuman primates that were fed high-cholesterol, high-fat diets to induce experimental atherosclerosis has demonstrated that aneurysms form only in animals maintained on atherogenic diets for prolonged periods of time. The cynomolgus monkey, in which diet-induced atherosclerosis produces destruction of the media, is much more prone to the development of aneurysms than the rhesus monkey, in which atherosclerotic destruction of the media rarely occurs. In cynomolgus monkeys, aneurysms developed in 13% of animals maintained on atherogenic regimens for more than 12 months. Histologic studies of these primate aneurysms showed evidence of aortic wall thinning with destruction of the medial lamellar architecture and of plaque atrophy [38].

Of particular note in these primate experiments is the relationship between plaque regression and aneurysm formation. In a controlled trial of cholesterol lowering, significant aneurysmal enlargement of the abdominal aorta was noted only in those monkeys undergoing atherosclerotic regression. Aneurysmal enlargement was associated with significant reduction in plaque volume and medial thickness in the abdominal aorta [39]. These data are consistent with the hypothesis that the atherosclerotic process plays a significant role in the pathogenesis of aneurysms and that plaque regression and medial thinning may be important factors in this process.

Others have reported aneurysm formation with experimental diet-induced atherosclerosis in several species of monkeys and canines [97, 99]. In these studies, aneurysms have been observed only after extended exposure to atherogenic regimens—suggesting that aneurysm formation occurs at a later stage in the atherosclerotic process. This is consistent with the observation that patients undergoing operation for abdominal aortic aneurysms tend to be approximately 10 years older than those undergoing operation for occlusive disease [100].

Summary

Atherosclerosis is a degenerative process of the arterial tree that has various local effects on the artery wall. Specific hemodynamic forces are important in plaque localization. Intimal plaque deposition is counterbalanced by compensatory artery wall responses, such as fibrous cap formation and artery enlargement. The fibrous cap sequesters the plaque from the arterial lumen and compensatory arterial enlargement serves to preserve a normal lumen caliber. Erosion of the fibrous cap may lead to ulceration, thrombosis, and embolization. Regression of plaque contents may be associated with release of proteolytic enzymes. Erosion of the artery wall may result in progressive aneurysmal enlargement. Stenoses may develop as a result of inadequate compensatory enlargement or excessive plaque deposition. Occlusion is usually caused by superimposed thrombosis. The simultaneous occurrence of differing rates of plaque deposition and differing types of artery wall responses engenders the variety and heterogeneity of the clinical manifestations of atherosclerosis. Further understanding of the cellular and molecular mechanisms underlying the atherosclerotic process will improve our ability to control the disease.

References

1. Ross R: The pathogenesis of atherosclerosis – an update, *N Engl J Med* 314:488–500, 1986.
2. Benditt EP, Barrett T, McDougall JK: Viruses in the etiology of atherosclerosis, *Proc Natl Acad Sci USA* 80:6386–6389, 1983.
3. Caro CG: Transport of 14c-4 cholesterol between intraluminal serum and artery wall in isolated dog common carotid artery, *J Physiol* 233:37P–38P, 1973.
4. Ross R, Harker L: Hyperlipidemia and atherosclerosis, *Science* 193:1094–1100, 1976.
5. Ross R, Glomset JA: The pathogenesis of atherosclerosis (first of two parts), *N Engl J Med* 295:369–377, 1976.
6. Ross R: George lyman duff memorial lecture. Atherosclerosis: a problem of the biology of arterial wall cells and their interactions with blood components, *Arteriosclerosis* 1:293–311, 1981.
7. Ip JH, Fuster V, Badimon L, Badimon J, Taubman MB, Chesebro JH: Syndromes of accelerated atherosclerosis: role of vascular injury and smooth muscle cell proliferation, *J Am Coll Cardiol* 15:1667–1687, 1990.
8. Schwartz SM, Heimark RL, Majesky MW: Developmental mechanisms underlying pathology of arteries, *Physiol Rev* 70:1177–1209, 1990.
9. Zarins CK, Taylor KE, Bomberger RA, Glagov S: Endothelial integrity at aortic ostial flow dividers, *Scan Electron Microsc* 3:249–254, 1980.
10. Taylor KE, Glagov S, Zarins CK: Preservation and structural adaptation of endothelium over experimental foam cell lesions. Quantitative ultrastructural study, *Arteriosclerosis* 9:881–894, 1989.
11. Reidy MA: A reassessment of endothelial injury and arterial lesion formation, *Lab Invest* 53:513–520, 1985.
12. Falcone DJ, Hajjar DP, Minick CR: Lipoprotein and albumin accumulation in reendothelialized and deendothelialized aorta, *Am J Pathol* 114:112–120, 1984.
13. Dzau VJ, Gibbons GH, Cooke JP, Omoigui N: Vascular biology and medicine in the 1990 s: scope, concepts, potentials, and perspectives, *Circulation* 87:705–719, 1993.
14. DiCorleto PE, Bowen-Pope DF: Cultured endothelial cells produce a platelet-derived growth factor-like protein, *Proc Natl Acad Sci USA* 80:1919–1923, 1983.
15. Hajjar DP, Pomerantz KB: Signal transduction in atherosclerosis: integration of cytokines and the eicosanoid network, *FASEB J* 6:2933–2941, 1992.
16. Pomerantz KB, Hajjar DP: Eicosanoids in regulation of arterial smooth muscle cell phenotype, proliferative capacity, and cholesterol metabolism, *Arteriosclerosis* 9:413–429, 1989.
17. Bond MG, Adams MR, Bullock BC: Complicating factors in evaluating coronary artery atherosclerosis, *Artery* 9:21–29, 1981.
18. Beere PA, Glagov S, Zarins CK: Experimental atherosclerosis at the carotid bifurcation of the cynomolgus monkey. Localization, compensatory enlargement, and the sparing effect of lowered heart rate, *Arterioscler Thromb* 12:1245–1253, 1992.
19. Armstrong ML, Heistad DD, Marcus ML, Megan MB, Piegors DJ: Structural and hemodynamic response of peripheral arteries of macaque monkeys to atherogenic diet, *Arteriosclerosis* 5:336–346, 1985.
20. Glagov S, Weisenberg E, Zarins CK, Stankunavicius R, Kolettis GJ: Compensatory enlargement of human atherosclerotic coronary arteries, *New Engl J Med* 316:1371–1375, 1987.

21. Zarins CK, Weisenberg E, Kolettis G, Stankunavicius R, Glagov S: Differential enlargement of artery segments in response to enlarging atherosclerotic plaques, *J Vasc Surg* 7:386–394, 1988.
22. Masawa N, Glagov S, Zarins CK: Quantitative morphologic study of intimal thickening at the human carotid bifurcation: Ii. The compensatory enlargement response and the role of the intima in tensile support, *Atherosclerosis* 107:147–155, 1994.
23. Masawa N, Glagov S, Zarins CK: Quantitative morphologic study of intimal thickening at the human carotid bifurcation: I. Axial and circumferential distribution of maximum intimal thickening in asymptomatic, uncomplicated plaques, *Atherosclerosis* 107:137–146, 1994.
24. Blair JM, Glagov S, Zarins CK: Mechanism of superficial femoral artery adductor canal stenosis, *Surgical Forum* 41:359–360, 1990.
25. Malinow MR: Experimental models of atherosclerosis regression, *Atherosclerosis* 48:105–118, 1983.
26. Wissler RW, Vesselinovitch D: Combined effects of cholestyramine and probucol on regression of atherosclerosis in rhesus monkey aortas, *Appl Pathol* 1:89–96, 1983.
27. Stary HC: Regression of atherosclerosis in primates, *Virchows Arch A Pathol Anat Histol* 383:117–134, 1979.
28. Clarkson TB, Bond MG, Bullock BC, McLaughlin KJ, Sawyer JK: A study of atherosclerosis regression in macaca mulatta. V. Changes in abdominal aorta and carotid and coronary arteries from animals with atherosclerosis induced for 38 months and then regressed for 24 or 48 months at plasma cholesterol concentrations of 300 or 200 mg/dl, *Exp Mol Pathol* 41:96–118, 1984.
29. Daoud AS, Jarmolych J, Augustyn JM, Fritz KE: Sequential morphologic studies of regression of advanced atherosclerosis, *Arch Pathol Lab Med* 105:233–239, 1981.
30. Blankenhorn DH, Nessim SA, Johnson RL, Sanmarco ME, Azen SP, Cashin-Hemphill L: Beneficial effects of combined colestipol-niacin therapy on coronary atherosclerosis and coronary venous bypass grafts, *JAMA* 257:3233–3240, 1987.
31. Brown G, Albers JJ, Fisher LD, Schaefer SM, Lin JT, Kaplan C, Zhao XQ, Bisson BD, Fitzpatrick VF, Dodge HT: Regression of coronary artery disease as a result of intensive lipid-lowering therapy in men with high levels of apolipoprotein b, *N Engl J Med* 323:1289–1298, 1990.
32. Buchwald H, Varco RL, Matts JP, Long JM, Fitch LL, Campbell GS, Pearce MB, Yellin AE, Edmiston WA, Smink RD Jr et al.: Effect of partial ileal bypass surgery on mortality and morbidity from coronary heart disease in patients with hypercholesterolemia. Report of the program on the surgical control of the hyperlipidemias (posch), *N Engl J Med* 323:946–955, 1990.
33. Zarins CK, Zatina MA, Glagov S: Correlation of postmortem angiography with pathologic anatomy: Quantitation of atherosclerotic lesions. In Bond MG, Insull W Jr, Glagov S, Chandler AB and Cornhill JF, editors: *Clinical diagnosis of atherosclerosis: quantitative methods of evaluation*, New York, 1983, Springer-Verlag, pp. 283–306.
34. Diethrich EB, Pauliina Margolis M, Reid DB, Burke A, Ramaiah V, Rodriguez-Lopez JA, Wheatley G, Olsen D, Virmani R: Virtual histology intravascular ultrasound assessment of carotid artery disease: the carotid artery plaque virtual histology evaluation (capital) study, *J Endovasc Ther* 14:676–686, 2007.
35. Prasad A, Cipher DJ, Prasad A, Mohandas A, Roesle M, Brilakis ES, Banerjee S: Reproducibility of intravascular ultrasound virtual histology analysis, *Cardiovasc Revasc Med* 9:71–77, 2008.
36. Pundziute G, Schuijf JD, Jukema JW, Decramer I, Sarno G, Vanhoenacker PK, Boersma E, Reiber JH, Schalij MJ, Wijns W, Bax JJ: Evaluation of plaque characteristics in acute coronary syndromes: Non-invasive assessment with multi-slice computed tomography and invasive evaluation with intravascular ultrasound radiofrequency data analysis, *Eur Heart J* 29(19):2373–2381, 2008.
37. Sangiorgi GM, Clementi F, Cola C, Biondi-Zoccai G: Plaque vulnerability and related coronary event prediction by intravascular ultrasound with virtual histology: "It's a long way to tipperary"? *Catheter Cardiovasc Interv* 70:203–210, 2007.
38. Zarins CK, Glagov S, Vesselinovitch D, Wissler RW: Aneurysm formation in experimental atherosclerosis: relationship to plaque evolution. [see comments], *J Vasc Surg* 12:246–256, 1990.
39. Zarins CK, Xu CP, Glagov S: Aneurysmal enlargement of the aorta during regression of experimental atherosclerosis. [see comments], *J Vasc Surg* 15:90–98, 1992, discussion 99–101.
40. Glagov S, Zarins C, Giddens DP, Davis J, Harry R: Atherosclerosis: What is the nature of the plaque?. In Strandness DE, Didisheim P, Clowes AW, Watson J, editors: *Vascular diseases: current research and clinical applications*, Orlando, FL, 1987, Grune and Stratton.
41. Glagov S, Zarins C, Giddens DP, Ku DN: Hemodynamics and atherosclerosis. Insights and perspectives gained from studies of human arteries, *Arch Pathol Lab Med* 112:1018–1031, 1988.
42. Zarins CK, Bomberger RA, Glagov S: Local effects of stenoses: increased flow velocity inhibits atherogenesis, *Circulation* 64:II221–II227, 1981.
43. Bassiouny HS, Zarins CK, Kadowaki MH, Glagov S: Hemodynamic stress and experimental aortoiliac atherosclerosis, *J Vasc Surg* 19:426–434, 1994.
44. Caro CG, Fitz-Gerald JM, Schroter RC: Atheroma and arterial wall shear. Observation, correlation and proposal of a shear dependent mass transfer mechanism for atherogenesis, *Proc R Soc Lond B Biol Sci* 177:109–159, 1971.
45. Robertson J: Oxygen requirements of the human arterial intima in atherogenesis, *Prog Biochem Pharmacol* 4:305, 1968.
46. Giddens DP, Zarins CK, Glagov S: Response to arteries to near-wall fluid dynamic behavior, *Appl Mech Rev* 43:S98–S102, 1990.
47. Zarins CK, Giddens DP, Bharadvaj BK, Sottiurai VS, Mabon RF, Glagov S: Carotid bifurcation atherosclerosis. Quantitative correlation of plaque localization with flow velocity profiles and wall shear stress, *Circ Res* 53:502–514, 1983.
48. Gerrity RG, Goss JA, Soby L: Control of monocyte recruitment by chemotactic factor(s) in lesion-prone areas of swine aorta, *Arteriosclerosis* 5:55–66, 1985.

49. Morton WA, Parmentier EM, Petschek HE: Study of aggregate formation in region of separated blood flow, *Thromb Diath Haemorrh* 34:840–854, 1975.
50. Fox JA, Hugh AE: Static zones in the internal carotid artery: correlation with boundary layer separation and stasis in model flows, *Br J Radiol* 43:370–376, 1970.
51. Ku DN, Giddens DP, Zarins CK, Glagov S: Pulsatile flow and atherosclerosis in the human carotid bifurcation: positive correlation between plaque location and low oscillating shear stress, *Arteriosclerosis* 5:293–302, 1985.
52. Ku DN, Giddens DP, Zarins CK, Glagov S: Pulsatile flow and atherosclerosis in the human carotid bifurcation. Positive correlation between plaque location and low oscillating shear stress, *Arteriosclerosis* 5:293–302, 1985.
53. Bassiouny HS, Zarins CK, Lee DC, Skelly CL, Fortunato JE, Glagov S: Diurnal heart rate reactivity: a predictor of severity of experimental coronary and carotid atherosclerosis, *J Cardiovasc Risk* 9:331–338, 2002.
54. Nerem RM, Levesque MJ, Cornhill JF: Vascular endothelial morphology as an indicator of the pattern of blood flow, *J Biomech Eng* 103:172–176, 1981.
55. Dewey CF Jr, Bussolari SR, Gimbrone MA Jr, Davies PF: The dynamic response of vascular endothelial cells to fluid shear stress, *J Biomech Eng* 103:177–185, 1981.
56. Karsch KR: Atherosclerosis – where are we heading? *Herz* 17:309–319, 1992.
57. Giddens DP, Khalifa AM: Turbulence measurements with pulsed doppler ultrasound employing a frequency tracking method, *Ultrasound Med Biol* 8:427–437, 1982.
58. Davies PF, Remuzzi A, Gordon EJ, Dewey CF Jr, Gimbrone MA Jr: Turbulent fluid shear stress induces vascular endothelial cell turnover in vitro, *Proc Natl Acad Sci USA* 83:2114–2117, 1986.
59. Gutstein WH, Farrell GA, Armellini C: Blood flow disturbance and endothelial cell injury in preatherosclerotic swine, *Lab Invest* 29:134–149, 1973.
60. Xu C, Zarins CK, Glagov S: Biphasic response of tropoelastin at the poststenotic dilation segment of the rabbit aorta, *J Vasc Surg* 36:605–612, 2002.
61. Lieber BB, Aenis M, Zhao Y, Wakhloo AK: Flow characteristics in a stented and non-stented side wall aneurysm model. *Advances in bioengineering*, New York, 1995, BED, ASME Publication, 31:379–380.
62. Khalifa AM, Giddens DP: Characterization and evolution poststenotic flow disturbances, *J Biomech* 14:279–296, 1981.
63. Ku DN, Chen C, Salam T: Neointimal hyperplasia thickness is inversely proportional to wall shear stress in ptfe grafts. *Advances in bioengineering*, New York, BED, 1995, ASME Publication, 31:175–176.
64. Coutard M, Osborne-Pellegrin MJ: Decreased dietary lipid deposition in spontaneous lesions distal to a stenosis in the rat caudal artery, *Artery* 12:182–198, 1983.
65. Bomberger RA, Zarins CK, Taylor KE, Glagov S: Effect of hypotension on atherogenesis and aortic wall composition, *J Surg Res* 28:402–409, 1980.
66. Bharadvaj BK, Mabon RF, Giddens DP: Steady flow in a model of the human carotid bifurcation. Part ii – laser-doppler anemometer measurements, *J Biomech* 15:363–378, 1982.
67. Ku DN, Giddens DP, Phillips DJ, Strandness DE Jr: Hemodynamics of the normal human carotid bifurcation: in vitro and in vivo studies, *Ultrasound Med Biol* 11:13–26, 1985.
68. Glagov S, Rowley DA, Kohut R: Atherosclerosis of human aorta and its coronary and renal arteries, *Arch Pathol* 72:82–95, 1961.
69. Chobanian AV: Pathophysiologic considerations in the treatment of the elderly hypertensive patient, *Am J Cardiol* 52:49D–53D, 1983.
70. Kannel WB, Schwartz MJ, McNamara PM: Blood pressure and risk of coronary heart disease: the framingham study, *Dis Chest* 56:43, 1969.
71. Robertson WB, Strong JP: Atherosclerosis in persons with hypertension and diabetes mellitus, *Lab Invest* 18:538–551, 1968.
72. Gifford RW Jr: Review of the long-term controlled trials of usefulness of therapy for systemic hypertension, *Am J Cardiol* 63:8B–16B, 1989.
73. Xu C, Zarins CK, Pannaraj PS, Bassiouny HS, Glagov S: Hypercholesterolemia superimposed by experimental hypertension induces differential distribution of collagen and elastin, *Arterioscler Thromb Vasc Biol* 20:2566–2572, 2000.
74. Bomberger RA, Zarins CK, Taylor KE, Glagov S: Effect of hypotension on atherogenesis and aortic wall composition, *J Surg Res* 28:402–409, 1980.
75. Bretherton KN, Day AJ, Skinner SL: Hypertension-accelerated atherogenesis in cholesterol-fed rabbits, *Atherosclerosis* 27:79–87, 1977.
76. Bomberger RA, Zarins CK, Glagov S: Resident research award: subcritical arterial stenosis enhances distal atherosclerosis, *J Surg Res* 30:205–212, 1981.
77. Hollander W, Madoff I, Paddock J, Kirkpatrick B: Aggravation of atherosclerosis by hypertension in a subhuman primate model with coarctation of the aorta, *Circ Res* 38:63, 1976.
78. Lyon RT, Runyon-Hass A, Davis HR, Glagov S, Zarins CK: Protection from atherosclerotic lesion formation by reduction of artery wall motion, *J Vasc Surg* 5:59–67, 1987.
79. Cozzi PJ, Lyon RT, Davis HR, Sylora J, Glagov S, Zarins CK: Aortic wall metabolism in relation to susceptibility and resistance to experimental atherosclerosis, *J Vasc Surg* 7:706–714, 1988.
80. Zarins CK, Bomberger RA, Taylor KE, Glagov S: Artery stenosis inhibits regression of diet-induced atherosclerosis, *Surgery* 88:86–92, 1980.
81. Xu C, Glagov S, Zatina MA, Zarins CK: Hypertension sustains plaque progression despite reduction of hypercholesterolemia, *Hypertension* 18:123–129, 1991.
82. McGill HC Jr: George lyman duff memorial lecture. Persistent problems in the pathogenesis of atherosclerosis, *Arteriosclerosis* 4:443–451, 1984.
83. Montenegro MR, Eggen DA: Topography of atherosclerosis in the coronary arteries, *Lab Invest* 18:586–593, 1968.
84. Tang C, Blatter DD, Parker DL: Accuracy of phase-contrast flow measurements in the presence of partial-volume effects, *J Magn Reson Imag* 3:377–385, 1993.

85. Granata L, Olsson RA, Huvos A, Gregg DE: Coronary inflow and oxygen usage following cardiac sympathetic nerve stimulation in unanesthetized dogs, *Circ Res* 16:114–120, 1965.
86. Beere PA, Glagov S, Zarins CK: Retarding effect of lowered heart rate on coronary atherosclerosis, *Science* 226:180–182, 1984.
87. Schroll M, Hagerup LM: Risk factors of myocardial infarction and death in men aged 50 at entry. A ten-year prospective study from the glostrup population studies, *Dan Med Bull* 24:252–255, 1977.
88. Dyer AR, Persky V, Stamler J, Paul O, Shekelle RB, Berkson DM, Lepper M, Schoenberger JA, Lindberg HA: Heart rate as a prognostic factor for coronary heart disease and mortality: findings in three Chicago epidemiologic studies, *Am J Epidemiol* 112:736–749, 1980.
89. Williams PT, Wood PD, Haskell WL, Vranizan K: The effects of running mileage and duration on plasma lipoprotein levels, *JAMA* 247:2674–2679, 1982.
90. Williams PT, Haskell WL, Vranizan KM, Blair SN, Krauss RM, Superko HR, Albers JJ, Frey-Hewitt B, Wood PD: Associations of resting heart rate with concentrations of lipoprotein subfractions in sedentary men, *Circulation* 71:441–449, 1985.
91. Ku DN, Glagov S, Moore JE Jr, Zarins CK: Flow patterns in the abdominal aorta under simulated postprandial and exercise conditions: an experimental study, *J Vasc Surg* 9:309–316, 1989.
92. Zarins CK, Glagov S: Aneurysms and obstructive plaques: Differing local responses to atherosclerosis. In Bergan JJ, Yao JST, editors: *Aneurysms, diagnosis and treatment*, New York, 1982, Grune and Stratton, Inc.
93. Busuttil RW, Abou-Zamzam AM, Machleder HI: Collagenase activity of the human aorta. A comparison of patients with and without abdominal aortic aneurysms, *Arch Surg* 115:1373–1378, 1980.
94. Menashi S, Campa JS, Greenhalgh RM, Powell JT: Collagen in abdominal aortic aneurysm: typing, content, and degradation, *J Vasc Surg* 6:578–582, 1987.
95. Brophy CM, Marks WH, Reilly JM, Tilson MD: Decreased tissue inhibitor of metalloproteinases (timp) in abdominal aortic aneurysm tissue: a preliminary report, *J Surg Res* 50:653–657, 1991.
96. Dobrin PB, Baker WH, Gley WC: Elastolytic and collagenolytic studies of arteries. Implications for the mechanical properties of aneurysms, *Arch Surg* 119:405–409, 1984.
97. DePalma RG, Koletsky S, Bellon EM, Insull W Jr: Failure of regression of atherosclerosis in dogs with moderate cholesterolemia, *Atherosclerosis* 27:297–310, 1977.
98. Zatina MA, Zarins CK, Gewertz BL, Glagov S: Role of medial lamellar architecture in the pathogenesis of aortic aneurysms, *J Vasc Surg* 1:442–448, 1984.
99. Strickland HL, Bond MG: Aneurysms in a large colony of squirrel monkeys (saimiri sciureus), *Lab Anim Sci* 33:589–592, 1983.
100. Clark ET, Gewertz BL, Bassiouny HS, Zarins CK: Current results of elective aortic reconstruction for aneurysmal and occlusive disease, *J Cardiovasc Surg (Torino).* 31:438–441, 1990.

Part II

Components of an Endovascular Practice

3 Training and Credentialing in Vascular and Endovascular Surgery

Stephen T. Smith and G. Patrick Clagett

The previous decade has seen explosive growth in technological advances in the endovascular arena. A partial list of these technologies would include carotid angioplasty and stenting, refinements in thoracic and abdominal endografts, and lower extremity angioplasty stenting, atherectomy, and mechanical thrombectomy. The field of vascular surgery has completely embraced these minimally invasive techniques and adapted its training paradigms accordingly. With the increasing complexity and breadth of endovascular interventions, vascular surgery has become a distinct surgery specialty. Reflecting this change, candidates for the Vascular Surgery Board examination of the American Board of Surgery (VSB-ABS) can sit for the examination after completion of an Accreditation Council for Graduate Medical Education (ACGME)-accredited vascular residency without previous certification in general surgery.

Vascular surgery is the specialty that deals with diagnosis and management of disorders of the arterial, venous, and lymphatic systems, exclusive of intracardiac and intracranial vessels [1]. A fully trained vascular surgeon should be a specialist who performs open surgery and endovascular interventions and has the expertise in vascular medicine to manage appropriate patients non-operatively. This expertise includes the skills to interpret non-invasive vascular lab studies.

S.T. Smith (✉)
Assistant Professor, Division of Vascular & Endovascular Surgery, Department of Surgery, University of Texas Southwestern Medical Center, Dallas, TX, USA

Training and Certification in Vascular Surgery

Because of the field's increasing complexity, having vascular surgery exposure during other residencies, such as general and cardiothoracic surgery, is no longer sufficient to acquire the appropriate judgment and skills necessary to practice vascular surgery. Completion of an ACGME-accredited vascular training program is necessary to achieve board certification in vascular surgery. Multiple training pathways have come about in an attempt to adapt to the various pressures facing vascular surgery training, including trainee's desire for shortened pathways, and vascular surgery's evolution as a distinct specialty. There are currently four ACGME-approved training pathways in vascular surgery [1]:

1. Traditional. This is the oldest but remains the most common method for obtaining vascular training. The candidate enters a 2-year ACGME-approved vascular residency following successful completion of a 5-year ACGME-approved general surgery training program.
2. Early Specialization. In the Early Specialization Program (ESP), the trainee completes 4 years of general surgery training followed by 2 years of vascular fellowship at the same ACGME-accredited facility. The selected candidate must be identified early so their program can be adapted such that the fourth year of training will be as a chief resident in general surgery. At this time, both the general and vascular surgery training must take place at the same institution. ESP graduates are eligible for both general and vascular surgery board certification.

T.J. Fogarty, R.A. White (eds.), *Peripheral Endovascular Interventions*,
DOI 10.1007/978-1-4419-1387-6_3,

3. Integrated. This pathway directly accepts graduating students from a Medical Doctor (MD) or Doctor of Osteopathic Medicine (DO) program into a 5-year vascular surgery training program. During the first 4 years, the trainee is exposed to 2 years of core general surgery and 2 years of vascular surgery. The final fifth year is devoted entirely to vascular surgery. Graduates of the integrated program are only eligible for board certification in vascular surgery.
4. Independent. This 6-year pathway includes 3 years of core general surgery training plus 3 years of vascular surgery training. The final year of the program serves as the chief resident responsibility on the vascular surgery service. All 6 years must be completed at the same ACGME-approved institution. Graduates from this pathway are only eligible for board certification in vascular surgery.

Specific Requirements for Vascular Surgery Residents

Vascular Surgery

The vascular surgery trainee should get broad exposure to open vascular surgery and is expected to have performed at least the minimum number of operations in each required area. The Residency Review Committee for Surgery (RRC-S) carefully evaluates and sets these requirements. The established minimum criteria for major open vascular reconstructive procedures include 30 abdominal vascular operations, 25 cerebrovascular, 45 peripheral, and 10 complex. In addition, the RRC-S guidelines set a minimum experience of 250 major vascular reconstructive cases that include open and endovascular operations. These are the 2008 recommendations but are continually reviewed and are subject to change.

Endovascular Interventions

All vascular surgery residents are expected to have sufficient experience to perform vascular catheter-based interventions. The RRC-S has recently updated the minimum numbers for endovascular cases, which includes 80 endovascular therapeutic procedures, 100 endovascular diagnostic procedures, and 20 endovascular aortic aneurysm repairs (EVAR). The experience should be balanced between the arterial and venous systems, with at least half of the diagnostic and 75% of the therapeutic procedures being performed on the arterial system [1]. The rationale for this is that venous interventions for dialysis grafts, and fistulas, and venous catheter placements should not constitute the major endovascular experience. Table 3.1 includes these requirements as well as guidelines for thoracic endovascular aortic repair (TEVAR) and carotid angioplasty and stenting (CAS).

Non-invasive Vascular Laboratory

Vascular surgery fellowship programs must include training in non-invasive vascular lab studies. This includes the traditional vascular lab, including arterial and venous ultrasound studies, and the ability to analyze and manipulate three-dimensional (3-D) computer tomography (CT) reconstructions. three-dimensional reconstructions have become integral to the planning and surveillance of endovascular interventions like EVAR, angioplasty, and stenting. Adequate training for vascular ultrasound must include basic ultrasound anatomy, physiology and physics, and clinical ultrasound application to the treatment of vascular disorders. A minimum number of supervised interpretations of vascular studies in key areas should be performed as recommended by the Inter-societal Commission for Accreditation of Vascular Laboratories (ICAVL) (Table 3.2).

Hospital Credentialing

New Vascular Graduates

Physicians applying for vascular surgery privileges should have completed an ACGME-accredited vascular fellowship. All current training paradigms discussed above provide 2 years of vascular and endovascular training in addition to a core general surgery

Table 3.1 Society for vascular surgery credentialing guidelines for endovascular procedures

	Number of cases	Number as primary operator
Endovascular diagnostic	100[a]	
Endovascular therapeutic	80[a]	
Endovascular aortic aneurysm repair (EVAR)	20[a]	
Thoracic endovascular aortic repair (TEVAR)	10 within 2 years or 25 EVARs plus full endovascular privileges[b,c]	12 EVARs as primary
Carotid stenting (CAS)	25, plus	Half as primary
	30 diagnostic cervicocerebral angiograms[d]	Half as primary

Adapted from Calligaro et al. [1], with permission.
[a] Residency review for surgery established minimums for training.
[b] Physicians performing TEVAR should be familiar with the perioperative management of aortic surgical patients and are expected to have experience in performing adjunctive procedures for TEVARs, including iliac conduits, femoral exposures and repairs, and carotid–subclavian bypasses.
[c] Pre-existing open thoracoabdominal privileges are not a requirement.
[d] Diagnostic and stenting procedures may both be counted if performed during the same procedure.

Table 3.2 Inter-societal commission for accreditation of vascular laboratories minimum guidelines for interpretation of vascular non-invasive studies

Non-invasive study	Minimum interpretations[a]
Peripheral arterial physiologic test	100
Peripheral arterial duplex scanning	100
Peripheral venous duplex scanning	100
Carotid duplex scanning	100
Transcranial duplex/Doppler scanning	100
Visceral vascular duplex scanning	75

[a] Physicians may seek privileges only in those areas where they have sufficient qualifications and training.

experience. The importance and increasing use of catheter-based interventions has been recognized by the ACGME through the RRC-S, which has made training in endovascular techniques a required component of vascular surgery training programs [2]. The need to develop increased expertise with endovascular procedures has led to the requirement for a minimum of 2 years of vascular surgery training. The endovascular training can be concentrated in 1 year or distributed evenly during the vascular fellowship. The minimum requirements of the RRC-S include 100 endovascular diagnostic cases, 80 endovascular therapeutic cases, and 20 EVARs. These should be distributed among the various vascular anatomic areas to establish competency in the treatment of patients with the complete breadth of vascular disease.

While there are no specific criteria for many subtypes of endovascular procedures such as subclavian stenting, mesenteric angioplasty and stenting, thrombolysis, percutaneous mechanical thrombectomy, and embolizations, two specific procedures deserve mention. Specific guidelines have been published for credentialing in thoracic endovascular aortic repair (TEVAR) [3]. In addition to adequate training and exposure to thoracic aneurysm patients, anyone performing TEVAR should have knowledge of the perioperative management of thoracic aorta patients and have experience with adjunctive procedures often required with TEVAR. These include iliac conduits, femoral exposure, carotid subclavian bypass, and carotid–carotid bypass [1]. Requirements for TEVAR include basic endovascular privileges with an experience of 25 EVAR, 12 of which should be as the primary operator. Credentials for open thoracic surgery are not a requirement for TEVAR privileges.

A multi-disciplinary statement on training and credentialing for carotid stenting was published in 2005 [4]. Carotid stenting with embolic protection (CAS) is a relatively new procedure with the largest randomized controlled trial comparing CAS to carotid endarterectomy (CREST trial) ongoing [5]. The minimum numbers of procedures to achieve competence are 30 diagnostic carotid arteriograms and 25 carotid stent procedures, both with at least half as the primary operator (Table 3.1). These multi-specialty guidelines also state that the diagnostic and stenting portions may both be counted if performed during the same procedure. In addition to the procedural skills, the trainee must gain competency in the cognitive and clinical skills as well as judgment regarding care of the patient with carotid bifurcation disease.

Credentialed Surgeons

Guidelines for vascular surgeons in practice are no different from those of vascular surgery residents entering practice. With rapidly advancing technology and new procedures, vascular surgeons should continue learning new procedures as the field evolves. Surgeons are expected to acquire proficiency in new procedures. For physicians trained in endovascular interventions, special training and certification may not be necessary. Credentialing for these new procedures and the training necessary will depend on the procedure's complexity and needs to be determined on a case-by-case basis.

Maintenance of Certification

The ABS has instituted a Maintenance of Certification (MOC) program that goes beyond the traditional recertification process [6]. It is designed to give diplomates a greater opportunity to assess their practice and demonstrate their commitment to lifelong learning and practice improvement. ABS diplomates are automatically enrolled in MOC upon certification or recertification in any specialty after July 1, 2005. The MOC program consists of four parts:

Part 1—*Professional standing* through maintenance of an unrestricted medical license, hospital privileges, and satisfactory references;

Part 2—*Lifelong learning* through continuing education and periodic self-assessment;

Part 3—*Cognitive expertise* based on performance on a secure examination;

Part 4—*Evaluation of performance* in practice through tools such as outcome measures and quality improvement programs and the evaluation of behaviors such as communication and professionalism.

For vascular surgeons maintaining their specialty certification, the ABS will allow evidence of professional standing, lifelong learning/self-assessment, and evaluation of performance in practice (Parts 1, 2, and 4) that are performed in compliance with one certificate to be credited toward any other certificates the diplomate may hold. Maintenance of certification in general surgery is not mandatory for the maintenance of vascular certification. The Society for Vascular Surgery has introduced the Vascular Education and Self-Assessment Program (VESAP) to meet MOC self-assessment requirements.

Turf Battles

The area of peripheral endovascular interventions is an evolving one in which multiple specialties have expertise, including cardiology, interventional nephrology, interventional radiology, and vascular surgery. As there is no central credentialing process, each hospital must make credentialing decisions independently. In general, no specialty should hold territory over any specific anatomic area or specific procedure. Rather, if a physician can document proper training and show acceptable outcomes, the hospital should approve the credentials for that procedure. Each specialty has a different focus, and thus has some areas of expertise that are not shared. The best situation may be one where physicians from different specialties can work together and "cross-train." However, the political realities and competition between specialties often make this working relationship difficult to achieve.

Summary

This is an exciting time in vascular surgery with the evolution of peripheral endovascular interventions. With expertise in both open surgery and endovascular techniques, the vascular surgeon has multiple tools to attack almost any vascular problem with which a patient may present. With each new technological advance, new vascular beds are amenable to minimally invasive treatment. Physicians must maintain proper training and ongoing experience to keep abreast of the latest advances.

References

1. Calligaro KD, Toursarkissian B, Clagett GP et al.: Guidelines for hospital privileges in vascular and endovascular surgery: recommendations of the society of vascular surgery, *J Vasc Surg* 47:1–5, 2008.
2. Creager MA, Goldstone J, Hirshfeld JW, Kazmers A, Kent KC, Lorell BH, Olin JW, Pauly RR, Rosenfield K, Roubin GS, Sicard GA, White CJ: ACC/ACP/SCAI/SVMB/SVS

clinical competence statement on vascular medicine and catheter-based peripheral vascular interventions: a report of the American College of Cardiology/American Heart Association/American College of Physicians Task Force on Clinical Competence (ACC/ACP/SCAI/SVMB/SVS writing committee on clinical competence on peripheral vascular disease), *J Am Coll Cardiol* 44: 941–957, 2004.
3. Hodgson KJ, Matsumura JS, Ascher E, Dake MD, Sacks D, Krol K et al.: SVS/SIR/SCAI/SVMB writing committee. Clinical competence statement on thoracic endovascular aortic repair (TEVAR) – multispecialty consensus recommendations. A report of the SVS/SIR/SCAI/SVMB Writing committee to develop a clinical competence standard for TEVAR, *J Vasc Surg* 46:858–862, 2006.
4. Rosenfield K, Cowley MJ, Jaff MR, Ouriel K, Gray W, Cates CU, Feldman T, Babb JD, Gallagher A, Green R, Kent KC, Roubin GS, Weiner BH, White CW: SCAI/SVMB/SVS clinical competence statement on carotid stenting: training and credentialing for carotid stenting – multispecialty consensus recommendations, a report of the SCAI/SVMB/SVS writing committee to develop a clinical competence statement on carotid interventions, *J Am Coll Cardiol* 45:165–174, 2005.
5. Hobson RW 2nd, Howard FJ, Roubin GS, Ferguson RD, Brott G, Howard G: CREST. Credentialing of surgeons as interventionalists for carotid artery stenting: experience from the lead-in phase of CREST, *J Vasc Surg* 40:952–957, 2004.
6. Maintenance of certification, American Board of Surgery web address: www.absurgery.org
7. Society for Vascular Surgery, web address: www.vascularweb.org

4 Assessment of Vascular Patients and Indications for Therapy

Christian de Virgilio and Tony Chan

Evaluation of the vascular patient requires a systematic approach that begins with the history and physical examination, generally followed by noninvasive studies to obtain a more quantitative estimation of the degree of vascular compromise. The decision to perform more invasive studies or to proceed to endovascular or open therapy must be individualized but is dependent in large part on the findings of the history, physical examination, and noninvasive studies [1]. The following sections outline the principles of vascular patient assessment and the indications for endovascular therapy.

History and Physical Examination of the Ischemic Lower Extremity

A thorough history and physical examination are essential components of the assessment of vascular patients. Risk factors for atherosclerosis, such as smoking, diabetes, hyperlipidemia, and familial predisposition, must be identified. Evidence of coronary or cerebrovascular involvement should be sought. In most instances, the status of the lower extremity vascular bed can be accurately defined by a carefully obtained history. The site of pathology can be further localized by a diligent physical examination. It is imperative to determine early whether the patient's complaints and presentation represent acute or chronic arterial insufficiency, as this greatly affects the timing of the intervention. Likewise, in patients with chronic arterial insufficiency it is imperative to distinguish between potentially limb-threatening and non-limb-threatening problems.

Chronic Arterial Insufficiency

Patients with chronic arterial insufficiency most often complain of pain in the lower extremity. The location, character, and duration of the pain provide vital information and help distinguish arterial disease from other causes of extremity pain. The pain of arterial insufficiency takes on one of two forms: intermittent claudication or ischemic rest pain. It is critical to identify patients with ischemic rest pain, as it is considered limb threatening; claudication by itself is not. Additional signs of critical ischemia are non-healing ulcers and gangrene.

The definition of *claudication* consists of three parts: (a) pain with exertion, which is (b) relieved by rest, and is (c) reproducible at the same distance or degree of effort each time. The pain is described as a cramping or aching lower extremity pain, usually in the calf, brought on by walking. Thigh and buttock claudication usually signifies aortoiliac disease. Associated impotence increases the likelihood of aortoiliac disease. Isolated calf claudication suggests disease in the superficial femoral artery (SFA), although aortoiliac disease occasionally is the cause. Isolated foot claudication is rare and is seen in patients with isolated tibioperoneal arterial disease, such as in Buerger's disease. The physical examination helps to make the distinction. Patients with aortoiliac disease

C. de Virgilio (✉)
Professor, Department of Vascular Surgery, Harbor-UCLA Medical Center and UCLA School of Medicine, Torrance, CA, USA

T.J. Fogarty, R.A. White (eds.), *Peripheral Endovascular Interventions*,
DOI 10.1007/978-1-4419-1387-6_4, © Springer Science+Business Media, LLC 1998, 2010

have diminished femoral pulses and bruits, those with isolated SFA disease have normal femoral pulses and diminished/absent popliteal pulses, and those with isolated tibioperoneal artery disease have normal femoral and popliteal pulses and absent distal pulses.

Additionally, there are other signs of chronic arterial ischemia which should be sought on examination. Calf muscle atrophy, loss of hair, and atrophy of the skin, skin appendages, and subcutaneous tissue are indicative of chronic ischemia. The skin takes on a shiny, scaly appearance. The fate of patients with claudication has been studied extensively. Only about 25% of claudicants will significantly deteriorate with respect to their walking distance [2]. The likelihood of deterioration is greatest in the first year after the diagnosis is established. Furthermore, the risk of limb loss at 5 years in patients with isolated claudication is very low, estimated at between 1 and 3% [2]. The best predictor of deterioration is the ankle brachial index (ABI) at initial presentation. Patients with an ABI less than 0.5 are twice as likely to progress to needing revascularization or amputation as those with an ABI more than 0.5 [2].

Differential Diagnosis

When assessing a patient for possible arterial insufficiency, it is important to remember that other disease processes can mimic arterial claudication. Osteoarthritis of the hip or knee joint can cause similar symptoms, but the pain is not reproducible at a predictable walking distance and not immediately relieved by rest. Osteophytic narrowing of the lumbar canal leading to neurospinal compression can be confused with aortoiliac disease, but the weakness is relieved by leaning over and worsened by increasing lumbar lordosis. Likewise, nerve root compression can potentially be confused with claudication. However, the character of the pain is sharper, more lancinating, and often radiates down the back of the leg. The pain is not typically reproducible at the same walking distance, and may be worse with sitting.

Critical Limb Ischemia

Critical limb ischemia (CLI) includes symptoms of ischemic rest pain, non-healing ulcer, and gangrene. *Ischemic rest pain* usually occurs at night, involves the foot, and in particular the metatarsals and toes. The pain is described as throbbing or cramping (not burning), may be associated with numbness, and is relieved by placing the foot in a dependent position. Patients typically describe waking up at night and having to dangle their feet over the edge of the bed. Alternatively, they will report that the symptoms are improved by standing up and ambulating. The patient may associate the walking with the improvement, and not recognize that it is the effect of gravity which increases extremity circulation while the patient is standing. In the most severe form of rest pain, patients literally have to sleep sitting up in a chair. The foot develops continuous rubor and dependent edema. In these circumstances, the findings can be misinterpreted as cellulitis. In addition, ischemic rest pain can be confused with the burning discomfort of diabetic neuropathy, though the latter is not relieved by dependency. The finding of marked foot pallor upon leg elevation for 2 min followed by a transition to a deep rubor on dependency (Buerger's sign) further supports severe ischemia and helps distinguish rest pain from other diagnoses. Some patients awaken with cramping in the calf at night, although this is not considered ischemic rest pain per se.

The extremities should be examined for the presence of *non-healing ulcers*. The location and appearance of the ulcers help to determine the etiology (venous, arterial, neuropathic). Ulcers over the medial malleolus, in association with leg edema, hyperpigmentation, and varicose veins, are classically venous stasis ulcers. The presence of healthy granulation tissue at the base of the ulcer confirms that the arterial blood supply is adequate. Ulcers due to arterial insufficiency are usually located on or between the toes and have a dull gray appearance without granulation tissue. Neuropathic ulcers present at pressure points, such as on the plantar surface over the first or second metatarsal head. They have a punched-out appearance with granulation tissue. Chronic osteomyelitis may concomitantly be present. A useful test to detect osteomyelitis is to gently probe the ulcer with a cotton tip applicator. If the tip comes in contact with bone, this finding has a high specificity for osteomyelitis (but low sensitivity). A monofilament probe should be used to confirm neuropathy. In addition to a low ABI less than 0.5, the risk of developing CLI is related to age and other risk factors. Patients with diabetes mellitus are at four times increased risk. Smokers are at three times increased risk, whereas patients older than 65 years of age and those with lipid abnormalities have a twofold higher risk [2].

Rutherford (REF) and Fontaine (REF) have provided useful classification systems for peripheral artery disease (PAD), ranging from an asymptomatic patient to major tissue loss (Table 4.1). When embarking on an intervention, it is important to document the degree of PAD using one of these systems.

Table 4.1 Classification systems for peripheral arterial disease

Rutherford classification of peripheral arterial disease		
Grade 0	Category 0	Asymptomatic
Grade 1	Category 1	Mild claudication
Grade 1	Category 2	Moderate claudication
Grade 1	Category 3	Severe claudication
Grade 2	Category 4	Ischemic rest pain
Grade 3	Category 5	Mild tissue ulceration
Grade 3	Category 6	Tissue loss/gangrene
Fontaine classification of peripheral arterial disease		
Stage I	Asymptomatic	
Stage IIa	Mild claudication (>200 m)	
Stage IIb	Moderate to severe claudication (≤200 m)	
Stage III	Ischemic rest pain	
Stage IV	Tissue loss or ulceration	

Acute Arterial Insufficiency

The presentation of acute arterial insufficiency is frequently dramatic. Sudden onset of severe extremity pain, pallor, and pulselessness may progress to paresthesia and paralysis (the so-called Five Ps). However, these five signs are not necessarily present in acute limb ischemia, so they cannot be used to grade the severity of the ischemia.

Three categories (with two subcategories) of severity of acute lower extremity ischemia have been adopted by the Inter-Society Consensus for the Management of Peripheral Arterial Disease (TASC II): viable, threatened, and irreversible (Table 4.2) [2]. A *viable* extremity (category I) has no continuing ischemic pain, no neurologic deficit, and adequate skin capillary return and there are clearly audible Doppler signals in a pedal artery [2]. A *threatened* extremity (category II) has more severe ischemia, but it is still reversible if prompt revascularization is achieved. Arterial Doppler signals are not clearly audible in the foot, although venous signals are present.

Table 4.2 TASC Classification of Aortoiliac Lesions

Type A lesion
- Unilateral or bilateral stenoses of CIA
- Unilateral or bilateral single short (<3 cm) stenosis of EIA

Type B lesions
- Short (<3 cm) stenosis of infrarenal aorta
- Unilateral CIA occlusion
- Single or multiple stenosis totaling 3–10 cm involving the EIA not extending into the CFA
- Unilateral EIA occlusion not involving the origins of internal iliac or CFA

Type C lesions
- Bilateral CIA occlusions
- Bilateral EIA stenoses 3–10 cm long not extending into the CFA
- Unilateral EIA stenosis extending into the CFA
- Unilateral EIA occlusion that involves the origins of internal iliac and/or CFA
- Heavily calcified unilateral EIA occlusion with or without involvement of origins of internal iliac and/or CFA

Type D lesions
- Infrarenal aortoiliac occlusion
- Diffuse disease involving the aorta and both iliac arteries requiring treatment
- Diffuse multiple stenoses involving the unilateral CIA, EIA, and CFA
- Unilateral occlusions of both CIA and EIA
- Bilateral occlusions of EIA
- Iliac stenoses in patients with AAA requiring treatment and not amenable to endograft placement or other lesions requiring open aortic or iliac surgery

From Norgren et al., [2] with permission.
CIA: common iliac artery; EIA: external iliac artery; CFA: common femoral artery; AAA: abdominal aortic aneurysm; TASC: Inter-Society Consensus for the Management of Peripheral Arterial Disease.

Category II is further divided into marginally threatened (IIa) and immediately threatened (IIb) ischemia. With *marginally* threatened ischemia, patients may complain of numbness and minimal sensory loss in the toes, without continuous pain [2]. *Immediately* threatened limbs have continuous ischemic pain with detectable loss of sensation above the toes, a continuing lack of all sensation in the toes, any motor loss, or a combination of these factors [2]. Patients with *irreversible* ischemia have profound sensory loss and muscle paralysis extending above the foot. Arterial and venous Doppler signals are absent, as is capillary refill. Muscle rigor or skin marbling may be present. Irreversible ischemia requires major amputation or results in permanent neuromuscular damage regardless of therapy [2].

It is important to differentiate between embolic and thrombotic causes of acute ischemia, as the etiology of the ischemia may have therapeutic implications. *Embolic* arterial occlusion should be suspected in patients who have no antecedent history of chronic arterial insufficiency. Pulse examination in the uninvolved extremities is often normal. A history of recent myocardial infarction or atrial fibrillation points to a cardiac source of the embolus. Bilateral toe gangrene in the face of good pedal pulses (blue toe syndrome) suggests an aortic source of the embolus, typically from an aortic aneurysm or an atherosclerotic plaque. *Thrombotic* arterial occlusion occurs most often in the setting of underlying progressive atherosclerosis. Volume depletion or a sudden drop in cardiac output may be contributing factors. The patient often reports a long-standing history of claudication or ischemic rest pain. Physical examination may reveal evidence of diffuse atherosclerosis with diminished pulses and bruits in the uninvolved extremities in addition to the findings of acute ischemia.

Noninvasive Studies

Following the history and physical examination, noninvasive studies are undertaken to provide a more objective and quantitative assessment of the degree of ischemia. The decision of which noninvasive tests to perform is dictated in part by the acuity and severity of the ischemia. The minimum assessment includes interrogation of the distal artery with continuous-wave handheld Doppler and measurement of the ankle–brachial index.

Continuous-Wave Doppler

A great deal of information can be gleaned from the audible signal of a continuous-wave nondirectional, handheld Doppler test. Normal arterial signals are biphasic or triphasic [3]. The first sound corresponds to high-velocity forward flow during systole. The second sound results from reversed flow during early diastole. Flow reversal occurs in high-resistance vascular beds (e.g., normal extremity arteries). Some vessels rely on continuous forward flow during diastole (e.g., internal carotid and renal arteries) and, as such, their resistance is low. The second sound is absent in these arteries. The third sound represents forward flow during late diastole.

In the presence of extremity ischemia, the distal arterial bed vasodilates, peripheral resistance falls, flow reversal ceases, and the second sound disappears. As ischemia worsens, the signal becomes monophasic or absent. In evaluating a patient with acute ischemia, complete absence of arterial signals correlates with a threatened or potentially irreversible ischemia and should prompt an attempt to elicit adjacent venous signals. A combination of an inaudible arterial and venous signals generally signifies irreversible ischemia.

Ankle–Brachial Index and Segmental Pressures

The ankle–brachial index (ABI) is obtained by measuring the highest pressure at the ankle using continuous-wave Doppler and dividing the result by the highest arm pressure. The normal ABI averages 1.1, and ranges from 1 to 1.2, as the pressure in the ankle is 12–24 mm greater than that in the arm in the supine position [3]. By definition, PAD is defined as an ABI more than 0.9. Segmental pressures are measured to further localize the site of obstruction. Segmental pressures are performed by sequentially placing a pneumatic cuff around the upper thigh, above the knee, around the calf, and at the ankle and measuring the pressure at each position. A pressure drop of more than 15 mmHg from one site to the next suggests that a hemodynamically significant stenosis is present in the artery with the lower pressure [3].

The ABI is an indicator of the presence of hemodynamically significant arterial disease. With a normal ABI, significant disease is unlikely. If the ABI is normal and the clinical index of suspicion remains high, the ABI should be repeated following exercise. The increased flow generated by exercise may accentuate the pressure drop across a fixed stenosis. ABI readings of more than 1.2 are also considered abnormal. Medial calcification, as seen in diabetics, results in noncompressible vessels and is one cause of spuriously elevated ankle pressures.

The degree of ABI diminution is related to the severity of the ischemia. The ankle pressure is reduced by at least 10 mmHg by a single 50% or greater *stenosis* and by 53 and 61 mmHg in the presence of an SFA and iliac *occlusion*, respectively [3]. Pressure drops of more than 50 mmHg suggest multilevel obstruction. In general, in patients with claudication the ABI is 0.59 ± 0.15, in patients with rest pain 0.26 ± 0.13, and in patients with gangrene 0.05 ± 0.08 [4]. By using the ABI and segmental pressures in combination with the history and physical examination one can determine the level of disease and estimate whether the lesion represents a stenosis or an occlusion. For example, a patient with unilateral thigh claudication, a diminished femoral pulse with a bruit, an ankle pressure of 100 mmHg, and an arm pressure of 120 mmHg (ABI 0.83) can be predicted to have an isolated iliac *stenosis.* Conversely, a patient with calf claudication and foot rest pain, absent femoral, popliteal, and pedal pulses, an ankle pressure of 30 mmHg, and an arm pressure of 120 mmHg (ABI 0.25) likely has both iliac and SFA *occlusions.*

Digital pressures are a valuable adjunct to the segmental pressure measurements. Digital pressures may enable the examiner to localize arterial disease to the pedal or digital arteries. When evaluating lower extremity ischemia, the digital pressure is particularly useful in diabetics, as medial calcification rarely involves the digital arteries. The normal toe pressure is 24–41 mmHg less than the brachial pressure, and the corresponding normal toe–brachial index is 0.89 ± 0.16 [4]. Toe pressures below 30 mmHg correlate with non-healing of toe ulcers or amputation sites [4].

Presently, the ABI remains the gold standard for assessing patient with suspected PAD. It permits establishment of the diagnosis, gives an objective assessment of disease severity, provides a baseline to follow the patient, and provides objective pre- and post-intervention documentation of whether the revascularization procedure has improved distal blood flow.

Pulse Volume Recording

The pulse volume recording (PVR) relies on air plethysmography to produce waveforms that correlate with pulsatile arterial flow. The PVR, which can be calibrated to provide a semiquantitative estimate of the degree of obstruction, is particularly useful in two settings. First, the toe PVR is helpful for determining the need for revascularization in the diabetic patient with a foot ulcer or gangrene who has a spuriously elevated ABI. The absence of pulsatile arterial flow on a PVR in such a patient indicates severe arterial obstruction. Second, the PVR is a valuable intraoperative tool. Performed immediately before and after an intervention (i.e., bypass, angioplasty), it can detect improvement or deterioration of the pulsatile arterial flow.

Transcutaneous Oximetry

Transcutaneous measurement of the oxygen pressure ($tcPO_2$) is another helpful tool when evaluating CLI. The $tcPO_2$ has been used to predict the healing of ischemic ulcers, determine the level of amputation, and predict the success of revascularization postoperatively [5, 6]. Like the PVR, $tcPO_2$ is valuable in the diabetic patient with a foot ulcer or gangrene and falsely elevated ankle pressures. One study found that ischemic ulcers were unlikely to heal when $tcPO_2$ measurements in the foot were less than 30 mmHg [7]. The ulcers healed when the $tcPO_2$ was at least 38 mmHg.

Duplex Ultrasonography

Duplex ultrasonography combines a real-time, high-resolution image of the vessel wall and lumen with Doppler signal analysis. The ultrasound image localizes the plaque and characterizes its morphology. It may also demonstrate abnormalities such as aneurysm formation, intraluminal thrombus, intraplaque hemorrhage, and dissection (Figs. 4.1and 4.2) [8, 9].

Analysis of the Doppler signal includes three components: spectral analysis, velocity waveforms, and color-flow imaging. *Spectral analysis* detects stenoses by identifying abnormalities in blood flow patterns. Stenoses from atherosclerotic plaques interrupt laminar flow and produce more random movements of blood cells [10]. These more random movements create spectra with a wide range of frequencies and amplitudes. Spectral broadening is the term used to describe the resultant wide frequency band. Specific criteria have been established for calculating the percent diameter reduction for carotid and lower extremity lesions

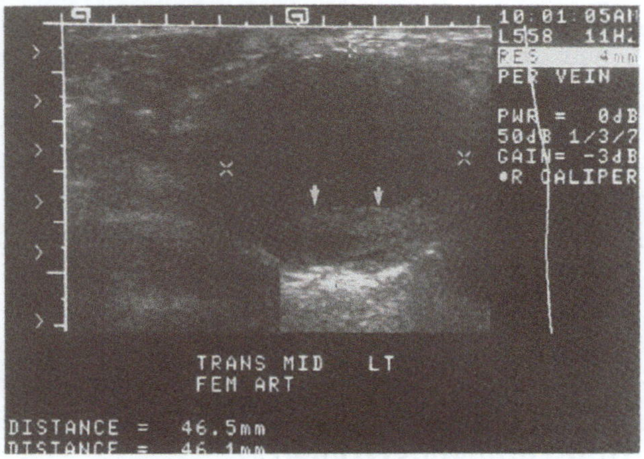

Fig. 4.1 Ultrasonography of *left* groin reveals a 4.6 × 4.6 cm common femoral artery aneurysm (*cursors*). Thrombus is visible posteriorly (*arrows*).

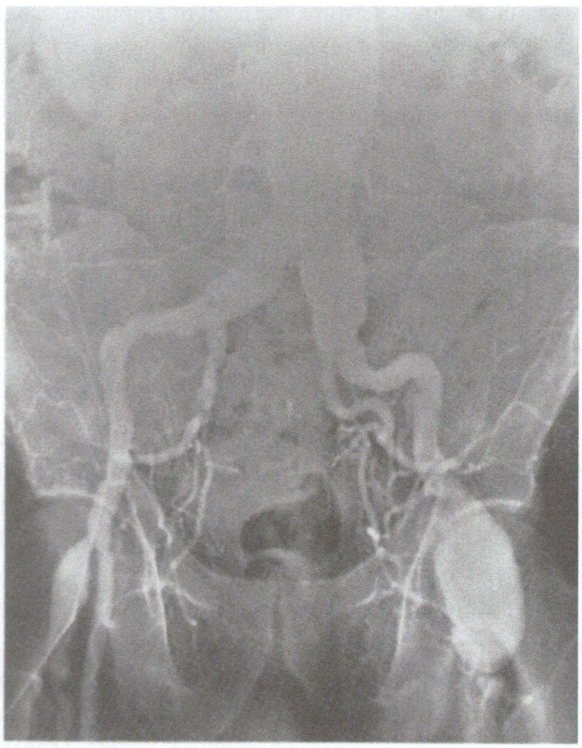

Fig. 4.2 Aortogram of same patient as in Fig. 4-1 demonstrates aneurysmosis. In addition to the *left* common femoral artery aneurysm, aortic, bilateral common iliac, and *right* superficial femoral artery aneurysms are present. The classic slow blood flow velocity makes angiographic assessment difficult.

based on spectral analysis of pulsed Doppler signals. For carotid stenosis, the criteria are based on the peak systolic frequency, end-diastolic frequency, and degree of spectral broadening [10]. For lower extremity stenosis, the velocity waveforms are adjuncts utilized in the analysis. The normal extremity artery has a triphasic waveform that corresponds to the audible Doppler signals previously described. In the presence of an arterial stenosis, peripheral resistance distally decreases, eliminating the flow reversal phase. With severe stenosis, the waveform *distal* to the stenosis becomes monophasic, with a low, rounded peak. The waveform *within* the stenosis, on the other hand, demonstrates a markedly increased peak systolic velocity. *Color-flow* imaging provides flow information of the entire image in real time. The specific information produced by the color includes the direction of flow and an estimate of the mean frequency. Color-flow imaging does not allow as precise calculation of the degree of stenosis as does spectral analysis [10]. The technique is particularly useful when scanning a long length of artery. Color changes that correspond to an increased frequency can be rapidly identified. The examiner can then focus the spectral analysis to that area. Color-flow imaging is also helpful when interrogating deeply located vessels, as the color makes it easy to distinguish vessels from adjacent structures. Recent studies suggest that Duplex ultrasound has a higher sensitivity and specificity for early atherosclerotic lesions in the SFA than the ABI. Early lesions in the SFA may not alter the ABI at rest. Early identification of PAD is important as this will allow earlier medical intervention.

The role of computed tomography (CT), magnetic resonance angiography, and CT angiography are discussed in detail in other chapters.

Indications for Intervention

Asymptomatic Peripheral Arterial Disease

Patients who are identified as having PAD based on an ABI more than 0.9 are candidates for medical intervention regardless of whether they are symptomatic. This is based on the fact that patients with PAD are at significantly increased risk of stroke and myocardial infarction. Medical intervention should include enrollment in a smoking cessation program, a lipid lowering program using statins, fibrates, and/or niacin to raise HDL-cholesterol levels and lower triglyceride levels, hypertension control, aggressive control of glucose in diabetic patients, and aspirin. Medical intervention in patients with PAD, even in the absence of symptoms, has been shown to lower the risk of cardiovascular events. Conversely, there is no evidence to support an endovascular intervention for an asymptomatic PAD (Rutherford category 0).

Symptomatic Peripheral Arterial Disease

In patients with symptomatic PAD, the decision to perform an endovascular intervention must be individualized. To make a proper decision, multiple factors must be taken into consideration. First, the indication for intervention must be clear to both the patient and the physician. Is the problem acute or chronic, and is it limb threatening or lifestyle limiting? In addition, the patient's overall risk for an intervention must be taken into consideration. The Rutherford category of PAD must be taken into consideration, as well as the type of TASC lesion. Emergent intervention is indicated for acute limb ischemia. Urgent intervention is indicated for chronic PAD in patients with Rutherford categories 4–6, as these patients are also at high risk for limb loss. Recently the Bypass versus Angioplasty in Severe Ischemia of the Leg (BASIL) Trial presented the results of their randomized study of 452 patients. Overall morbidity at 30 days and all-cause mortality at 6 months were higher in the bypass first arm. However, at 2 years patients in the bypass first arm had better amputation-free survival and lower all-cause mortality. Patients in the bypass first arm had a lower reintervention rate as well [11].

For patients with Rutherford categories 2 and 3, an intervention is based more on improving lifestyle, and as such the role of intervention is more controversial. Prior to intervention, careful consideration must be given to three factors. First, one must consider whether medical management options have been or should be maximized. In addition to smoking cessation and a walking program, cilostazol, a phosphodiesterase III inhibitor, has been shown to improve walking distance. Cilostazol has salutary antiplatelet, vasodilator, and metabolic effects in patients with PAD. Second, it is important to assess the degree of lifestyle impairment, such as a patient who cannot work because of the walking disability. Finally, the proposed procedure and anesthetic approach must be placed into the context of the patient's medical risk. A patient's cardiac risk during general anesthesia can readily be calculated using the revised cardiac index (score 0–6), which includes a history of coronary artery disease, history of heart failure, insulin-dependent diabetes, history of a cerebrovascular event, creatinine > 2 mg/dl, and high-risk surgery (open aortic). In patients without CLI on presentation, factors such as a history of smoking more than 40 pack-years, a history of diabetes, an initial ankle pressure less than 70 mmHg, an initial ABI less than 0.5, toe pressure less than 40 mmHg, and a significant drop in ABI during follow-up are predictive of a future need for intervention [12]. Conversely, in one series, no patient with an initial ABI of 0.7 or more required amputation over a 6.5-year follow-up [13].

Life expectancy of the patient and associated comorbid conditions also comprise essential information. Lower extremity atherosclerosis is a marker for diffuse atherosclerosis. In one study the 5-year mortality in patients with an initial ABI of less than 0.5 was 50% [14]. Most of the deaths were due to myocardial infarction or stroke. Therefore, particular attention should be paid to eliciting signs of concomitant symptomatic coronary and carotid disease.

Prior to embarking on endovascular intervention the physician must determine how amenable the lesion is to the treatment plan and the probable long-term outcome. The TASC II consensus statement offers guidelines for treatment depending on the pattern of disease. The endovascular approach is the treatment of choice for TASC A aortoiliac and femoral popliteal lesions and is preferred for TASC B lesions. For TASC D lesions, open surgery remains the procedure of choice. For TASC C lesions, open surgery is recommended for good-risk patients and the endovascular approach for higher risk patients (Table 4.3).

Although open bypass procedures overall have declined, current perspectives still regard open bypass as the gold standard procedure for infrainguinal disease [15]. As the BASIL trial has demonstrated, patients who are medically fit for open surgery and who have good vein conduits (either from the leg or the arm) have better long-term outcomes. It must be remembered, though, that patients with critical limb ischemia (ischemic rest pain, non-healing ulcer, or gangrene) typically have multilevel disease and may not be medically optimal candidates for extensive open bypasses. Thus adequate revascularization in many

Table 4.3 The TASC Classification System for Femoropopliteal Disease

TASC type A
- Single stenosis ≤10 cm in length
- Single occlusion ≤5 cm in length

TASC type B
- Multiple lesions each ≤5 cm (stenoses or occlusions)
- Single stenosis or occlusion ≤15 cm not involving the infrageniculate popliteal artery
- Single or multiple lesions in the absence of a continuous tibial vessel to improve inflow for a distal bypass
- Heavily calcified occlusion ≤5 cm long
- Single popliteal stenosis

TASC type C
- Multiple stenoses or occlusions totaling >15 cm in length, with or without heavy calcification
- Recurrent stenoses or occlusions that need treatment after two endovascular interventions

TASC type D
- Chronic total occlusion of the common femoral artery or SFA >20 cm in length involving the popliteal artery
- Chronic total occlusion of popliteal artery and proximal trifurcation vessels

From Norgren et al., [2] with permission.
TASC: Inter-Society Consensus for the Management of Peripheral Arterial Disease.

patients may require multilevel endovascular interventions or a combined endovascular and open surgical approach.

References

1. Rutherford R: Evaluation and selection of patients for vascular surgery. In Rutherford R, editor: *Vascular surgery*, Philadelphia, 2005, Saunders.
2. Norgren L, Hiatt W, Dormandy J et al.: Inter-society consensus for the management of peripheral arterial disease (TASC II), *J Vasc Surg* 45(suppl S):S5–S67, 2007.
3. Sumner D: Objective diagnostic techniques: the role of the vascular laboratory. In Rutherford R, editor: *Vascular surgery*, Philadelphia, 1989, Saunders.
4. Kinney EV, Bandyk DF, Towne JB: The vascular laboratory in clinical care: part I, *Surg Rounds*, 765–777, 1991.
5. Osmundson PJ, Rooke TW, Hallett JW: Effect of arterial revascularization on transcutaneous oxygen tension of the ischemic extremity, *Mayo Clin Proc* 63:897–902, 1988.
6. White RA, Nolan L, Harley D et al.: Noninvasive evaluation of peripheral vascular disease using transcutaneous oxygen tension, *Am J Surg* 144:68, 1982.
7. Cina C, Kastamouris A, Megerman J et al.: Utility of transcutaneous oxygen tension measurements in peripheral arterial occlusive disease, *J Vasc Surg* 1:362–369, 1984.
8. Zierler RE: Physiologic basis of hemodynamic measurement. In White R, Hollier L, editors: *Vascular surgery: basic science and clinical correlations*, Philadelphia, 1994, Lippincott.
9. Flanigan DP, Ballard JL, Robinson D et al.: Duplex ultrasound of the superficial femoral artery is a better screening tool than ankle-brachial index to identify at risk patients with lower extremity atherosclerosis, *J Vasc Surg* 47:789–792, 2008.
10. Dougherty MJ, Hallett JW Jr, Naessens JM et al.: Optimizing technical success of renal revascularization: the impact of intraoperative color-flow duplex ultrasonography, *J Vasc Surg* 17:849–857, 1993.
11. Adam AJ, Beard JD, Cleveland T, Bell J, Bradbury AW, Forbes JF et al.: BASIL trial participants: bypass versus angioplasty in severe ischaemia of the leg (BASIL): multicentre, randomised controlled trial, *Lancet* 366:1925–1934, 2005.
12. Walsh DB, Cronenwett JL: Natural history of atherosclerosis in the lower extremity, carotid, and coronary circulations. In White RA, Hollier LH, editors: *Vascular surgery: basic science and clinical correlations*, Philadelphia, 1994, Lippincott.
13. Jelnes R, Gaardsting O, Jensen KH et al.: Fate in intermittent claudication: outcome and risk factors, *BMJ* 293:1137, 1986.
14. O'Riordan DS, O'Donnell JA: Realistic expectations for the patient with intermittent claudication, *Br J Surg* 78:861, 1991.
15. Beard JD: Which is the best revascularization for critical limb ischemia: endovascular or open surgery? *J Vasc Surg* 48(6 suppl):11S–16S, 2008.

Anesthesia Techniques for Endovascular Surgery

5

Maurice Lippmann, Inderjeet Singh Julka, and Clinton Z. Kakazu

In the United States each year there are about 15,000 deaths directly related to abdominal aortic aneurysms (AAA) [1]; 62% may die outside the hospital from rupture of their aneurysms; the overall mortality is 90% [2]. In the year 1984 in patients with ruptured aneurysms, hospitals lost some $24,000 per patient [3]. If repaired electively, 2,000 patients were saved per year and annual costs were $50 million in 1984 [4]. Elective repair is indicated when aneurysms are 5 cm in diameter or greater and may lead up to 20% mortality if the patients have comorbid diseases [5, 6], Now add thoracic aneurysms, aortic dissections, and transections to the picture and the same as stated previously can be staggering.

Open repair of abdominal aortic aneurysms (AAA) and thoracic aortic aneurysms (TM) as well as thoracic dissection and transections is associated with significant morbidity and mortality. Endovascular stent–graft repair of these conditions is a new alternative to conventional open surgical repair of this pathologic disease state [7]. In 1968, Dotter first suggested this new technique [8]. Further interest in endovascular aortic aneurysm repair (EVAAR) was further increased due to the first report in 1991 by Parodi et al. [9]. This new technique was developed in an effort to reduce morbidity and mortality associated with open repair [10], which in turn would theoretically lessen or decrease postoperative cardiopulmonary complications in comparison to open repair. This new evolving technique is aimed at a less disruptive approach toward repair of these disease entities.

Because the surgical approach is from the peripheral groin area, the surgeon needs to gain control of the femoral and iliac arteries which makes this approach easier for the surgeon. In addition to this new surgical approach one must consider which anesthetic technique would be most beneficial to the patient and their outcomes. This chapter focuses on several anesthetic techniques that the anesthesiologist can institute, for example, general anesthesia (GA), regional anesthesia which includes continuous epidural or spinal anesthesia, a combination of both, or local anesthesia with monitored anesthesia care (MAC) which also includes intravenous analgesics/sedatives. Choice of anesthetic technique may depend to a great extent on the patient's coexisting morbidities (Table 5.1). In the discussion on anesthesia techniques the discussion will include the specifics of each and the pros and cons of each option.

As anesthesiologists it should be our goal to provide the safest and least invasive means of anesthesia/analgesia. Given the fact that the EVAAR is a newer advancement in vascular surgery, there is also an associated learning curve accompanying it in regard to a surgeon and anesthesiologist skill and comfort level. This can influence indirectly anesthetic management that may be instituted. A surgeon's unfamiliarity with EVAAR often requires the institution of general anesthesia. As the comfort level is increased with EV MR, the feasibility of local anesthesia with intravenous sedation (MAC) becomes apparent. A shift was seen toward almost exclusive use of this local anesthesia technique at an institution described by deVirgilio et al. [10].

M. Lippmann (✉)
Professor, Department of Anesthesiology, Harbor/UCLA Medical Center, Torrance, CA, USA

T.J. Fogarty, R.A. White (eds.), *Peripheral Endovascular Interventions*,
DOI 10.1007/978-1-4419-1387-6_5, © Springer Science+Business Media, LLC 1998, 2010

Table 5.1 Common coexisting diseases in the elderly

Anemia
Cardiac conduction abnormalities
Chronic obstructive pulmonary disease
Congestive heart failure
Coronary artery disease
Diabetes mellitus
Hypertension
Peripheral vascular disease
Renal insufficiency
Previous coronary artery bypass and/or valve surgery
Osteoarthritis
Rheumatoid arthritis

Local Anesthesia

Using the local anesthetic technique lends itself to be extremely advantageous not only in the elderly high-risk patients but also in traditional patients. Local anesthesia with the administration of analgesics and sedatives as adjunctive medications while monitoring the patient's vital signs (MAC) is simple and appropriate in these patients. This technique offers cardiopulmonary morbidity reduction especially in patients with multiple system diseases (Table 5.1). Lippmann and White et al. [11–13] performed several studies on patients having AAA repair and TAA repair. They determined in both studies that using a local anesthetic along with analgesics and sedatives offered very good outcomes in a population that was extremely of high risk. They concluded that repair of AAAs and TAAs, dissections and transections, using this new endovascular technique combined with local anesthesia and MAC in the elderly patient offers extremely great advantages over open repair and general anesthesia. Analgesic drugs and sedatives can often be minimized [14, 15] (Tables 5.2 and 5.3), and blood loss and replacement is reduced. There is also less stress afforded to the patient, who then can ambulate and eat earlier postoperatively. Analgesia post-procedure can also be reduced and cardiopulmonary complications are much fewer. In-hospital stay is also reduced to 1–2% days post-procedure compared to open repair (4–7 days) resulting in decreased cost. The aforementioned techniques, local anesthesia and MAC, are now accompanied at our institution by performing ilioinguinal–iliohypogastric nerve blocks by the authors as an adjunctive modality using 0.25% bupivacaine (20 cc) in each groin area. This addition would often lessen the amount of local anesthetic used by the surgeon. In a recent study by Lippmann and Kakazu [14] they determined exactly the reduction made when the surgeon uses local anesthetic in the groin with 0.5% lidocaine without epinephrine (Table 5.4).

The articles and studies mentioned above using local anesthesia with analgesics/sedation and MAC afford tremendous advantages. Lippmann and White [11–13] also determined that by using this anesthetic technique, the anesthesiologist can also converse with the patient during the operation, informing the patient as to what is occurring during the procedure and thereby assuring patient comfort.

Still another advantage to local anesthesia with MAC is that the anesthesiologist can more easily detect adverse reactions to contrast agents or anaphylactoid reactions from other medications, thereby treating the patients more rapidly [15]. Several other authors have also used local anesthesia as their anesthetic technique of choice. In a study by Henretta et al. [16]. consisting of 47 patients it was concluded that endovascular treatment of MAs with local anesthesia is feasible and can be performed safely in their patient population. They also compared their study with previous studies and found equivalent, if not improved results. The study by

Table 5.2 Abdominal aortic aneurysm repair

	Age	Height (cm)	Weight (kg)	Midazolam (mg)	Fentanyl (mcg)	Lidocaine (cc) 0.5% plain	Blood loss (cc)	Auto vac (cc)	Blood replacement (unit)	Hespan (cc)	Fluids (cc) plasmalyte
Mean	73	171	81.2	1.66	256	49.6	703	475	0.23	531	1,781
High	92	188	159.0	8.00	750	100.0	3,400	3,150	4.00	2000	5,000
Low	23	140	42.0	0.00	25	10.0	50	0	0.00	250	250
Median	74	173	81.0	1.00	250	60.0	600	365	0.00	500	1,600
± SD	12	11	18.3	1.74	159	29.4	516	546	0.70	184	846

Modified from White et al. [13], with permission of Elsevier, Inc.

Table 5.3 Thoracic aortic aneurysm repair

	Age	Height (cm)	Weight (kg)	Midazolam	Fentanyl (mcg)	Blood loss (cc)	Auto vac (cc)	Blood replace-ment (unit)	Hespan	Plasmalyte fluid (cc)
Mean	73	169	77	1	263	671	561	0	498	1,712
High	92	203	110	4	750	3,000	3,000	2	2,000	3,000
Low	54	147	33	0	0	100	100	0	0	300
Median	75	168	79	0	250	450	450	0	500	1,750
±SD	9	14	18	1	152	671	671	1	345	753

Table 5.4 Comparison of no block versus ilioinguinal–iliohypogastric block [a]

	No block	ILIH block
Mean local (mL)	87.9	49.5
P-value	0.00006	
Mean local (mL/kg)	1.08	0.67
P-value	0.0004	

[a]Local lidocaine 0.5% given during surgery.

Bettex et al. [17] also concluded that using local anesthesia was a safe technique in patients for endovascular repair of infrarenal MAs offering several advantages over the other two methods being general anesthesia or regional anesthesia. These advantages included simplicity, more stable hemodynamics, reduced consumption in ICU and hospital beds, reduced use of vasoactive agents, and a more favorable fluid balance. Because of the nature of the disease, rupture is always a potential hazard and conversion to an open procedure is a possibility with this new surgical innovation. If a retroperitoneal conduit needs to be performed and should the need arise, converting local with MAC anesthesia to a general anesthesia is very easily accomplished. Of course a team approach to the entire process is quite necessary for good outcomes. Lippmann and White [11] in 2001 published a paper including the title "Fast Track" Anesthesia. The use of this phrase was first introduced as an approach to decreasing the time to achieve tracheal extubated after cardiac surgery [18]. To achieve this goal, early studies emphasized the importance of using short-acting intravenous agents as well as minimizing the total dose of opioid analgesics administered during the perioperative period [18–21]. Based on these studies local anesthesia with MAC is our choice of anesthesia in this high-risk group of patients. This technique together with peripheral nerve blocks and infiltration or installation of the local anesthesia is becoming more widely used as adjunctives to general anesthesia as well as MAC technique. The quote "preemptive" use of local anesthetics [22] facilitates recovery by providing both intraoperative and postoperative analgesia [23]. Anesthetic and analgesic sparing effects of local anesthetics when administered before incision allow patients to be maintained at a "lighter" plane of anesthesia (or sedation) during surgery, contributing to a faster, smoother emergents and more rapid return to baseline function status [22]. General anesthesia and regional anesthetics can be avoided by using a combination of local anesthetics, IV sedative/analgesic drugs as part of an awake technique [24] for other invasive procedures such as endovascular stent grafting of aortic aneurysms, dissections, as well as transections. This technique also decreases the incidence and severity of postoperative pain by reducing the need for both parenteral and oral opioid analgesics in the postoperative period and therefore enabling earlier patient ambulation and discharge.

Still another benefit of using local anesthesia with MAC was demonstrated by Lippmann et al. [25] in a case report depicting an extremely morbid obese male patient weighing over 350 pounds with a body mass index of 73.3 and having multiple comorbidities, having a large abdominal aortic aneurysm. Not wishing to administer a general anesthetic to this patient because of his comorbidities plus his excessive weight the patient did extremely well throughout the entire procedure under the local anesthetic MAC technique. The outcome was excellent [25]. Another benefit to using local anesthesia and MAC is due to the fact that our surgeon has the expertise in the use of intravascular ultrasound (IVUS) in all our patients to measure all aspects of the aorta and its side branches and to visualize the pathology via the exposed femoral and iliac vessels. This precludes the use of a transesophageal echocardiogram (TEE), which some surgeons use but

Table 5.5 Advantage and disadvantages of transesophageal echocardiogram versus intravascular ultrasound

Intravascular ultrasound	Transthoracic echocardiogram
Advantages	
Better clarity and resolution	Direct vascular access not required
Better visualization of side-branch anatomy	Ability to visualize the heart (preload, ejection fraction, valvular anatomy, and regional wall motion abnormalities)
Visualization of entire aorta (abdominal and thoracic) including its main tributaries (iliac artery and femoral artery)	
General anesthesia *not* required	
Disadvantages	
Requires direct vascular access to perform ultrasound	Inability to visualize a portion of the aortic arch
Vascular perforation, rupture, or dissection	Inability to visualize aorta beyond the diaphragm
Additional intraluminal hardware	Requires GA

necessitates the patient being administered an endotracheal tube general anesthetic. Both modalities have pros and cons (Table 5.5).

Anesthesia Techniques to Aid Proximal Deployment of the Stent–Graft in TAAs

In order to assist the surgeon during the deployment of a thoracic stent–graft a surgeon may need to have the patient's (cardiac) status placed in an asystolic mode. The anesthesiologist has several options. The first being a pacing wire [26] placed peripherally to the heart in order to cause the heart to fibrillate for the amount of time it takes the surgeon to deploy the stent–graft. The other method is using the drug adenosine. Adenosine is a natural purine nucleoside used primarily by cardiologist at a low dose (6–12 mg) as an anti-arrhythmia agent to slow down superventricular tachycardia (SVT). It is rapidly inactivated by red blood cells and vascular endothelial cells. The half-life of adenosine in human plasma is less than 10 s at therapeutic doses [27]. Therefore, cardiac standstill can be reached when large doses are given as a bolus injection. Life threatening events after adenosine appear to be rare [28]. Minor side effects are common in the awake patient studies that have been performed [29] using adenosine in endovascular stent deployment in the thoracic aortic aneurysm cases. The authors ascertain that adenosine's onset is usually within 7–8 s at high doses when administered through a peripheral vessel and quicker if given through a central line because it reaches the myocardium immediately, although we do not employ central lines in our patients anymore. Because adenosine is broken down so rapidly by red blood cells and vascular endothelium its offset is not only rapid but also dose dependent (Table 5.6). Transient cardiac asystole aids endovascular stent–graft deployment by causing a brief cessation in the cardiac propulsive force, thus preventing distal device migration within the thoracic aorta. Once the endovascular device is in proper position and confirmed by fluoroscopy, optimal adenosine dose for deployment, which usually takes less than 20 s, may be achieved by an 18–36 mg dose. This translates into a weight-based dose range of 0.2–0.5 mg/kg administered through a peripheral IV. Although rapidly metabolized, larger adenosine doses (0.5 mg/kg or greater) produce a statistically significant longer asystole duration. Constant communication with the surgeon maximizes the window of opportunity for stent deployment during asystole; with the goal of minimizing the adenosine dose. While the common side effects are self-limiting, no patient required eternal defibrillation and/or pacing. The authors of the study [30] also noted the side effects in the 45 patients that were studied (Table 5.7). It should be noted that the asystole produced with adenosine is not reduced by the drug Atropine. The

Table 5.6 Asystole duration according to adenosine dose

Dose (mg)	Patients ($n = 45$)	Asystole duration ± SD (s)	*P*-value [a]
18 [b]	18	11.6 ± 5.5	0.0009
36	45	18.8 ± 8.8	0.0009

[a] A *P*-value <0.01 was considered significant.
[b] Second dose, given if needed.

Table 5.7 Adenosine side-effect profile (in 45 patients)

Side effect	Patients affected (no.)
Hypotension	45
Dizziness	9
Palpitations	8
Facial flushing	5
Light headedness	4
Shortness of breath	3
Nausea	2
Thump in the chest	0

adverse side effects of adenosine are usually very transient. It should also be noted by the anesthesiologist that if a patient has asthma, upper respiratory disease states, and/or a history of bronchopulmonary disease, the use of adenosine may be hazardous to the patient and may cause bronchoconstriction after intravenous implementation. The rescue drugs are either theophylline or aminophylline. The anesthesiologist must be cautious when administering adenosine to patients with asthma and so forth. The bolus injection maybe more advantageous than the use of controlled ventricular fibrillation, because adenosine is cerebral protective [31] and cardioprotective [32].

The use of anesthetic technique of local anesthesia with monitored anesthesia care (MAC) plus the implementation of the ilioinguinal/iliohypogastric nerve blocks for endovascular repair of both AAAs and TAAs can also be used in stent–graft repair of peripheral vascular surgeries such as iliac artery stenosis cases with the same good outcomes.

For carotid artery stenting the anesthetic technique is also simple to administer, except that one does need to perform the groin block since the surgeon will perform his procedure through a percutaneous puncture to do the IVUS and insert the stent. A little local anesthetic in the skin is sufficient along with manual doses/fentanyl. It is extremely important to keep these patients fully awake and responsive to commands.

General Anesthesia for Endovascular Aortic Surgery

As previously discussed, monitored anesthesia care (MAC) with local anesthesia is our first preference for providing anesthetic care in patients undergoing endovascular aortic aneurysm repair (EVAAR). In our review of cases, the overall incidence of general anesthesia (GA) for over 400 thoracic and 1,600 abdominal EVAAR was less than 1 and 2%, respectively. While the reasons requiring GA may be predicted and obvious at the start of the case, there are instances where conversion to GA necessitates a quick and rapid, albeit smooth response and induction. In some cases, MAC is not an option, particularly in patients who are hemodynamically unstable or suffered major trauma and/or cases where an adjunctive procedure is required. Other reasons requiring GA are based upon a tripartite agreement between all parties involved: (1) the patient, (2) the surgeon, and (3) the anesthesiologist.

Patient refusal is an absolute contraindication for MAC with local anesthesia or regional anesthesia (RA) technique. GA is then necessitated. Patient's preconceived notions and expectations make MAC less attractive. Societal, cultural, ethnical [33], and personal ideologies, or a combination thereof, play a major role in patient's acceptance and tolerance. The inform consent process for an anesthetic in which they will be awake during the operation evokes great fear and anxiety for some. Other concerns that limit patient selection for administering a MAC or RA are cognitive impediments. Everything from foreign language and other communication barriers such as deafness and dementia poses problems from a patient standpoint.

It may also be a challenge to convince a less experienced surgeon unfamiliar with endoluminal techniques to accept conscious sedation. As surgical experience and device refinement improves, however, acceptance for MAC with local anesthesia will likely be the norm. Just within the past decade endovascular surgery has seen an explosive increase in the development and use as new technological advancements have changed treatment paradigms for aneurismal repair. Hence, the surgical learning curve is steep. But until the operative time is shorter than the reasonable duration for a patient to remain still, MAC will be difficult to perform. Patient's intolerance despite adequate sedation manifests as agitation, complaints, and frequent movement during longer operative times. Often, the time burden is due to ischemic pain from the distal femoral arterial clamp. Ischemic pain in the lower extremity manifests as a gradual rise in blood pressure and heart rate that becomes refractory to sedatives, analgesics and even vasodilators and antihypertensive agents [34].

Patients describe leg cramps expressing the urgency to stretch their leg, and often wiggle and fidget in effort to become more comfortable. Also frequent patient movement, more commonly in the elderly, is seen in those that have lower back pain or prior back surgery. The hard operation table makes it difficult for them to get comfortable.

During our initial learning curve, operative times were longer (1.5 times our current length) and nearly every patient received a GA. In fact, during our first 500 EVAAR cases 100% received a GA. As new delivery systems are introduced unfamiliarity may also create longer operative times.

More importantly the anesthesiologist must be willing to accept an awake patient. Comfort levels are undermined with less experience surgeons who require longer operative times. MAC requires more effort on the anesthesiologist part: to placate the patient, tend to the surgeon, follow the critical events of the procedure, all the while monitoring essential vital signs. With MAC and local anesthesia there is an element of patient unpredictability. GA virtually guarantees the absence of patient movement throughout the entire case, whereas in MAC and sedation the ability to control against patient movement, especially during critical moments of stent deployment, is lost.

The categorization of patients in whom MAC will not be tolerated is useful. Preoperative screening helps predict which patients will likely require a GA. In our review of over 2,000 cases, both thoracic and abdominal EVAAR, factors necessitating a GA can be based on absolute and relative indications (Table 5.8).

Table 5.8 Indications of general anesthesia for endovascular aortic aneurysm repair

Absolute
Patient refusal for MAC or RA
Hemodynamically unstable
Major trauma with evidence of end-organ impairment
Iliac vessel conduit
Relative
Cognitive impairment
Language barrier
Need for TEE
Small and tortuous iliac and femoral vessels
Reversible organ impairment

The feasibility of performing MAC and local anesthesia technique relies on a classical approach to the aorta via the femoral arteries. Its superficial nature, yet being a major blood vessel having a relatively large diameter to allow passage of the delivery systems, makes it minimally invasive and, therefore, ideal for MAC and local anesthesia supplementation. The possibility of utilizing a MAC and local anesthesia technique, however, becomes less feasible once it is determined that access to the aorta is limited by small and/or tortuous external iliac and femoral arteries, usually secondary to atherosclerotic disease. Smaller vessel size is also found more commonly in elderly, petite, female patients. Several alternatives are available when passage of the delivery system is limited due to severely diseased femoral or iliac vessels, which include balloon angioplasty, local endarterectomy, and an alternative access site usually retroperitoneal dissection for iliac conduit placement. When balloon angioplasty fails to provide adequate dilation or local endarterectomy is not an option, a synthetic conduit is sutured to the common iliac through which the delivery system is placed in the aorta.

Discussion with the surgeon in the preoperative period and review of the CT scan screen for patients requiring a retroperitoneal dissection for iliac conduit placement. A retroperitoneal dissection is estimated to be necessary in up to 20% of cases [35]. In preselected cases where a high probability of an iliac conduit is required, GA is selected due to surgical invasiveness, painful stimulation, and patient's intolerance of retroperitoneal dissection under local anesthesia. Often, however, an unanticipated discrepancy of limited vessel to device size ratio necessitates a conversion from MAC and local anesthetic technique to GA. GA for retroperitoneal dissection and iliac conduit is selected not only for patient comfort but also for optimal anesthetic conditions because greater blood loss, longer procedure time, and increased complications have been reported [35].

Besides retroperitoneal incision and iliac conduit placement, other adjunctive procedures related to EVAAR may require GA. It has been estimated in one series that 21% needed left subclavian–carotid transposition to provide for an adequate proximal fixation site [36]. In our experience, adjunctive procedures are becoming increasingly common.

Advantages of a General Anesthetic

There are many advantages of GA for abdominal and thoracic EVAAR. Failure of MAC or RA usually requires hastily conversion to GA. The ability to titrate parental anesthetic drugs and provide a smooth hemodynamic induction is compromised. Performing a GA prior to surgical incision avoids a scenario where rapid bolus of multiple anesthetic drugs in successive fashion to facilitate intubation results in wide hemodynamic fluctuations. GA allows for better control and predictability of operative conditions: less patient movement, less concerns of recall, less intraoperative psychological and post-traumatic stress [37]. Moreover, performance of a GA at the onset gives the anesthesiologist peace of mind from the start of the case, knowing that he/she is prepared for the worst.

Some of the unpleasant side effects of adenosine-induced cardiac arrest (Table 5.8) such as loss of consciousness and palpitations are averted by a GA [38]. Of our 200 cases using adenosine cardiac arrest, none required cardiopulmonary resuscitation with antiarrhythmic drugs or transcutaneous cardiac pacemaker. If prolonged asystole or malignant arrhythmia requiring resuscitation occurred, then GA would be most suitable when performing advanced cardiac life support.

GA allows the anesthesiologist to perform transesophageal echosonography (TEE), which may provide important information of the heart and aneurysm. TEE allows assessment of contractility, valve function, regional wall motion, and presence of pericardial fluid. Severity and degree of retrograde dissection with aortic valve involvement leading to acute aortic insufficiency can be diagnosed with TEE [39–41]. Also, TEE aids in accurate stent–graft placement by determination of branching points and location of an intimal tear [39]. Cardiac and volume status is managed optimally with appropriate administration of IV fluids [42, 43], vasopressors, and anesthetic drugs. Pericardial fluid representing blood may have serious consequences which if diagnosed by TEE may mitigate some of the deleterious effects. Left undetected acute cardiac tamponade results in hemodynamic compromise and sudden cardiovascular collapse. In cases where the dissection leads to a subacute, more insidious pericardial effusion detection is paramount. Hemodynamic goals are contrary to aortic dissection; in tamponade, high normal heart rates, maintenance systemic vascular resistance (SVR), preload, and contractility are important. All of which are in direct conflict of acute dissection management.

The major advantage with GA for EVAAR is during massive and sudden blood loss. There is better management and control of precipitous hemodynamic decline with earlier response to blood and fluid replacement. The anesthesiologist is not distracted by managing other aspects of patient care. Focus and attention in its entirety is directed at blood and fluid replacement. In rapid and massive blood loss, the clinical situation quickly turns from bad to worst. Critical seconds lost could mean the difference in morbidity and mortality. With an aortic rupture, MAC sedation progresses to confusion and abruptly to obtundation due to cerebral hypoperfusion secondary to low blood pressure or severe anemia. Other possible causes of cognitive decline may be a result of inadvertent carotid artery occlusion, thromboembolism, or anesthetic overdose. Whatever the cause of mental status deterioration, vigilance by the anesthesiologist is required to manage the situation. If patient confusion prohibits the progress of surgery or if it limits the ability to protect his/her airway, intervention by securing an airway usually with an endotracheal tube becomes necessary.

A major disadvantage of RA is resultant sympathectomy, which if combined with massive surgical blood loss, treatment may be refractory to fluid and vasopressor drugs. In patients with ischemic heart disease, RA may exacerbate regional myocardial dysfunction through vasodilatation, hypotension, and decreased coronary perfusion pressure [44]. Another important advantage of GA over neuroaxial RA is the avoiding risk of epidural hematoma. While the estimated incidence of epidural hematoma following a spinal or epidural anesthetic is low, 1:220,000 and 1:150,000, respectively [45], the possible complication of paralysis is devastating. Risk of epidural hematoma is increased [46] with antiplatelet (i.e., ticlopidine [ticlid], clopidogrel) and anticoagulant drugs (i.e., heparin, warfarin [coumadin], and enoxaparin). These drugs are commonly administered to patients suffering from peripheral vascular disease. Moreover, heparin is utilized as an anticoagulant of choice intraoperatively. For appropriate management of perioperative use of antiplatelets and anticoagulants, refer to American Society of Regional Anesthesia Guidelines [46].

Disadvantages of a General Anesthetic

The advantages have to be weighed against the disadvantages of GA for EVAAR. While it is argued that better control of hemodynamics can be achieved with GA, it is accepted that laryngoscopy and endotracheal intubation are associated with increase in blood pressure, heart rate, and arrhythmias. In hypertensive patients the hemodynamic response to intubation varies widely depending on their perioperative control and laryngoscopic time [47]. Conversely, maneuvers to blunt the hemodynamic response such as fentanyl premedication, lidocaine and/or esmolol IV on induction, and limiting laryngoscope time to less than 15 s may lessen the possibility of aortic rupture, dissection, and myocardial ischemia [48]. More importantly, assuring complete anesthesia prior to intubation is the most efficacious way to limit BP increase.

While the surge in blood pressure and heart rate is transient and short lived, the potential consequences are nonetheless very real. It has been shown in a case report that rupture may occur [49]. The advent of the laryngeal mask airway may mitigate the hemodynamic problems associated with endotracheal stimulation; however, it does not provide definitive airway control and poses limits in the amount of positive pressure ventilation [50]. These problems may be magnified in trauma patients with pulmonary contusion requiring higher airway pressure or patients with restrictive lung disease.

The argument against GA requirement is due to the less invasive nature of EVAAR. With less invasiveness there is less hemodynamic fluctuations, minimal skin incision(s), less blood loss, shorten surgical times, and avoidance of aortic cross-clamp. Compared to traditional open repair, there is an association with less hemodynamic instability [51].

Risk of postoperative nausea and vomiting is lessened by avoiding GA. Patients also tend to maintain normothermia without GA inhibition of the thermoregulatory center [52]. Maintaining body temperature is important. Unintentional hypothermia increases the risk of myocardial ischemia, angina, and hypoxemia during the early postoperative period [53]. RA, however, does not guarantee against hypothermia; it produces both peripheral and central inhibition of thermoregulatory control. In fact, hypothermia during major conduction anesthesia may be as severe as that during GA [52].

While the type of anesthesia (GA versus RA) has not been shown to increase the incidence of postoperative cognitive delirium [54], it has important considerations for patients undergoing EVAA because of higher rates of major complications [55]. Risk factors for developing postoperative cognitive delirium are congruent to those presenting for EVAAR including advanced age; ASA classification status III–IV; and hearing, visual, cognitive, and functional impairment. Postoperative delirium may mask an intraoperative stroke and lead to a delay in detection and diagnosis postoperatively.

Preoperative Evaluation

A thorough and careful preoperative evaluation of the patient is paramount, because major morbidity and mortality are related to affected organ systems and comorbid conditions. Coexisting disease of patient's with abdominal and thoracic aneurysm is multiple and occur with high incidences (Table 5.9). The anesthetic plan should incorporate the aneurismal management with consideration of the other disease entities. Younger patients usually present with traumatic aortic transactions and/or dissections and are without significant coexisting disease. However, trauma patients may have other associated injuries related to the chest and thorax such as rib fractures, flail chest, hemothorax, pneumothorax, pulmonary contusion, and myocardial injury such as myocardial ischemia, tamponade, contusion, and valvular abnormalities. Consideration and workup of injuries outside the chest and thorax of particular importance for the anesthesiologist involve the airway and cervical spine.

Associated comorbidities found in order of frequency are hypertension (55–70%) coronary artery disease (50%), chronic obstructive pulmonary disease (30%), angina (25%), and congestive heart failure (10%). The overall reported incidence of perioperative hypertension in patients with aortic aneurysm varies from 57% to as high as 70% depending on the study and BP criteria used [56, 57].

Table 5.9 Considerations in evaluating end-organ damage to the various organs

Heart
1. History relating to angina and exercise tolerance
2. Physical examination of ventricular lift or S3 heart sound
3. Laboratory studies including electrocardiogram, chest film, echocardiogram, stress test with or without echocardiogram, radionuclide imaging
Brain
1. History relating to transient ischemic attack and stroke
2. Physical examination evaluating for carotid bruit and retinopathy
3. Laboratory studies
4. Radiological studies, including a carotid Doppler ultrasound
Kidneys
1. History of weakness, lethargy, or accelerated hypertension
2. Physical examination evaluating for acute hypertension and edema
3. Laboratory studies including creatinine and electrolyte levels

From Martin and Shanks [113], with permission of Elsevier.

Blood Pressure Evaluation, Monitoring, and Treatment

Perioperative hypertension, being a systemic disease and defined as blood pressure (BP) >160/90, warrants evaluation of major end organs: the brain, heart, and kidneys (Table 5.9). BP evaluation should include measurements in both arms. Variations occur up to 20 mmHg between each arm, with the right arm being greater than the left arm 60% of the time in patients with peripheral vascular disease and coronary artery disease [58]. Moreover, in patients with prior thoracic EVAAR presenting for endoleak repair, right arm pressures are expected to exceed left arm pressures because of occlusion of the left subclavian origin by the stent–graft.

In emergent and/or urgent cases with aortic dissection or unstable aneurysm for EVAAR, intraoperative BP control is equally important as preoperative BP control [59]. While various agents may be used, our preference is an afterload reducing agent, such as nitroglycerin or sodium nitroprusside in combination with a chronotropic and ionotrophic reducing agent, such as esmolol. This modality offers several advantages, namely, rapid onset without prolonged duration, a reduction of intraluminal aneurismal pressure by lowering systemic vascular resistance (SVR), and decreasing the shearing force by reduction in contractility. Beta blockade decreases the systolic ejection slope of the left ventricle (i.e., d*p*/d*t*), which decreases the shearing force on the aortic wall [60].

Vasodilators, such as nitroglycerin or nitroprusside, given alone widen the pulse pressure by dropping the diastolic pressure and actually may increase the likelihood of rupture [61]. Moreover, given alone reflex tachycardia promotes shearing forces on the intimal layer which may possibly expand the dissection. Other parenteral treatment options are listed in Table 5.10.

Induction of General Anesthesia

The goals of GA induction are (1) establish and secure airway; (2) maintain hemodynamic stability by avoiding hypertension and tachycardia; and (3) provide adequate oxygenation and ventilation. Induction of GA is a critical time during EVAAR. Wide swings in blood pressure can be deleterious for a patient. Whereas, hypotension may precipitate myocardial ischemia, hypertension may lead to aortic rupture and dissection. Many IV induction agents can be utilized to achieve loss of consciousness and facilitate airway procurement, all the while providing hemodynamic stability. Less emphasis should be placed on what drug is used, but rather how the drug is used. Nevertheless, our first preference for induction of GA is etomidate or a reduced dose of propofol. Etomidate, an imidazole-derived sedative–hypnotic, is known for its hemodynamic stability with maintenance of blood pressure and heart rate. Its major disadvantage is it causes myoclonus, and a propensity for postoperative nausea and vomiting. Propofol can be associated with a reduction in SVR, particularly in rapid boluses and at higher doses >2–3 mg/kg [62]. Moreover, it causes myocardial depression, which further leads to blood pressure decline that can be exacerbated in the debilitated and volume depleted [62]. Uncontrolled hypertensive patients are volume depleted and have autonomic instability. SVR reduction secondary to IV induction, whether by propofol or etomidate, is

Table 5.10 Intravenous antihypertensive drugs, classification, and effects

Direct arterial and venous dilators	
Nitroglycerin reduction	Venous: arterial dilator causing preload
Sodium Nitroprusside	Arterial: venous dilator causing afterload reduction [63–65]
Calcium channel antagonist	
Nicardipine	Systemic vascular resistance (SVR)/total peripheral resistance reduction [66]
Beta antagonist	
Esmolol	Beta 1-selective blockade causing reduced heart rate and contractility [67, 68]
Labetolol	Non-selective alpha and beta blockade causing reduced heart rate, contractility, and SVR [69]
Alpha antagonist	
Phentolamine	Non-selective alpha blockade causing reduced SR
Angiotensive-converting enzyme inhibitor	
Enalaprilat	Indirectly reduce SVR, long-acting agent [70]
Selective dopamine 1 receptor agonist	
Fenoldopam	SVR reduction, renal blood flow, and sodium excretion increase, with maintainence of normal heart rate [71]

poorly compensated. In patients who have poor ejection fractions or present with aortic valve involvement, a narcotic induction with fentanyl (7–10 mcg/kg) may reduce SVR indirectly by inhibition of catecholamine release and it causes slight bradycardia. But the important advantage, however, is that fentanyl does not cause myocardial depression.

Maintenance of General Anesthesia

GA maintenance is usually carried out with a volatile agent in an air/oxygen mixture or 100% oxygen, a cardiovascular stable muscle relaxant, and intermittent bolus or infusion of a narcotic. The concentration of oxygen is dependant on the patients' intrinsic lung disease and systemic oxygen requirement. Nitrous oxide is avoided for several reasons: (1) it expands closed air spaces (may expand a pneumothorax in trauma cases); (2) limits the amount of FiO_2 that can be delivered; and (3) causes significant myocardial depression in combination with narcotics, especially in patients with myocardial dysfunction.

Desflurane, a volatile gas, is touted for its low blood gas solubility coefficient allowing for rapid changes in anesthesia depth and quick emergence. This provides ease of titration in affording the anesthesiologist to trend the inspiratory concentration to the blood pressure and depth of anesthesia. The major concerns are that its pungent odor may irritate the airways leading to bronchoconstriction and sympathomimetic stimulation leading to increase in heart rate with rapid changes in blood gas concentrations.

Sevoflurane, a volatile gas, is touted not only for its low blood gas solubility coefficient but also for its bronchodilating properties. This clear advantage makes it the volatile agent of choice in patients with reactive airway disease.

Isoflurane, a volatile gas structurally related to desflurane, may also produce tachycardia to a lesser degree. It reduces SVR to a greater extent than any other volatile gas per given concentration.

Narcotics are titrated intraoperatively based on perceived need and selected on their pharmacokinetic and pharmacodynamic properties. Our practice is to avoid morphine, due to its potential histamine release and that in accumulated doses it leads to a prolonged half-life. Meperidine, structurally related to atropine, is also avoided due to its propensity to cause tachycardia.

Because MAC and local are our first preference for anesthetic management of EVAAR, extenuating disease processes are usually present to indicate GA. For this reason, a majority of our patients remain intubated at the conclusion of surgery. Usually, if at the end of a case, the same conditions(s) for which intubation was indicated still exist, then extubation is contraindicated. Extubation criteria must be strictly followed.

Summary

In conclusion, GA with endotracheal intubation is definitive anesthetic management. The type of anesthetic management is based on factors such as surgical invasiveness and comfort levels of the surgeon, patient, and anesthesiologist alike. The decision to perform GA is often obvious at the start of the case. If MAC with local is undertaken, the anesthesiologist must always be prepared for a conversion to a general anesthetic. This conversion, if performed smoothly, should be a seamless transition. Constant communication during the case between the surgeon and anesthesiologist provides early warning signs that give clues to when GA becomes indicated. A team approach optimizes patient care and case management from the surgical and anesthesia standpoint.

Regional Anesthesia and Analgesia for Endovascular Stent Grafting

Endovascular surgery is becoming the surgical procedure of choice for disorders such as thoracic and abdominal aortic aneurysms often allowing access to inoperable high-risk patients. Various regional anesthetic approaches can be used at the neuroaxial level safely in properly selected candidates as a sole technique or as an adjunct to general anesthesia. Techniques described have included single shot spinals, continuous spinal catheters, epidural catheters, and combined spinal epidural techniques (CSE). A single shot or bolus technique involves a single injection of medication through a needle into the spinal or an epidural space with the effect lasting for a specific duration depending upon the agent(s) used. Alternatively, a continuous technique involves placement of a catheter into the epidural space or subarachnoid space for repetitive injection or ongoing infusion.

A detailed history and physical examination should ascertain the feasibility of administration of regional anesthetic without problems. One should look to rule any evidence of coagulopathy, use of herbal medications, hypovolemia, septicemia, congestive heart failure, ability of patient to tolerate positioning in light of coexisting diseases. Local skin infection should be ruled out at the site of needle insertion. Concomitant injuries should also be assessed specially in trauma cases, namely, spine injuries.

While the only absolute contraindication is the lack of patient consent, a few relative contraindications exist, namely, uncorrected hypovolemia, which can lead to shock and cardiovascular collapse due to sympathectomy with local anesthetics, increased ICP due to attendant risk of brain stem herniation, coagulopathy which can lead to bleeding and hematoma formation. Meningomyelocele, spina bifida, scoliosis, and previous spine surgeries may also complicate insertion and successful outcomes due to anatomical abnormalities. In neurologic disorders such as multiple sclerosis, use of regional anesthesia is controversial; however, it has been successfully conducted with lower doses of local anesthetics [72, 73], Aortic stenosis, a heart valve condition where maintenance of systemic vascular resistance is critical for optimal cardiac output, may be one such disorder where regional anesthetic should be carefully considered.

Since the autonomic fibers are thinner than the sensory nerve fibers, autonomic block will occur inevitably before any sensory blockade is achieved with local anesthetics; hypotension is likely to precede a good sensory block. Motor nerve fibers are the thickest and hence hardest to block, hereby requiring higher concentrations of local anesthetic to cause loss of motor function. Motor block is often required to achieve a static surgical field.

Performance of all techniques of neuroaxial anesthesia requires good patient positioning and alertness on the patient's part, which is often difficult in critically ill or intubated patients. An alert patient can warn the anesthesiologist of any paresthesias, the report of which should signal anesthesiologist to halt and withdraw the needle to prevent nerve damage. If the situation allows, the patient can be placed in the sitting, supine, or lateral position with flexion of the spine which requires considerable patient cooperation. Flexion of the spine produces opening of the interspinous spaces, allowing easier access for needle placement.

Low thoracic and high lumbar catheters can effectively provide anesthesia and analgesia for endovascular stent placement as the area of the femoral triangle is the most common approach to gain access to the femoral artery for most procedures.

Common local anesthetics used are lidocaine, bupivacaine, and ropivacaine. Opioids include morphine, fentanyl, and sufentanil. Mechanism of action of local anesthetic drugs is to block transmission of signaling through nerve fibers [74–78] whereas opioids modulate signaling at the level of substantia gelatinosa within the spinal chord by acting on opioid receptors [79–84].

While factors like positioning and baracity (specific gravity of the substance divided by specific gravity of the CSF) of the local anesthetic solutions alters the spread of local anesthetics in the CSF and can aid in directing the spinal blockade to required areas, they have no effect on the spread of local anesthetic in the epidural space. Block height and intensity are a function of volume and concentration of local anesthetics used [85, 86].

Epidural Anesthesia

Epidural anesthesia involves placing a catheter in between the dura and the ligmantum flavum using a loss of resistance to saline or air technique. Fluoroscopic guidance can help facilitate placement if the patient can lie in a prone position. Contrast injected through the needle or catheter can help confirm the location in the epidural space. Once a catheter is fed through the placement needle into the epidural space about 3–4 cm it is secured to the skin with transparent adhesive tape or dressings to allow follow-up examination of the site and secure the catheter in place. Prior to utilization of the catheter a test dose should be administered to check if the location is not subarachnoid or intravascular [87].

Inserted epidural catheters can then be used to deliver intraoperative anesthesia and also postoperative analgesia using bolus/continuous infusion of dilute concentration of local anesthetics or opioids or a combination of both for several days.

Local anesthetic should be administered slowly to achieve the appropriate sensory level and allow time for recovery from the sympathetic blockade by allowing the cardiovascular system to adjust to the reduction in systemic vascular resistance. Intravenous fluids (crystalloids) can be administered if permitted by the patient's clinical condition to prevent drop in blood pressure by increasing the preload or else temporization of hemodynamic status can be achieved with short-term use of vasopressors such as phenylephrine or ephedrine.

Spinal Anesthesia

This type of regional anesthesia involves injection of anesthetics and opioids or mixtures of both into the subarachnoid space in the cerebrospinal fluid (CSF). This causes a fast and dense sensory and motor blockade at the spinal level.

Combined Spinal–Epidural Anesthesia

In combined spinal–epidural (CSE) anesthesia, a spinal injection is performed followed up by insertion of epidural catheter which is attempted at the same or different vertebral level. This combination provides the benefit of fast and dense block of a spinal anesthetic plus the capability to provide analgesia after the surgery. Since the epidural catheter cannot be tested as the exam is masked by the previous profound blockade produced by the spinal injection, it could occasionally lead to failure in the postoperative period to provide epidural analgesia.

Postoperative Management

Catheters can safely remain in place for 2–4 days with little risk infection [88–91]. A good follow-up wound check should be done daily through a transparent dressing. Monitoring the progress of continuous infusion with neuroaxial catheters should include vital signs including verbal or facial pain scores, bedsides pulse oximetry and neurological checks. Level of activity, ability to use incentive spirometry, quality of sleep, need and extent of usage of breakthrough pain medication, and return of bowel function can help estimate the effectiveness of therapy. Side effects such as pruritis, nausea, emesis, confusion, somnolence, respiratory depression, motor weakness, hypotension, urine retention should be watched for and treated. Arterial blood gases can be useful to indicate patient respiratory status.

We recommend following American Society of Regional Anesthesiologists (ASRA) guidelines for anticoagulation and regional anesthesia for insertion and removal of catheters [92].

A laboratory study of patients PT/PTTIINR should be done before pulling the catheter out as patients may be on anticoagulation and under increased risk for a spinal hematoma formation. Of note, these laboratory values do not identify anticoagulation in patients receiving low molecular weight heparin. In fact, it may be normal. In such circumstances, waiting for the effect of the low molecular heparin to wear off may be the only option [93, 94]. Time required to withdraw these indwelling catheters then depends upon the dose and type of anticoagulant used.

Advantages of Regional Anesthesia

Although general anesthesia was initially the preferred technique for endovascular repairs, over time the regional techniques have become increasingly utilized. They may have benefits to the endovascular patients in both reduction in the stress response to surgery and improved myocardial performance. Regional anesthesia can be associated with reduction of the hypercoagulable states and thromboembolic complications after vascular surgery which results in a lower incidence of thrombus formation [95].

Epidural analgesia has been demonstrated to have several other benefits in the postoperative period. These include reduced incidence of postoperative respiratory infections due to improved pulmonary toilet, reduced incidence of postoperative myocardial infarction, improved gastrointestinal motility, and early return of function can be attributed due to unopposed parasympathetic activity secondary to sympathetic blockade and reduction in opiate medication use.

Use of epidural analgesia during surgery is associated with reduced blood transfusion requirements during surgery [96, 97]. Complications associated with intubation and mechanical ventilation are avoided using regional anesthesia. Other advantages of regional anesthesia over general anesthesia include a shorter postoperative hospital stay. It also offers greater reduction in stress response [98–100] and better pain relief than with parental opioids [101]. Improved graft patency in vascular surgery has also been reported as compared to general anesthesia [100, 102]. Despite all these advantages, no survival benefit has been proven for high-risk patients.

Disadvantages of Regional Anesthesia

Often administration of regional anesthetics is precluded due to emergent nature of the surgery as it requires time, patient cooperation, and a hemodynamic stability. Also, vascular patients may be receiving anticoagulants that cannot be readily reversed. This increases the risk for development of an epidural hematoma. Not only the difficulty in positioning patients for administration of anesthesia but also the inability to lay supine may discourage this technique. Awareness of surrounding and pain evokes fear and anxiety especially during placement of invasive lines,

Foley catheters and monitors may be objectionable to the patient. General anesthesia may eventually be required if there is respiratory insufficiency or compromise due to a high spinal, excessive sedation, massive blood loss, or conversion to an open surgical repair. Patients with history of difficult airway should have their airways secured in advance so as to avoid emergent situations.

Location of fluoroscopic equipment around the head and upper thorax can impede quick access to patients' airway. Strict hemodynamic control may not be possible under regional secondary to a profound sympathectomy.

Post-dural puncture headache (PDPH) can occur when dura is punctured during placement or due to catheter migration which leads to CSF leak. The patient usually complains of occipitofrontal postural headache in the absence of meningeal signs [103, 104]. This can be treated conservatively or with an epidural blood patch [105, 106]. Nerve and spinal chord injury is a possibility. Hence some authors recommend placement in an awake state.

Other rare but possible devastating complications include epidural abscess. The onset is slow and presenting symptoms include fever, malaise, rigors, and back pain [107–109]. Epidural hematoma is likely in patients being anticoagulated or in the presence of alcoholism and liver disease [110–112]. Onset is sudden with sharp, radicular back and leg pain. Spinal infarction is rare with a predisposition in patients with arteriosclerosis and hypotension. Onset is sudden with weakness and paralysis. MRI can be done to rule out the presence of collection, blood, or infarction [110]. If MRI is not immediately available a CT myelogram can be sought to look for any extradural compression. An early neurosurgical consult should be sought to rule out any necessity for surgical intervention.

Summary

Regional anesthesia is a viable alternative to either MAC or general anesthesia and can be used to provide intraoperative and continued postoperative analgesia by injection of anesthetics or insertion of subarachnoid or epidural catheters. Often choices depend on weighing the advantages and disadvantages against the patient's clinical condition, surgical requirements, and the anesthesiologist's ability to perform these techniques.

References

1. National Center for Health Statistics. Vital Statistics of the United States, 1988: Mortality. Part A. Washington, DC: US Dept. of Health and Human Services, DHHS Publication (PHS 91-1101):1991.
2. Ingoldby CJ, Wujanto R, Mitchell JE: Impact of vascular surgery on community mortality from ruptured aortic aneurysms, *Br J Surg* 73:551, 1986.
3. Breckwoldt WL, Mackey WC, O'Donnell TF Jr: The economic implications of high-risk abdominal aortic aneurysms, *J Vasc Surg* 13:798, 1991.
4. Pasch AR, Ricotta JJ, May AG et al.: Abdominal aortic aneurysm: The case for elective resection, *Circulation* 70(suppl 1):1–1, 1984.
5. McCombs PR, Roberts B: Acute renal failure following resection of abdominal aortic aneurysm, *Surg Gynecol Obstet* 148:175, 1979.
6. Gardner RJ, Gardner NL, Tarnay TJ et al.: The surgical experience and a one to sixteen year follow-up of 277 abdominal aortic aneurysms, *Am J Surg* 135:226, 1978.
7. Dake MD, Miller DC, Semba CP, Mitchell RS, Walker PJ, Liddell RP: Transluminal placement of endovascular stent-grafts for the treatment of descending thoracic aortic aneurysm, *N Engl J Med* 331:1729–1734, 1994.
8. Dotter CT: Transluminally-placed coilspring endoarterial tube grafts: long-term patency in canine popliteal artery, *Invest Radiol* 4:329–332, 1969.
9. Parodi JC, Palmaz JC, Barone NO: Transfemoral intraluminal graft implantation for abdominal aortic aneurysms, *Ann Vasc Surg* 5:491–499, 1991.
10. deVirgilio C, Romero L, Donayre C, Meek K, Lew RJ, Lippmann M et al.: Endovascular abdominal aortic aneurysm repair with general versus local anesthesia: a comparison of cardiopulmonary morbidity and mortality rates, *J Vasc Surg* 36:988–991, 2002.
11. Lippmann M, White R, Walot I, Lee J, Kopchok G: Fast Trac anesthesia minimizes hospital stay after abdominal and thoracic endovascular aortic aneurysm repair, *Anesthesiology* 95:A30, 2001.
12. Lippmann M, White R, Lee J, Kopchok G, Wu Y, Walot I: Endovascular repair of descending thoracic aortic aneurysms using "Fast Track" MAC anesthesia, *Anesth Analg* 93:SCA 1–SCA 11, 2002.
13. White RA, Donayre CE, Walot I, Lippmann M et al.: Endovascular exclusion of descending thoracic aortic aneurysms and chronic dissections: Initial clinical results with the Aneurx device, *J Vasc Surg* 33:927–934, 2001.
14. Kakazu C, Lippmann M, Donayre C, White R: Regional nerve block reduces local anesthetic requirement for endovascular aortic aneurysm repair, *Anesthesia*, (A-378) October 2007.
15. Ginsburg R, Lippmann M: Anaphylactoid reactions to radio-opaque contrast media, *Br J Anesth* 88:879–880, 2002.
16. Henretta JP, Hodgson KJ, Mattos MA, Karch LA, Hurlbert SN, Sterback Y et al.: Feasibility of endovascular repair of abdominal aorta aneurysms with local anesthesia with intravenous sedation, *J Vasc Surg* 29:793–798, 1999.
17. Bettex DA, Lachat M, Pfammatter T, Schmidlin O, Turina MI, Schmid ER: To compare general epidural and local anesthesia for endovascular aneurysm repair (EVAR), *Eur J Vasc Endovas Surg* 21:179–184, 2001.
18. Cheng DC, Karski J, Peniston C, Raveendran G, Asokumar B, Caroll J et al.: Early tracheal extubation after coronary artery bypass graft surgery reduces costs and improves resource use. A prospective, randomized, controlled trial, *Anesthesiology* 85:1300, 1996.
19. Chen DC: Fast track cardiac surgery: implications in postoperative care, *J Cardiothorac Vasc Anest* 12:72–79, 1998.
20. Cheng DC, Wall C, Peraghlo RA, Bruce J, Naylor C: Hospital re-admission within 1 year after surgery, *Anesthesiology* 89:A23, 2000.
21. Nora CT, Dodek C, Torjman MC, White PF: The effect of anesthetic technique on the hemodynamic response and recovery profile in coronary revascularization patients, *Anesth Analg* 81:900–910, 1995.
22. Tverskoy M, Cozacov C, Ayache M, Bradley EL Jr, Kissen I: Postoperative pain after inguinal herniorrhaphy with different type of anesthesia, *Anesth Analg* 70:29–35, 1990.
23. Ding Y, White PF: Post-herniorrhaphy pain in outpatients after pre-incision ilioinguinal-hypogastric nerve block during monitored anesthesia care, *Can J Anaesth* 42:12–15, 1995.
24. Sa Rego M, Watcha MF, White PF: The changing role of monitored anesthesia care in the ambulatory setting, *Anesth Analg* 85:1020–1036, 1997.
25. Lippmann M et al.: An alterative technique for the morbidly obese patient undergoing endovascular repair of an

abdominal aortic aneurysm, *Anesth Analg* 97:981–983, 2003.
26. Kahn RA, Marin ML, Hollier L, Parsons R, Griepp R: Induction of ventricular fibrillation to facilitate endovascular stent graft repair of thoracic aortic aneurysms, *Anesthesiology* 88:534–536, 1998.
27. Pennell OJ, Mahmood S, Ell PJ, Underwood SR: Bradycardia progressing to cardiac arrest during adenosine thallium myocardial perfusion imaging in occult sino-atrial disease, *Eur J Nucl Med* 21:1702, 1994.
28. Moser GH, Schrader J, Oeussen A: Turnover of adenosine in plasma of human and dog blood, *Am J Physiol* 256(4 Pt 1):C799–C806, 1989.
29. Kakazu CZ, Lippmann M, Hancock O, Oonayre C, White RA: Adenosine-induced transient cardiac asystole in the awake elderly patient for endovascular thoracic aortic aneurysm repair, *Anesth Analg* 102:S–64, 2006.
30. Lippmann M et al.: Adenosine's usefulness in vascular surgery, *Tex Heart Inst J* 34:258–259, 2007.
31. Rudolphi KA, Keil M, Hinze HJ: Effect of theophylline on ischemically induced hippocampal damage in mongolian gerbils: a behavioral and histological study, *J Cereb Blood Flow Metab* 7:74–81, 1987.
32. Ely SW, Berne RM: Protective effects of adenosine in myocardial ischemia, *Circulation* 85:893–904, 1992.
33. Ezri T, Sessler D, Weisenberg M et al.: Association of ethnicity with the minimum alveolar concentration of sevoflurane, *Anesthesiology* 107(1):9–14, 2007.
34. Gielen MJM, Stienstra R: Tourniquet hypertension and its prevention: A review, *Reg Anesth* 16:191–194, 1991.
35. Lee WA, Berceli SA, Huber TS et al.: Morbidity with retroperitoneal procedures during endovascular abdominal aortic aneurysm repair, *J Vase Surg* 38:459–463, 2003, discussion 464–465.
36. Cambria RP, Brewster DC, Lauterbach SR et al.: Evolving experience with thoracic aortic stent graft repair, *J Vase Surg* 35:1129–1136, 2002.
37. Lennmarken C, Bildfors K, Enlund G et al.: Victims of awareness, *Acta Anaesthesiol Seand* 46:229, 2002.
38. Kakazu C, Lippmann M, Hancock D, Donayre C, White R, Adenosine-Ind cardiac arrest for endovascular thoracic aortic aneurysm stent placement in the elderly patient. Anesth Analg 102:S-64, 2006.
39. Practice guidelines for perioperative transesophageal echo cardiography: report by the American Society of Anesthesiologists and the Society of Cardiovascular Anesthesiologists Task Force on Transesophageal Echocardiography. Anesthesiology 84:986–1006, 1996.
40. Swenson JD, Harkin C, Pace NL et al.: Transesophageal echocardiography: an objective tool in defining maximum ventricular response to intravenous fluid therapy, *Anesth Analg* 83:1149–1153, 1996.
41. Goarin JP, Cluzel P, Gosgnach M et al.: Evaluation of transesophageal echocardiography for diagnosis of traumatic aortic injury, *Anesthesiology* 93: 1373–1377, 2000.
42. Erbel R, Engberding R, Daniel W et al.: Echocardiography in diagnosis of aortic dissection, *Lancet* 1:457–461, 1989.
43. Cheung AT, Savino JS, Weiss SJ et al.: Echocardiographic and hemodyna IC indexes of left ventricular preload in patients with normal and abnormal ventricular function, *Anesthesiology* 81:376–387, 1994.
44. Saada M, Duval AM, Bounet F et al.: Abnormalities in myocardial segment wall motion during lumbar epidural anesthesia, *Anesthesiology* 71:32, 1989.
45. Tryba M: Epidural regional anesthesia and low molecular weight heparin [in German], *Anasthesiol Intensivmed Notfallmed Schmerzther*, 28:181, 1993.
46. Regional anesthesia in the anti-coagulated patient – defining the risks. American Society of Regional Anesthesia Consensus Statement 2002.
47. Maguire AM, Kumar N, Parker IL et al.: Comparison of effects of remifentanil and alfentanil on cardiovascular response to tracheal intubation in hypertensive patients, *Br J Anaesth* 86:90–93, 2001, Abstract.
48. Edwards ND, Alford AM, Dobson PMS et al.: Myocardial ischemia during tracheal intubation and extubation, *Br J Anaesth* 73:57–539, 1994, Abstract.
49. Padro JM, Caralps JM, Garcia J, Aris A: Spontaneous rupture of the ascending aorta, *J Cardiovasc Surg (Torino)* 29:109–110, 1988.
50. Devitt JR, Wenstone R, Noel AG et al.: The laryngeal mask airway and positive-pressure ventilation, *Anesthesiology* 80:550, 1994.
51. Salartash K, Stembergh WC 3rd, York JW, Money SR: Comparison of transabdominal AAA repair with endovascular AAA repair, *J Endovasc Surg* 4:62–65, 1997.
52. Miller RD: *Miller's anesthesia*, vol. 1, ed. 6, Philadelphia, 2005, Elsevier, Chap. 40.
53. Frank SM, Beattie C, Christopherson R et al.: Unintentional hypothermia' associated with postoperative myocardial ischemia. The perioperative ischemia randomized anesthesia trial study group, *Anesthesiology* 78:468–476, 1993.
54. Marcantonio ER, Goldman L, Orav EJ et al.: The association of intraoperative factors with the development of postoperative delirium, *Am J Med* 105: 380–384, 1998.
55. Marcantonio ER, Goldman L, Mangione CM et al.: A clinical prediction for delirium after elective noncardiac surgery, *JAMA* 271:134–139, 1994.
56. Goldman L, Caldera DL: Risks of general anesthesia and elective operation in the hypertensive patient, *Anesthesiology* 50:285–292, 1979.
57. Solomonson MD, Johnson ME, Ilstrup D: Risk factors in patients having surgery to create an arteriovenous fistula, *Anesth Analg* 79:694–670, 1994.
58. Frank SM, Norris EJ, Christopherson R, Beattie C: Right-and-left-arm blood pressure discrepancies in vascular surgery patients, *Anesthesiology* 17:529–548, 1991.
59. McNulty SE: Preoperative evaluation of hypertension (anesthetic implications in patients with coronary disease), *Anesthesiol Clin North Am* 17:549–565, 1999.
60. Khan LA, Nair CK: Clinical, diagnostic, and management perspectives of aortic dissection, *Chest* 122(1):311–328, 2002.
61. Meredith JW, Hoth N: Thoracic Trauma: When and How to Intervene, *Surg Clin North Am* 87(1):95–118, 2007.
62. Lippmann M, Kakazu C: Hemodynamics with propofol: Is propofol dangerous in classes III-V patients? *Anesth Analg* 103:260, 2006.

63. Francis GS: Vasodilators in the intensive care unit, *Am Heart J* 121:1875–1878, 1991.
64. Fung HL: Clinical pharmacology of organic nitrates, *Am J Cardiol* 72:9C–13C, 1993.
65. Murphy C: Hypertensive emergencies, *Emerg Med Clin North Am* 13:973–1007, 1995.
66. Sorkin EM, Clissold SP: A review of its pharmacodynamic and pharmacokinetic properties, and therapeutic efficacy, in the treatment of angina pectoris, hypertension and related cardiovascular disorders, *Drugs* 33:296–345, 1987.
67. Gray RJ: Managing critically ill patients with esmolol. An ultra short-acting beta-adrenergic blocker, *Chest* 93:398–403, 1998.
68. Lowenthal DT, Porter RS, Saris SD et al.: Clinical pharmacology, pharmacodynamics and interactions with esmolol, *Am J Cardiol* 5:8F, 1985.
69. Lund-Johansen P: Pharmacology of combined alpha-beta-blockade. Haemodynamic effects of labetalol, *Drugs* 28(suppl A):A3–A14, 1984.
70. Levy JH: Treatment of peri operative hypertension, *Anesthesiol Clin North Am* 17:567–579, 1999.
71. Goldberg ME, Cantillo J, NemiroffM S et al.: Fenoldopam infusion for treatment of postoperative hypertension, *J Clin Anesth* 5:386–391, 1993.
72. Warren TM, Datta S, Ostheimer GW: Lumbar epidural anesthesia in a patient with multiple sclerosis, *Anesth Analg* 61:1022–1023, 1982.
73. Siemkowicz E: Multiple sclerosis and surgery, *Anaesthesia* 31:1211–1216, 1976.
74. Hille B: The pH-dependent rate of action of local anesthetics on the node of Ranvier, *J Gen Physiol* 69:475–496, 1977.
75. Hille B: Local anesthetics: hydrophilic and hydrophobic pathways for the drug-receptor reaction, *J Gen Physiol* 69:497–515, 1977.
76. Ritchie JM, Ritchie BR: Local anesthetics: effect of pH on activity, *Science* 162:1394–1395, 1968.
77. Chernoff OM, Strichartz GR: Tonic and phasic block of neuronal sodium currents by 5-hydroxyhexano-2',6'-xylide, a neutral lidocaine homologue, *J Gen Physiol* 93:1075–1090, 1989.
78. Ulbricht W: Kinetics of drug action and equilibrium results at the node of Ranvier, *Physiol Rev* 61:785–828, 1981.
79. Wang JK, Nauss LA, Thomas JE: Pain relief by intrathecally applied morphine in man, *Anesthesiology* 50:149–151, 1979.
80. Yaksh TL, Rudy TA: Analgesia mediated by a direct spinal action of narcotics, *Science* 192:1357–1358, 1976.
81. Duggan AW, North RA: Electrophysiology of opioids, *Pharmacol Rev* 35:219–281, 1983.
82. Atweh S, Kuhar M: Autoradiographic localization of opiate receptors in rat brain, *Brain Res* 124:53–67, 1977.
83. Samii K, Chauvin M, Viars P: Postoperative spinal analgesia with morphine, *Br J Anaesth* 53:817–820, 1981.
84. Cousins MJ, Mather LE, Glynn CJ et al.: Selective spinal analgesia, *Lancet* 1:1141–1142, 1979.
85. Greene NM: Distribution of local anesthetic solutions within the subarachnoid space, *Anesth Analg* 64:715, 1985.
86. Stienstra R, Veering BT: Intrathecal drug spread: Is it controllable? *Reg Anesth Pain Med* 23:347, 1998.
87. Moore DC, Batra MS: The components of an effective test dose prior to epidural block, *Anesthesiology* 55:693, 1981.
88. Scott DA, Beilby OS, McClymont C: Postoperative analgesia using epidural infusions of fentanyl with bupivacaine. A prospective analysis of 1,014 patients, *Anesthesiology* 83:727, 1995.
89. Liu SS, Allen HW, Olsson GL: Patient-controlled epidural analgesia with bupivacaine and fentanyl on hospital wards: Prospective experience with 1,030 surgical patients, *Anesthesiology* 88:688, 1998.
90. Wigfull J, Welchew E: Survey of 1057 patients receiving postoperative patient-controlled epidural analgesia, *Anaesthesia* 56:70, 2001.
91. Burstal R, Wegener F, Hayes C et al.: Epidural analgesia: prospective audit of 1062 patients, *Anaesth Intensive Care* 26:165, 1998.
92. The second consensus conference on neuroaxial anesthesia and anticoagulation. American Regional anesthesia and Pain medicine. www.asra.com
93. Hynson JM, Katz JA, Bueff HU: Epidural hematoma associated with enoxaparin, *Anesth Analg* 82:1072, 1996.
94. Horlocker TT, Wedel DJ: Neuraxial block and low-molecular-weight heparin: Balancing perioperative analgesia and thromboprophylaxis, *Reg Anesth Pain Med* 23(suppl 2):164, 1998.
95. Tuman KJ, McCarthy RJ, March RJ et al.: Effects of epidural anesthesia and analgesia on coagulation and outcome after major vascular surgery, *Anesth Analg* 73:696, 1991.
96. Blake DW: The general vs. regional anesthesia debate: time to re-examine the goals, *Aust N Z J Surg* 65:51, 1995.
97. Neilsen KK, Andersen K, Asbjorn J et al.: Blood loss during transurethral resection of the prostate: a comparison of epidural and general anesthesia [abstract], *Int Urol Nephrol* 19:287, 1987.
98. Breslow MJ, Parker SD, Frank SM et al.: Determinants of catecholamine and cortisol responses to lower extremity revascularization. The PIRA T Study Group, *Anesthesiology* 79:1202–1209, 1993.
99. Christopherson R, Beattie C, Fran SM et al.: Perioperative morbidity in patients randomized to epidural or general anesthesia for lower extremity vascular surgery. Perioperative Ischemia Randomized Anesthesia Trial Study Group, *Anesthesiology* 79: 422–434, 1993.
100. Christopherson R, Glavan NJ, Norris EJ et al.: Control of blood pressure and heart rate in patients randomized to epidural or general anesthesia for lower extremity vascular surgery. Perioperative Ischemia Randomized Anesthesia Trial (PIRAT) study group, *J Clin Anesth* 8:578–584, 1996.
101. Block BM, Liu SS, Rowlingson AJ et al.: Efficacy of postoperative epidural analgesia: a meta-analysis, *JAMA* 290:2455–2463, 2003.
102. Tuman KJ, McCarthy RJ, March RJ et al.: Effects of epidural anesthesia and analgesia on coagulation and outcome after major vascular surgery, *Anesth Analg* 73: 696–704, 1991.

103. Lybecker H, Djernes M, Schmidt JF: Postdural puncture headache (PDPH): Onset, duration, severity and associated symptoms, *Acta Anaesthesiol Scand* 39: 605, 1995.
104. Denny N, Masters R, Pearson D et al.: Postdural puncture headache after continuous spinal anesthesia, *Anesth Analg* 66:791, 1987.
105. Gormley JB: Treatment of postspinal headache, *Anesthesiology* 21:565, 1960.
106. Safa-Tisseront V, Thormann F, Malassine P et al.: Effectiveness of epidural blood patch in the management of post-dural puncture headache, *Anesthesiology* 95:334, 2001.
107. Schmidt RD, Markovchik V: Nontraumatic spinal cord compression, *J Emerg Med* 2:189, 1992.
108. Hlavin ML, Kaminski HJ, Ross JS et al.: Spinal epidural abscess: a ten-year perspective, *Neurosurgery* 27:177, 1990.
109. Danner RL, Hartman BJ: Update of epidural abscess: 35 cases and a review of the literature, *Rev Infect Dis* 9:265, 1987.
110. Boukobza M, Guichard JP, Boissonet M et al.: Spinal epidural hematoma: Report of 11 cases and review of the literature, *Neuroradiology* 36:456, 1994.
111. Dickman CA, Shedd SA, Spetzler RF et al.: Spinal epidural hematoma associated with epidural anaesthesia: complications of systemic heparinization in patients receiving peripheral vascular thrombolytic therapy, *Anesthesiology* 72:947, 1990.
112. Mattie H et al.: Nontraumatic spinal epidural and subdural hematomas, *Neurology* 37:1351, 1987.
113. Martin DE, Shanks GE: Strategies for the preoperative evaluation of the hypertensive patient, Anesthesiol Clin North Am 17:529–548, 1999.

6 Intraprocedural Monitoring for Endovascular Procedures

Ali Khoynezhad and G. Matthew Longo

Peripheral (non-cardiac) endovascular interventions have penetrated the field of vascular surgery, and it is the standard of care in many occasions. Compared to traditional open peripheral operations, the minimal access and image-guided interventions have many advantages including shorter hospital stay and faster patient recovery. However, the interventions remain a high-risk procedure due to patients advanced age and significant comorbidities such as coronary artery disease and chronic renal and pulmonary disease. Procedure-specific factors further modulate the preexisting risk factors and may add further complications during the procedure and in the postprocedural period. For example, in patients undergoing thoracic endovascular aortic repair (TEVAR), specific complications such as spinal cord injury and stroke are the focus of intraprocedural neurophysiologic monitoring, because neurological deficits remain of the most devastating complications after peripheral endovascular interventions.

Every patient undergoing a peripheral endovascular intervention will have a series of intraprocedural monitoring. The goal of the monitoring is early detection of abnormalities in physiologic parameters and their rapid correction. In a few instances (such as with cerebrospinal fluid pressure monitoring during TEVAR), the monitoring device is also an important therapeutic option [1]. The monitoring tools have to be less invasive, accurate, efficient, and cost-effective. Probably as important as the patient's outcome is the proficiency of the involved physicians to interpret the collected data in a timely fashion. This includes a high index of suspicion and anticipation of upcoming complications, cognitive skills to diagnose the adverse outcome with understanding of limitations of the monitoring device, and knowledge of the skills necessary to most efficiently treat the physiologic abnormality or complication. Misinterpretation of monitored data may happen with more sophisticated monitoring devices and will render the monitoring device futile and even harmful to the patients. In case of pulmonary artery catheter, the most common complication remains the misinterpretation of data altered by various physiologic and anatomic parameters. This underscores the importance of competency in putting the pieces of the puzzle together and filtering out inaccurate data. Therefore a sound working knowledge of intraprocedural monitoring devices is crucial for physicians performing peripheral endovascular interventions and represents the aim of this chapter. The monitoring devices have been divided into general anesthetic monitoring, special anesthetic monitoring, and neurophysiologic monitoring used for TEVAR and carotid interventions.

General Monitoring

The general anesthetic monitoring of the patient during a procedure is done either by the surgeon/interventionalist or a member of the anesthesiology team. The areas routinely assessed while the intervention is occurring include electrocardiogram (ECG) monitoring, pulse oximetry temperature, capnography if the patient is intubated, and arterial blood pressures.

A. Khoynezhad (✉)
Associate Professor, Director of Aortic and Arrhythmia Surgery, Division of Cardiothoracic and Vascular Surgery, Department of Surgery, Creighton University Medical Center, Omaha, NE, USA

T.J. Fogarty, R.A. White (eds.), *Peripheral Endovascular Interventions*,
DOI 10.1007/978-1-4419-1387-6_6, © Springer Science+Business Media, LLC 1998, 2010

Electrocardiography

Continuous ECG monitoring is routinely performed in the intra- and postoperative setting. It is non-invasive, inexpensive, widely available, and requires minimal training for monitoring and interpretation. Real-time information regarding cardiac rate and rhythm is provided. This tool is invaluable for maintaining heart rate control in the vasculopath. In situations of tachycardia or bradycardia, prompt assessment of the situation can ensue followed by an appropriate therapeutic maneuver to improve cardiac perfusion and output. The ability to monitor the cardiac rhythm also provides an important tool. Rhythm changes can often signal cardiac ischemia or abnormalities in the patient's volume status. Continuous ECG monitoring can also detect ST- or T-wave changes which may signal a cardiac ischemic event. The sensitivity is low with typical two-lead continuous ECG, but this can be improved using a five-lead system. More sensitive tools for monitoring cardiac ischemia will be discussed later.

Pulse Oximetry

Pulse oximetry, utilizing a photosensor, estimates the difference between the oxygenated and deoxygenated blood to calculate the saturation of arterialized blood (oxyhemoglobin saturation) [2]. The difference is calculated through utilization of the different measured wavelengths of oxyhemoglobin (660 nm, red) and reduced hemoglobin (940 nm, infrared). The ratio of transmittance of each varies based on the percentage of oxyhemoglobin. Similar to ECG, it is standard of care in monitoring in any setting. It is non-invasive, inexpensive, widely available, and requires minimal training for monitoring and interpretation. A number of factors can limit the effectiveness of pulse oximetry including abnormal hemoglobins (methemoglobin, carboxyhemoglobin), impaired local perfusion due to peripheral vascular disease or vasoconstrictors or hypotension, high pO_2s, fingernail polish and body paint. Ultimately, the pulse oximeter can signal cardiopulmonary deterioration before it becomes clinically apparent. Caution should be applied in monitoring patients with partial respiratory insufficiency, as poor ventilation may be missed in the face of optimal oxygenation, until the patients decompensate. The application of near-infrared cerebral and tissue oximetry will be discussed later.

Temperature

Core body temperature measurements are essential in the basic monitoring armamentarium [2]. Hypothermia is very common in patients undergoing endovascular procedures. The movement of a patient's core temperature outside of the normal ranges can result in a number of complications. Hypothermia may contribute to platelet dysfunction, surgical site infection, arrhythmias, electrolyte imbalances, metabolic acidosis, and altered metabolism. Hyperthermia can cause tachycardia, insensible fluid losses with increased fluid requirements, and an increased metabolic rate. The importance of thermoregulation in hypothermic patients using external body warmers and warm fluid/medication administration has been appreciated by anesthesiologists and has been included in core quality measurement and assessments.

Capnography

Capnography measures the changes of CO_2 concentration during the ventilatory cycle. Utilizing either mass spectroscopy or infrared light absorption to detect CO_2, the practitioner can see the peak CO_2 concentration which is often equated to the end-tidal CO_2 [2]. This is trended on a breath-to-breath basis and is a sensitive method to detect acute changes in end-tidal CO_2. This can be utilized to assess tracheal intubation and ventilation adequacy, CO_2 production, and respiratory gas exchange. Sudden decreases in the peak CO_2 concentration can suggest increased dead space (for example, pulmonary embolus), hypoventilation, airway obstruction, or leak in the ventilatory circuit. Increases in the peak CO_2 are often due to hypermetabolic states. The ability to use capnography can reduce the need for arterial blood gases.

Arterial Blood Pressure

If constant monitoring of blood pressure is necessary, this can be accomplished by directly placing a catheter in an artery. Compared to the oscillometric method, direct blood pressure monitoring is more accurate and continuous. It is the preferred method for patients undergoing peripheral endovascular interventions. Usually, the radial, brachial, or femoral artery is chosen. Complications are rare in experienced hands and include thrombosis, dissection, distal malperfusion, and infection [3].

Blood pressures measured intra-arterially tend to be elevated systolically the more peripheral the artery, and depressed diastolically. However, the mean pressure remains relatively constant. Therefore targeting antihypertensive therapies based on mean arterial pressure is appropriate in the majority of patients. As with any direct pressure tools, direct arterial pressure monitoring is subject to inaccuracies due to calibration, zeroing, and positioning errors. This method of monitoring is utilized in patients requiring frequent blood draws, those who may lose substantial amounts of blood, patients requiring precise blood pressure control, and those needing inotropic support.

Recently, the arterial pressure waveform has been used to assess intravascular volume status in ventilated patients. Furthermore, continuous beat-to-beat calculation of stroke volume and cardiac output (CO) and its correlation to thermodilution CO has been increasingly studied in cardiac surgical literature [4]. Further validation studies will be needed to integrate this exciting technology into daily practice.

Advanced Cardiopulmonary Monitoring

Central Venous Catheter

There is no level 1 evidence for routine use of central venous catheter in monitoring patients with peripheral vascular disease. However, it is routinely used in high-risk patients and/or patients with coronary artery disease and right or left ventricular dysfunction. Placement of the central line in internal jugular or subclavian vein (and less commonly transfemoral into iliac veins) is a routine procedure with very low morbidity. This should be preferably done using duplex ultrasound-guided technique to reduce the possibility of arterial puncture and dilatation or pneumothorax. This technique is of special value in patients with previous multiple central venous access lines (such as patients with hemodialysis lines, chemotherapy lines, and pacemaker lines) and in patients with low intravascular volume and collapsed venous lumen.

Central venous pressure (CVP) monitoring is commonly used to assess intravascular fluid shifts (and/or blood loss) and right ventricular preload. The latter approximates the left ventricular preload in patients with normal valvular and right ventricular function and is one of the four independent determinants of cardiac output based on the Frank–Starling relationship [5]. Further indications for use of central venous catheter monitoring are in patients with poor peripheral vascular access and in prolonged procedures where multiple intraprocedural blood draws are necessary. It also serves as a secure route for (hyperosmolar) drug administration and an access for placement of pulmonary artery catheterization and transvenous pacing. If rapid transfusion or intraprocedural administration of large quantities of fluid is indicated, a 14-gauge peripheral intravenous access will allow a higher flow rate given its shorter length and less resistance.

As with arterial pressure monitoring, CVP is subject to inaccuracies due to calibration, zeroing, and positioning errors. For more accurate pressure monitoring, the CVP should be measured at the end of expiration to reduce interference of intrathoracic pressure variation [6]. Given the variability of intrathoracic vascular pressure, no change in CVP less than 4 mmHg should be considered as clinically significant [7]. For purposes of clinical decision making, one should rely on CVP trends rather than strict reliance on isolated instantaneous values. There are many other pitfalls that can affect accuracy of CVP in detecting right ventricular preload. In patients with tricuspid or mitral valve regurgitation or stenosis, patients with right ventricular dysfunction, and patients with primary and secondary pulmonary hypertension, the accuracy of the monitoring tool is significantly reduced. Therefore, although CVP is a good proxy of right ventricular preload in most patients, it cannot be used in isolation as an indicator of hypo- or hypervolemia [8]. In these patients, an evaluation of other physiologic parameter of intravascular volume status is indicated. For similar reasons, a physician should not treat the patient based on abnormal CVP, if other physiologic markers indicate good tissue perfusion status.

Pulmonary Artery Catheter

The pulmonary artery catheter (PAC) has been the most scrutinized monitoring device. It has been slandered in recent years because of clinical studies showing that mortality was not reduced and can, in fact, be higher in patients with PAC [9, 10]. There are two fundamental problems with such criticism: first, the PAC is solely a monitoring tool and not a therapeutic device. When used in patients with poor prognosis due to untreatable problems, the PAC is not the cause of the mortality, it is merely a messenger. Blaming and "killing the messenger" would be futile in such a condition. Second, mortality rates are not an appropriate criterion to evaluate a monitoring tool; they are used to assess therapeutic options.

PAC is indicated in high-risk patients with advanced pulmonary or valvular or coronary artery disease to obtain necessary data that would assist with clinical decision making. PAC should not be used, if a less-invasive (and more cost-effective) monitoring device can reliably reproduce the information provided by the catheter. Besides the morbidities associated with central venous catheter placement, the PAC can produce self-limiting atrial and ventricular arrhythmias. During advancement of the PAC and in patients with left complete bundle branch block, the tip of the catheter may cause (temporary) complete atrioventricular block that may require cardiac pacing. The most feared complication is pulmonary artery rupture due to overzealous inflation of the balloon in the distal pulmonary artery bed. This maneuver is especially worrisome in anticoagulated patients with pulmonary artery hypertension. This will be associated with a sudden and persistent drop in pulmonary artery occlusion pressure. Treatment includes withdrawal and re-inflation of the balloon to tamponade/infarct that pulmonary artery bed, reversal of anticoagulation, reduction of pulmonary artery pressure with nitric oxide or epoprostenol, and cardiothoracic surgical consultation. However, by using a standard insertion technique and avoidance of high-risk maneuvers, the complications associated with PAC are minimal.

The most common complication of PAC is not associated with the insertion but rather with accurate interpretation of the obtained data. Understanding the limitations of the monitoring parameters in the face of abnormal physiologic and anatomic variables is crucial for the treating physician. PAC provides a series of information including pulmonary artery occlusion pressure (PAOP), mixed-venous artery saturation (SvO_2), and a series of hemodynamic parameters associated with thermodilution CO. In a patient with normal valvular function and absent pulmonary artery hypertension, PAOP is a proximate of left ventricular end-systolic pressure or preload of the left ventricle. Intraprocedural increase of such pressure is unspecific markers of hypervolemia, diastolic dysfunction, or left ventricular dysfunction associated with cardiac ischemic. Intraprocedural reduction in PAOP is a sensitive monitor for hypovolemia, hemorrhage, or systemic allergic reactions. The aforementioned pitfalls of CVP monitoring apply here as well. In every fourth patient, a true "wedge" pressure is unobtainable due to pulsatility of the balloon tip. In these patients, the pulmonary artery diastolic pressure should be used as a surrogate. A similar strategy should be used in anticoagulated patients or those with pulmonary artery hypertension to reduce the possibility of pulmonary artery rupture.

The oxygen saturation measured at the tip of the PAC is used to evaluate the balance of systemic oxygen delivery and oxygen delivery uptake (DO_2/VO_2). In a steady state, the tissue oxygen consumption is approximately 20–25% of the DO_2, making for a VO_2 in the pulmonary artery of about 75%. Acute intraprocedural changes signify either reduction of oxygen delivery due to reduced CO, poor systemic oxygen content (decreased hemoglobin or systemic saturation), or increased tissue oxygen demands (infection, shivering, hyperthermia, inadequate sedation, or relaxation). Therefore all intraprocedural interventions are logically aimed to meet a balanced DO_2/VO_2. Central venous oxygen saturation may substitute PAC-assisted SvO_2 only if multiple measurements are averaged. Due to significant differences and variability of oxygen saturation in the superior and inferior vena cava, a single measurement of SvO_2 through a central venous catheter may differ as much as 10% compared to a PAC-assisted SvO_2 [11].

In addition to SvO_2, PAC measures/calculates a series of hemodynamic parameters. CO is derived by the thermodilution method (Fick principle). Continuous cardiac output PAC is preferred for monitoring cardiac output because it is more accurate than intermittent bolus injection PAC [12]. Cardiac index is a preferred way for evaluating changes in the CO. The intraprocedural utility of derived (calculated) values such as stroke volume index, ventricular stroke work index, systemic (and pulmonary) vascular resistance index, and oxygen delivery is limited. In rare conditions, they may be used to differentiate intraprocedural cardiogenic shock versus hypovolemic (hemorrhagic) and vasogenic (anaphylaxis and neurogenic) shock. These cardiovascular and oxygen transport parameters, however, can be extremely valuable in critically ill patients in the intensive care unit.

Transesophageal Echocardiography

Transesophageal echocardiography (TEE) is a useful real-time monitoring tool of cardiac function. It provides real-time assessment of left ventricular wall motion abnormalities (as a sign of acute ischemia), valvular abnormalities such as acute evidence of mitral regurgitation (a sign of posterolateral wall cardiac ischemia), evidence of pericardial effusion and tamponade physiology, accurate assessment of right and left ventricular preload, evaluation of diastolic and systolic function of both ventricles, and much more. While there is no prospective trial supporting the use of TEE in patients undergoing peripheral endovascular procedures, there is accumulating evidence to support the use of TEE for high-risk patients with cardiac, pulmonary, or aortic pathologies.

Complications associated with TEE are rare. The most feared complication is associated with improper placement and repositioning causing esophageal perforation. Erosions in the pharynx, esophagus, and stomach are not uncommon but self-limiting and rare in experienced hands. TEE is similar to the PAC—highly operator—and interpreter-dependant. It is useful in intubated patients and its use is limited in spontaneously breathing patients.

Intraprocedural monitoring with TEE for patients with ischemic heart disease is the most accurate tool for detection of intraprocedural cardiac ischemia. A short axis view at the level of both the left ventricular papillary muscles can detect coronary artery ischemia in any of three major coronary distributions. In patients with questionable thoracic aortic dissection, TEE has a specificity and sensitivity of 98% in detection of type A or B dissection [13]. TEE and the duplex mode can be helpful in detecting primary and secondary entry sites in type B aortic dissection. This information is of special value for endovascular repair and coverage of large entry sites that are typically located in the proximal descending thoracic aorta.

Advanced Vascular Monitoring

A number of modalities are utilized in the operating room to assess the anatomic and/or hemodynamic success of peripheral endovascular interventions. The primary tools utilized in the operating room or angiography suite consist of angiography, intravascular ultrasound, duplex ultrasonography, and pull-back pressures with gradient calculation.

Angiography

The primary modality for the evaluation and performance of endovascular procedures is contrast angiography. This involves gaining access to the vascular system through the puncture of a vessel. At this point, a variety of contrast agents can be utilized through direct injection into the vessels desired for imaging. Angiography provides intraprocedural imaging with demonstration of the vascular anatomy. It allows determination if an intervention is warranted, the selection of devices for treatment, imaging during the intervention, and documentation of the success or failure of the procedure [14].

At the beginning of the procedure, access is typically obtained via the common femoral, axillary, or brachial vessels. In rare circumstances, popliteal, tibial, aortic, or carotid access is utilized. A contrast agent is then injected and used to guide wires and catheters to the vessels and pathology in question. This imaging will allow the visualization of dissections, aneurysms, stenotic lesions and ulcers, arteritis, and embolic disease. Once the desired vessel is imaged, the extent of the lesion, as well as the non-diseased vessel luminal diameter, is obtained. The appropriate device for intervention is then selected. Angiograms guide the procedure. Immediately post-intervention, the success can be evaluated with completion images. Besides the apparent success of the procedure, perforations, dissections, emboli, endoleaks, vessel thrombosis, spasm, and recoil can be appreciated. Complications associated with angiography include contrast nephropathy, radiation exposure (both to the patient and health-care providers), and issues associated with vascular access.

A useful adjunct when treating occlusive disease is the use of pull-back pressures or arterial gradients [15]. A trans-stenotic gradient of 10 mmHg or greater is considered an indication for intervention. Pharmacologic agents, either 100–200 μg/mL of nitroglycerine or 30–60 mg of papaverine, can be directly injected into the vessel. This stimulates vasodilatation in an effort to identify a hemodynamically significant stenosis. Transduction of the pressures across the lesion in question is then taken under hyperemic condition, and once again, a 10 mmHg or greater difference is considered significant.

Although angiography has demonstrated its usefulness and is widely considered the "gold standard" for intraoperative monitoring and evaluation, it has limitations and potential complications. The images obtained are two dimensional; thus the operator needs to be able to take the information and apply it to a three-dimensional vessel [16]. Artifact related to both magnification and thrombus can also lead to misinterpretation of visual data. Difficulties related to spatial and contrast resolution can negatively impact the quality of images.

Intravascular Ultrasound

Intravascular ultrasound (IVUS) is catheter-based ultrasound imaging that provides a 360° cross-sectional image [17]. IVUS is utilized in the periphery, abdominal and thoracic aorta, and vena cava. With respect to the peripheral arteries, the length, morphology, and pathology of a lesion can be precisely assessed through intraluminal cross-sectional imaging. The measurement of the vessel diameter is utilized for balloon sizing. Post-angioplasty the vessel is re-imaged, and the luminal gain is reassessed. If a stent is required, the decision is made at this time. The post-angioplasty lesion is re-sized and an appropriately sized stent is chosen. After a stent is placed, IVUS evaluates the stent–vessel wall apposition as well as the adequacy of stent deployment [18].

With respect to peripheral interventions, IVUS has proven most useful for aortic interventions. IVUS's primary use with abdominal aortic endografting involves assessment of the suitability of the vessel for endografting, through determination of the length of fixation sites, confirmation of cannulation of the contralateral gate, and the presence of atherosclerotic lesions and thrombus. Also, the vessel diameters at the proximal and distal fixation sites are ascertained allowing appropriate graft selection. During placement of the graft, the use of IVUS has been shown to decrease or eliminate the use of contrast agents and reduce fluoroscopy time. After placement of the graft, IVUS interrogation demonstrates renal and internal iliac artery patency, the presence of an endoleak, and adequacy of stent deployment. With respect to the thoracic aorta, IVUS is helpful for sizing (Fig. 6.1), reducing the use of contrast agents and fluoroscopy time, and post-deployment evaluation, much in the same way it is utilized in the abdominal aorta. IVUS has proven particularly helpful when dealing with thoracic dissections. The areas assessed by IVUS include the proximal and distal extent of the dissection, location of primary and secondary entry sites, measurement of the size of the aorta, and the relationship of the aortic branches to the true and false lumen of the dissection.

Once the intervention has begun, IVUS is critical to confirming that wire placement is within the true lumen of the vessel. IVUS is very helpful in establishing primary endpoints of endovascular treatment after the stent graft deployment (complete exclusion of primary intimal tear and stagnation of blood flow in the false lumen) [19] and can be utilized to confirm that the blood supply is intact to the major branches off the aorta [20].

IVUS has also proven adept at imaging the vena cava for bedside caval filter placement. In the critically ill patient that cannot be moved or the patient that cannot tolerate contrast agents due to kidney function, IVUS allows visualization of the renal veins at the bedside. The distance from the renal veins to the access site is ascertained, the filter is then positioned based on this measurement, and deployed. The vena cava is then either re-imaged with IVUS to confirm placement, or placement is confirmed with an abdominal radiograph.

Use of IVUS (and TEE) may contribute significantly to our understanding of stroke during TEVAR or carotid stenting. IVUS is used to assess the risk of stroke by visualizing calcifications and loose atheromas in the thoracic aorta. IVUS and TEE very accurately detect major thoracic aortic calcification

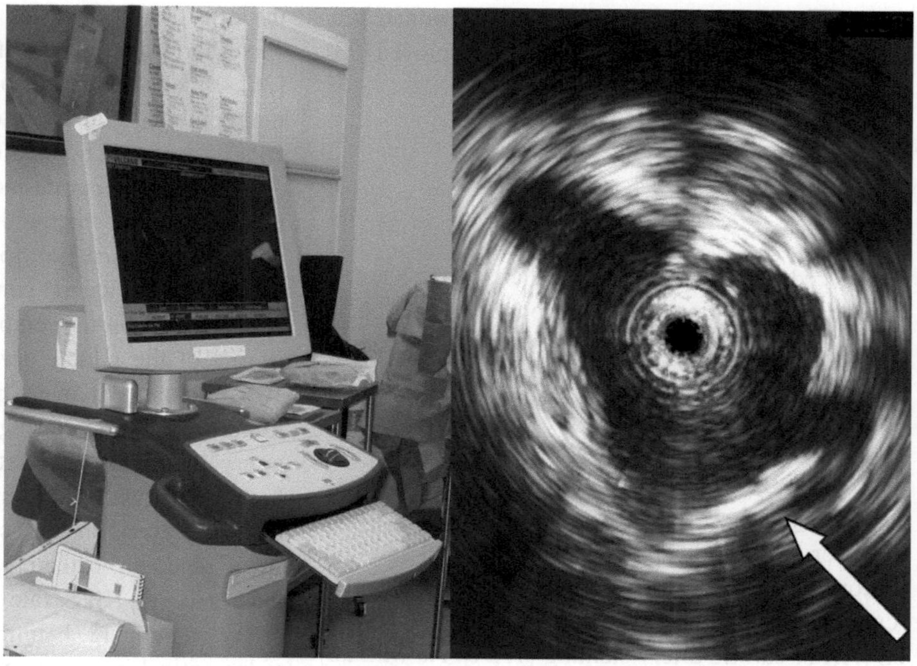

Fig. 6.1 Intravascular ultrasound revealing grade 4–5 aorta

as classified by Katz and colleagues [21]. The areas with grade 4 and 5 calcification should be carefully approached using wires and catheters to reduce the possibility of embolization [1]. The presence of an unchanged aortic lesion at the end of the peripheral endovascular procedure is a reasonable assurance that a major embolization has not happened from the screened source before the endovascular procedure [20].

Duplex Ultrasonography

In patients with chronic kidney disease where a physician wishes to limit nephrotoxic contrast material or in an attempt to limit radiation exposure to both the patient and the medical team, duplex ultrasonography has been utilized to guide endovascular procedures [22]. In this situation, the physician has to be comfortable using and interpreting real-time duplex images. An experienced registered vascular technologist (RVT) is also of utmost importance. The RVT needs a thorough understanding of the lower extremity arterial anatomy. Furthermore, this individual must have demonstrated accuracy with duplex imaging, which is confirmed by other diagnostic modalities.

The performance of duplex-guided procedures includes pre-procedure arterial mapping, and the individual performing the preprocedural mapping ideally will be the same individual assisting with the duplex-guided intervention. During the procedure, when performed on the lower extremities, a L7-4 MHz probe is usually most useful. Imaging is limited to the length of the ultrasound probe. Standard fluoroscopy provides a wider field of view, thus wires and catheters can be advanced faster; with duplex guidance, slower, more deliberate movements are required to achieve adequate visualization. Care also needs to be taken with regard to checking guidewire placement during advancement of stents and balloons. However, duplex imaging can provide multiple views of a vessel and hemodynamic information that is not readily apparent with angiography. Duplex allows the assessment of the hemodynamic impact of dissections and vessel recoil; it also allows accurate vessel sizing for balloons and stents. Occasionally, the duplex-guided procedure needs to be supplemented with a contrast study. Most duplex studies need to be performed with an ipsilateral puncture and antegrade approach, unless contrast is utilized to cross the aortic bifurcation. Joint prostheses can prevent adequate imaging via duplex ultrasonography, and thus require a contrast study. Furthermore, heavy calcifications can prevent adequate imaging. If more than 1 cm of the vessel cannot be insonated, an alternative imaging modality should be employed [23].

Advanced Neurologic Monitoring

Postprocedural neurological deficits are one of the most devastating complications after peripheral endovascular procedures. The goal of intraprocedural neurologic monitoring is early recognition of ischemic neurological insult, reduction of the intraprocedural risk, and to promptly initiate targeted therapy. There is no level 1 evidence to support neurophysiologic monitoring during peripheral endovascular procedures. However, there are many single-institutional and non-randomized studies (level III) supporting such interventions especially in high-risk patients undergoing TEVAR or carotid artery stenting [1, 24]. As with any other sophisticated monitoring device, the sole presence of these monitoring devices will be futile and possibly harmful. It will require the cognitive skills and accurate interpretation of the data and its integration with physiological parameters to translate into improved outcome. TEVAR or carotid stenting under local/regional anesthesia has the advantage that the patient can be directly observed for neurologic deterioration and asked to follow certain commands for neurological monitoring purposes. However, if general anesthesia is chosen or preferred, following monitoring tools have been helpful in early detection of stroke and paraplegia/paraperesis. The utility of IVUS and TEE as a helpful tool in monitoring and potentially reducing intraprocedural cerebral embolic events were discussed earlier.

Transcranial Doppler

Advancing wires and catheters in the aorta and its calcified branches are known to dislodge significant amounts of atherosclerotic emboli. The initial studies on cholesterol embolization following catheterization of the aortic arch come from the cardiology literature. In autopsy series, catheter-related embolization was reported in 30% of patients [25]. Recently, transcranial Doppler ultrasound (TCD) has been used to evaluate the effect of guidewires and catheters in the transverse aorta after diagnostic left heart catheterization [26]. Braekken and coworkers [26] reported cerebral microembolic signals detected by the TCD in up to 86% of the study population.

TCD is an accurate monitoring tool for the detection of cerebral microemboli in a patient population with an increased risk for strokes. It is non-invasive and has no associated complications. The TCD probe is positioned on the temporal bone window for monitoring of the middle cerebral artery. Approximately 10% of patients may not have adequate bone windows to allow TCD monitoring. The mean middle cerebral artery blood flow velocities, pulsatility indices, and high-intensity transient signals (HITS) are recorded and displayed on the screen. TCD is very helpful in selecting catheters, wires, and maneuvers that have a lower HITS rate during TEVAR and carotid artery stenting [27]. Intraprocedural monitoring provides critical information regarding the occurrence of cerebral microemboli and adequacy of cerebral blood flow [28].

Careful attention should be given to TCD data during portions of the operation likely to affect the cerebral circulation, either by changes in blood flow or the number of HITS. This will provide an insight into pathogenesis of postprocedural cerebral events [24]. The significance of cerebral microemboli detected as HITS is found in their association with cognitive impairment [29]. Since postoperative stroke seems to be a perpetual risk of TEVAR and carotid artery stenting, TCD monitoring is poised to become a more widespread tool in analyzing the cause of stroke in these procedures.

Cerebral Oximetry

Cerebral oximetry is based on near-infrared spectroscopy and provides important information about regional cerebral tissue oxygenation (rSO_2) as an absolute value and as a real-time trend. The probes are placed on either side of patient's forehead, where the near-infrared light from its light source penetrates the first 3–4 cm of skull and brain tissue, providing mixed arterial and venous regional brain oxygenation. Over a range of 45–85%, the accuracy of the trended rSO_2 is 2.9% and the accuracy of the absolute value is ±5%

[30]. There are also probes available to be placed on the peripheral organ in regions of interest. Similar to pulse oximetry, cerebral oximetry is void of any side-effects or complications. Given its non-invasiveness and proven usefulness in many cardiovascular conditions, it is thought to become a standard of care in neurophysiologic monitoring.

Although cerebral oximetry has been most extensively researched in open cardiovascular and aortic surgery [31, 32] the literature in peripheral endovascular procedures is growing [33–35]. It has been a non-invasive indicator of ischemia and embolic stroke during carotid artery lesion catheterization and cerebral hyperperfusion after carotid stenting [34, 35]. In patients with abdominal aortic or iliac aneurysm who will need bilateral iliac artery coverage or coiling, near-infrared oximetry has been helpful in monitoring pelvic ischemia [33].

Cerebrospinal Fluid Pressure Monitoring

Intraoperative hypotension, hypovolemia, and decreased spinal cord perfusion pressure precipitate ischemia of the spinal cord and are thought to be the etiology of immediate paraplegia that may present in patients undergoing (thoracic) aortic operations [36, 37] Cerebrospinal fluid (CSF) pressure monitoring and drainage have been shown to lower the incidence of spinal cord ischemia, by improving CSF perfusion pressure [38]. The evidence for CSF monitoring comes mostly from open surgical repair of thoracic aortic pathologies. However, many lessons learned from the pathophysiology of SCI in open repairs are useful in the treatment of patients undergoing TEVAR. The pathogenesis of SCI after endovascular repair differs from open surgery in that there is no sustained aortic occlusion and thus no interruption in blood flow to the distal aorta. Consequently, reperfusion injury may not be an issue [36]. The severity of SCI after TEVAR can range from monoparesis or paraperesis to paraplegia or quadriplegia. The presentation can be immediate, usually readily apparent postoperatively. Possible mechanisms for immediate SCI after TEVAR might include graft coverage of critical intercostal arteries and postoperative hypotension causing inadequate spinal cord perfusion pressure [1, 36].

Spinal cord protective measures during TEVAR include CSF drainage and prevention of hypotension, all aiming at improved CSF perfusion pressure [1]. They are recommended in high-risk patients with the following characteristics: female gender, abdominal aneurysm (repaired or not), covered (or planned coverage of) internal iliac arteries (including need for iliac artery conduit) and planned left subclavian coverage, and long-segment coverage of the lower portion of the descending thoracic aorta [1]. The CSF pressure is kept at 10 mm of water or lower, while the mean arterial blood pressure is kept high to maintain a spinal column perfusion pressure above 65–70 mmHg throughout the procedure (Fig. 6.2). These measures have shown to reverse the changes in evoked potentials during stent deployment and decrease the postprocedural spinal cord injury rate after TEVAR [39, 40]; 10 mL of CSF

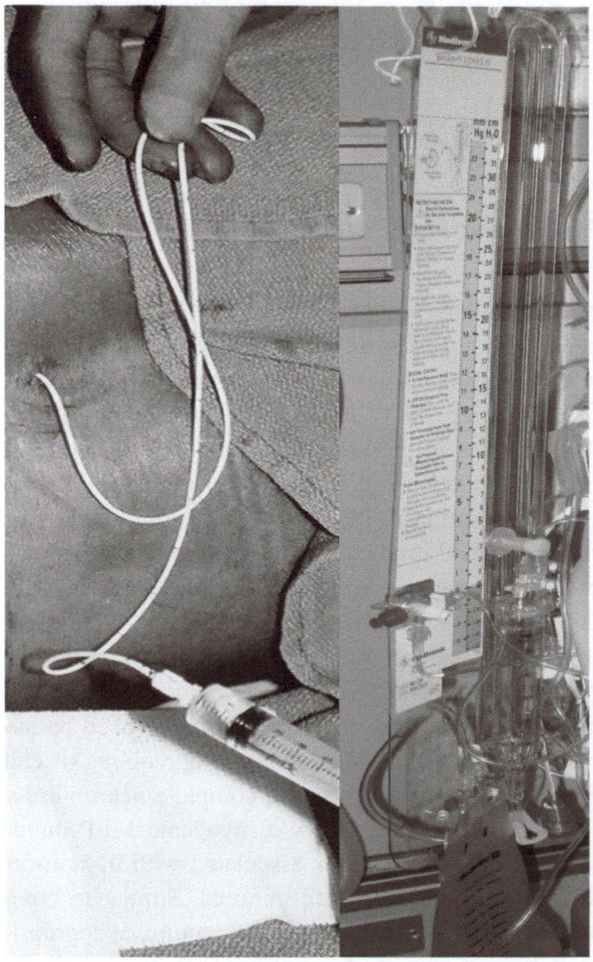

Fig. 6.2 CSF drain setup in ICU

is drained if the CSF pressure exceeds 10 mL of H_2O and this maneuver may be repeated up to 5 times/h. The goal is to reduce CSF pressure, improve perfusion pressure, and reduce the chance of brain stem herniation by removing a large quantity of CSF. The CSF drains are usually kept for 24–48 h, but may stay longer if the patient is hemodynamically unstable. These strategies contribute significantly to the full recovery observed in some patients presenting with delayed presentation of neurological deficits [36]. Some cases of spinal cord injury respond to augmentation of blood pressure alone [41, 42]. Complications associated with CSF catheters are low in experienced hands. The most feared complications are brain stem herniation, meningitis, and spinal column or cerebral hematoma. The two former can be significantly reduced by following the aforementioned recommendations and limiting the amount of CSF drainage in a certain time intervals, while the latter can be reduced by avoiding antiplatelet or antithrombotic treatment at the time of insertion and removal of the CSF catheter. Svensson and colleagues had no catheter-related complication in a series of 99 patients [43].

Motor-Evoked Potential Monitoring

Myogenic motor-evoked potential (MEP) is a sensitive tool to estimate cord motor neuron function, and thereby the anterior spinal artery perfusion adequacy during TEVAR. Electric stimulation of the motor cortex in the brain produces MEP at the level of a peripheral nerve (neurogenic) or muscle (myogenic). Variation in the latency and amplitude of the recorded MEP implies ischemia in the anterior spinal column. Myogenic MEP has been FDA approved in 2003 for intraoperative neurophysiologic monitoring of patients undergoing descending thoracic and thoracoabdominal aortic surgery. It is more sensitive and predictive compared to somatosensory-evoked potentials [44]. Myogenic MEP monitoring requires special anesthetic techniques because complete neuromuscular blockade will not allow a myogenic MEP monitoring. The complications associated with intraprocedural MEP monitoring are minimal. Similar to other advanced monitoring tools, it will require an appropriately trained operator to identify MEP changes during TEVAR.

References

1. Khoynezhad A, Donayre CE, Bui H, Kopchok GE, Walot I, White RA: Risk factors of neurologic deficit after thoracic aortic endografting, *Ann Thorac Surg* 83(2):S882–S889, 2007, discussion S890-2.
2. Buhne W, Rossaint R: Perioperative management and monitoring in anaesthesia, *Lancet* 362:1839–1846, 2003.
3. Gardner RM: Direct arterial pressure monitoring, *Curr Anaesth Crit Care* 1:239–246, 1990.
4. Mayer J, Boldt J, Wolf MW, Lang J, Suttner S: Cardiac output derived from arterial pressure waveform analysis in patients undergoing cardiac surgery: validity of a second generation device, *Anesth Analg* 106(3):867–872, 2008.
5. Pinsky MR: Hemodynamic monitoring in the intensive care unit, *Clin Chest Med* 24:549–560, 2003.
6. Schmitt EA, Brantigen CO: Common artifacts of pulmonary artery and pulmonary artery wedge pressures: recognition and management, *J Clin Monit* 2:44–52, 1986.
7. Nemens EJ, Woods SL: Normal fluctuations in pulmonary artery and pulmonary capillary wedge pressures in acutely ill patients, *Heart Lung* 11:393–398, 1982.
8. Leibowitz AB: More reliable determination of central venous and pulmonary artery occlusion pressures: does it matter? *Crit Care Med* 33:243–244, 2005.
9. Yu DT, Platt R, Lamken PN et al.: Relationship of pulmonary artery catheter use to mortality and resource utilization in patients with severe sepsis, *Crit Care Med* 31:2734–2741, 2003.
10. Connors AF, Speroff T, Dawson NV et al.: The effectiveness of right heart catheterization in the initial care of critically ill patients, *JAMA* 276:889–897, 1996.
11. Dueck MH, Kilmek M, Appenrodt S et al.: Trends but not individual values of central venous oxygen saturation agree with mixed venous oxygen saturation during varying hemodynamic conditions, *Anesthesiology* 103:249–257, 2005.
12. Boldt J, Menges T, Wollbruck M et al.: Is continuous cardiac output measurement using thermodilution reliable in the critically ill patient? *Crit Care Med* 22:1913–1918, 1994.
13. Shiga T, Wajima Z, Apfel CC et al.: Diagnostic accuracy of transesophageal echocardiography, helical computed tomography, and magnetic resonance imaging for suspected thoracic aortic dissection: systematic review and meta-analysis, *Arch Intern Med* 166(13):1350–1356, 2006.
14. Murray KK, Hawkins IF: Angiography of the lower extremities in atherosclerotic vascular disease. Current techniques, *Surg Clin North Am* 72(4):767–789, 1992.
15. Kinney TB, Rose SC: Intraarterial pressure measurements during angiographic evaluation of peripheral arterial disease: techniques, interpretation, applications, limitations, *AJR Am J Roentgenol* 166(2):237–284, 1996.
16. Green NE, Chen SY, Messenger JC, Groves BM, Carroll JD: Three-dimensional vascular angiography, *Curr Prob Cardiol* 29(3):104–142, 2004.
17. Lee JT, White RA: Basics of intravascular ultrasound: an essential tool for the endovascular surgeon, *Semin Vasc Surg* 17(2):110–118, 2004.

18. Lee JT, Fang TD, White RA: Applications of intravascular ultrasound in the treatment of peripheral vascular disease, *Semin Vasc Surg* 19(3):139–144, 2006.
19. Khoynezhad A, Donayre CE, Kopchok G, Walot I, Omari BO, White RA: Mid-term results of endovascular treatment of complicated acute type B aortic dissection. Accepted for publication, *J Thor Cardiovasc Surg* 138:625–31, 2009.
20. Song TK, Donyare CE, Kopchok GE, White RA: Intravascular ultrasound use in the treatment of thoracoabdominal dissections, aneurysms, transections, *Semin Vasc Surg* 19(3):145–149, 2006.
21. Katz ES, Tunick PA, Rusinek H et al.: Protruding aortic atheromas predict stroke in elderly patients undergoing cardiopulmonary bypass: experience with intraoperative transesophageal echocardiography, *J Am Coll Cardiol* 20(1):70–77, 1992.
22. Ahmadi R, Ugurluogli A, Schillinger M, Katzenschlager R, Sabeti S, Minar E: Duplex ultrasound guided femoropopliteal angioplasty: initial and 12-month results from a case controlled study, *J Endovasc Ther* 9(6):873–881, 2002.
23. Ascher E, Marks NA, Hingorami AP, Schuteer RW, Mutyala M: Duplex-guided endovascular treatment for occlusive and stenotic lesion of the femoral-popliteal arterial segment: a comparative study in the first 253 cases, *J Vasc Surg* 44(6):1230–12327, 2006.
24. Ackerstaff RG, Suttorp MJ, van den Berg JC et al.: Prediction of early cerebral outcome by transcranial Doppler monitoring in carotid bifurcation angioplasty and stenting, *J Vasc Surg.* 41(4):618–624, 2005.
25. Ramirez G, O'Neill WM Jr, Lambert R, Bloomer HA: Cholesterol embolization: a complication of angiography, *Arch Intern Med* 138(9):1430–1432, 1978.
26. Braekken SK, Endresen K, Russell D, Brucher R, Kjekshus J: Influence of guidewire and catheter type on the frequency of cerebral microembolic signals during left heart catheterization, *Am J Cardiol* 82(5):632–637, 1998.
27 Rubartelli P, Brusa G, Arrigo A et al.: Transcranial Doppler monitoring during stenting of the carotid bifurcation: evaluation of two different distal protection devices in preventing embolization, *J Endovasc Ther* 13(4):436–442, 2006.
28. Khoynezhad A, Kruse MJ, Donayre CE, White RA: Use of transcranial doppler ultrasound in endovascular repair of a type B aortic dissection, *Ann Thorac Surg* 86(1):289–291, 2008.
29. Russel D: Cerebral microemboli and cognitive impairment, *J Neurol Sci* 203–204:211–214, 2002.
30. Kim MB, Ward DS, Cartwright CR, Kolano J, Chlebowski S, Henson LC: Estimation of jugular venous O_2 saturation from cerebral oximetry or arterial O_2 saturation during isocapnic hypoxia, *J Clin Monit Comput* 16(3):191–199, 2000.
31. Murkin JM, Adams SJ, Novick RJ, Quantz M, Bainbridge D, Iglesias I, Cleland A, Schaefer B, Irwin B, Fox S: Monitoring brain oxygen saturation during coronary bypass surgery: a randomized, prospective study, *Anesth Analg* 104(1):51–58, 2007.
32. Kouchoukos NT, Mauney MC, Masetti P, Castner CF: Single-stage repair of extensive thoracic aortic aneurysms: experience with the arch-first technique and bilateral anterior thoracotomy, *J Thorac Cardiovasc Surg* 128(5):669–676, 2004.
33. Unno N, Inuzuka K, Yamamoto N, Sagara D, Suzuki M, Konno H: Preservation of pelvic circulation with hypogastric artery bypass in endovascular repair of abdominal aortic aneurysm with bilateral iliac artery aneurysms, *J Vasc Surg* 44(6):1170–1175, 2006.
34. Horie N, Kitagawa N, Morikawa M, Kaminogo M, Nagata I: Monitoring of regional cerebral oxygenation by near-infrared spectroscopy in carotid arterial stenting: preliminary study, *Neuroradiology* 47(5):375–379, 2005.
35. McCleary AJ, Nelson M, Dearden NM, Calvey TA, Gough MJ: Cerebral haemodynamics and embolization during carotid angioplasty in high-risk patients, *Br J Surg* 85(6):771–774, 1998.
36. Carroccio A, Marin ML, Ellozy S, Hollier LH: Pathophysiology of paraplegia following endovascular thoracic aortic aneurysm repair, *J Card Surg* 18(4):359–366, 2003.
37. Khoynezhad A, Bello R, Smego DR, Nwakanma L, Plestis KA: Improved outcome after repair of descending and thoracoabdominal aortic aneurysms using modern adjuncts, *Interact CardioVasc Thorac Surg* 4:574–576, 2005.
38. Safi HJ, Campbell MP, Miller CC 3rd, Iliopoulos DC, Khoynezhad A, Letsou GV et al.: Cerebral spinal fluid drainage and distal aortic perfusion decrease the incidence of neurological deficit: the results of 343 descending and thoracoabdominal aortic aneurysm repairs, *Eur J Vasc Endovasc Surg* 14(2):118–124, 1997.
39. Mitchell RS, Miller DC, Dake MD, Semba CP, Moore KA, Sakai T: Thoracic aortic aneurysm repair with an endovascular stent graft: the "first generation", *Ann Thorac Surg* 67(6):1971–1974, 1999.
40. Weigang E, Hartert M, Siegenthaler MP, Beckmann NA, Sircar R, Szabo G et al.: Perioperative management to improve neurologic outcome in thoracic or thoracoabdominal aortic stent-grafting, *Ann Thorac Surg* 82(5):1679–1687, 2006.
41. Cheung AT, Pochettino A, McGarvey ML, Appoo JJ, Fairman RM, Carpenter JP et al.: Strategies to manage paraplegia risk after endovascular stent repair of descending thoracic aortic aneurysms, *Ann Thorac Surg* 80(4):1280–1288, 2005.
42. McGarvey ML, Mullen MT, Woo EY, Bavaria JE, Augoustides YG, Messe SR et al.: The treatment of spinal cord ischemia following thoracic endovascular aortic repair, *Neurocrit Care* 6(1):35–39, 2007.
43. Svensson LG, Crawford ES: Aortic dissection and aortic aneurysm surgery: clinical observations, experimental investigations, and statistical analyses. Part II, *Curr Probl Surg* 29(12):913–1057, 1992.
44. Dong CC, MacDonald DB, Janusz MT: Intraoperative spinal cord monitoring during descending thoracic and thoracoabdominal aneurysm surgery, *Ann Thorac Surg* 74(5):S1873–S1876, 2002.

Safety Considerations for Endovascular Surgery

7

George E. Kopchok

The continuing evolution of endovascular techniques and instrumentation has enhanced the armamentarium available to vascular surgeons. The majority of endovascular procedures are minimally invasive with reduced risk and morbidity for the patient. However, imaging techniques, endovascular instrumentation, and delivery devices may introduce environmental safety concerns that were not present in conventional surgery. In this regard, it is essential that operating room personnel become knowledgeable about potential hazards and appropriate precautions that are necessary to create a safe work environment for themselves, as well as the patient.

As with most surgical procedures, adequate visualization allows for precise evaluation, treatment, and postprocedural assessment. For endovascular surgery, the majority of visualization and imaging is achieved through fluoroscopic radiation. Fluoroscopic imaging in the endovascular suite may introduce new or prolonged radiation exposure risks not normally associated with vascular surgery. Other hazards associated with the endovascular suite may include laser exposure and increased blood contact resulting from patient catheterization. This chapter reviews the considerations relevant to reduce risks and produce a safe utilization of endovascular suites.

G.E. Kopchok (✉)
Director, Vascular Surgery Research Laboratory, Department of Vascular Surgery, Los Angeles Biomedical Research Institute, Harbor-UCLA Medical Center, Torrance, CA, USA

History

The X-ray was first discovered, accidentally, by Wilhelm Roentgen [1]. Roentgen was investigating the conduction of cathode rays (electrons) through a large, partially evacuated glass tube known as Crookes' tube (Fig. 7.1a). On November 8, 1895, Roentgen was working in his laboratory in Wurzburg University and was completely enclosing his Crookes' tube with black photographic paper to visualize the effects of the cathode rays. A plate of fluorescent material (barium platinocyanide) was laying on a bench several feet away from the Crookes' tube. When the enclosed tube was excited, Roentgen noticed that the barium platinocyanide began to fluoresce. The intensity of the fluorescence increased as the barium platinocyanide was brought closer to Crookes' tube, leaving little doubt as to the origin of the stimulus. Based on this initial observation, Roentgen began a feverish investigation of this "X-light" by interposing different materials, including his hand, between the Crookes' tube and the fluorescing plate. He reported his findings to the scientific community near the end of 1895. Roentgen quickly recognized the value of his discovery to medicine and produced the first medical X-ray film, one of his wife's hand. For his work he received the first Nobel Prize given in physics in 1901.

A few months after Roentgen's original paper announcing the discovery of X-rays, the first X-ray-induced fatality in the United States was reported in 1904 by Thomas A. Edison. Edison, who invented the fluoroscope in 1898, was experimenting with new fluorescent materials, including two materials that are still used today. However, he discontinued his X-ray research when his assistant and friend, Clarence Dally, received severe X-ray burns of both arms that

T.J. Fogarty, R.A. White (eds.), *Peripheral Endovascular Interventions*,
DOI 10.1007/978-1-4419-1387-6_7, © Springer Science+Business Media, LLC 1998, 2010

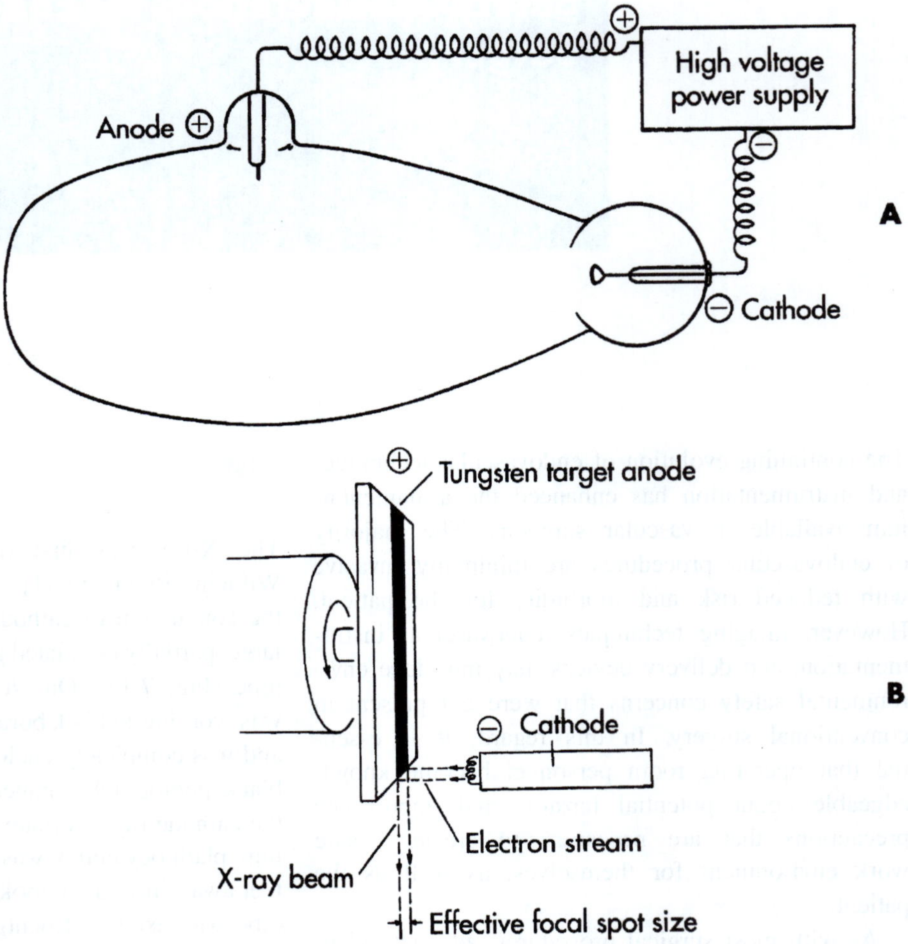

Fig. 7.1 **a**, Original Crookes' tube used by Wilhelm Roentgen to study conduction of cathode rays (electrons). These experiments led to the accidental discovery of X-rays. **b**, Modern rotating disk used to produce X-rays. The production of X-rays from electrons is very inefficient; most of the energy loss is in the form of heat. By rotating the anode, heat is kept to a minimum

eventually required amputation. Dally died in 1904 and is considered the first X-ray fatality in the United States. By 1910, X-ray exposure and safety parameters were developed. Shortly thereafter, new imaging techniques and protective wear reduced exposure, thus leading to a new emphasis for radiation control and safety.

Fluoroscopic Image Production

Fluoroscopic imaging is defined as a radiologic examination using fluorescence for observation of a transient image. The two major components of image-intensified fluoroscopy are the X-ray tube and image intensifier (Fig. 7.2). The X-ray tube (much like the original Crookes' tube) contains two major parts, the cathode, which serves as the source of the electrons, and the anode, which acts as the target for the electrons. As the stream of high-velocity electrons hit the target (i.e., anode), most of their energy is transformed into heat, but a small part is transformed into X-rays, which can be directed onto a patient and image intensifier (Fig. 7.1b). When the X-rays are directed toward the patient, most are absorbed by the dense structures, such as bone, whereas some pass through and strike the image intensifier's phosphor. This layer of fluorescent material absorbs the X-rays and converts the energy into different levels of light photons that are directly proportional to the intensity of incident energy. The light photons then impact a photocathode, causing electrons to be given off in direct proportion to the intensity of the fluorescent light. The electrons are then accelerated and focused onto a smaller electrostatic layer called an output phosphor. The output phosphor is hundreds of times brighter than the input phosphor because of its smaller size and the additional energy given to the electrons through acceleration. The output phosphor is then viewed, usually with a

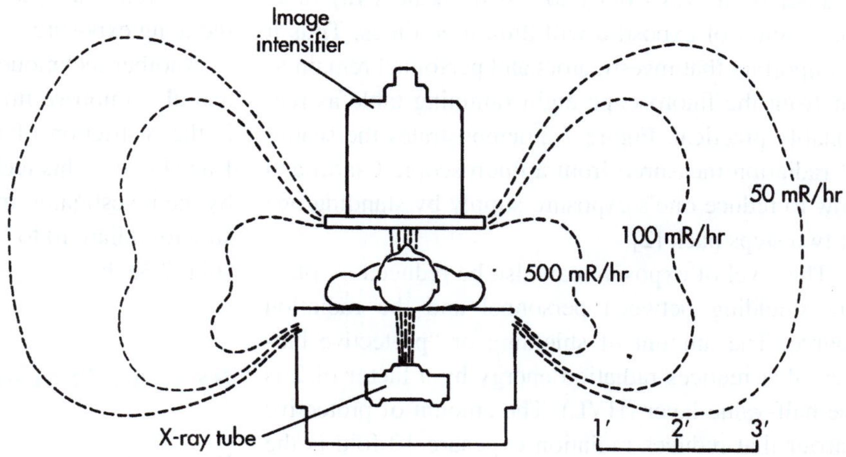

Fig. 7.2 Fluoroscopic intensifier demonstrating the position of the X-ray tube and image intensifier. Also illustrated are the approximate X-ray exposures at 1, 2, and 3 ft. It is important to realize that X-ray exposure decreases with the square of the distance from the source

television camera, and displayed on a high-resolution black and white monitor.

Radiation Safety

The unit of radiation exposure from X-rays is the roentgen (R). A roentgen is defined as the amount of radiation that will produce 2.1×10^9 ion pairs in 1 cm^3 of air. For diagnostic imaging such as fluoroscopy, exposure rate is measured in roentgens per minute (R/min). The absorbed radiation dose is referred to as a rad, which refers to the absorption of 100 erg (10^{-5} J) of energy per gram of mass. A more useful unit used to measure the biologic effects in humans is rem (rad equivalent in man). Rems are commonly used to record and monitor human exposure to radiation. Total annual background radiation for individuals without occupational exposure to X-rays is about 125 millirems (mrem).

The knowledge that any exposure to radiation is injurious to human tissue has led to the development of maximum permissible dose (MPD) guidelines. The MPD is defined as the maximum dose of radiation that, in light of present knowledge, would not be expected to produce significant radiation effects. The guidelines have steadily dropped in the last 60 years. In 1931 the MPD was 50 rems/year. In 1936 and 1948 the MPD was dropped to 30 and then 15 rems/year. In 1958 the MPD was again dropped to the current standard of 5 rems/year for any person over the age of 18. The whole body exposure of 5 rems/year applies to the head, neck, trunk, lens of the eye, blood-forming organs, and gonads. A higher MPD is allowed for less sensitive parts of the body such as the hands (75 rems), skin (15 rems), and forearms (30 rems).

The three major principles of radiation protection are *time, distance,* and *shielding*. The radiation dose to an individual is directly proportional to the duration of exposure (i.e., exposure = exposure rate × time). During fluoroscopic procedures it is important that the investigator only activates the foot pedal when the X-ray image is needed. The investigator should always try to pulse the fluoroscopic foot switch to limit overall exposure. For example, many short pulses of exposure can be used to watch a balloon angioplasty while the balloon is stationary and inflated. Many fluoroscopic systems have an optional pulse mode, which can pulse the fluoroscopy at 3–30 pulse/s. This can be used during non-critical maneuvers to reduce the amount of exposure. Systems that do not have the pulse feature often have a "low-dose" option that can also reduce the amount of exposure during non-critical maneuvers. Exposure should also be used only when the investigator is actually viewing the video monitor. Most systems have an image-hold program which maintains the last image for the investigator's review. There is no need to leave the fluoroscope activated to view a static image. Fluoroscopic equipment is required to have an audible 5-min timer to remind the physician that a considerable amount of imaging time has elapsed.

The distance between the radiation source and personnel should also be kept at the maximum. As with many energy sources, radiation exposure decreases with the square of the distance (inverse square law).

If a person moves from 1 to 3 ft from an X-ray tube, the amount of exposure will drop nine times. Thus it is important that investigators and personnel remain as far from the fluoroscope and examining table as reasonably practical. Figure 7.2 demonstrates the scatter of radiation measured from a fluoroscopic C-arm and how to reduce one's exposure simply by standing one or two steps back [2].

The level of exposure can also be reduced by placing shielding between personnel and the radiation source. The amount of shielding or "protective barrier" that reduces radiation energy by a factor of 2 is the half-value layer (HVL). The amount of protective barrier that reduces radiation exposure 10-fold is the tenth value layer (TVL). These values are used to rate the protective apparel used during radiographic imaging. Current protective aprons consist of a lead and tin mixture that optimizes energy absorption and comfort. Protective aprons come in two thicknesses, 0.25- and 0.50-mm lead equivalent [3]. Absorption of X-rays is nonlinear with respect to the thickness of shielding. Overall, the 0.5-mm equivalent apron provides approximately 90% reduction in radiation exposures. The 0.25-mm apron provides only a 75% reduction and is therefore usually limited to pediatric procedures or used as a back for wraparound aprons. The exact amount of protection offered by lead aprons will vary with the kilovolts peak (kVp) used for patient imaging. The higher the kVp, the lower the protection. Protective aprons should be examined radiographically every 3 months and repaired or discarded if leakage is confirmed. Aside from lead aprons, it is also suggested that personnel wear thyroid shields and lead glasses to minimize exposure to these sensitive areas. Other protective screens such as ceiling-mounted transparent lead glass screens can be very effective at reducing exposure.

Another technique that can reduce radiation scatter and also improve image quality is collimation, which is the restriction of the radiation beam by moveable lead shields. This technique, which is often underused by the investigator, minimizes the field of view (exposure to radiation) to only the area of visual importance (Fig. 7.3a, b).

Personnel Monitoring

Personnel who are routinely involved with fluoroscopic procedures or other forms of radiation exposure should be monitored to determine the total amount of exposure. The most common monitoring device is the film badge. The film badge contains a film that is sensitive to ionizing radiation. Film badges must be worn on the front, outside of the protective apron, at the level of the shoulders or neck. The badges should be exchanged and processed every month. State and federal regulations require that personnel be given monthly reports summarizing their monthly, quarterly, cumulative annual, and cumulative lifetime exposure. As mentioned above, adults should receive far less than the recommended MPD of 5 rems/year.

Pregnancy

Pregnancy can greatly alter the tolerable level for safe exposure to radiation. This is of obvious importance for personnel, as well as potential patients. When

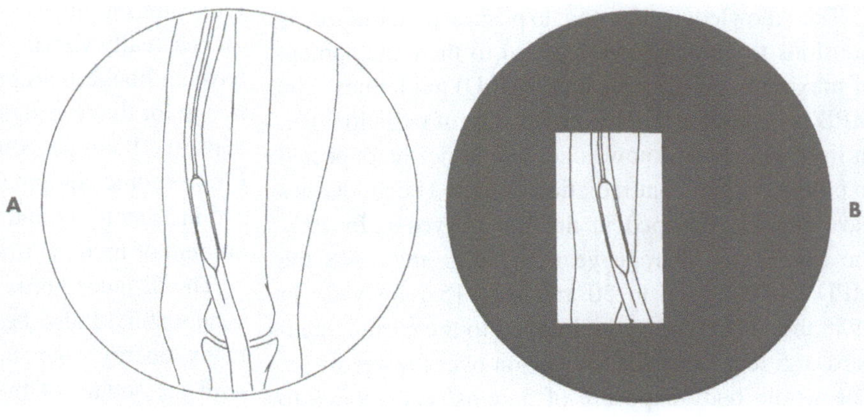

Fig. 7.3 **a**, Typical fluoroscopic image in which collimation is not being used. **b**, Same fluoroscopic image as seen in (**a**), except collimation has been used to reduce the amount of scattered radiation and improve image quality

personnel become pregnant, it is important that they discuss their options with a supervisor. The MPD for a fetus is 500 mrem for the period of pregnancy. Most personnel in a fluoroscopic imaging room receive less than 500 mrem/year. Therefore, by simply reviewing the individual's records, it may be decided that she could safely continue working in an exposed area. Exposure at the waist, under a protective apron, will not normally exceed 10% of the whole body value measured outside of the apron. Pregnant personnel who decide to continue their work should wear a second monitoring badge under the protective apron at the level of the waist to further measure the fetal exposure. If possible, personnel should be offered a temporary position in a nonexposed area.

Inadvertent irradiation of a pregnant patient should be avoided if at all possible. The fetus is at greatest risk to radiation during the first month of pregnancy and oftentimes, the patient may be unaware of pregnancy at this time. Under normal conditions, radiographic procedures should not be performed on any pregnant patient unless the health of the mother or fetus would be directly compromised. The International Commission on Radiological Protection (ICRP) suggests that women of childbearing years only be exposed to lower abdominal or pelvic area radiographic examination during the 10-day interval after the onset of menstruation.

Laser Physics

LASER is an acronym for "light amplification by stimulated emission of radiation." The theoretic principles of the lasing process were first described by Albert Einstein in 1917 [4]. In the paper entitled "Quantum Theory of Radiation," he described the process of stimulated emission. This theory combined with other work was the basis for awarding Einstein the Nobel Prize in physics in 1921.

Before one can understand the concept of stimulated emission, an understanding of spontaneous emission is required. Under normal conditions, atoms interact with photons and absorb their energy by elevating an electron from a lower energy orbit to a higher energy orbit. This process will only occur when an atom interacts with a photon that has enough energy to elevate an electron one outer orbit. An atom with an electron in the elevated energy state, "excited atom," quickly releases the energy in the form of a photon as the electron returns to its normal orbit. The wavelength and energy of the emitted photon correspond to the differences between the higher and lower energy orbits. This process, because it occurs naturally in all matter, is called spontaneous emission (Fig. 7.4).

Lasers work by a process known as stimulated emission. The process begins when atoms (or molecules) are excited from an external source. When one excited atom returns to its normal state, it emits a photon (Fig. 7.5), which interacts with a second excited atom. The photon is not absorbed by the second excited atom. It causes the atom to drop back to its normal state and emits two photons with identical characteristics (the incident photon and its original). The two photons proceed to stimulate two more excited atoms, which emit 4, then 8, 16, 32, and so on, identical photons. The photons are identical in wavelength, phase, and amplitude. This process is called stimulated emission and is the basis for laser energy.

Laser light has three unique characteristics: the light is monochromatic, directional, and coherent.

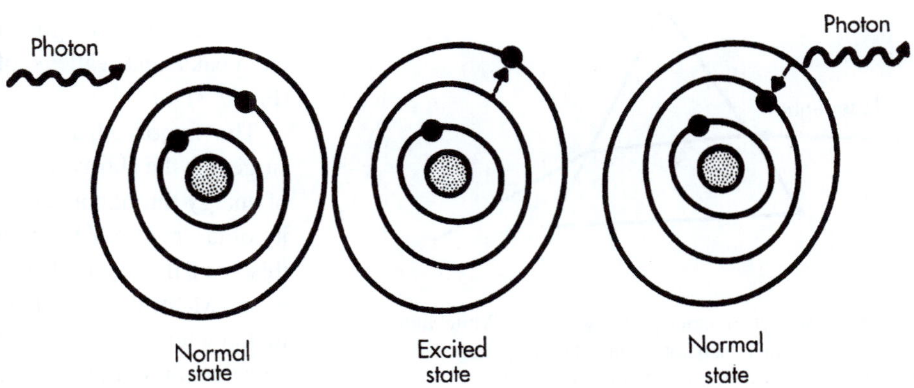

Fig. 7.4 Spontaneous emission. An atom absorbs the energy of a photon by elevating an electron to a higher orbit and then spontaneously releases the energy as a second photon

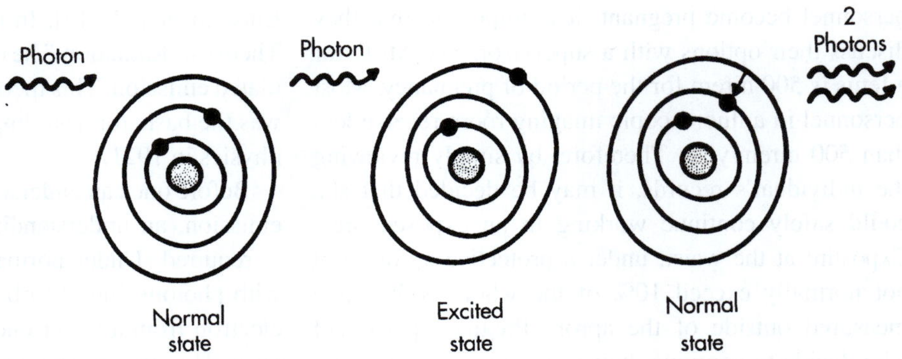

Fig. 7.5 Stimulated emission. When an atom in the excited state is struck by a photon, it will be stimulated to return to its normal state and in the process emit two identical photons

Monochromaticity means that the laser light consists of a particular wavelength or a very narrow range of wavelengths. If the wavelength of laser energy is in the visible range, between 350 and 1,400 nm, it will have a color corresponding to its particular wavelength. Normal white light from a source such as a lamp contains the entire spectrum of wavelengths of visible light. When the light is passed through a prism, the individual wavelengths are separated to produce the characteristic colors in the pattern of a rainbow. When laser energy is passed through a prism, because of the select wavelength distribution, only one wavelength or color is visible (Fig. 7.6). Lasers that operate above the visible wavelengths (>1,400 nm) are known as infrared lasers. Lasers that operate below the visible spectrum (<350 nm) are called ultraviolet lasers.

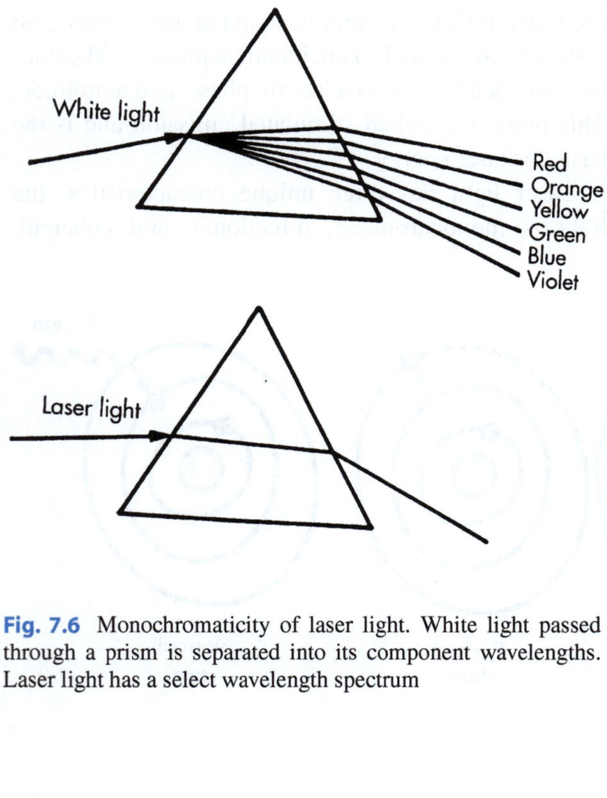

Fig. 7.6 Monochromaticity of laser light. White light passed through a prism is separated into its component wavelengths. Laser light has a select wavelength spectrum

Laser light is also described as directional. Directionality or collimation means that the laser energy is released in a highly concentrated, parallel beam with minimal amounts of light spread. As an example, light emitted from a light bulb is not directional and spreads so that it lights up the whole room. In contrast, laser light emitted in a dark room only illuminates a very small spot. Spread of laser energy is so minimal that a point source aimed at the Moon will only spread to a circle approximately one-half mile in diameter on the Moon's surface [5].

The third unique property of laser energy is that it is coherent. According to the wave theory of electromagnetic radiation, the waveform of laser energy can be characterized according to the wavelength, amplitude, and frequency. Amplitude is the vertical height of the wave, wavelength (λ) is the distance between two successive wave peaks, and frequency (f) is the speed of light (c) divided by the wavelength ($f = c/\lambda$). The light waves emitted from a normal lamp are incoherent in that the waveforms have different amplitudes and different wavelengths. The wavelengths are not aligned spatially as to peaks and valleys of the waveform. Laser energy is coherent in that all of the waveform amplitudes, wavelengths, and temporal distribution of the peaks and valleys of the curves are the same (Fig. 7.7).

The major advantage of lasers for endovascular surgery is the ability to precisely deliver a large amount of energy through a very small conduit. For the majority of lasers (Nd:YAG, holmium:YAG, excimer, argon) this is easily accomplished by using fiberoptic waveguides. Most fibers are made from quartz and will vary in diameter, flexibility, and shape according to the laser wavelength and clinical application. The efficiency of

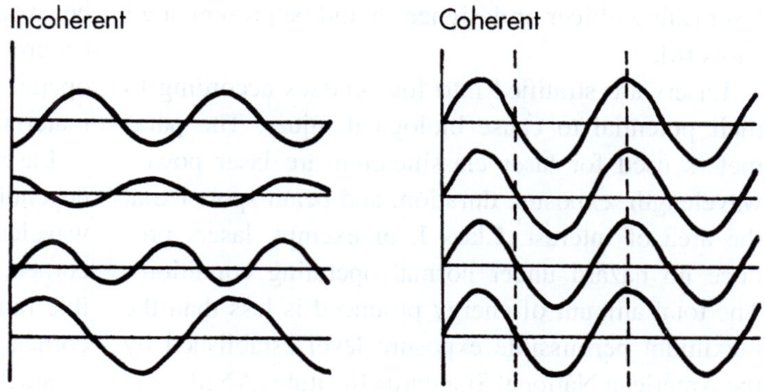

Fig. 7.7 Incoherent waveforms of normal light vs. coherent waveforms of laser light

energy transmission through a fiber varies with wavelength of the light, the diameter, and the quality of the fiber. On transmission through the fiber, the collimated laser light bounces from side to side as it travels through the fiber. This change of direction causes the laser light to diverge 10–15° as it exits the fiber tip (Fig. 7.8). The divergence property can be used to vary the power density (watts/area) and resultant tissue effects (cutting or coagulating) by changing the distance between the fiber tip and the tissue.

When laser energy interacts with the tissue, it may be absorbed, transmitted, scattered, or reflected. Laser–tissue interactions depend on how the laser energy is dissipated and the absorption coefficients of the tissue for the particular wavelength. When tissue absorption occurs, the laser energy produces variable effects depending on the type of interaction. These include laser photochemical effects (chemical bond disruption), laser fluorescence (reemission of photons), or photothermal changes (heat-producing vibration and collision of atoms).

Laser Safety

Establishment of a laser protocol, facility specifications, procedure approvals, in-service training sessions, and continuing education for personnel is essential to maintain a safe environment. Personnel must be trained in operating procedures and precautions to prevent personal injury and property damage. Only laser-certified personnel should be permitted to set up, to use, and to discontinue use of laser equipment. Although laser radiation can cause eye damage, skin burns, and combustion of flammable materials, these hazards can easily be avoided by a carefully planned program.

The physician and all key operating room personnel should be fully versed with an understanding of laser physics, appropriate nomenclature regarding laser energy, and laser–tissue interactions [6, 7]. The physician user is ultimately responsible for selecting the wattage, choosing an appropriate lens or fiber, and ensuring safe laser use for each procedure; however, a

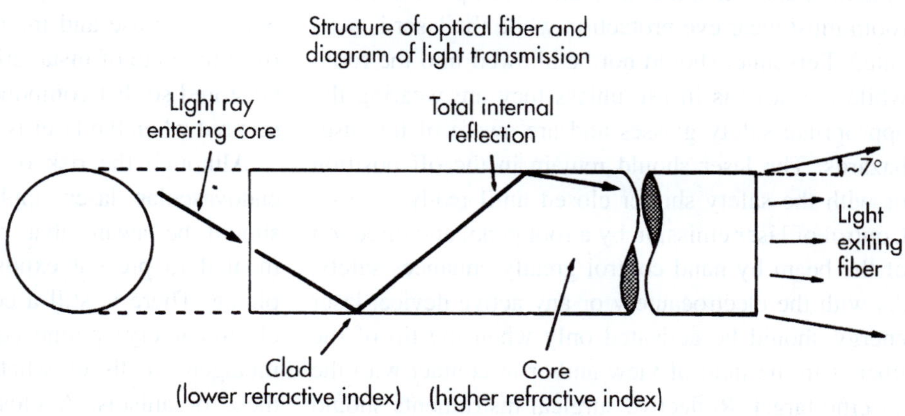

Fig. 7.8 Transmission through the optic fiber causes the laser light to bounce from side to side, thus losing its coherent property. This also causes the light to diverge at an angle of 10–15° from the tip of the fiber

laser safety officer or designee should be present at all cases [8].

Lasers are stratified into four classes according to their potential to cause biological injury. The parameters used for laser classification are laser power, wavelength, exposure duration, and beam spot size at the area of interest. Class I, or exempt, lasers produce no hazard under normal operating conditions. The total amount of energy produced is less than the maximum permissible exposure level established by the American National Standards Institute (ANSI), and therefore no special facility or safety precautions are needed. Class II lasers are low-power lasers that do not present a visual hazard resulting from a normal aversion response. The eye normally closes approximately 0.25 s when exposed to a noxious stimulus. This response avoids eye damage from a class II laser. Class III lasers operate with maximum power output (<2.5 mW/cm^2). These lasers present a hazard if viewed through collecting optics but present no hazard if viewed momentarily with the unaided eye. Class III lasers can damage the eyes if viewed directly but present no hazard to the skin. Class IV denotes high-power laser systems that are hazardous to the eyes, skin, and flammable material from a direct or diffusely reflected beam. Facility requirements vary with the class of laser being used. Generally, class IV lasers are used in surgical applications, and therefore operating facilities must be set up in accordance with requirements for this classification [7, 9].

Class IV laser procedure and operating rooms must have all windows covered with nontransparent barriers to prevent the inadvertent passage of laser light. All doors must be closed, and access to the room should be restricted while the laser is activated. Visible warning signs, which have flashing lights to signify that the system is activated, are mandatory. All persons in the room must wear eye protection while the laser is activated. Personnel should not be allowed into the room while the laser is in use unless they are wearing the appropriate safety glasses and are aware of the laser hazards. The laser should remain in the off position or with the safety shutter closed until ready for use. Control of laser emission by a foot pedal and direction of the beam by hand control greatly enhances safety. As with the electrocautery or any active device, laser energy should be activated only when the tip of the fiber is in the field of view and/or in contact with the specific target. Reflective surgical instruments should be avoided and reflective surfaces in the laser procedure room minimized. Moist sponges in the open operating fields can prevent combustion of dry or paper materials.

Laser energy can affect different parts of the eye depending on which structure absorbs the particular wavelength. The three areas of most concern are the cornea, lens, and retina. Laser energy outside the visible range (<350 and >1,400 nm) is absorbed by the cornea and lens. Exposure to this energy can produce cataracts and corneal scarring. Laser energy in the visible wavelength is focused by the cornea and lens onto the retina and causes up to 100,000× amplification of radiant exposure [9]. Careless misdirection of the laser light even at low powers can result in instantaneous burning of the retina and consequent blindness in the visual field corresponding to the burn spot. As mentioned in the preceding paragraph, everyone in the operating room, including the patient, must have appropriate eye wear during the procedures. For the CO_2 laser, clear plastic or glass lenses with side guards are adequate, while wet gauze can be used to protect an anesthetized patient's eyes. Green lenses (nontransparent to 1,060 nm) are required for the Nd:YAG laser and amber lenses (nontransparent to 488–515 nm) are necessary to absorb the green or blue light of the argon laser. Other lasers with different wavelengths require specific lenses for eye protection as recommended by the manufacturer.

The most frequent cause of laser injury in industrial environments is electrical accidents. Laser systems frequently require large power supplies with potential for fatal shock. Electrical outlets with safety switches should be carefully positioned when the laser is installed. Adequate warning signs and in-service training are essential to prevent inadvertent accidents. Maintenance is to be performed by trained technicians only. Laser use and maintenance should be recorded from the date of installation. The laser system should be stored so that components and the ignition key are secured when the laser is not being used.

Although the risk of airborne contaminants with endovascular laser applications is minimal, users should be aware that precautions must be implemented to prevent exposure and inhalation of laser plume. There is still a controversy whether laser (or electrocautery) plume contains viable cancer and/or mutagenic cells or whether laser exposure destroys these organisms. A closed-system smoke evacuator should be used if exposure to laser plume is likely to occur. Dangerous by-products may also be released from inorganic materials. Plastic bottles, drapes, instruments, polytetrafluoroethylene (PTFE) prosthetic materials, and tubing may emit poisonous gases if exposed to laser energy.

Blood Exposure

No current description of endovascular suite safety can be complete without mentioning the risk of blood exposure. Although one may dismiss blood exposure as minimal risk because of the "noninvasive" environment, the potential for blood exposure still exists. Maneuvers that reduce the risk of exposure are a benefit to both health-care workers and patients.

Several studies of general surgical procedures have shown a correlation between the duration of an operation and the potential for blood contamination, as well as a strong correlation between blood loss and contamination [10, 11]. Telford et al. [10] reported on two categories of contamination: injuries and blood exposure. They found that, under stringent monitoring by a study nurse, cuts to at least one surgical team member occurred during 2.6% of the operations, and needle sticks occurred during 13% of operations. Most of the cuts in this study occurred during hand-to-hand passing of knives from the surgeon to the scrub nurse, whereas most of the needle sticks occurred during suturing. The same study monitored effectiveness of double gloving to control blood exposure to the hands. They found that 11.5% of single-gloved personnel had hand contamination, whereas only 1.2% of double-gloved personnel had contamination during procedures that lasted more than 2 h and resulted in more than 100 ml of blood loss, personnel who single- or double-gloved had a hand contamination of 40 and 9%, respectively.

Endovascular surgical techniques should greatly reduce blood exposure because of shorter procedure times and less blood loss. However, the use of indwelling arterial sheaths and catheters presents a new exposure modality. Because of arterial pressures, the simple misdirection of a three-way stopcock or flush with a syringe can contaminate a person several feet away. Protective clothing for personnel near the operating field should include fluid-resistant gowns, eye guards, or face shields, and double gloving if the procedure lasts longer than 1 h. Personnel who might be within 3–4 ft of the access site would also be advised to wear protective eye wear. Needles are routinely used for arterial access. When a needle or any sharp instrument is exchanged, care must be taken not to drop or toss the sharp object toward the scrub nurse. The safest mode of exchange is to set the needle or sharp instrument down, allowing the other person to pick it up.

References

1. Bushong SC: *Radiologic science for technologists*, St. Louis, 1984, Mosby.
2. Nissen SE: Principles of radiographic imaging. In Roubin GS, Califf RM, O'Neill WW et al. editors: *Interventional cardiovascular medicine*, New York, 1994, Churchill Livingstone.
3. Geise RA, Hunter DW: Personnel exposure during fluoroscopy procedures, *Postgrad Radiol* 8:162–173, 1988.
4. Einstein A: Zur Quantem Theorie dr Strahlung, *Phys Zeit* 18:121, 1917.
5. Hallmark C: *Lasers, the light fantastic*, Blueridge Summit, PA, 1979, TAB Books.
6. Arndt KA, Noe JM, Northam BC: Laser therapy—basic concepts and nomenclature, *J Am Acad Dermatol* 5: 649–654, 1981.
7. American National Standards Institute: American national standard for the safe use of lasers, [ANSI] Z 130.1, New York, 1980, the Institute.
8. American National Standards Institute: American national standard for the safe use of lasers in health care facilities, [ANSI] Z 136.3, New York, 1988, the Institute.
9. A guide for the control of laser hazards, Cincinnati, 1981, American Conference of Governmental Industrial Hygienists.
10. Telford GL, Quebbeman EJ: Assessing the risk of blood exposure in the operating room, *Am Pract Infect Cont* 6(21):351–356, 1993.
11. Quebbeman EJ, Telford GL, Wadsworth K et al.: Risk of blood contamination and injury to operating room personnel, *Ann Surg* 214:614–620, 1991.

Part III

Facilities and Equipment for Endovascular Intervention

Endovascular Intervention Suite Design

8

Irwin Walot and Joe P. Chauvapun

The need for a sound structural design, in this modern age of endovascular intervention, is paramount. With the forever evolving technology, it is often difficult to keep up with the latest trends in room design. There are, however, several key basic factors that remain unchanged in the design venue. Availability for your core operating room equipment which includes a scrub sink, anesthesia equipment, substerile area for the autoclave, and ample equipment storage area is required. In order to fulfill the dual role of an operating arena and an imaging suite, the modern endovascular suite must be outfitted with a state-of-the-art imaging system.

General Considerations

There have been major shifts in angiographic equipment since the initial publication of this text. Medical imaging has shifted away from analog imaging (photographic film) to increasingly sophisticated digital imaging equipment. This shift initially involved image review and archival, with images being acquired with analog imaging chains for digital conversion and storage, but has now extended to the entire imaging chain. In angiographic equipment, there has been a shift away from hybrid analog/digital systems (with large glass image intensifiers coupled to video cameras) to high-resolution digital systems utilizing digital flat panel detectors (in various sizes). Larger detectors cover larger fields of view but are more expensive.

Current equipment purchase must also include hardware and software integration to allow studies to be archived and displayed in full resolution on a picture archiving and communication system (PACS) and for studies to be archived and distributed on inexpensive digital media such as DVD-ROM. Where there is an existing PACS (hospital or existing clinic), equipment purchases should be vetted by the PACS administrator to ensure compatibility and determine whether information systems architecture must be upgraded (may involve additional costs that must be factored into the purchase price).

Portable System Versus Fixed Imaging System

The choices of room design and equipment still come down to price and space. In the setting of limited space and limited budget, portable equipment will always win out. Portable "C" arms with excellent road mapping capability, sophisticated post-processing software packages, and radiation dose control utilizing pulsed fluoroscopic imaging are available from several manufactures. These units are now available with flat panel detectors and can transmit images to a PACS system. They can be configured with "on table" controls and motorized options. Used in conjunction with radiolucent, "floating" surgical tables (also available from several different manufactures) the combination makes for a sophisticated endovascular imaging solution that can be used in any reasonably sized operating room,

I. Walot (✉)
Professor, Department of Radiology, Harbor-UCLA Medical Center, Torrance, CA, USA

T.J. Fogarty, R.A. White (eds.), *Peripheral Endovascular Interventions*,
DOI 10.1007/978-1-4419-1387-6_8, © Springer Science+Business Media, LLC 1998, 2010

does not require a control room or additional construction, and has the further advantage of being able to be completely pulled out the way during surgical interventions.

If space and budget are not major constraints, purpose-designed and built combination angiographic/operating room suites provide the optimal solution. Although it may be possible to install angiographic equipment in smaller spaces, a procedure room should be at least 500 ft^2 with high (10 ft or greater) ceilings. Room design cannot focus only on the imaging equipment. The procedure room must also be designed in such a way as to simplify transfer of patients and accommodate anesthesia personnel and equipment. Our operative room schematic is demonstrated in Fig. 8.1. The major radiographic equipment manufacturers can provide complete "turnkey" proposals encompassing design, construction, and equipment installation or a dedicated design firm can be hired to oversee the process. In either case, modern design/visualization software allows computerized models of the room to be produced to show how well the chosen equipment will fit the room, how workflow will occur once the equipment is in place, and determine if the room size/configuration will impose equipment limitations. In addition, choosing designers/contractors with experience in the design and installation of radiographic facilities should ensure that the installation meets the individual state occupational and safety requirements—including air turnover and radiation shielding requirements (plans must generally be submitted to the state for review and approval prior to the start of construction).

Fixed angiographic equipment is available in monoplane and biplane designs. Biplane configurations are more expensive to purchase and install and are more difficult to operate. They are not generally required for peripheral interventions but are helpful in intracranial and cardiac procedures. Current equipment designs allow for rotational angiography/3d reconstruction as an option. Although occasionally helpful (particularly in intracranial procedures), the angiograms can be cumbersome to acquire and the optional capability can be expensive. Manufacturers often have several

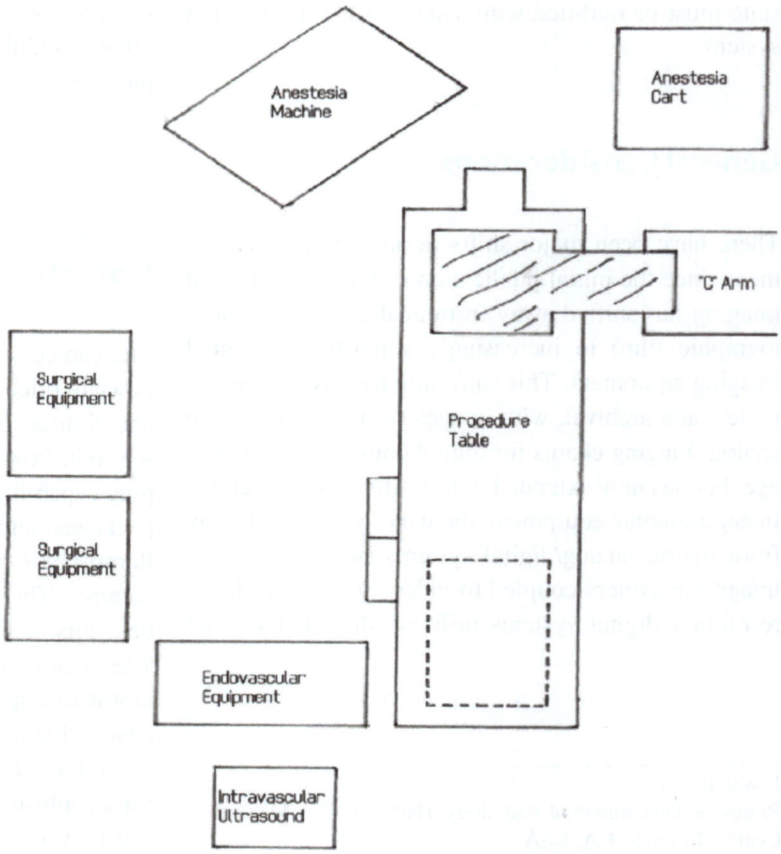

Fig. 8.1 Schematic of our endosuite

different angiographic table designs available for the same imaging chain, with possible options including stepping tables, tilting tables, tables which can oblique the patient, and tables that pivot (the last option can be particularly useful in aiding patient transfer in small rooms). One problem that we have encountered is that the weight of patients has generally increased over time and that the table weight limits have not always kept pace.

Current equipment design for single plane suites generally dictates a "C" arm configuration with a base that can be floor mounted or ceiling mounted (one manufacturer is offering a new positioner that has a flexible mounting base allowing for multiple degrees of freedom, but experience is limited at this time). Ceiling mounting can allow for more versatile patient/equipment positioning as the "C" arm mounting itself is track mounted and can move within the room (floor mounted units are fixed in place). There are trade-offs for the added flexibility that ceiling mounting offers; in that there must be sufficient room above the ceiling for equipment and cabling and there is also considerable additional engineering and construction cost involved. It can be more difficult to isolate and stabilize ceiling-mounted equipment. The additional "track" occupies ceiling space that can be otherwise used to mount other equipment and ceiling mounting requires that additional care be taken to ensure that the "C" arm does not collide/interfere with other ceiling-mounted equipment such as lights, fluoroscopic monitors, radiation shields, and contrast injectors (Figs. 8.2 and 8.3).

In-room display monitors can be ordered in several overhead "crane" configurations with up to eight

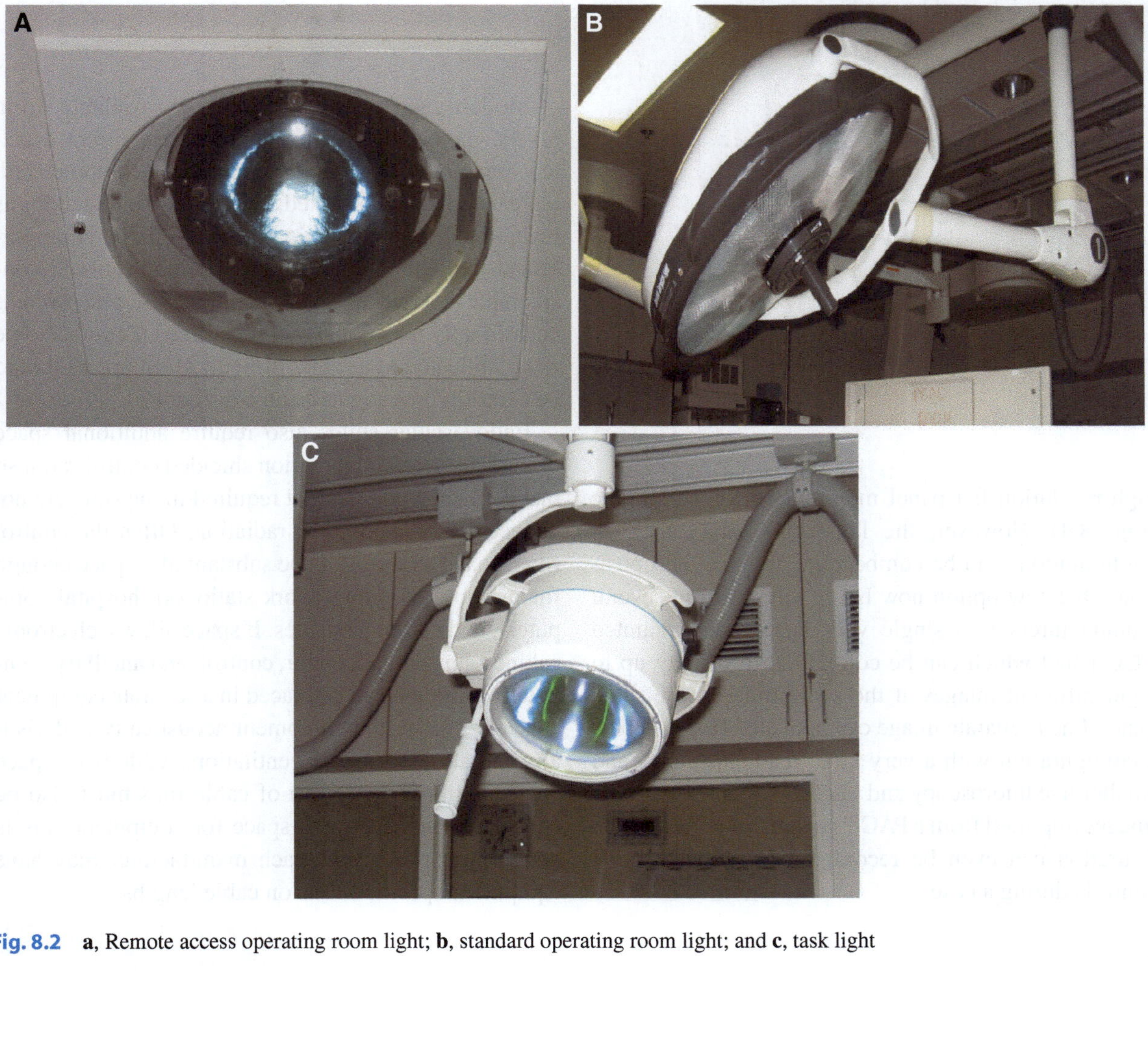

Fig. 8.2 **a**, Remote access operating room light; **b**, standard operating room light; and **c**, task light

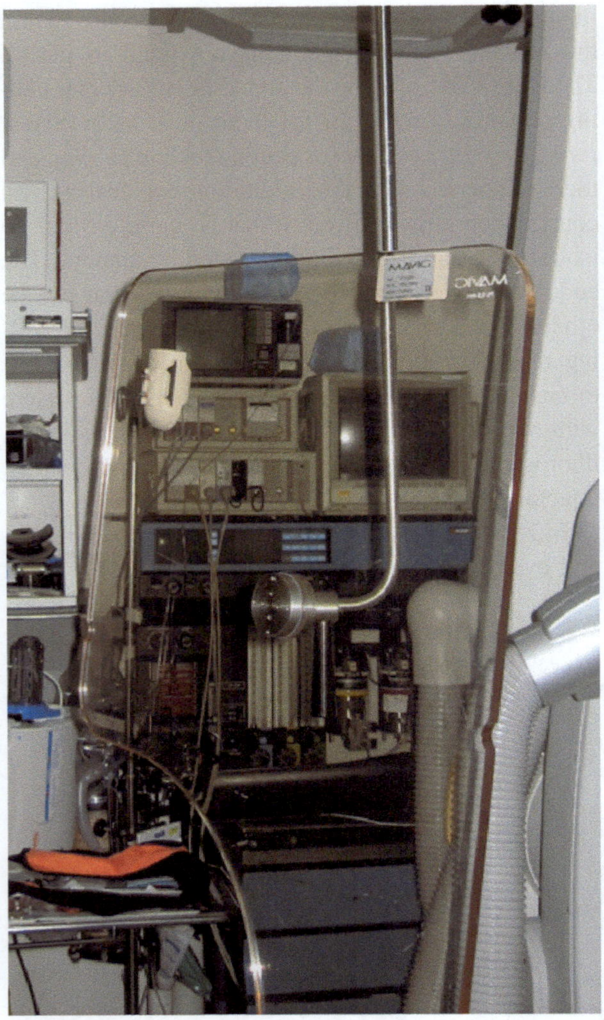

Fig. 8.3 Ceiling-mounted radiation shield

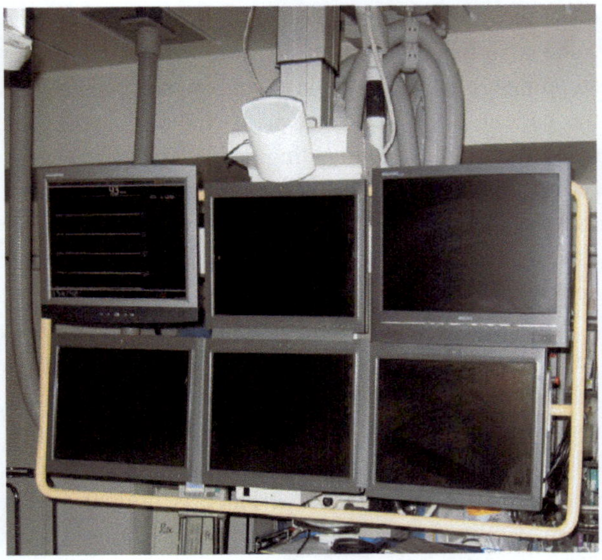

Fig. 8.4 In-room display monitors can be ordered in several overhead "crane" configurations with six high-resolution flat panel monitors on a single crane

high-resolution flat panel monitors on a single crane (Fig. 8.4). However, the larger 6/8 panel monitor configurations can be cumbersome to move and position. One new option now being offered from several manufacturers is a single very large crane-mounted LCD panel which can be configured to display up to eight different images at the same time on the same panel. Each separate image can be scaled (for instance, a configuration with a very large roadmap image and smaller live fluoroscopy and vital sign images and even images imported from a PACS system), and image configuration can even be reconfigured from table-side controls during a case.

Modern angiographic equipment available from all the major equipment manufacturers offers excellent imaging chains. The equipment is computerized, increasingly sophisticated, and offers many options including 3d reconstruction and even limited computerized tomographic capability. Options can add considerable cost to equipment purchases, and even if occasionally useful may not be utilized if cumbersome or complicated to use and difficult to set up, so should be carefully investigated and considered.

Endovascular suites also require additional space for a scrub area and radiation shielded control room so that personnel who are not required in the suite are not unnecessarily exposed to radiation. Often the control room space required can be substantial—space enough for multiple monitors, work station(s), hospital computers, and control consoles. If space allows, electronic cabinets housing generator, control, and ancillary computer equipment can be placed in a separate equipment closet to isolate the equipment acoustically and visually and allow for better ventilation. Aside from space considerations, the length of cable runs must also be considered in selecting a space for equipment closets and control rooms and each manufacturer may have equipment-specific limits on cable lengths.

Monitoring Equipment

The anesthesia department should be consulted early during the design process. Generally, the anesthesiologist will want to position the anesthesia machine and associated equipment near the head of the patient. This requires that the "C" arm base be positioned in such a way as to leave sufficient room for the anesthesiologist and ancillary equipment near the head of the procedure table and to allow for the most efficient placement of medical gas, suction, and electrical outlets. Although ceiling-mounted racks for anesthesia equipment seem like a good idea, in our experience, the anesthesiologists tend to keep most equipment on mobile carts for ease of maintenance, service, and restocking, and the ceiling-mounted racks are often underutilized. For patients undergoing procedures with conscious sedation and without anesthesiologist, monitoring equipment should parallel that available in the intensive care unit. Again, such equipment must be considered in the design process in terms of space, positioning, and cabling.

Contrast Injectors

Contrast injectors are comprised of a control unit and injector head. The two components can be combined in a single mobile cart (which can be manually positioned for each case) or the two components can be separated with the control unit placed in the control room or on the procedure room wall and the injector head ceiling mounted on a track or at the end of an articulated arm to save valuable floor space. The injector head can also be mounted on the angiographic table, although this is not generally recommended, particularly when the table is designed to automatically step. Table-mounted injector heads can contribute to "cable clutter" around the table and pose an obstacle when transferring patients. Contrast injectors should be considered in the design phase of the project as mounting hardware and electrical wiring conduits must be installed and cable runs calculated. Different injectors may have different cabling and electrical requirements to properly electrically sync with the angiographic equipment.

Equipping the Endovascular Suite

Integrating the modern equipments into the endovascular suite is no small task. The basic tools for interventions which include sheaths, catheters, wires, stents, and balloons must be readily available for the interventionist. However, due to limited storage availability, acquisition of appropriate mixed equipment is necessary. In addition to the basic equipment noted one may need to integrate the use of intravascular ultrasound (IVUS), lasers, angiojet into the armentarium of diagnostic and therapeutic tools. Keep in mind, however, your available premium equipment space.

Ergonomics in the Endovascular Suite

Ergonomics is the science of integrating the physical environment and the workers limitation to the task performed. In the United States, work-related musculoskeletal disorders are the most prevalent work place injuries. Prolonged standing as we experience in endovascular suite could lead to sore feet, general muscular fatigue, stiffness in the neck and shoulders, and lower back pain. Adjunctively, with the use of lead apron, the musculoskeletal burden incrementally increases.

Working in an endovascular suite like all standing jobs becomes problematic when we are restricted to limited body positions. This is often due to the layout of modern workstation and controls. The lack of flexibility in choosing a body position contributes discomfort in the short term and eventually leads to severe and chronic health problems in the long run.

A well-designed endovascular suite would allow the surgeon to choose from a variety of work position and change between them frequently. The optimum working height is 5–10 cm below working height. A portable foot rest would also allow the surgeon and the work staff the ability to shift body weight from one leg to the other. Aside from a quality footwear, the endovascular suite could incorporate anti-fatigue mats into the flooring design.

One other consideration is the monitor's positioning in the endovascular suite. Neck extension and forward head posturing is often required by the surgeon during the endovascular intervention. This has been associated with neck discomfort and disease. Well-designed monitor placement should allow for multiple positioning of the monitors to account for the appropriate working height of the surgeon.

The storage system within the endovascular suite should be required to have an "easy-reach" system. Retrieval of frequently used equipment should be efficient and time saving. A well-designed storage system in the endovascular suite could be cost saving when it comes to occupational safety and efficiency of the workforce.

Angioscopy: Instrumentation, Techniques, and Applications

9

Arnold Miller and Juha P. Salenius

Angioscopy is the only imaging technology that allows direct in vivo visualization of the interior of blood vessels in real-life colors. This capability to detect and quantify endoluminal findings and delineate subtle variations of the different normal and abnormal endoluminal states has only begun to be appreciated. The evolution and clinical application of the endoluminal techniques in the treatment of occlusive arterial disease and the performance of the distal bypass to the tibial and pedal arteries have highlighted the deficiencies of the arteriogram in providing accurate and clinically relevant information regarding the endoluminal state.

The main obstacle to the expanding role of angioscopy in modern vascular surgery remains the necessity to remove all blood from the visual field within the lumen of the vessel to obtain good endoluminal visualization. Blood is opaque to all light. To achieve complete removal of blood is not always easy. It requires skill and an understanding of the available instrumentation and techniques required for the different procedures.

Acceptance of angioscopy as an essential part of the armamentarium of the vascular surgeon based solely on the ability to demonstrate clear *superiority* with regard to outcome ignores the obvious benefits of direct intraluminal observation in normal and diseased states. These include the recognition of new or previously unappreciated intraluminal pathologies and their correlation with clinical outcome, as well as the use of the angioscope for evaluating technical success of surgical procedures and the new interventional procedures. In addition, angioscopy has proven to be an excellent educational tool for teaching surgical technique. Most reported studies defining the role of angioscopy in the treatment of vascular disease have focused on infrainguinal bypass surgery, thromboembolectomy, carotid endarterectomy, vascular access surgery, and percutaneous coronary and peripheral arterial angioscopy [1–16]. It should be appreciated that endoscopic vascular surgery is still in its infancy and remains one of the exciting and challenging areas of exploration in vascular surgery.

Since 1987, we have attempted to explore and optimize angioscopic techniques and instrumentation and to critically assess the role of angioscopy in clinical practice. In this chapter, we describe the basic instrumentation, the principles of irrigation, and our current techniques of angioscopy for vascular surgery.

Angioscopic Equipment

Flexible angioscopes in current clinical use range in external diameter from 0.5 to 3.0 mm. They consist of bundles of flexible glass fibers (3,000 to as many as 30,000 or more) of various types and refractive indexes (clear glass or quartz) coherently arranged and covered by an outer coating or *cladding,* which ensures undistorted light and image transmission (Fig. 9.1). The number of fiber bundles ("pixels") and the lensing systems are the main factors responsible for the resolution of the angioscopic image; the more fibers there are, the more the pixels and the higher the resolution. The fiber bundles are organized into those for imaging and those conducting light. At the distal end

A. Miller (✉)
Attending Vascular Surgeon, Department of Surgery, MetroWest Medical Center, Natick, MA, USA

T.J. Fogarty, R.A. White (eds.), *Peripheral Endovascular Interventions*,
DOI 10.1007/978-1-4419-1387-6_9, © Springer Science+Business Media, LLC 1998, 2010

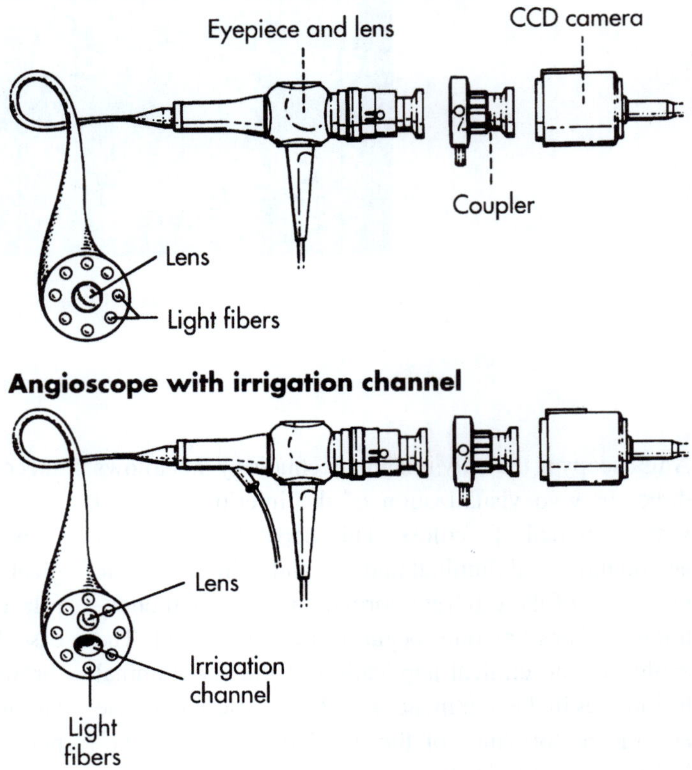

Fig. 9.1 Anatomy of an angioscope (from Miller and Jepsen [23], with permission of Elsevier)

of the angioscope a convex lens is fitted to capture the light emitted from the viewed intraluminal object and to refocus the "image" onto the mosaic of fibers of the optical bundle (see Table 9.1 for a list of angioscopic equipment).

Table 9.1 Angioscopy equipment

Angioscopes
0.5- to 3.0-mm outer diameter
Steerability (120° in two directions)
Working/irrigation channel
Reusable/disposable
Dedicated irrigation pump
Light source
Camera (chip, CCD)
High-resolution monitor
Documentation
Patient record, paperprint, slides
Video (VHS, U-matic) and microphone
Programmable character generator
Computerized processing and storing
Endovascular tools
Valvulotome
Endoluminal microinstrumentation
Occlusion devices
Angioscopy cart

Because the fiber bundles are coherently arranged, this image is faithfully reproduced at the opposite end of the optical bundle, where it may be magnified by an eyepiece and viewed directly or transmitted directly to a computer-controlled display (CCD) chip video camera and viewed as an image on a high-resolution monitor (or attached to any other camera lens system). This has been an important advance in the clinical application of angioscopy because it allows the procedure to be visualized as an enlarged image, avoiding all problems of maintaining a sterile field in the operating room or angiography suite. To inject sufficient light for transmission through the small volume of fiber bundles available in the modern angioscope for satisfactory intraluminal viewing, a very intense and focused cold light source is used, most usually derived from quartz–halogen or xenon arc lamps with energy of 250–300 W.

The definitive clinical angioscope may consist of only the flexible light fibers or include hollow channels of 0.3–1.0 mm, allowing irrigation at the distal tip of the angioscope or for use as a working channel for special intraluminal instrumentation. Steering the distal tip of some special angioscopes 120° in two directions is possible. This is usually mechanical and is facilitated by thin cables that extend along the surface of the angioscope sheath. Such specialized features, hollow channels, or steering mechanisms increase the external diameter of the angioscope and the overall rigidity of the instrument. Inclusion of these special features into a particular angioscope is always a compromise between the resolution and light intensity (i.e., total number of fiberoptic bundles) and the external diameter of the angioscope.

For percutaneous applications, particularly in the coronary arteries, an occlusion balloon either built-in at the distal part of the endoscope (Mitsubishi Cable Industries, Ltd, Tokyo, Japan, and Advanced Cardiovascular Systems, Santa Clara, CA) or integrated with a guidewire catheter system (Baxter, Irvine, CA) may allow brief periods of antegrade occlusion of the blood flow essential to successful angioscopy.

Currently, both reusable and disposable angioscopes are available for routine clinical use. In general, the optics of the reusable angioscopes has a better resolution. However, with modern fiberoptic and imaging technologies the resolution of both types of angioscope is adequate for clinical application. The choice for the individual surgeon depends on the circumstance, volume of procedures, and economics. The availability of a particular angioscope for clinical use is limited by the necessity for gas sterilization, a fairly lengthy procedure after each use. On a busy vascular service, a large number of angioscopes may be required for routine application.

Immediately after use, the reusable angioscope should be rinsed with water to remove all blood and cleaned in accordance with the manufacturer's instructions. Excessive kinking must be avoided to prevent breakage of the optical glass fibers. Gas sterilization is performed with ethylene oxide at a temperature of 55°C for a maximum of 105 min followed by aeration for 12 h in a special aeration chamber. Before gas sterilization a venting cap is attached to allow escape of air from within the endoscope and to prevent sheath rupture.

The adequacy of the irrigation system is crucial to consistent high-quality endoscopic studies, with volumes of irrigation fluid safe for routine clinical use. The venous infusion bag, an inflatable pressure cuff device, is only useful in a few special circumstances. A dedicated roller pump for irrigation, with adjustable high and low flow rates, is the cornerstone of the irrigation necessary for consistent clearing of all the blood from the relevant vessel.

Standard medical-grade video (i.e., VHS or U-matic) and audio equipment (e.g., a directional microphone) is used to record relevant parts of the angioscopy procedure, allowing repeated review of the procedure and the unique intraoperative findings. A character generator provides patient and study identification. Hard copy is useful to present the intraoperative findings. Paperprints may be included immediately in patient records or with computer technology stored in an electronic database for later processing.

Storage of the equipment on a dedicated mobile cart minimizes the complexity of all the electronic equipment, which once adjusted reduces the entire operation to a single on/off switch. It also facilitates transfer of the equipment between operating rooms or even several institutions. Finally, it reduces the required storage space and minimizes the risk of damage to the equipment.

Basic Techniques of Angioscopy

Principles of Saline Irrigation

The fundamental problem with vascular endoscopy remains the necessity to clear blood from the visual field. In the intraoperative setting, complete isolation of the vascular segment may be obtained by isolating the segment of the vasculature to be visualized between arterial clamps and removing the blood by flushing with a clear saline solution. This is standard practice during surgery for blood vessels in the suprainguinal and abdominal vasculature, during carotid surgery, and during venous thrombectomy. In the infrainguinal region, only proximal control by occluding the antegrade blood flow is necessary. The retrograde blood flow from collaterals is cleared by flushing these vessels or grafts with clear saline solution.

The intraarterial injection of CO_2 [17] for blood displacement, although promising, remains an experimental technique. Unlike saline, the gas is compressible; thus the delivery of CO_2 requires a special injector that delivers a precise volume of CO_2 over a prolonged injection time. A standard angiographic contrast injector may compress the gas with an explosive delivery.

Lack of appreciation of the factors governing successful saline irrigation and the difficulty in achieving the flow rates necessary for irrigation during angioscopy have delayed the incorporation of angioscopy as a routine procedure in the practice of vascular surgery. Unlike angiography, where a sufficient concentration of contrast medium mixing with the blood allows high-quality angiograms, during angioscopy the intraluminal blood must be totally replaced by a clear column of fluid. A small volume of red cells causes blurring of the visual field, and the image appears to be out of focus. Addition of any more blood makes meaningful visualization impossible.

Certain requirements are necessary to achieve a clear column of fluid in the vessels or grafts being studied by angioscopy (summarized in Table 9.2). All antegrade blood flow, from both the main inflow vessel and collaterals, needs to be prevented; otherwise, blood flowing in the same direction as the irrigation fluid will join the irrigation fluid and a clear fluid column will never be established. At surgery this usually entails proximal clamp occlusion of the native arteries or graft.

Table 9.2 Principles of irrigation for intraoperative angioscopy

Aim

- To establish and maintain a *column of clear fluid* within the vessel

Requirements

- No antegrade flow in the main vessel or collateral vessels
- Initial fluid bolus of large volume and high flow rate to establish column of clear fluid
- Subsequent small volume and low flow rate, with pressure in excess of backflow pressure, to maintain clear fluid column

From Miller et al. [18], with permission of Elsevier.

To clear all blood and establish the clear fluid column, a bolus of fluid, injected at a high flow rate and large volume, is necessary. The more rapidly the column of fluid can be established, the less the total fluid will be needed for the angioscopic study [18]. Once the column of fluid is established, it can be maintained by irrigating at a much lower flow rate and smaller volume. This prolongs the time that visualization is possible and minimizes the total volume of irrigation fluid used.

The practical problem in achieving these flow rates is the small size of the irrigation catheters necessary for intraoperative use. Inflating a standard venous transfusion pressure cuff device to between 400 and 450 mmHg, around a single liter of saline in a plastic container, allows a maximum flow rate of approximately 150 ml/min [18]. As the saline container empties and alters its shape, despite maintaining the pressure in the pressure cuff inflated to between 400 and 450 mmHg, the flow rate decreases. With the addition of various irrigation catheters, there is a further decrease in the flow rate. From our experimental [18] and clinical [19–21] experience the flow rates achieved with the pressure cuff device are inadequate for routine intraoperative angioscopy except in very limited circumstances. Furthermore, there is no control over the flow rate. The flow rate cannot be varied, and the exact volume of fluid being injected into the patient is difficult to monitor until termination of the procedure, when the pressure cuff is removed, and the saline bag examined.

Together with the Olympus Corporation (Lake Success, NY), we developed a dedicated irrigation pump (Angiopump; Fig. 9.2) for angioscopy. This pump is designed to provide flow rates between 10 and 400 ml/min and to generate a maximum pressure of 2,000 mmHg at the pump head. The pump provides for the selection of two independent flow rates, a high flow rate, or *bolus,* and a low flow rate, or *maintenance.* These flow rate settings are variable and independent of each other and may be adjusted either before or during the procedure. The flow rate is controlled remotely with a foot pedal, allowing switching back and forth

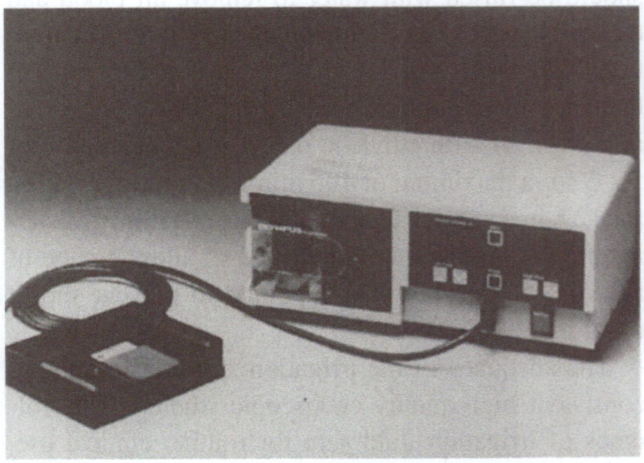

Fig. 9.2 Dedicated irrigation pump (Angiopump, Olympus Corporation) controlled with foot pedal. High and low flow rates may be set independently. Safety features include bubble detector and monitor to measure total volume infused

from bolus to maintenance so that, after the column of clear fluid is established, it may be maintained at all times in the vessel under examination [18].

A serious concern when infusing fluid intraarterially into a relatively restricted outflow tract at high flow rates is that excessively high intraarterial pressures may be generated, which could damage either the intimal lining or inner layer of the arterial wall even to the extent of complete rupture. In our experimental and clinical studies we have shown this not to be a problem, provided the vessel is not totally occluded or the irrigation is ceased as soon as clearing of the visual field [18–20, 22] occurs.

The most significant limitation of angioscopy is the volume of irrigation fluid that can safely be infused into a particular patient. In our experience during intraoperative angioscopy the volumes of fluid routinely required for irrigation with the dedicated irrigation pump, less than half a liter, have not been excessive [19, 20, 22]; provided the patient is carefully monitored, such volumes are safe even in the elderly and ill population typically undergoing infrainguinal bypass surgery. Furthermore, no increased patient morbidity or mortality in the intraoperative, perioperative, or early postoperative (<30 days) periods could be demonstrated, even in patients with the highest preoperative cardiovascular risk status [22]. The irrigation fluid volumes necessary for successful completion angioscopy are safe, provided the anesthetist is aware that angioscopy is to be performed, runs the patient "dry" until the angioscopy is completed, and includes the irrigation fluid in the calculations of the patient's total fluid requirements.

Techniques of Angioscopy

We have previously described in detail the basic techniques for intraoperative angioscopy [23]. The standard equipment and technique for setting up in the operating room are shown in Fig. 9.3. For each angioscopic application we use a standard method of angioscopic examination. The following general principles are important to achieve consistently good studies, maintain safety, and avoid complications:

1. To avoid inducing spasm in the native artery or vein, choose an angioscope for the procedure smaller than the lumen of the smallest vessel to be intubated

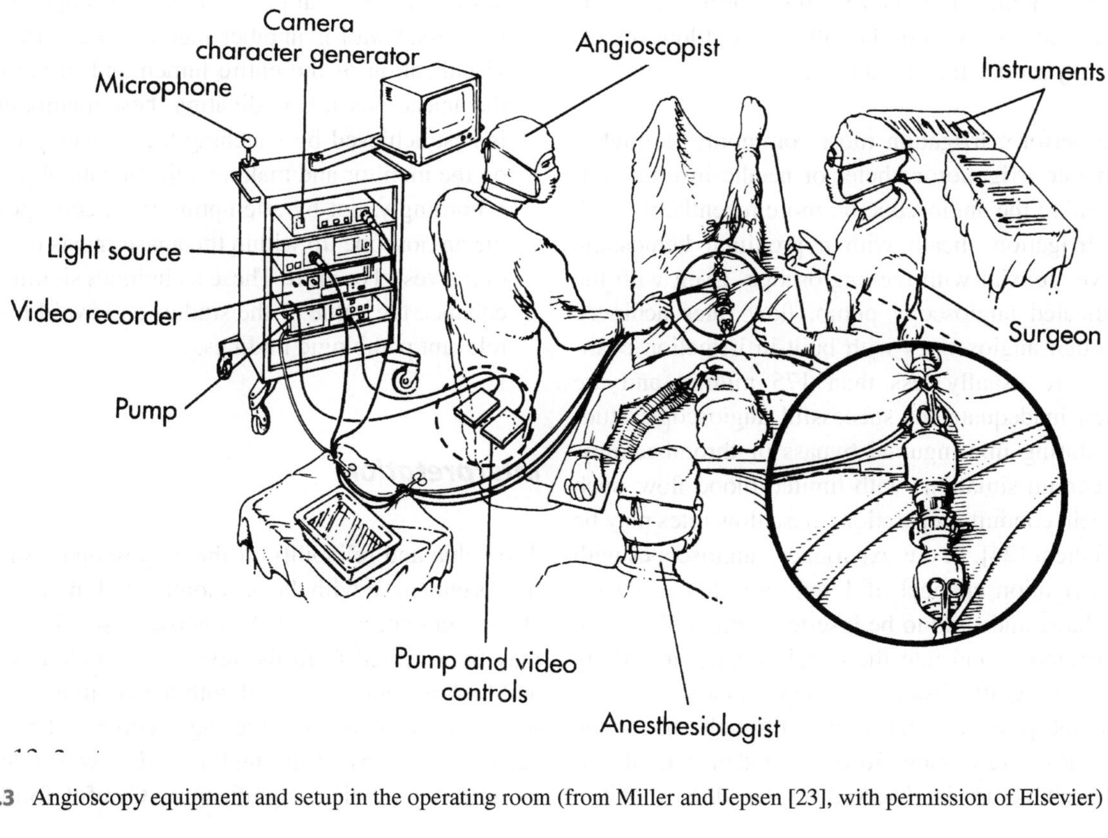

Fig. 9.3 Angioscopy equipment and setup in the operating room (from Miller and Jepsen [23], with permission of Elsevier)

and pass it through these vessels only in the presence of flowing blood or irrigation fluid. Passage of an angioscope occupying almost the entire lumen of the vessel or passage in a vessel emptied of all blood or irrigation fluid may result in intense, irreversible vasospasm.

2. To minimize the irrigation fluid volume and optimize the duration of angioscopic imaging, do the following:

   a. Perform angioscopy on withdrawal whenever possible.
   b. During completion angioscopy for bypass grafts, occlude the artery just proximal to the distal anastomosis whenever possible. This reduces the size of the outflow tract and the likelihood of any blood mingling with the clear column of irrigation fluid.
   c. Whenever possible, reduce the retrograde flow or prevent it from flowing into the clear fluid column. In bypass grafts, when withdrawing the angioscope from the distal artery and anastomosis and moving it into the graft, occlude the distal end of the graft between the fingers or use a fine "bulldog" clamp to trap the column of clear fluid within the graft. During thrombectomy, external compression of the inflow or outflow vessels may reduce the blood flow.

3. We perform irrigation most commonly through a separate irrigation catheter or needle inserted collateral to the angioscope or, more recently, through an irrigation sheath with a proximal hemostatic valve, coaxial with the angioscope. Even with the dedicated angioscopy pump, flow rates achieved through angioscopes with built-in irrigation channels are usually less than 175 ml/min and are often inadequate for successful angioscopic studies during infrainguinal bypass or thrombectomy. In certain situations with limited blood flow, such as vein conduit preparation, these flow rates may be sufficient [24]. In our experience, angioscopes with an irrigation channel of 1 mm are almost always too large and rigid to be inserted through the distal anastomosis and into the distal artery, particularly in bypass grafts distal to the popliteal arteries.
4. Do not pass the angioscope through the native vessels or graft unless flowing blood or normal vessel architecture is observed on the video monitor. A "white out" of the image means that the angioscope is abutting an obstruction; insertion should be halted and the angioscope withdrawn a few centimeters. If the obstruction remains and the freely flowing blood is not seen, further insertion of the angioscope must be performed under direct vision. This avoids injury to the vessels or the anastomotic structures, even if it means using more irrigation fluid, and prevents "buckling" of the optical fibers with irrepairable damage to the angioscope.
5. Visualize the entire lumen of the vessels being studied to ensure completeness of the angioscopy study. This may be achieved using a steerable angioscope or manipulating a nonsteerable angioscope. Steerable angioscopes not only enhance the quality of the angioscopic study but are much easier to manipulate intraluminally than the standard nonsteerable angioscope. Although useful in the femoropopliteal and larger tibial vessels, their large size precludes use in many of the more distal bypass grafts. For the smaller nonsteerable angioscopes, rolling or torquing the angioscope between the plantar surfaces of the thumb and index finger allows rotation of the angioscope and the entire vessel circumference to be visualized. Direct manipulation on the distal end of the angioscope through the vessel wall is another method of ensuring full visualization of the entire lumen and in particular the anastomosis. Coordinating these manipulations is best achieved by watching the images produced on the monitor and making adjustments of position accordingly, not by attempting to directly position the angioscope tip within the anastomosis or lumen of the vessel or graft. These techniques significantly enhance the value of the studies and avoid missing relevant pathologic findings.

Interpretation

The value and reliability of the angioscopic examination is enhanced with the development of interpretative skills and experience of the endoscopist. These skills may be acquired from the review of previous studies and findings but are refined with the continued critical review and evaluation of the angioscopic findings after each study. Many of the findings are new, subtle, and of uncertain clinical significance. Careful follow-up and correlation with the clinical course will eventually establish the significance of these findings.

It is especially important to appreciate that the angioscope in its current form is a qualitative instrument. The accurate assessment of size of an angioscopic image on the video monitor remains problematic. Magnification of the image changes with the distance of the angioscope lens to an object; the closer the lens to the object, the larger the image [5]. This makes much of the interpretation of the angioscopic images subjective and the significance of many of the more subtle endoluminal findings difficult to assess, even with a large amount of experience. Methods to quantitate the angioscopic image would substantially enhance the value of angioscopy.

Clinical Applications

Indications

Our current indications for angioscopy are summarized in Table 9.3. The usefulness and varied applications of angioscopy depend in the main on the ingenuity and creativity of the individual surgeon. We conceptualize and use the angioscope as an adjunctive tool to see inside vessels so that rational and informed clinical and surgical decisions can be made with "objective" findings. We do not rely simply on "experience."

Table 9.3 Indications for angioscopy of peripheral vessels

Diagnostic
Monitoring of surgical interventional procedures
Bypass, endarterectomy, thrombectomy, embolectomy, vascular access, preparation of renal transplants, and valvuloplasty for venous insufficiency
Angioplasty, atherectomy, stenting, and endoluminal grafting
Lesions responsible for anginal syndromes
Endoscopic findings and graft failure
Therapeutic
Surgical
Endoluminal vein graft preparation (valvulotomy and tributary occlusion)
Catheter-directed thrombectomy or embolectomy
Percutaneous
Thrombolysis
Assisted interventions (angioplasty, atherectomy, stenting, and endoluminal grafting)

Initially, we used angioscopy as a simple alternative or adjunct to the operative angiogram as a means to avoid or correct technical errors. However, we soon appreciated that the rich and detailed endoluminal information not only provides a sensitive and accurate method for the detection of technical errors but also allows continual assessment of technical proficiency. It has become an excellent teaching tool, improving and refining surgical technique of the surgeon and resident staff. Angioscopy has also identified new or previously unappreciated endovascular pathologies that have enhanced our understanding of the pathogenesis of graft failure [25] and fostered the development and design of new instrumentation for intraluminal manipulations such as valve cutters, tributary occluders, and various grabbing and cutting intraluminal instruments [21, 24, 26, 27].

Infrainguinal Bypass Grafting

Angioscopy plays a significant role in infrainguinal bypass grafting. It allows preparation of the best-quality vein conduit available, irrespective of the configuration of the vein graft or the source of the vein. We have shown that whereas the incidence of unsuspected endoluminal pathology of the saphenous vein [20] is between 10 and 20%, in arm veins [28] it is much more frequent, between 60 and 70% of arm veins harvested for grafting. It also allows the application of the minimal surgical techniques for the in situ vein graft and monitoring of the entire bypass graft after completion of the surgery, including the conduit, distal anastomosis, and distal artery, to assess technical success of the surgery.

Vein Conduit Preparation

Reversed Vein. We monitor all reversed veins for quality control and the detection of endoluminal defects. This may be performed ex vivo or after completion of the distal anastomosis. The advantage of examining the vein ex vivo is that no irrigation fluid enters the patient's circulation.

Nonreversed Vein. After harvesting the nonreversed vein, the angioscope is introduced through an irrigation sheath into the proximal portion of the vein;

the valvulotome, a modified Mills retrograde valvulotome, is introduced from the distal end of the vein. Irrigation fluid to distend the vein is provided through the sheath. Angioscopically directed valvulotomy proceeds smoothly, coordinating the movements of the valvulotome and angioscope so that the valvulotome is visualized at all times and guided to cut each valve leaflet accurately. This is performed ex vivo with no irrigation fluid entering the patient's circulation.

In Situ Vein Conduit Preparation

Open Technique. Our open technique of angioscopically directed valvulotomy with variations used, depending on clinical preference or circumstance, is shown in Fig. 9.4. The greatest advantage of this technique is that it allows the accurate ligation of the tributaries before valvulotomy and thereby minimizes the volume of irrigation fluid needed; it also simplifies angioscopically directed valvulotomy. In general, the greater saphenous vein is completely exposed through a single continuous incision. The inflow and outflow arteries are dissected out, and the patient is systemically heparinized in a dosage of 0.5–1.5 mg/kg according to the surgeon's preference. Thereafter, the proximal end of the vein is divided and the saphenofemoral junction oversewn. The saphenous vein is likewise mobilized several centimeters distal to the distal arterial anastomotic site and ligated distally. The first proximal valve is invariably located close to the saphenofemoral junction and can be identified by gentle eversion of the vein and excised with scissors under direct vision. The vein is then gently distended with warm irrigation fluid (a balanced salt solution with normalized pH containing papaverine hydrochloride, 60 mg/500 ml, and heparin sodium, 2,000 IU); and the flexible shaft of the valvulotome, with the blunt bullet-shaped introducer in place, is passed from the distal end to protrude through the proximal open end of the vein graft. The introducer is removed and replaced by the appropriate-sized cutting valvulotome head, and the valvulotome is withdrawn into the proximal vein. The angioscope is then introduced into the proximal end of the vein and the valvulotome visualized. The vein is flushed clear of blood, and the fluid is allowed to escape at the end of the vein opposite to that of the irrigation catheter. The valvulotome is gradually withdrawn under constant angioscopic visualization, avoiding all tributaries, and maneuvered accurately onto the center of each valve leaflet. Ideally, each leaflet is cut by a single pull on the valvulotome shaft. The valvulotome is then repositioned on the opposite valve leaflet, and the procedure is repeated throughout the length of the vein graft.

Semiclosed Techniques. The aim of semiclosed techniques is to minimize the size of the wound necessary to harvest and prepare the vein. Various techniques have been described. Mehigan described the technique of tributary ligation through small stab incisions at the same time as endoluminal valvulotomy [24]. Others have modified the technique with preoperative vein and tributary mapping [29, 30]. These mapped tributaries are then ligated before valvulotomy through small stab incisions.

Exposure and mobilization of the arteries and the greater saphenous vein at the anticipated sites of proximal and distal anastomosis are similar to the open technique described in the preceding section. Generally, location and ligation of side branches are performed concurrently with valvulotomy. This reduces the volume of irrigation fluid required for the procedure. Others complete the valvulotomy and then ligate the marked-out tributaries. Side branch visualization from the interior of the saphenous vein is readily accomplished, since on the video monitor a branch site is characterized by a dimple in the side wall of the vein, from which often a thin stream of blood exudes if the irrigation stream is set at a low flow rate or discontinued. As each side branch is visualized, the valvulotome is positioned so that it points to the exact opening. The angioscope light transilluminates the skin of the leg at that point and a small marking on the skin is made. The side branch can also be located both visually and by palpation of a vein, inside of which the tip of the valvulotome can be felt pointing to the exact orifice of the side branch. The side branch is thereby pinpointed and can be ligated with minimal mobilization of the vein, preserving the in situ character of the operation.

When the angioscope and valvulotome have reached the most distal aspect of the vein, all valves having been incised, a completion study to ensure that all valves have been cut is performed as the angioscope is slowly withdrawn. Each valve site is again inspected for completeness of incision and for incompetence.

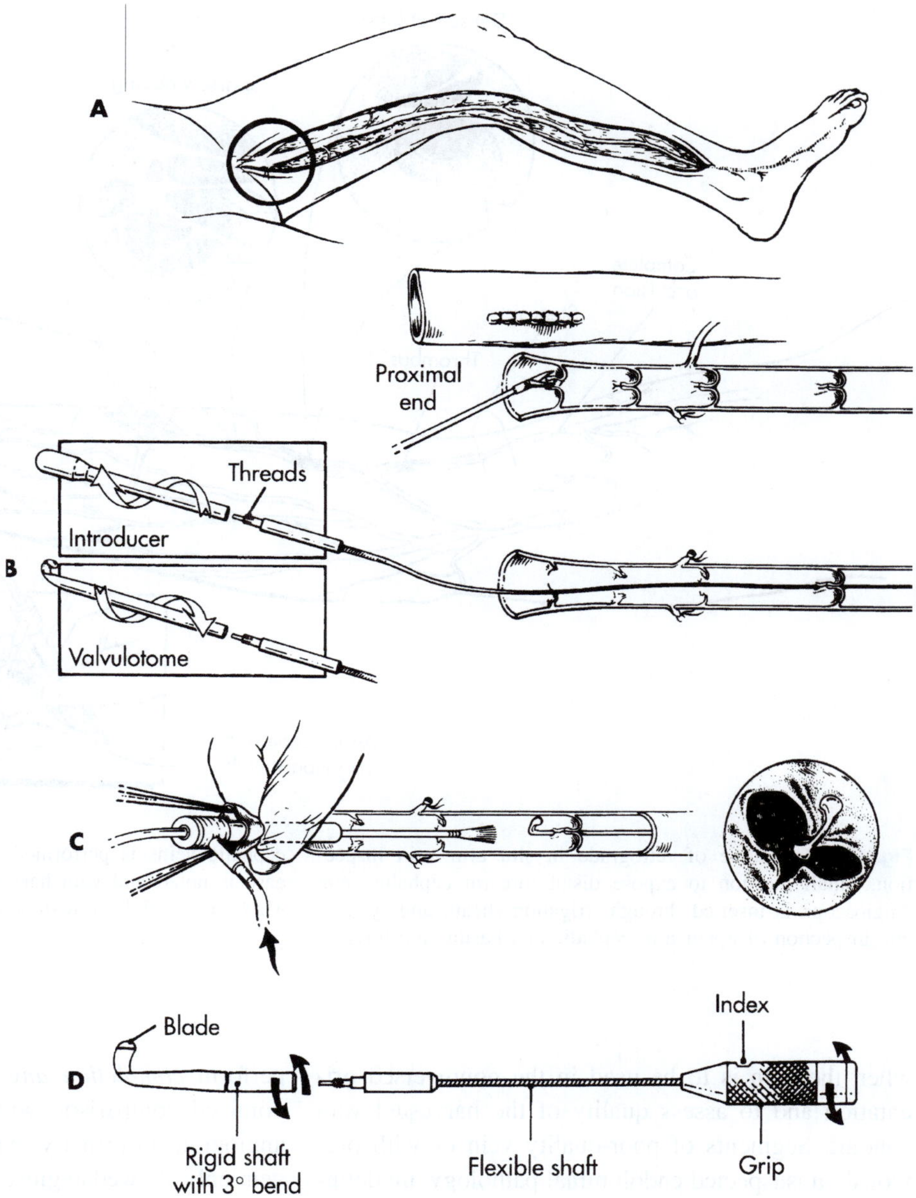

Fig. 9.4 Angioscopically directed valvulotomy. **a**, Saphenous vein is completely exposed and tributaries ligated. Patient is heparinized and vein transected at both ends. Vein is gently distended with papaverine–heparin saline solution, and the first proximal valve is excised with scissors. **b**, Valvulotome with introducer in place is passed through vein from distal end to protrude through proximal end of vein. Introducer is replaced with appropriately sized valvulotome. **c**, Valvulotome is withdrawn under constant angioscopic direction steering past the tributary orifices and accurately cutting each valve leaflet. **d**, Valvulotome (from Miller et al. [21], with permission of Elsevier)

After removal of the angioscope, the proximal and distal anastomoses are performed in the usual fashion.

Our preferred technique is a combination of the open and semiclosed techniques. The entire vein is exposed through short interrupted skin incisions and all tributaries ligated or clipped with hemoclips. Valvulotomy is then performed. Using modern retractors and laparoscopic techniques, the length of the skin incisions is minimized. Closed techniques for the complete endoluminal in situ vein preparation, angioscopic valvulotomy and coil occlusion of tributaries, are currently in trial [31].

Arm Vein Preparation with Angioscope for Bypass Grafting

Angioscopy is performed in all instances after the vein harvesting and before implantation of the graft with angioscopes ranging from an outer diameter from 0.8 to 2.2 mm. When the quality of the vein is in question, we perform an in situ examination of the arm veins before any extensive vein dissection and exposure (Fig. 9.5) [28]. It allows directed harvesting of only the appropriate segments of available vein conduit. The angioscope is routinely used for valve lysis

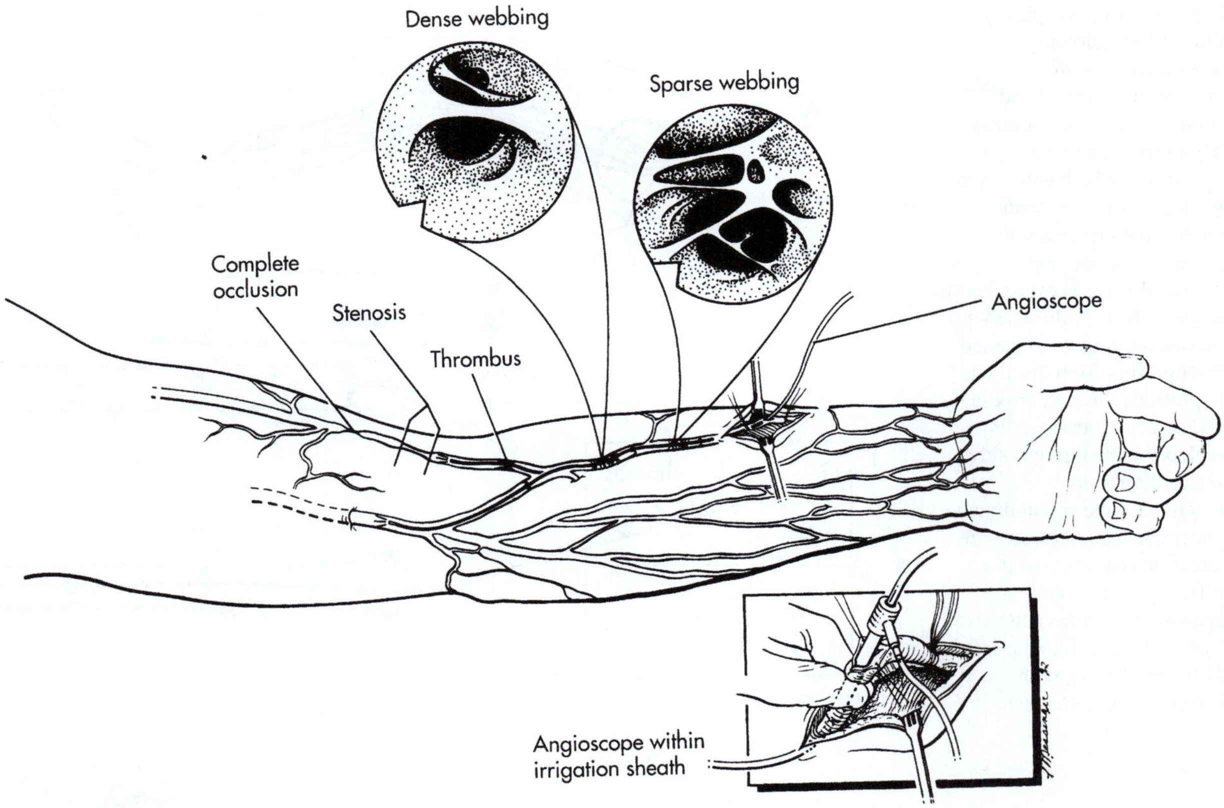

Fig. 9.5 Technique of retrograde in situ arm vein inspection. Small incision to expose distal forearm cephalic vein. Angioscope is inserted through irrigation sheath and systematic inspection of upper arm cephalic and basilic and forearm cephalic veins is performed. All segmental intraluminal disease is noted and vein harvest is planned accordingly (from Marcaccio et al. [28], with permission of Elsevier)

when the vein is to be used in the nonreversed orientation and to assess quality of the harvested vein conduit. Segments of poor-quality vein or with previously unsuspected endoluminal pathology are delineated and marked for "upgrading." Angioscopically directed upgrading of the vein conduit can be done by endoluminal repair, such as cutting sparse endoluminal strands and fine webs with a retrograde valvulotome, removal of endoluminal thrombus, or vein patch angioplasty in a region of stenosis; where a segment of vein is unusable because of dense webbing or stricture or thrombus, the entire diseased segment is excised. The normal segments can then be spliced together to attain a conduit of adequate length. Such upgrading significantly improves arm vein bypass graft patency [28].

Although the value of routine intraoperative monitoring of bypass grafts is still unresolved, we routinely perform *completion angioscopy.* A prospective randomized comparison with completion intraoperative angiogram in primary bypass grafts using saphenous vein only showed angioscopy to be more sensitive and specific in detecting technical abnormalities, particularly in the vein conduit and anastomosis [32]. We perform intraoperative angiography when the distal circulation is not well delineated on the preoperative angiogram or if there is some concern regarding the exact anatomy of the distal runoff circulation. The technique is shown in Fig. 9.6, wherein the in situ or nonreversed vein tributaries are left long at the proximal part of the vein conduit for access of the angioscope and irrigation catheters. In the reversed and occasionally in the nonreversed vein, the completion angioscopy is done through the open end of the vein graft after first completing the distal anastomosis.

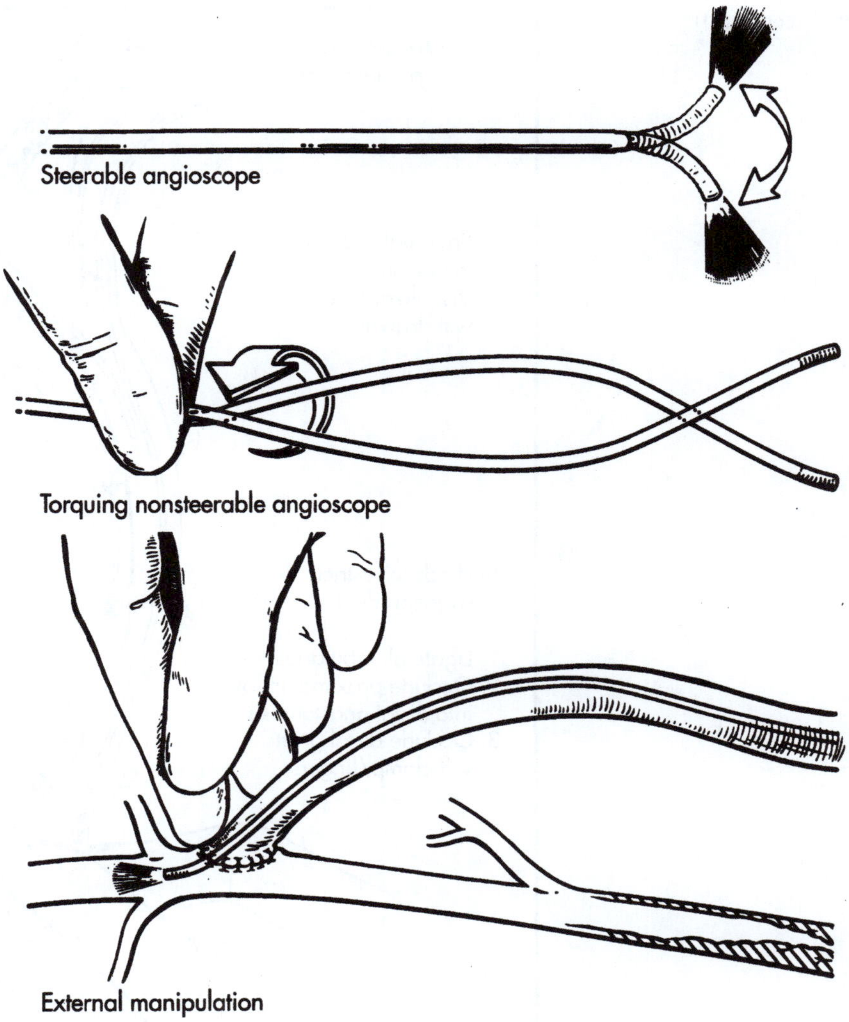

Fig. 9.6 Technique of the completion angioscopy. **a**, Inspection of anastomotic region with distal outflow artery and methods to enhance angioscopic visualization (from Miller and Jepsen [23], with permission of Elsevier). **b**, Each valve site and ligated side branch are inspected for completeness while the angioscope is slowly withdrawn

Angioscopy for Carotid Endarterectomy

After standard carotid endarterectomy the arteriotomy is closed from both ends. Before completion of the suture line the shunt, if used, is removed. The angioscope, preferably with a built-in irrigation channel, is inserted into endarterectomized vessels without removal of the clamps. Irrigation is provided with flow rates of approximately 100 ml/min (high flow) and 50 ml/min (low flow). The force of the irrigant stream directed toward the end point of the reconstruction clearly establishes whether the intima at the distal end point is sufficiently attached. The angioscope is passed gently up the internal carotid artery until the distal occlusion clamp is visualized and then gently withdrawn. Small intimal flaps can be removed by microbiopsy forceps; or if significant residual plaque or flaps need to be removed, the arteriotomy is reopened and the defect corrected. Endoscopy also allows inspection of the external and common carotid arteries [14, 15, 33].

Vascular Access Surgery

The techniques for angioscopy during vascular access surgery are similar to the techniques for intraoperative angioscopy during infrainguinal bypass grafting. Suitable angioscopes range from 0.8 to 2.2 mm in external diameter (Olympus Corporation). We seldom use an angioscope with an irrigating channel; they

Fig. 9.6 (continued)

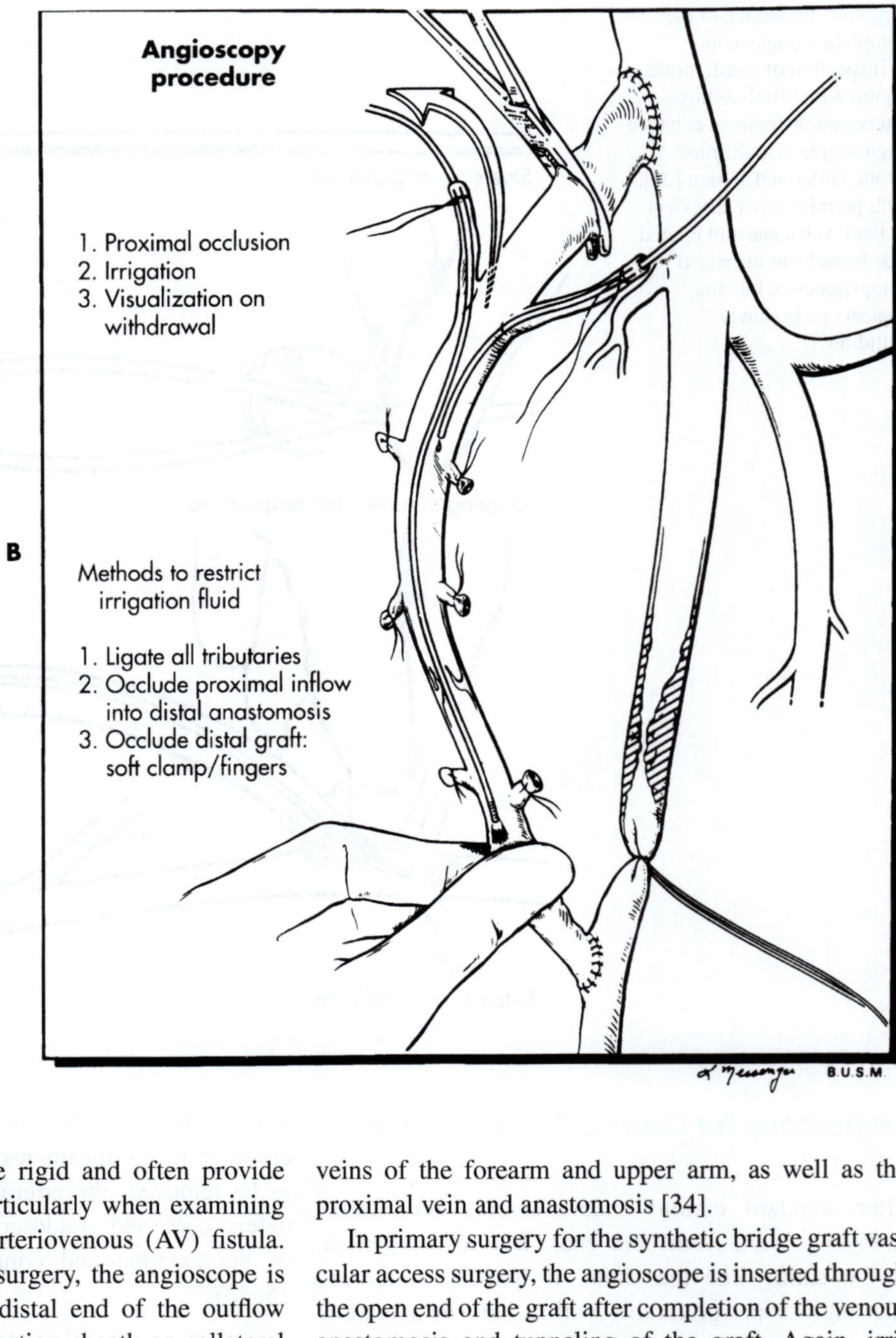

tend to be larger and more rigid and often provide an inadequate flow rate, particularly when examining the arterial inflow of the arteriovenous (AV) fistula. For autogenous AV fistula surgery, the angioscope is inserted through the open distal end of the outflow vein, either through an irrigation sheath or collateral to an irrigation catheter, where an in situ vein inspection is performed similar to that described for arm vein harvesting in infrainguinal bypass grafting [28]. In the failing or occluded autogenous AV fistula, the angioscope is introduced into the vein at a site where the cause of failure is most likely determined either by clinical examination or preoperative fistulogram. The angioscope is introduced in both antegrade and retrograde directions, allowing inspection of the runoff veins of the forearm and upper arm, as well as the proximal vein and anastomosis [34].

In primary surgery for the synthetic bridge graft vascular access surgery, the angioscope is inserted through the open end of the graft after completion of the venous anastomosis and tunneling of the graft. Again, irrigation is provided either with an irrigation sheath or collateral catheter. The outflow vein and the anastomosis are inspected. The techniques of angioscopy unique for revision surgery in synthetic bridge grafts are illustrated in Fig. 9.7 [35]. A small skin incision is made, usually at the apex of the loop graft. A few centimeters of the synthetic graft are freed up, sufficient to allow placement of fine occluding clamps after reestablishing flow. Rummel tourniquets are placed to prevent

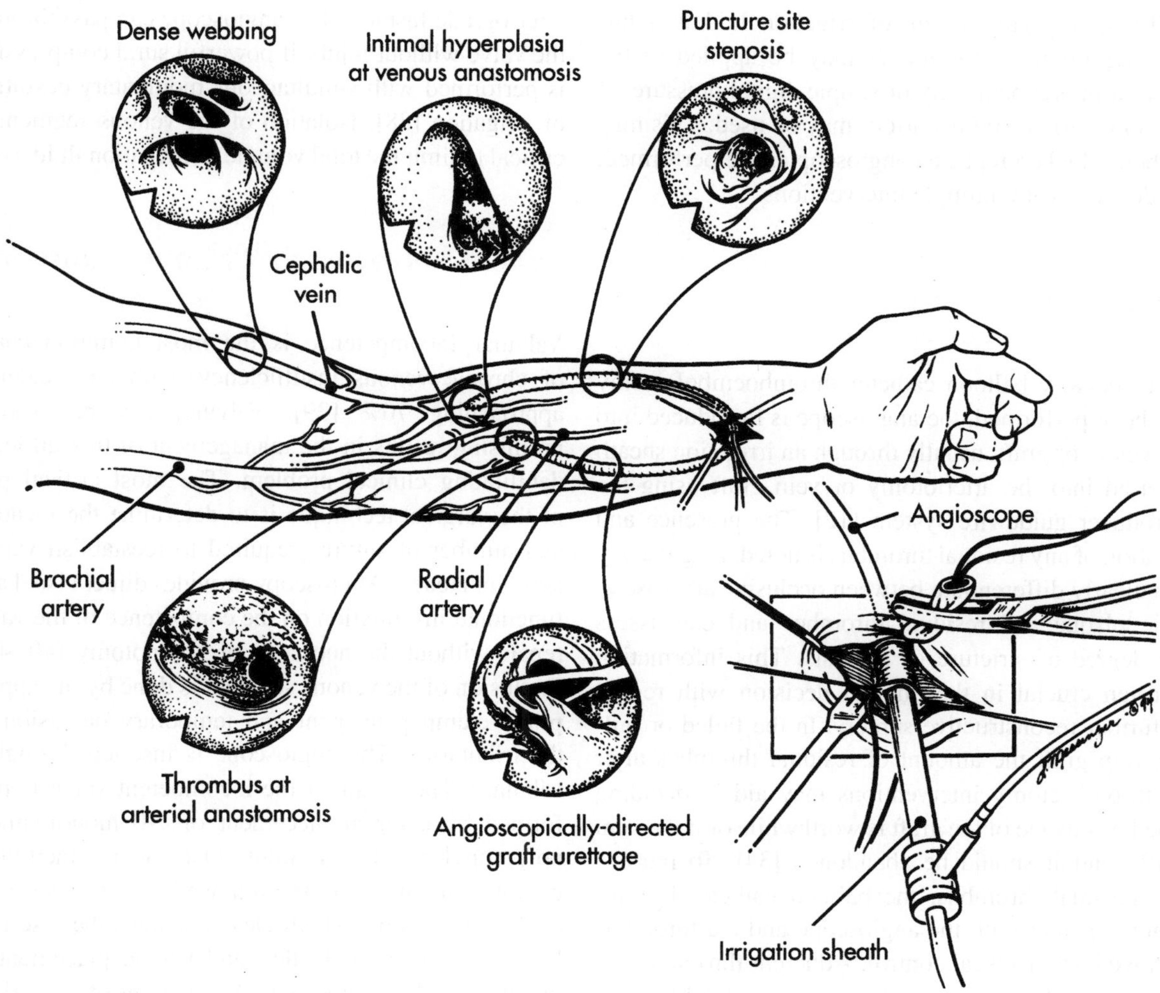

Fig. 9.7 Technique of angioscopy to evaluate a failed vascular access graft. Angioscope, inserted through a small skin incision and a transverse graft arteriotomy, is directed toward venous and arterial anastomoses to evaluate the graft, both anastomoses, and native vessels. If additional sites of pathology are localized, direct limited exposures are facilitated by the light of the angioscope shining through the skin. Occlusive lesions can be removed under direct vision using a Kevorkian-Young curette (from Hölzenbein et al. [35], with permission. © International Society of Endovascular Specialists)

leakage of irrigation fluid around the angioscope after insertion. A transverse incision is made in the anterior wall of the graft. Thrombectomy of the venous limb is generally performed first to take advantage of the lack of bleeding from the occluded arterial limb. The arterial limb is approached only after completion of all manipulations on the venous limb. The angioscope is then introduced through an irrigation sheath and passed through the graft, through the anastomosis, and into the runoff vein. The extent and location of any endoluminal pathology, completeness of the thrombectomy, or other endoluminal intervention are determined. Repeat angioscopic examination after each manipulation may be performed. On occasion, the light of the angioscope shining through the skin may serve as a guide to direct further exposure of the graft or autogenous vessel at the site of a particular abnormality. This allows much of the revision surgical procedure to be performed through separate small skin and graft incisions, limits surgical exposure of the graft and extent of the surgery, and eliminates the need for general anesthesia. In addition, to monitor thrombus removal with the various thrombectomy catheters, angioscopy may be used to direct removal of the excessively thickened intimal lining causing stenosis of the graft with a curette or any other interventional device.

To minimize the volume of irrigation fluid used during angioscopy, a tourniquet may be applied to the upper arm preoperatively or simple digital pressure on the upper arm or inflow artery may be used. This may be helpful when repeated angioscopies are performed, particularly with multiple interventions.

Thromboembolectomy

After Fogarty balloon catheter thromboembolectomy has been performed, the angioscope is introduced into the vessel or graft, usually through an irrigation sheath inserted into the arteriotomy or vein graft using the introducer guidewire system [12]. The presence and location of any residual thrombus is noted. Angioscopy can clearly differentiate between occlusive atherosclerotic plaque and residual thrombus and can assess the degree of stricture or stenosis. This information is often crucial in the clinical decision with regard to further reconstructive surgery. In the failed or failing vein graft the amount of residual thrombus after all thrombectomy interventions may aid in deciding whether salvage of the graft is worthwhile or if the vein graft conduit should be abandoned [34]. To retrieve any residual thrombus, the balloon catheter is reinserted together with the angioscope and the thrombus removed under visual control. Adherent thrombus can be removed from the vessel wall with special balloon catheters or directly with various endoluminal microforceps. Using an occlusion balloon, the occluded limb of an aortofemoral bypass graft may be safely thrombectomized and the cause of the occlusion, most commonly an anastomotic stenosis, corrected through a small groin incision [36].

Venous Thrombectomy

Angioscopy has been used for monitoring completeness of venous thrombectomy [37]. After the disobliteration of the iliac and femoral veins via transfemoral thrombectomy, the proximal common iliac vein is isolated with a proximal occlusion catheter and large tributaries isolated and controlled. Antegrade angioscopy is performed until the occlusion catheter is observed and the venous thrombectomy completed. When indicated, the proximal femoral vein can be examined in a retrograde fashion. The angioscope can pass through the valve without injury if powerful sural compression is performed with simultaneous momentary cessation of irrigation [38]. Isolation of the venous segment is critical to limit the total volume of irrigation fluid used.

Venous Valve Repair Without Venotomy

Valvular incompetence is the most common cause of chronic venous insufficiency, with an incidence approaching 70% [39]. Valvuloplasty has shown promising results in the management of this difficult, debilitating clinical problem. The most critical part of the surgical technique is to determine the location and number of sutures required to reestablish valvular competence. Angioscopy provides direct visual and functional information on the competence of the valve repair without the necessity of a venotomy [40, 41]. Exclusion of the venous segment is done by the appropriate clamp placement and temporary occlusion of the tributaries. The angioscope is inserted through a tributary. The repair of the incompetent valve is performed by external placement of 7-0 monofilament polypropylene sutures. Suture placement is facilitated by transillumination of the vein wall by the light source of the angioscope, which clearly defines the insertion lines of each valve leaflet, and needle placement is directed by the angioscope. Assessment of the valvular competence is done after placement and tying of each suture, using the irrigation fluid infused through the angioscope to oppose the valve leaflets.

Percutaneous Applications of Angioscopy

Depending on the size of angioscope, introducer sheaths from 6 to 9 Fr can be used. Percutaneous angioscopy may be performed through a direct antegrade needle stick of the superficial femoral artery just below the bifurcation of common femoral artery using the introducer sheath [11, 13, 16] or a small angioscope [<1 mm outer diameter (OD)] through an angioplasty catheter passed over the aortic bifurcation into the contralateral superficial femoral artery. The angioscope is guided to the endoluminal lesions identified on fluoroscopy using standard contrast studies. Placing a radiopaque marker on the tip of the angioscope is useful. Proximal occlusion can be achieved by using a sheath large enough to occlude the superficial femoral artery, external compression of the femoral artery, or an angioplasty balloon inflated proximal to the angioscope. Irrigation is through the sheath or angioplasty catheter with the variable flow of between 300 and 400 ml/min using the dedicated angioscopy irrigation pump. To minimize the irrigation fluid requirements, a tourniquet may be applied below the knee joint to reduce the collateral circulation.

Summary

Since performing our first clinical angioscopy, we have performed intraoperative angioscopy during more than 1,500 revascularization procedures. Our clinical studies have been directed to systematically evaluate this technology and evaluate its place in the modern practice of vascular surgery. As outlined in this chapter, angioscopy is a useful clinical tool for the modern practicing vascular surgeon. It provides endoluminal information on the vasculature remote from the surgical site and exposed vessels, which enhances the intraoperative decision-making process. Angioscopy has proven a most valuable tool for monitoring the technical success of reconstructive surgery, for quality control of the graft conduit, and for providing a reliable method to assess the effectiveness of endoluminal surgery and interventions.

References

1. Vollmar J, Storz L: Vascular endoscopy, *Surg Clin North Am* 54:111–122, 1974.
2. Towne J, Bernhard V: Vascular endoscopy: an adjunct to carotid surgery, *Stroke* 8:569–571, 1977.
3. Towne J, Bernhard V: Technique of intraoperative endoscopic evaluation of occluded aortofemoral grafts following thrombectomy, *Surg Gynecol Obstet* 148:87–89, 1979.
4. Shure D, Gregoratos G, Moser K: Fiberoptic angioscopy: role in the diagnosis of chronic pulmonary artery obstruction, *Ann Intern Med* 103:844–850, 1985.
5. Spears J, Marais H, Serur J et al.: In vivo coronary angioscopy, *J Am Coll Cardiol* 1:1311–1314, 1983.
6. Grundfest W, Litvack F, Sherman T et al.: Delineation of peripheral and coronary detail by intraoperative angioscopy, *Ann Surg* 202:394–400, 1985.
7. Grundfest W, Litvack F, Glick D et al.: Intraoperative decisions based on angioscopy in peripheral vascular surgery, *Circulation* 78(suppl I):113–117, 1988.
8. Sherman T, Litvack F, Grundfest W et al.: Coronary angioscopy in patients with unstable angina pectoris, *N Engl J Med* 315:913–919, 1986.
9. Seeger J, Abela G: Angioscopy as an adjunct to arterial reconstructive surgery: a preliminary report, *J Vasc Surg* 4:315–320, 1986.
10. Mehigan J, Olcott C: Videoangioscopy as an alternative to intraoperative arteriography, *Am J Surg* 152:139–145, 1986.
11. Beck A: Percutaneous angioscopy. First reports on percutaneous transluminal angioplasty and local lysis under angioscopic conditions, *Radiologe* 27:555–559, 1987.
12. White G, White R, Kopchok B et al.: Angioscopic thromboembolectomy: preliminary observations with a recent techique, *J Vasc Surg* 7:318–325, 1988.
13. Lee G, Morelli R, Long J et al.: Combined laser-thermal and atherectomy treatment of peripheral arterial occlusion: documentation by angioscopy and angiography, *Am Heart J* 118:1324–1327, 1989.
14. Mehigan J, DeCampli W: Angioscopic control of carotid endarterectomy. In Ahn SS, Moore WS, editors: *Endovascular Surgery*, ed. 2, Philadelphia, 1992, WB Saunders.
15. Raithel D, Kasprzak P: Angioscopy after carotid endarterectomy, *Ann Chir Gynaecol* 81:192–195, 1992.
16. Dietrich E, Yoffe B, Kiessling J et al.: Angioscopy in endovascular surgery: recent technical advances to enhance intervention selection and failure analysis, *Angiology* 43:1–10, 1992.
17. Silverman S, Mladinich C, Hawkins I et al.: The use of carbon dioxide gas to displace flowing blood during angioscopy, *J Vasc Surg* 10:313–317, 1989.
18. Miller A, Lipson W, Isaacson J et al.: Intraoperative angioscopy: principles of irrigation and description of a new dedicated irrigation pump, *Am Heart J* 118:391–399, 1989.
19. Miller A, Campbell D, Gibbons G et al.: Routine intraoperative angioscopy in lower extremity revascularization, *Arch Surg* 124:604–608, 1989.
20. Miller A, Stonebridge P, Jepsen S et al.: Continued experience with intraoperative angioscopy for monitoring infrainguinal bypass grafting, *Surgery* 109:286–293, 1991.
21. Miller A, Stonebridge P, Tsoukas A et al.: Angioscopically directed valvulotomy: a new valvulotome and technique, *J Vasc Surg* 13:813–821, 1991.
22. Kwolek C, Miller A, Stonebridge P et al.: Safety of saline irrigation for angioscopy: results of a prospective randomized trial, *Ann Vasc Surg* 6:62–68, 1992.
23. Miller A, Jepsen S: Technique of intraoperative angioscopy in lower extremity revascularization. In Bergan J, Yao J, editors: *Techniques in arterial surgery*, Philadelphia, 1990, WB Saunders.
24. Mehigan J: Angioscopic preparation of the in situ saphenous vein for arterial bypass technical considerations. In White G, White R, editors: *Angioscopy: vascular and coronary applications*, St. Louis, 1989, Mosby.

25. Miller A, Jepsen S, Stonebridge P et al.: New angioscopic findings in graft failure after infrainguinal bypass grafting, *Arch Surg* 125:749–755, 1990.
26. Stierli P, Aeberhard P: Angioscopy-guided semi-closed technique for in site bypass with a novel flushing valvulotome: early results, *J Vasc Surg* 15:546–548, 1992.
27. White G, White R, Kopock G et al.: Endoscopic intravascular surgery removes intraluminal flaps, dissections, and thrombus, *J Vasc Surg* 11:280–288, 1990.
28. Marcaccio E, Miller A, Tannenbaum G et al.: Angioscopically directed interventions improve arm vein bypass grafts, *J Vasc Surg* 17:994–1004, 1993.
29. La Muraglia G, Cambria R, Brewster D et al.: Angioscopy facilitates a closed technique for in-situ vein bypass, *J Vasc Surg* 12:601–604, 1990.
30. Maini B, Andrews L, Salimi T et al.: A modified, angioscopically assisted technique for in situ saphenous vein bypass: impact on patency, complications, and length of stay, *J Vasc Surg* 17:1041–1049, 1993.
31. Rosenthal D, Cickson C, Rodriguez FL et al.: Infrainguinal endovascular in situ saphenous vein bypass: ongoing results, *J Vasc Surg* 20:389–395, 1994.
32. Miller A, Marcaccio E, Tannenbaum G et al.: Comparison of angioscopy and angiography for monitoring infrainguinal bypass grafts: results of a prospective randomized trial, *J Vasc Surg* 17:382–398, 1992.
33. Gaunt M, Naylor A, Ratliff D et al.: Role of completion angioscopy in detecting technical error after carotid endarterectomy, *Br J Surg* 81:42–44, 1994.
34. Hölzenbein T, Miller A, Tannenbaum G et al.: Role of angioscopy in reoperation for the failing or failed infrainguinal vein bypass graft, *Ann Vasc Surg* 8:74–91, 1994.
35. Hölzenbein T, Miller A, Gottlieb M et al.: The role of routine angioscopy in vascular access surgery, *J Endovasc Surg* 2:10–25, 1995.
36. White J, Haas K, Comerota A: An alternative method of salvaging occluded suprainguinal bypass grafts with operative angioscopy and endovascular intervention, *J Vasc Surg* 18:922–931, 1993.
37. Vollmar J, Hutschenreiter S: Vascular endoscopy for venous thrombectomy. In Ahn SS,Moore WS editors: *Endovascular surgery*, ed. 2, Philadelphia, 1992, WB Saunders.
38. Woelfle K, Bruijnen H, Zuegel N et al.: Technique and results of vascular endoscopy in arterial and venous reconstructions, *Ann Vasc Surg* 6:347–356, 1992.
39. Raju S, Fredericks R: Valve reconstruction procedures for nonobstructive venous insufficiency: rationale, techniques, and results in 107 procedures with two- to eight-year follow-up, *J Vasc Surg* 7:301–310, 1988.
40. Gloviczki P, Merrell S, Bower T: Femoral vein valve repair under direct vision without venotomy: a modified technique with use of angioscopy, *J Vasc Surg* 14:645–648, 1991.
41. Welch H, McLaughlin R, O'Donnell T Jr: Femoral vein valvuloplasty: intraoperative angioscopic evaluation and hemodynamic improvement, *J Vasc Surg* 16:694–700, 1992.

Duplex-Guided Balloon Angioplasty from the Carotid to the Plantar Arteries

10

Enrico Ascher, Anil Hingorani, and Natalie Marks

Over the last 12 years, our group has explored advantages and limitations of preoperative duplex arteriography of lower extremities as a sole imaging modality [1, 2]. This experience has taught us that duplex scanning offers multiple unique features such as (1) arterial visualization regardless of its patency, (2) imaging of the arterial wall, (3) real-time visualization in the presence of limb motion, (4) up to five times magnification, (5) instant precise measurements, and (6) readily available various hemodynamic parameters such as flow direction, velocity, and waveform. These distinctive features have manifested into the use of duplex imaging for guidance of various venous and arterial therapies such as endovenous procedures and thrombin injection of pseudoaneurysms and have helped to establish the field of interventional vascular ultrasound.

The preliminary experiments with transcutaneous ultrasound in the guidance of infrainguinal arterial procedures reported by Ahmadi et al. [3] and Ramaswami et al. [4] were the impetus for us to further extend this approach. The implementation of this exciting and novel technique approach for endovascular interventions at our institution proved to be viable, safe, and effective. Over the last 5 years we were able to complete duplex-guided lower extremity angioplasties of femoral–popliteal arterial segment in 360 cases, infrapopliteal arteries in 80 cases, and infrainguinal arterial bypasses in an additional 47 cases [5–9]. In addition, we successfully used duplex-guided interventions to treat 40 non-maturing or failing upper extremity arteriovenousfistulas [10, 11].

E. Ascher (✉)
Director, Division of Vascular Surgery, Department of Surgery, Maimonides Medical Center, NY, USA

Duplex-assisted balloon angioplasties and stenting of 41 internal carotid arteries represent yet another unique application of this approach [12, 13]. Herein, we describe our experience with these procedures.

Infrainguinal Arterial Angioplasty

Preoperative Evaluation

In our institution, arterial balloon angioplasty is offered to patients based on the results of preoperative duplex imaging only. Preoperative duplex arteriography in our Intersocietal Commission for the Accreditation of Vascular Laboratories (ICAVL) accredited vascular laboratory is performed by experienced registered vascular technologists (RVT) and includes assessment of pattern and extent of occlusive disease in the femoral–popliteal arterial segment as well as infrapopliteal arteries. Aortoiliac stenoses are ruled out by analysis of the common femoral artery (CFA) spectral waveform. Biphasic or monophasic waveform of the CFA warrants duplex assessment of the aortoiliac segment. Those with triphasic waveform in the CFA do not require further evaluation. Patients with significant ipsilateral suprainguinal stenoses undergo adjunctive iliac balloon angioplasty.

The Intersociety Consensus (TASC) classification can be used for morphological description of femoral–popliteal lesions. The length of the occluded and stenotic lesions is measured knowing that a L7-4 MHz probe foot has a length of 4 cm and by adding lengths of isolated images or by marking the beginning and end of the lesion on the skin using duplex image and measuring it with a tape.

T.J. Fogarty, R.A. White (eds.), *Peripheral Endovascular Interventions*,
DOI 10.1007/978-1-4419-1387-6_10, © Springer Science+Business Media, LLC 1998, 2010

Technique

It is essential that duplex-guided procedures be performed by experienced RVT with an extensive expertise in preoperative duplex arteriography. Guidance of balloon angioplasty procedures requires the technologist to be gowned and gloved and the duplex scanner's keyboard covered by a sterile film. We routinely used an HDI 5000 scanner with SonoCT feature (Philips Medical Systems, Bothell, WA). A variety of scan heads inserted into a sterile plastic sleeve with coupling gel were used to insonate the arteries according to the anatomic location and depth. Generally, the arteries on the thigh and calf (1–4 cm deep) are being assessed with a 7-4 MHz linear probe. More superficial (<1 cm deep) arterial structures at the ankle and foot can be insonated by a 15-7 MHz compact linear "hockey stick" probe. The addition of a curved 5-2 MHz transducer is necessary for visualization of deeper arterial segments including the distal superficial femoral artery (SFA) and above-the-knee popliteal artery (PA).

All duplex-guided procedures in our institution were performed in the operating room under local anesthetic infiltration of the puncture site and light sedation. One of the distinct differences of the proposed technique is the possibility to perform the majority of the procedures via an ipsilateral puncture. The ipsilateral approach for infrainguinal interventions has several advantages: (1) it is shorter and therefore easier to manipulate endovascular devices, (2) it avoids potential difficulties and complications of aortoiliac disease and variable anatomy, (3) and prevents potential complications associated with contralateral groin puncture. Additionally, duplex guidance helps avoid dissections, posterior wall puncture, bleeding, and other potential problems associated with blind arterial puncture.

Ipsilateral CFA access is possible in the majority of cases. In our experience with 360 femoral–popliteal angioplasties, 328 (91%) cases were performed via ipsilateral CFA while contralateral cannulation was necessary in the remaining 32 cases (9%). Contralateral CFA access required fluoroscopy (alone in six cases and with 10–20 ml of contrast in the remaining 26 cases) for the ipsilateral common iliac artery cannulation. Contraindications to antegrade ultrasound-guided CFA puncture are high bifurcation and/or deep location (≥3 cm from the skin).

After successful ipsilateral CFA cannulation, a guidewire is directed into the proximal SFA, across the diseased segment(s) and parked at the tibioperoneal trunk or one of the tibial arteries under duplex guidance. In cases of contralateral CFA access, fluoroscopy is used to cross the aortic bifurcation. After the guidewire is identified by duplex in the ipsilateral proximal CFA, the procedure should be continued with duplex guidance as described above.

In cases of femoral and/or popliteal occlusions, a directional catheter supporting the guidewire is pointed against the wall, 3–5 mm proximal to the occlusion, to initiate subintimal dissection. Wire loop formation is confirmed by duplex imaging. The advancement of the wire through the occlusion is followed to the patent arterial segment identified by the presence of color signal in the lumen. Reentry attempts should be initiated within the first 1–2 cm after flow reconstitution to minimize the length of angioplasty. The arterial segment with the least amount of calcification and thinnest intima-media layer should be preferably chosen for reentry. If the guidewire fails to enter the true lumen after several attempts, the directional catheter should be advanced and pointed toward the lumen for additional wire support. Reentry efforts are usually cautiously continued to prevent extension of the dissection plane to the popliteal artery below the knee. We make every effort to spare the outflow artery for possible femoral–popliteal bypass in the case of subintimal angioplasty failure. After the guidewire enters the true arterial lumen, its position is confirmed with color flow imaging in both longitudinal and transverse views.

The diseased segment(s) is then balloon-dilated under duplex guidance (Figs. 10.1, 10.2, 10.3, 10.4,

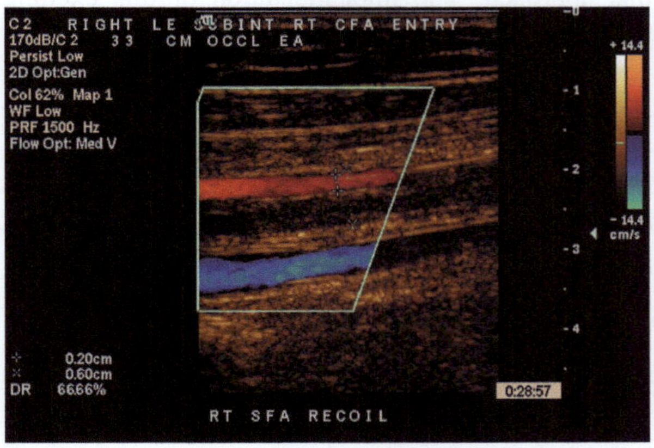

Fig. 10.1 Intraoperative color image of the distal superficial femoral artery after subintimal angioplasty demonstrates significant plaque recoil creating moderate (66.66%) stenosis

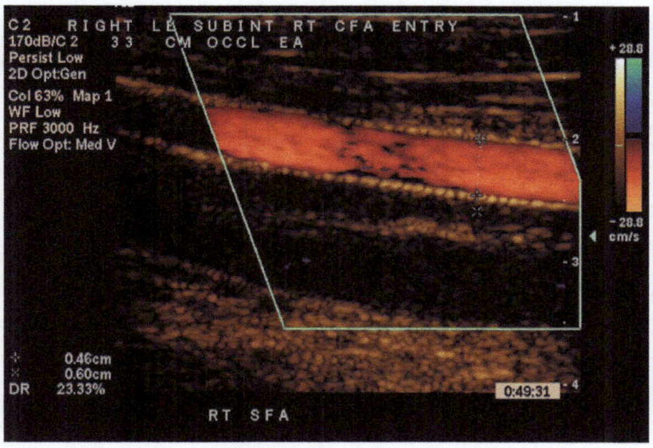

Fig. 10.2 Intraoperative color image of the superficial femoral artery depicted in Fig. 10.1 after placement of self-expandable stent. Residual stenosis (23.33%) created by the recoiled plaque is not significant after stent placement

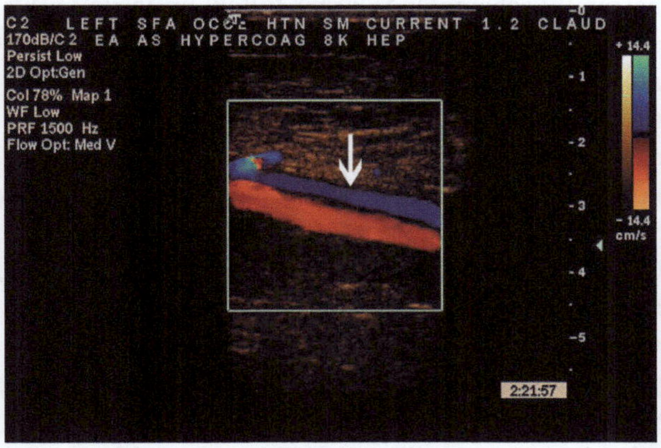

Fig. 10.3 Intraoperative color image of the superficial femoral artery after subintimal angioplasty demonstrated long arterial dissection (*arrow*). Dissection is confirmed by bidirectional flow pattern with antegrade flow (*red*) in the true arterial lumen and retrograde flow (*blue*) in the false lumen

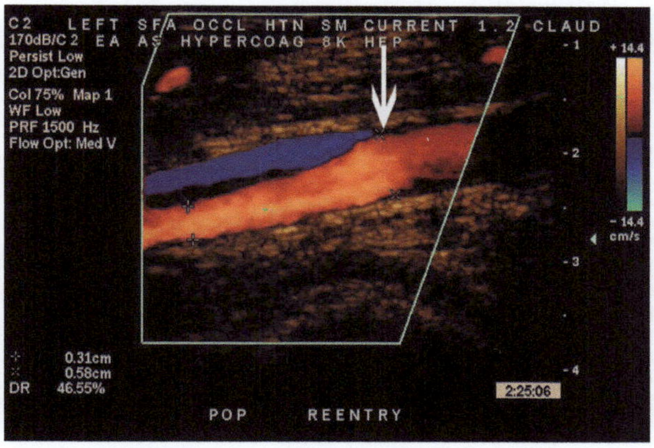

Fig. 10.4 Intraoperative color image of the popliteal artery depicted the origin (*arrow*) of the arterial dissection shown in Fig. 10.3. This dissection creating 46.55% diameter reduction originated at the point of the wire reentry to the true arterial lumen

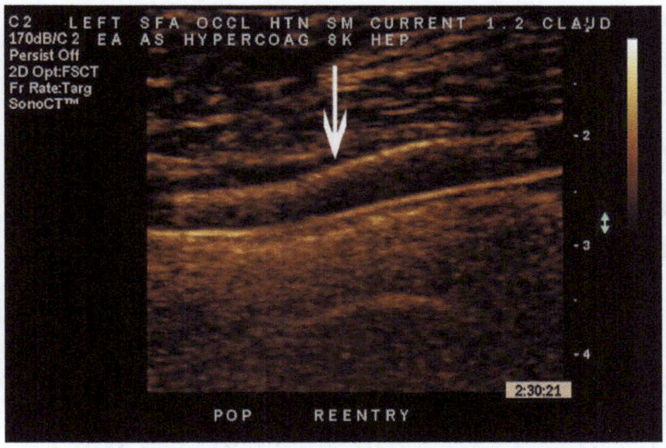

Fig. 10.5 Intraoperative B-Mode image of the self-expandable stent (*arrow*) placed in the popliteal artery to seal the beginning of the long arterial dissection

10.5, and 10.6). Balloon diameter and length can be chosen according to direct arterial measurements obtained by duplex. Duplex image magnification (up to five times) and small error of the measurements (0.1 mm) provide precise measurements of the arterial diameter as well as lumen and wall thickness and therefore eliminate over- or under-sizing of balloons and stents.

A detailed duplex examination of the entire treated segment should be performed following removal of the balloon angioplasty catheters to identify possible areas of residual disease, thrombi, plaque dissection, or recoil. Residual disease and plaque recoils are identified as luminal defects partially obstructing the flow. Partial or occlusive arterial thrombi have an anechoic intraluminal appearance. Dissections can be diagnosed by identification of bidirectional flow pattern or divided flow with clearly different velocities as shown by color Doppler. All suspected abnormalities are carefully evaluated by direct diameter reduction measurement on color and/or power images as well as spectral analyses including peak systolic velocities (PSV) ratios. Luminal defects of >30% diameter reduction with PSV ratio ≥2 across the stenosis can be treated by placement of self-expanding stents under duplex guidance. Significant technical defects were treated with a variety of stents (from one to five per case) in 233/342 cases (68%) in our series. Finally,

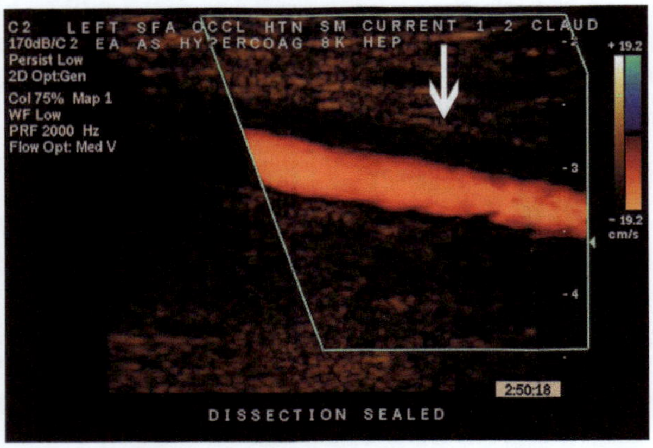

Fig. 10.6 Intraoperative color image of the same superficial femoral artery segment depicted in Fig. 10.3 after stent placement at the origin of dissection in the popliteal artery. No flow noted in the false arterial lumen at this time, former dissection is thrombosed (*arrow*)

infrapopliteal arteries are insonated to reassure the absence of embolization or thrombosis.

Technical Success and Predictors of Technical Failure of Femoral–popliteal Duplex-Guided Balloon Angioplasty

The overall technical success in our experience was 95% (342/360 cases), while it was 100% for TASC class A and B lesions, 96% (236/245 cases) for TASC class C lesions, and 74% for TASC class D lesions (26/35 cases) ($p < 0.0001$). Of the 17 cases where subintimal SFA/PA duplex-guided balloon angioplasty (DGBA) failed, only 2 (12%) were successfully completed under fluoroscopic-guidance. Comparison of multiple risk factors such as age, presence of diabetes (12%), CRI (11%), a combination of both diabetes and CRI (13%), or hemodialysis (38%) revealed that only hemodialysis was a statistically significant predictive factor of technical failure for duplex-guided subintimal angioplasties with $p < 0.04$.

Thromboembolic Complications

It was encouraging to note that some of the complications associated with balloon angioplasty, such as embolization or thrombosis, could be accurately identified by duplex examination and successfully corrected under duplex guidance. Completion duplex scans of the treated segment and infrapopliteal arteries were identified in 10 (2.9%) cases as thromboemboli. The proximal thrombus end was located at the below-the-knee popliteal artery in two cases, tibioperoneal trunk in seven cases, and peroneal artery in the remaining case. Six of these cases were treated with duplex-guided suction thrombectomy and intra-arterial pulse-sprayed infusion of thrombolytic agent and the remaining four cases resolved after thrombolysis only.

Follow-Up, Patency, and Limb Salvage

Arterial duplex scans are routinely performed before hospital discharge and during follow-up visits in our office at 1 month after the procedure and every 3–4 months thereafter. Severe recurrent stenoses are identified by arterial diameter reduction ≥70% measured and local PSV step-up of >3. The absence of color or power in the arterial lumen documents total occlusion.

The mean duration of follow-up was 12 ± 8.3 (range 1–41) months. Six-month patency rates by log rank analysis for TASC class A, B, C, and D lesions were 90, 74, 71, and 64%, respectively. Twelve-month patency rates for TASC class A, B, C, and D lesions were 90, 59, 52, and 46%, respectively. Overall limb salvage rates were 94 and 90% at 6 and 12 months, respectively (two amputations).

Adjunctive Infrapopliteal Balloon Angioplasty

Endovascular interventions for the infrapopliteal vessels are not widely accepted as the standard of care [14–16]. The reluctance to treat tibial vessels originates mostly from the limited patency rates achieved with this technique and uncertain long-term results. We believe that infrapopliteal balloon angioplasty may be beneficial in several settings: (1) run-off improvement during balloon angioplasty of femoral–popliteal arterial segment, (2) in patients with critical ischemia and multiple co-morbidities unsuitable for bypass surgery, and (3) in patients with inadequate autogenous vein for bypass surgery.

Our overall experience with infrapopliteal angioplasties included 80 arteries in 54 cases (15% of all infrainguinal arterial balloon angioplasty cases). All infrapopliteal angioplasties were attempted after completion of more proximal femoral–popliteal procedures in order to improve the run-off. Seventy cases (88%) had arterial stenoses (48 tibioperoneal trunks, 10 peroneal arteries, seven posterior tibial arteries, and five anterior tibial arteries). The remaining 10 cases (12%) had arterial occlusions (four tibioperoneal trunks, five peroneal arteries, and one anterior tibial artery). Low-profile balloons of an appropriate diameter (2–4 mm) and length were used for the infrapopliteal angioplasties. The diseased arterial segments are balloon-dilated starting from the most distal lesion.

A careful completion infrapopliteal duplex examination should be performed in each case for detection of possible plaque recoils, dissections, or distal thromboemboli. Hemodynamically significant plaque recoils (diameter reduction of >30%, a peak systolic velocity step-up of >2, or both) can be successfully treated with cutting balloons. Immediate technical success was achieved in 77 of 80 treated infrapopliteal arteries, for an overall success rate of 96%. Failure of the wire to cross two stenotic peroneal lesions and one occlusion of the peroneal artery accounted for the remaining three failure cases. Residual defects after angioplasty were documented in 10 (13%) of 77 infrapopliteal arteries. However, none of these cases was hemodynamically significant by duplex criteria. The 6- and 12-month patency rates of balloon-dilated infrapopliteal arteries were 78 and 66%, respectively.

Duplex-Guided Angioplasty of Infrainguinal Arterial Bypass Grafts

The long-term patency of lower extremity bypasses and limb salvage rates are significantly dependent upon diagnosis and timely repair of recurrent stenoses [17–19]. Modern duplex scanners provide reliable diagnostic information by identification of the exact location and degree of bypass stenosis. Endovascular treatment of failing bypasses has been proved to have comparable results and postprocedure patency rates as compared to a surgical approach [20–26]. While fluoroscopic-guidance for these treatments is considered standard, one of the major limitations of balloon angioplasty procedures under fluoroscopic-guidance is lack of hemodynamic information.

Duplex guidance offers several indispensable technical advantages. Measurements of graft and arterial depth and diameter and precise localization of the stenotic lesions in reference to the anastomotic sites facilitate the best access site selection for the procedure. Direct visualization of the access site assures accurate entry of the arterial puncture needle and prevention of dissections, posterior wall bleeding, and other arterial injuries. This technique is especially beneficial in obese patients and patients with previously operated groins in whom pulse identification becomes more difficult.

Patient Population

Forty-seven duplex-guided balloon angioplasty procedures were performed in 36 patients in our institution. Primary interventions were performed in 31 cases, first redo angioplasties in 11 cases, second redo angioplasties in three cases, third redo in one case, and fourth redo in the remaining case. Nineteen patients (53%) had renal insufficiency (serum creatinine level ≥1.5 mg/dl). Of the 47 attempted balloon angioplasties included in this study, 36 (77%) were performed in vein grafts and 11 (23%) were in polytetrafluoroethylene (PTFE) grafts. Nineteen autologous grafts were CFA to PA (7) and infrapopliteal (12) bypasses, 11 were SFA to PA (4) and infrapopliteal (7) bypasses, and the remaining six were PA to PA (3) and infrapopliteal (3) bypasses. Of the 11 prosthetic grafts, one was a femoral–femoral bypass, seven were CFA to popliteal (4) and infrapopliteal (3) bypasses, and the remaining three were superficial femoral artery to popliteal bypasses. Bypass operations were performed from 3 to 78 months prior to the current procedure (mean 28 ± 21 months).

Preoperative Evaluation

Diagnosis of a failing graft was made based on preoperative duplex scans performed during routine office follow-up visits in our vascular laboratory. The follow-up graft duplex scan protocol included insonation of the entire bypass conduit, infrainguinal inflow and outflow arteries for at least a 3 cm length proximal and distal to the anastomotic sites. After color and/or power imaging in longitudinal plane, the following points were evaluated with spectral analysis: proximal artery, proximal anastomosis, proximal, mid- and distal bypass conduit, distal anastomosis, and distal artery. Any areas of color aliasing created by elevated velocities were also assessed for calculation of PSV step-up ratios in order to estimate the degree of stenosis. Biphasic or monophasic waveform detected in the inflow artery warranted insonation of the more proximal ipsilateral arteries extended up to the ipsilateral common iliac artery. Graft duplex scans identified at least one severe stenosis along the bypass conduit or in the native inflow and/or outflow arteries in all cases. Stenosis was characterized as severe when local diameter reduction was measured to be ≥70% on color or power image and the corresponding PSV step-up across the lesion was ≥3. Twenty-two balloon angioplasties (47%) were performed on a single stenosis, while the remaining 25 cases (53%) had a mean of 2.9 ± 1 stenoses (range 2–5). The most significant stenotic lesion was found to be at the proximal inflow artery in eight cases, bypass conduit in 26 cases, and distal outflow artery in the remaining 13 cases. The highest PSV at the areas of stenosis were recorded and compared before and after the procedure. Additionally, we routinely measure preoperative bypass volume flows (VF) × 3 in all cases and report the mean value. VF is automatically calculated by the scanner's software using color duplex image and spectral analysis at the non-tapered bypass segment with Doppler angle adjusted at 60° and with the sample volume equal or larger than the lumen outlined by the calipers.

Technique

All procedures were performed using the same technique as described above for the arterial infrainguinal duplex-guided balloon angioplasties. Overall, ipsilateral arterial access was possible in 34 cases (72%) and the remaining 13 cases required a contralateral femoral puncture. The femoral artery (15 ipsilateral and 13 contralateral) was used as an access site in 28 cases. The remaining 19 balloon angioplasty procedures were carried out through direct graft puncture (10 venous and 9 PTFE). Duplex scanning was the only imaging tool used to visualize and manipulate all endovascular instrumentation during the 34 procedures (72%) performed via the ipsilateral access. Five of 13 (38%) cases with contralateral CFA punctures in patients with elevated serum creatinine (≥1.5 mg/dl) did not require contrast use for the cannulation of their ipsilateral iliac artery which was completed with fluoroscopic-guidance only.

In all cases, the guidewire supported by a directional catheter of appropriate caliber was advanced from the ipsilateral femoral artery through the bypass conduit to the distal outflow artery under direct duplex visualization.

Duplex measurements of bypass or arterial diameter and lesion extension allowed the precise selection of balloons caliber and lengths. Cutting balloons used in 25 (48%) cases allowed us to successfully treat recoiling lesions.

Thorough completion duplex exams followed the removal of balloon angioplasty catheters in all cases. Sagittal and transverse planes of scanning were used for identification of residual stenoses or recoils. A unique feature of a real-time ultrasound image is hemodynamic monitoring of the intervention. Spectral waveform and PSV ratios are essential for assessment of hemodynamic significance of dissections or recoils. Technical success was defined as patency and absence of diameter reduction areas with a PSV ratio ≥2 along the bypass as well as inflow and outflow arteries. Whenever a PSV ratio ≥2 was registered suggesting residual stenosis or recoil >50%, repeat inflations of larger balloons (if allowed by the adjacent arterial or bypass diameter) or cutting balloons were applied to the corresponding location.

Bypass VF measurements were obtained immediately following completion of the procedure as described above for preoperative measurements. VF average value ± SD as well as ranges were recorded and compared with the preoperative data. There was no intraoperative contrast arteriograms performed after duplex-guided balloon angioplasty procedures in these patients (Figs. 10.7, 10.8, and 10.9).

Intraoperative Technical Success

Overall technical success in our experience was 98% (46/47 cases). One technical failure was encountered in the case of a popliteal-to-plantar vein bypass where

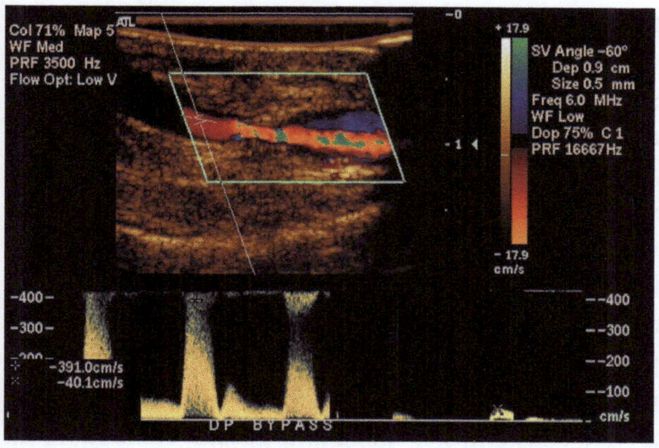

Fig. 10.7 Doppler spectral analysis obtained at the distal femoral to dorsalis pedis artery vein bypass graft demonstrated critical stenosis by PSV step-up ratio of 9.8 (391 cm/s over 40 cm/s)

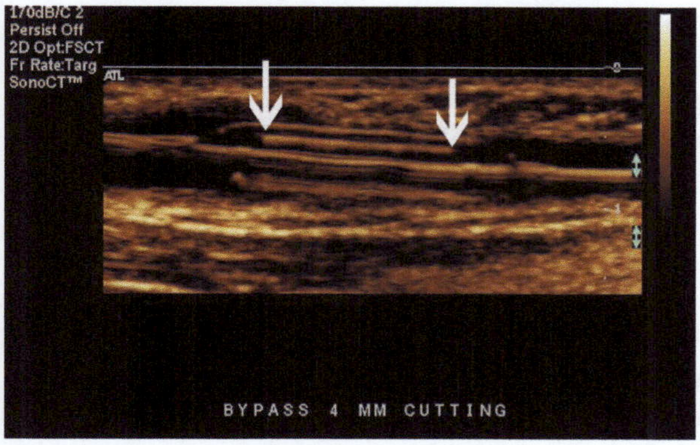

Fig. 10.8 Fully inflated cutting balloon (4 mm diameter × 15 mm length) placed across the stenosis depicted in Fig. 10.1. *White arrows* point to the balloon's blade

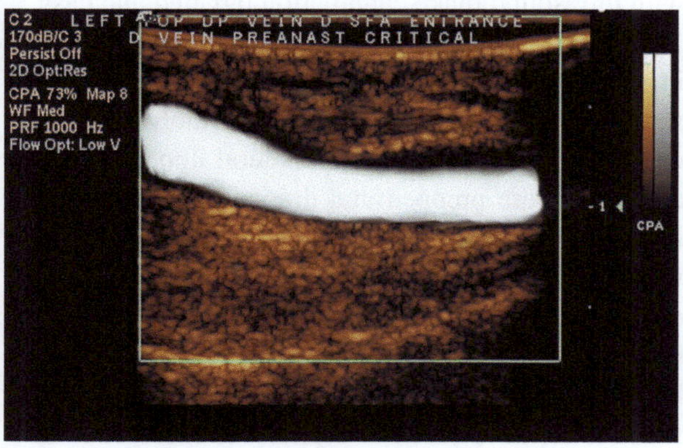

Fig. 10.9 Power Doppler image of the same location taken after balloon deflation and removal demonstrated complete stenosis resolution and absence of luminal defects in the bypass

the plantar artery anastomosis stenosis could not be crossed with the guidewire due to extreme tortuosity. Two cases of the inflow SFA dissections after balloon angioplasty were successfully treated by placement of self-expanding stents under duplex guidance. We did not use stents along the bypass conduit in any of these 47 cases.

Early Postoperative Complications

The overall local complication rate was 4% (two cases). In one case, the vein bypass developed a pseudoaneurysm at the site of rupture by a cutting balloon, which was repaired by patch angioplasty. In the second case, the patient was on Coumadin and had a persistent CFA pseudoaneurysm at the puncture site and required open repair after two unsuccessful thrombin injection attempts.

Duplex-Measured Hemodynamic Parameters

PSV obtained at the tightest stenosis level decreased in all 46 successful cases from a preoperative 408 ± 148 (range 191–807) cm/s to 97 ± 29 (range 53–152) cm/s after angioplasty procedures ($p < 0.0001$). Conversely, bypass VF in all cases increased from a preoperative 66 ± 38 (range 9–144) ml/min to postoperative 137 ± 72 (range 52–900) ml/min ($p < 0.0001$).

Patency and Limb Salvage Rate

The average follow-up was 29 ± 14 (range 3–46) months. Overall 6- and 12-month primary patency rates were 70 and 50%, respectively. Of the 10 patients whose procedures were performed via direct vein bypass access, 3 (30%) developed restenosis at the puncture site.

Duplex-Guided Angioplasty of Failing or Non-maturing Arteriovenous Fistulas

Arteriovenous (AV) hemodialysis access fistulas are known to be predisposed for development of multiple stenoses and eventual failure during their lifetime

[27–29]. Patency and functional ability of autologous AV fistulas have a tremendous influence on quality of life and survival for dialysis-dependent patients with chronic renal failure. Over the last decade, endovascular interventions have become the primary treatment option and almost entirely replaced surgical repair of failing or non-maturing permanent dialysis accesses [30–32]. Although contrast administration may not be harmful for individuals on hemodialysis, patients with borderline renal function and non-maturing AV accesses present a therapeutic challenge [33, 34]. Additionally, an allergy to contrast material makes the endovascular treatment option in some of these patients more challenging.

Despite very high flow creating a substantial current, real-time imaging facilitates accurate positioning and monitoring of the balloon location, in relation to the stenosis. Real-time Doppler spectral analysis assures confirmation of hemodynamic significance of the stenosis after balloon deflation, the presence of recoil, and the need for stenting. Residual stenoses due to elastic recoil were detected in 6 of 11 (55%) cases in this series. These recoiling lesions were successfully treated with cutting balloons in four cases, larger diameter conventional balloon in one case, and self-expanding stent implanted in the remaining case.

Patients

We performed 40 duplex-guided balloon angioplasties of autologous AV fistulas in 32 patients with chronic renal insufficiency. These were 17 males and 15 females with a mean age of 68.5 ± 10.3 (range 38–85) years. The 40 fistulas included 27 radial–cephalic, 12 brachial–cephalic, and one brachial–basilic. Of these, 17 accesses were failing and 23 were non-maturing fistulas in patients who were not yet on dialysis.

Preoperative Evaluation

Diagnosis of failing or non-maturing AV access was established based on a combination of physical examination (decreased thrill, present pulse), dialysis success (prolonged dialysis, suboptimal creatinine clearance, prolonged post-dialysis bleeding), and results of duplex scanning. Distinctive flow patterns such as very high velocities (often ≥ 500 cm/s) and major turbulence inherent to arteriovenous accesses present a diagnostic challenge for duplex surveillance. Although sonographic criteria indicating AV access abnormalities remain inconsistent, contemporary high-resolution ultrasound scanners and growing technical expertise among vascular technologists have established duplex scanning as a very reliable diagnostic tool in the detection of failing or non-maturing AV accesses. Duplex criteria defining compromised AV access included the presence of severe stenoses (>70%) measured on color image and confirmed by PSV ratio of ≥3 in the inflow artery, anastomosis, along the access conduit, or in the outflow vein. VF measurements were routinely obtained in a non-tapered fistula segment, at least 3 cm away from the anastomosis using the same method as described for infrainguinal bypasses. B-mode imaging of the entire fistula added information regarding the presence of luminal webs and "frozen" venous valves creating flow obstruction. The highest PSVs at the most significant stenosis were recorded and compared with postprocedure values. The mean number of stenoses was 1.9 ± 1.1 (range 1–5 per AV access).

Technique

Duplex-guidance of AV access interventions has multiple and distinctive advantages. Real-time visualization of an AV access stenoses and skin marking make possible identification of the most advantageous access site. This choice is made with consideration of multiple factors such as stenoses locations in relation to the anastomosis, fistula diameter, depth and tortuosity, and flow direction. Superficial location and direct visualization with ultrasound make cannulation targeted and easy.

The first 10 cases were performed in the operating room and the remaining 30 in the outpatient office setting. After the patient was comfortably positioned on the operating table, the ipsilateral upper extremity and neck were prepped and draped in the usual sterile manner. A Philips HDI 5000 scanner with SonoCT was feature used for all cases was placed on the side of intervention providing good monitor visibility for both the surgeon and the vascular technologist; the keyboard was covered with a sterile plastic cover. We found it useful to have two scan heads enclosed in sterile plastic and simultaneously available on the field due to anatomic and hemodynamic features inherent to an AV access. A CL 15-7 MHz transducer was used for insonation of superficial structures (<2 cm deep) and an L 7-4 MHz probe was used for deeper (≥2 cm) objects and for measurements of very high velocities present in the AV access.

We were able to complete all procedures via ipsilateral access under local anesthesia. All AV accesses were cannulated under duplex guidance at least 5 cm away from the most proximal stenosis. We attempted to select the access site proximal to the stenosis to use high AV access blood flow as an ally for wire manipulation through tortuosity. Unfortunately, this was possible in only three cases (8%). Two other cases required placement of two access sheaths in opposing directions to address venous and arterial stenoses. The remaining 35 cases were accessed via distal fistula puncture and the stenoses were addressed in a retrograde fashion.

Guidewire and then balloon catheter passage and inflation were performed under duplex guidance. Duplex measurements of arterial/venous lumen diameter adjacent to the stenosis assisted in determining balloon diameters. High-resolution B-Mode duplex images of the arterial and venous wall allow precise selection of proper diameter and length of balloons and stents. We found proper selection of balloons to be extremely important in prevention of AV access and vein overextension and avoidance of rupture while providing adequate dilation of stenotic areas. Ultrathin, symmetry, or sterling balloons of various sizes (3–8 mm) were used.

All cases had intraoperative completion duplex scans prior to access sheath removal. Adequacy of procedures was confirmed by the absence of residual stenoses on color and/or power image and measurements of VF and PSV ratios.

Technical Success

All procedures were completed under duplex guidance alone. One patient with small (3–4 mm in diameter) deep (2 cm from the skin level) brachial–basilic AV fistula had a completion contrast arteriogram which confirmed duplex findings. There were no intraoperative or postoperative local complications in these patients. Eight recoiling lesions (20%) were successfully treated with cutting balloons [35]. One additional patient (2.5%) with brachial–cephalic fistula and recoiling lesion at the junction of cephalic and axillary veins required duplex-guided placement of a self-expandable stent.

Comparison of Pre- and Postprocedure Duplex-Measured Hemodynamic Parameters

The mean preoperative PSVs obtained at the most significant stenosis was 563 ± 100 (range 370–760) cm/s and 200 ± 74 (range 62–354) cm/s after the procedure ($p < 0.0001$). Mean preoperative VF was 411 ± 279 (range 50–980) ml/min and 935 ± 360 (range 370–1,520) ml/min after balloon angioplasty ($p < 0.01$).

Complications and Mortality

One patient had a focal venous rupture with minimal bleeding controlled by manual pressure for 30 min. There were no 30-day mortalities; one patient with multi-organ failure expired 4 months after AV access angioplasty.

Duplex-Assisted Internal Carotid Artery Angioplasty

Superficial location of the cervical carotid arteries and up to five times magnification provided by contemporary duplex scanners result in exceptional clarity and detail resolution of ultrasound images. Duplex scanning of the carotid arteries has established itself as a reliable preoperative imaging modality for evaluation of degree, location, and extent of carotid stenoses in the neck [36, 37].

Hypothetically, the combination of clear-cut duplex images and real-time spectral analyses can offer data superior to the arteriography during multiple steps of the carotid balloon angioplasty and stenting (CBAS) procedure, including (1) selection of exact balloons and stents diameter and length, (2) exact position of the balloons and stents regardless of the artifacts created by the patient's breathing and movements, (3) confirmation of the apposition of the stent to the arterial wall, and (4) hemodynamic and B-mode verification of the procedure success.

Conversely, duplex insonation of the aortic arch is restricted by the chest wall anatomy, and fluoroscopic-guidance is necessary for manipulation of the wires and catheters in the aorta as well as cannulation of the aortic branches. One more maneuver requiring fluoroscopy is cerebral protection devices placement in the intracranial internal carotid artery (ICA).

The combination of both imaging modalities allowed us to perform a series of 41 duplex-assisted CBAS procedures described in the following section.

Patient Population

Forty patients who presented with severe (>70%) ICA stenoses underwent 41 carotid angioplasty and stenting procedures in our institution. Twenty-seven lesions (66%) were primary, 11 (27%) were recurrent stenoses after carotid endarterectomy (CEA), and the remaining three (7%) were restenoses after prior ICA angioplasties; 15 stenoses were symptomatic (37%).

There were 27 males (68%) and 13 females (32%) with a mean of 73 ±10 (range 44–92) years in this group. Twenty-four patients (59%) had elevated serum creatinine levels (≥1.5 mg/dl) and two additional patients had a history of allergy to the contrast material.

Preoperative Imaging

Carotid duplex mapping was the only pre-procedure imaging modality. The duplex mapping protocol included: (1) ICA stenosis degree measurements in sagittal and transverse planes using representative color and/or power images, (2) measurements of disease-free distal common carotid artery (CCA) and ICA lumen, (3) measurements of the plaque extension, (4) identification of severe tortuosity of the cervical ICA (angulation of >90°), and (5) reporting the CCA and ICA calcifications.

Technique

We performed all cases in the operating room with an ATL HDI 5000 scanner (Phillips Medical Systems, Bothell, WA) with SonoCT feature. A linear 7-4 MHz probe was chosen to insonate the CFA, CCA, and its branches. A digital mobile fluoroscopic imaging system with road-map capabilities was used in all cases. The duplex scanner was positioned contralateral to the C-arm at the patient's head; the monitor was turned to reassure the best visibility by the interventionist. It is absolutely crucial for the vascular technologist providing duplex imaging during this procedure to have extensive experience in duplex scanning of the carotid arteries and understanding of various carotid arterial pathologies, as well as their effect on duplex findings. One should not attempt or continue duplex guidance of the CBAS procedure unless the images of the diseased arterial segment and the carotid bifurcation are unquestionably excellent. ICA disease with severe arterial calcification creating shadows covering the lumen for >5 mm should not be treated with duplex-assisted CBAS.

The retrograde cannulation of the CFA was achieved under direct duplex visualization. Manipulation of the guidewire in the iliac arteries, abdominal, and thoracic aorta was performed with fluoroscopic assistance. The Bern selective angiographic catheter (Boston Scientific Corp) or Vitek cerebral catheter (Cook Inc, Bloomington, IN) was used in this series for selective catheterization of the ipsilateral CCA. After guidewire was visualized in the CCA by duplex, it was directed into the external carotid artery (ECA) using the same directional catheter. The next step was a Glidewire wire exchange for a stiff Amplatz (Boston Scientific Corp) wire to allow introduction of a 6F Shuttle SL introducer sheath (Cook Inc), which was positioned in the CCA about 2–3 cm proximal to the carotid bifurcation. All described maneuvers in the neck were completed with duplex visualization alone. The Filterwire embolic protection system (Boston Scientific Corp) was also negotiated into the distal cervical ICA beyond the stenosis under ultrasound-guidance. Further advancement of the filter, its placement and deployment 4–6 cm distal to the ICA stenosis was guided by fluoroscopy.

The next step was duplex-guided dilation of the ICA lesion with a 3 or 4 mm monorail balloon. Following this step, a biliary monorail Wallstent (Boston Scientific Corp) was positioned across the stenosis and deployed under ultrasound visualization A larger balloon (5 or 6 mm in diameter) was inflated once or twice to improve its apposition against the wall and eliminate any residual stenosis. Postprocedure completion Duplex scan confirmed: (1) wide patency of the native and stented CCA and ICA segments, (2) adequate stent apposition, and (3) absence of dissections, flaps, thrombi, or other potential abnormalities. Completion ICA arteriograms with a small amount of contrast material were performed as per the surgeon's preference for medicolegal reasons and correlation with duplex results.

Intraoperative Technical Findings

Completion duplex scans confirmed technical success in all cases. Aortic arch arteriograms were necessary to assist with difficult ipsilateral CCA cannulations in seven (17%) cases. Completion ICA arteriograms were obtained in 26 (63%) cases with 10–15 ml of contrast (Magnavist, Berlex Laboratories, Wayne, NJ, in four cases; Visipaque, Amersham Health, Princeton, NJ, in 22 cases) to validate the duplex findings. Adequate stent apposition and stenosis dilation were achieved in all cases. Biplanar postprocedural cerebral arteriograms performed in 30 patients (73%) for medicolegal reasons did not reveal any defects.

Postprocedure Mortality and Morbidity

There were no early (30-day) postprocedure mortalities. One patient had an ipsilateral stroke (2.4%) with almost complete clinical recovery in 4 months (mild residual hand weakness). This event occurred during the second balloon inflation in the stent. Nevertheless, intraoperative biplanar cerebral arteriogram did not reveal any abnormalities in this patient.

Follow-Up

All patients were advised to have duplex scans performed in our vascular clinic every 6 months after a CBAS procedure. The mean follow-up after duplex-assisted CBAS was 21 ± 14 (range 6–46) months. One patient developed restenosis at 9 months in the proximal end of the stent and underwent repeat duplex-assisted CBAS.

Summary

Unquestionably, duplex-guided arterial interventions are particularly beneficial for patients with allergies to contrast material and for those with chronic renal insufficiency. As vascular surgeons perform more endovascular procedures, they will have increased exposure to the deleterious effects of radiation [38]. Unfortunately, these effects are cumulative and permanent and may cause a delayed onset of symptoms. Our experience with the diverse duplex-guided and duplex-assisted vascular interventions leads us to believe that the duplex-guided angioplasties are safe, beneficial, and effective. The potential of these techniques grows exponentially with the advent of new and improved technology and the positive impact on patient care shows great promise. We anticipate that some of these procedures will eventually be performed in the vascular laboratory or in an office practice setting.

Acknowledgments Special acknowledgement for editorial assistance to Anne Ober.

References

1. Ascher E, Hingorani A, Markevich N, Costa T, Kallakuri S, Khanimoy Y: Lower extremity revascularization without preoperative contrast arteriography: experience with duplex ultrasound arterial mapping in 485 cases, *Ann Vasc Surg* 16(1):108–114, Epub 2002 Jan 17.
2. Ascher E, Hingorani A, Markevich N, Yorkovich W, Schutzer R, Hou A, Jacob T, Nahata S, Kallakuri S: Role of duplex arteriography as the sole preoperative imaging modality prior to lower extremity revascularization surgery in diabetic and renal patients, *Ann Vasc Surg* 18(4):433–439, July 2004.
3. Ahmadi R, Ugurluoglu A, Schillinger M, Katzenschlager R, Sabeti S, Minar E: Duplex ultrasound-guided femoropopliteal angioplasty; initial and 12-month results from a case controlled study, *J Endovasc Ther* 9(6):873–881, December 2002.
4. Ramaswami G, Al-Kutoubi A, Nicolaides AN, Dhanjil S, Vilkomerson D, Ferrara-Ryan M, Stansby G: Angioplasty of lower limb arterial stenoses under ultrasound guidance: single-center experience, *J Endovasc Surg* 6(1):52–58, February 1999.
5. Ascher E, Marks NA, Schutzer RW, Hingorani AP: Duplex-guided balloon angioplasty and stenting for femoropopliteal arterial occlusive disease: an alternative in patients with renal insufficiency, *J Vasc Surg* 42(6):1108–1113, December 2005.

6. Ascher E, Marks NA, Hingorani AP, Schutzer RW, Mutyala M: Duplex-guided endovascular treatment for occlusive and stenotic lesions of the femoral-popliteal arterial segment: a comparative study in the first 253 cases, *J Vasc Surg* 44(6):1230–1237, 2006.
7. Ascher E, Hingorani AP, Marks NA: Duplex-guided angioplasty of lower extremity arteries, *Perspect Vasc Endovasc Ther* 19(1):23–31, March 2007.
8. Ascher E, Marks NA, Hingorani AP, Schutzer RW, Nahata S: Duplex-guided balloon angioplasty and subintimal dissection of infrapopliteal arteries: early results with a new approach to avoid radiation exposure and contrast material, *J Vasc Surg* 42(6):1114–1121, December 2005.
9. Marks NA, Hingorani AP, Ascher E: Duplex-guided balloon angioplasty of failing infrainguinal bypass grafts, *Eur J Vasc Endovasc Surg* 32(2):176–181, August 2006.
10. Marks N, Ascher E, Higorani AP: Treatment of failing lower extremity arterial bypasses under ultrasound guidance, *Perspect Vasc Endovasc Ther* 19(1):34–39, March 2007.
11. Marks N, Ascher E, Hingorani AP: Duplex-guided repair of failing or nonmaturing arterio-venous access for hemodialysis, *Perspect Vasc Endovasc Ther* 19(1):50–55, March 2007.
12. Ascher E, Hingorani AP, Marks N: Duplex-assisted internal carotid artery balloon angioplasty, *Perspect Vasc Endovasc Ther* 19(1):41–47, March 2007.
13. Ascher E, Marks NA, Schutzer RW, Hingorani AP: Duplex-assisted internal carotid artery balloon angioplasty and stent placement: a novel approach to minimize or eliminate the use of contrast material, *J Vasc Surg* 41(3):409–415, March 2005.
14. Dorros G, Jaff MR, Dorros AM, Mathiak LM, He T: Tibioperoneal trunk (outflow lesion) angioplasty can be used as primary treatment in 235 patients with critical limb ischemia: five-year follow-up, *Circulation* 104:2057–2062, 2001.
15. Kudo T, Chandra FA, Ahn SS: The effectiveness of percutaneous transluminal angioplasty for the treatment of critical limb ischemia: a 10-year experience, *J Vasc Surg* 41(3):423–435, discussion 435, March 2005.
16. Clair DG, Dayal R, Faries PL, Bernheim J, Nowygrod R, Lantis JC 2nd, Beavers FP,, Kent KC: Tibial angioplasty as an alternative strategy in patients with limb-threatening ischemia, *Ann Vasc Surg* 19(1):63–68, January 2005.
17. Nguyen LL, Conte MS, Menard MT, Gravereaux EC, Chew DK, Donaldson MC, Whittemore AD, Belkin M: Infrainguinal vein bypass graft revision: factors affecting long-term outcome, *J Vasc Surg* 40(5):916–923, November 2004.
18. Bandyk DF, Bergamini TM, Towne JB, Schmitt DD, Seabrook GR: Durability of vein graft revision: the outcome of secondary procedures, *J Vasc Surg* 13(2):200–208, February 1991.
19. Sullivan TR Jr, Welch HJ, Iafrati MD, Mackey WC, O'Donnell TF Jr: Clinical results of common strategies used to revise infrainguinal vein grafts, *J Vasc Surg* 24(6):909–917, December 1996.
20. Calligaro KD, Syrek JR, Dougherty MJ, Rua I, McAffee-Bennett S, Doerr KJ, Raviola CA, DeLaurentis DA: Selective use of duplex ultrasound to replace preoperative arteriography for failing arterial vein grafts, *J Vasc Surg* 27(1):89–94, January 1998.
21. Dougherty MJ, Calligaro KD, DeLaurentis DA: The natural history of "failing" arterial bypass grafts in a duplex surveillance protocol, *Ann Vasc Surg* 12(3):255–259, May 1998.
22. van der Heijden FH, Legemate DA, van Leeuwen MS, Mali WP, Eikenboim BC: Value of duplex scanning in the selection of patients for percutaneous transluminal angioplasty, *Eur J Vasc Endovasc Surg* 7(1):71–76, January 1993.
23. Bandyk DF, Mills JL, Gahtan V, Esses GE: Intraoperative duplex scanning of arterial reconstructions: fate of repaired and unrepaired defects, *J Vasc Surg* 20:426–433, 1994.
24. Rzucidlo EM, Walsh DB, Powell RJ, Zwolak RM, Fillinger MF, Schermerhorn ML, Cronenwett JL: Prediction of early graft failure with intraoperative completion duplex ultrasound scan, *J Vasc Surg* 36(5):975–981, November 2002.
25. Avino AJ, Bandyk DF, Gonsalves AJ, Johnson BL, Black TJ, Zwiebel BR, Rahaim MJ, Cantor A: Surgical and endovascular intervention for infrainguinal vein graft stenosis, *J Vasc Surg* 29(1):60–70, January 1999.
26. Carlson GA, Hoballah JJ, Sharp WJ, Martinasevic M, Maiers Yelden K, Corson JD, Kresowik TF: Balloon angioplasty as a treatment of failing infrainguinal autologous vein bypass grafts, *J Vasc Surg* 39(2):421–426, February 2004.
27. USRDS: Excerpts from the United States Renal Data System 1998 annual data report. Incidence and prevalence of ESRD. *Am J Kidney Dis* 32(suppl 1):S38–49, 1998.
28. Beathard GA, Settle SM, Shields MW: Salvage of the nonfunctioning arteriovenous fistula, *Am J Kidney Dis* 33:910–916, 1999.
29. Vorwerk D: Percutaneous interventions to support failing hemodialysis fistulas and grafts, *Kidney Blood Press Res* 20:145–147, 1997.
30. Cavagna E, D'Andrea P, Schiavon F, Tarroni G: Failing hemodialysis arteriovenous fistula and percutaneous treatment: imaging with CT, MRI and digital subtraction angiography, *Cardiovasc Intervent Radiol* 23:262–265, 2000.
31. Dougherty MJ, Calligaro KD, Schindler N, Raviola CA, Ntoso A: Endovascular versus surgical treatment for thrombosed hemodialysis grafts: a prospective, randomized study, *J Vasc Surg* 30(6):1016–1023, 1999.
32. Hingorani A, Ascher E, Kallakuri S, Greenberg S, Khanimov Y: Impact of reintervention for failing upper-extremity arteriovenous autogenous access for hemodialysis, *J Vasc Surg* 34(6):1004–1009, December 2001.
33. Parfrey PS, Griffiths SM, Barrett BJ, Paul MD, Genge M, Withers J, Farid N, McManamon PJ: Contrast material-induced renal failure in patients with diabetes mellitus, renal insufficiency, or both. A prospective controlled study, ***N Engl J Med*** 320(3):143–149, January 19, 1989.
34. Lautin EM, Freeman NJ, Schoenfeld AH, Bakal CW, Haramati N, Friedman AC, Lautin JL, Braha S, Kadish EG, Sprayregen S: Radiocontrast-associated renal dysfunction: incidence and risk factors, *Am J Roentgenol* 157(1):49–58, July 1991.
35. Singer-Jordan J, Papura S: Cutting balloon angioplasty for primary treatment of hemodialysis fistula venous stenoses:

preliminary results, *J Vasc Interv Radiol* 16(1):25–29, January 2005.
36. Wain RA, Lyon RT, Veith FJ et al: Accuracy of duplex ultrasound in evaluating carotid artery anatomy before endarterectomy, *J Vasc Surg* 27(2):235–242, discussion 242–244, 1998.
37. Roth SM, Back MR, Bandyk DF, Avino AJ, Riley V, Johnson BL: A rational algorithm for duplex scan surveillance after carotid endarterectomy, *J Vasc Surg* 30(3): 453–460, 1999.
38. Lipsitz EC, Veith FJ, Ohki T, Heller S, Wain RA, Suggs WD, Lee JC, Kwei S, Goldstein K, Rabin J, Chang D, Mehta M: Does the endovascular repair of aortoiliac aneurysm pose a radiation safety hazard to vascular surgeons?, *J Vasc Surg* 32(4):704–710, 2000.

Intravascular Ultrasound Imaging

11

George E. Kopchok and Rodney A. White

The application of ultrasound in medical diagnosis has increased considerably due to the miniaturization of ultrasonic transducers and overall compatibility and ease of use. Current intravascular ultrasound (IVUS) catheters provide real-time, high-resolution, cross-sectional imaging in vessels with dimensional accuracy. IVUS can delineate wall morphology, lesion consistency and length, as well as the exact location of visceral or aortic branch orifices. Concomitant rapid expansion of minimally invasive endovascular therapies continues to add new roles for IVUS. In addition to diagnostic information, IVUS can assist clinicians in choosing appropriate endovascular devices and appropriate deployment sites and guidance. IVUS also allows real-time post-procedural assessment of efficacy on intervention. Further acceptance and implementation relies on effectiveness of IVUS in improving outcomes and minimizing peri- and post-procedural complications, as compared to alternative imaging modalities. This chapter reviews the design and function of available IVUS catheters, imaging techniques, and therapeutic utility in peripheral endovascular interventions.

Catheter Design and Function

The first IVUS prototypes were used to measure intracardiac dimensions and cardiac motion in the 1950s, utilizing A-mode transducers fixed to large intraluminal catheters [1, 2]. Various devices (A-, B-, and M-mode) were developed for both intravascular and transesophageal imaging of vascular structures, but it was not until the early 1970s that intraluminal, cross-sectional imaging of vessels was reported using a multielement array transducer [3–6]. To obtain a 360° cross-sectional image, the ultrasound beam must be scanned through a full circle and the beam direction and deflection on the display synchronized. This can be achieved by mechanically rotating the imaging element or by using electronically switched arrays.

Current multiple-element (phase array) IVUS catheters use frequencies in the range of 10–30 MHz. The plane of imaging is perpendicular to the long axis of the catheter and provides a full 360° image of the blood vessel. A problem of the early phased array devices was the electronic noise caused by the multiple wires within the catheter itself, since each of the elements was an independent mini-transducer needing its own connections. This problem was later overcome by the incorporation of a miniature integrated circuit at the tip of the catheter, which provided sequenced transmission and reception without the need for numerous electrical circuits traveling the full length of the catheter (Fig. 11.1). In addition to reducing the electronic noise, this modification simplified the manufacturing complexity and improved the flexibility of the catheter. One problem of these imaging catheters, common to all high-frequency ultrasound devices to some extent, is the inability to image structures in the immediate vicinity of the transducer (i.e., in the "near field"). Because the imaging crystals in a phased array configuration are in almost direct contact with the structure being imaged, a bright circumferential artifact known as the *ring down* surrounds the catheter.

G.E. Kopchok (✉)
Director, Vascular Surgery Research Laboratory, Department of Vascular Surgery, Los Angeles Biomedical Research Institute, Harbor-UCLA Medical Center, Torrance, CA, USA

T.J. Fogarty, R.A. White (eds.), *Peripheral Endovascular Interventions*,
DOI 10.1007/978-1-4419-1387-6_11, © Springer Science+Business Media, LLC 1998, 2010

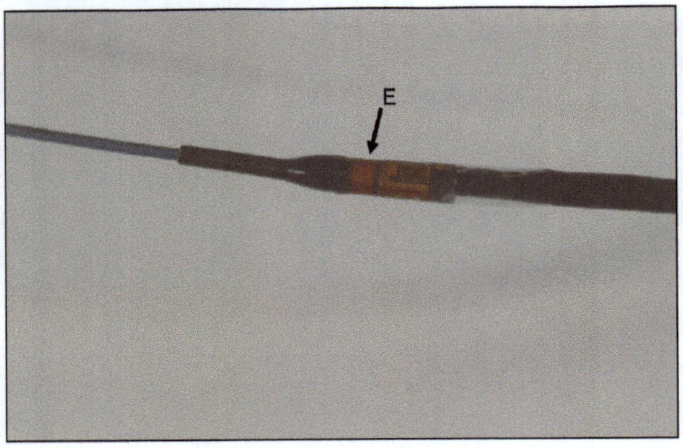

Fig. 11.1 Phased array catheter (8.2F) co-axial over a 0.035-in. guidewire. The gold-colored band contains 64 imaging elements (E) arranged circumferentially around the tip of the catheter (Visions PV8.2F catheter, Volcano Therapeutics, Rancho Cordova, CA, USA.)

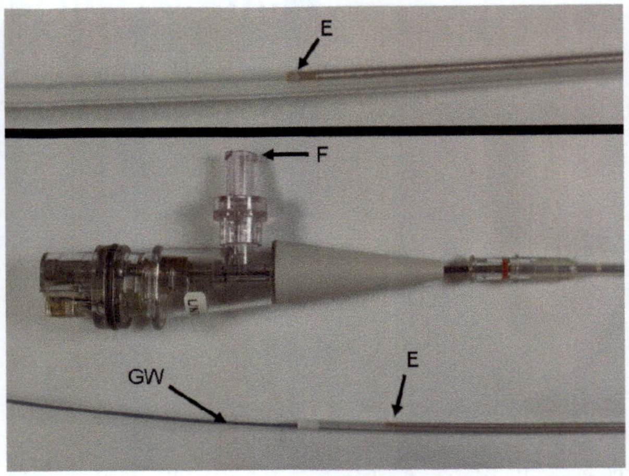

Fig. 11.2 *Top*, Mechanically rotating catheter demonstrating the imaging element (E) in the catheter lumen. *Bottom*, note how the imaging element can share the lumen with the guidewire (GW). This produces an imaging artifact that can mask a small part of the image. Also note the flush (F) port to maintain a fluid-filled chamber (Atlantis PV catheter, Boston Scientific, Natick, MA, USA.)

The ring-down artifact can be electronically removed, but structures within the masked region will not be imaged. Multielement phase array devices use a central guidewire channel, which offers the advantage of being quickly advanced over standard guidewires and good tractability. Phased array devices are generally more flexible and require minimal preparation prior to use. Recent advances in computer technology have combined with phase array image processing to produce real-time color flow or "Chromaflo" (Volcano, Rancho Cordova, CA, USA) imaging [7]. This program compares sequential axial images (up to 30 frame/s) and records any differences in the position of echogenic blood particles between images. A larger difference is interpreted as a greater flow rate. The software colorizes the flow accordingly and displays the results in axial and longitudinal views. Although the color differential may be substantial, actual flow velocities cannot be measure with this technique.

Mechanical IVUS catheters rotate a small transducer located at the tip of the catheter using a flexible, high-torque cable that extends the length of the device (Fig. 11.2). Catheters using a rotating transducer direct the signal at less than 90° from the catheter's long axis. This produces a cone-shaped ultrasound image of the vessel slightly forward in front of the transducer assembly. Rotating transducer devices utilize ultrasound frequencies between 10 and 30 MHz, although some experimental devices using frequencies up to 45 MHz have produced excellent images of human arteries in vitro. In the rotating transducer the ring-down region or near-field zone of the beam image loss is less than phase array, because they operate in a small saline filled chamber or lumen [8].

In mechanical type catheters it is necessary for the guidewire to pass along the side of the imaging assembly. This produces a guidewire artifact that occupies approximately 15° of the image cross section. New catheters have been developed to avoid this artifact. In these catheters the guidewire lumen serves a dual purpose. The guidewire is used to gain catheter access across a lesion or area of treatment (Fig. 11.2). Once the catheter is in place, the guidewire is withdrawn from the catheter lumen and the IVUS transducer advanced through the same lumen. The IVUS transducer can be moved up and down the length of the catheter lumen to interrogate artery. When the IVUS interrogation is completed, the transducer is withdrawn and the guidewire re-advanced through the working lumen. The IVUS catheter can then be withdrawn, leaving the guidewire in position. When using mechanical devices, the catheter lumen and guidewire channel must be flushed manually with saline to ensure a bubble-free fluid medium within the imaging chamber. Repeated, low-pressure manual irrigations may be necessary to clear all bubbles from the system.

Imaging Techniques

Access

The IVUS catheters should be introduced through a standard vascular access sheath (5F–9F) either percutaneously or via an arteriotomy or venotomy, as a hemostatic sheath will reduce blood loss and prevent catheter damage during insertion. In most situations, a retrograde femoral puncture provides access to the entire aorta and aortoiliac segments, since IVUS catheters are available in lengths up to 125 cm and are flexible. Percutaneous brachial or axillary puncture can also be used when appropriate.

Image Acquisition

Mechanical and phased array IVUS catheters are available in the range of 2.9F–9F diameter. Smaller diameter catheters use higher ultrasound transducer frequencies which have a greater resolution but decreased depth of beam penetration into adjacent tissues. Larger diameter catheters operate in lower frequencies which have less resolution but greater depth of penetration. Most of the IVUS catheters can be passed over standard guidewires (0.014–0.035 in. diameter) that are pertinent to the procedure being performed, both in guidewire diameter and in catheter frequency, as well as in overall French size.

Rotational Orientation

On-screen image orientation, although not crucial in the diagnosis, can be helpful for image interpretation. The image can be easily electronically rotated by pushing a button on the IVUS machine. The investigator should avoid rotating the catheter, especially in tortuous anatomy. The best way to identify vessel orientation is to use known anatomical landmarks. For example, as the catheter crosses the aortic bifurcation, the IVUS display can be electronically rotated such that the common iliac arteries are positioned side-by-side, in a correct anatomical location. Occasionally this anatomical arrangement is not true, especially in tortuous, dilated vessels, and the alignment must be checked against other parameters. The location of anterior visceral vessels, i.e., celiac, superior mesenteric, and the renal vein, is also useful when imaging in the abdominal aorta. For the iliac bed, the posterior-medial position of the internal iliac artery orifices can be utilized to adjust angulations.

Longitudinal Gray-Scale Imaging

A longitudinal gray-scale image is an option on most of the newer IVUS units. The longitudinal image is obtained by mechanically withdrawing the catheter through the vessel at a controlled rate. The cross-sectional images are then stacked by the processing unit and rotated 90° to produce a longitudinal view, very similar to an angiogram, of the vessel. Theoretically, distances can then be measured from one point to another. Unfortunately, this option is currently limited to cardiac applications due to the slow speed of current pull-back devices. Newer pull-back mechanisms need to be developed by the manufacturers, to pull the catheters over longer distances, at slightly greater speeds, for most peripheral endovascular procedures.

An important feature of 2D longitudinal reconstruction is that it displays an image of the entire length of the vessel, similar to contrast angiography. However, rather than only the luminal profile that contrast angiography provides, the 2D reconstruction provides detailed cross-sectional wall morphology alongside the longitudinal image. A tract ball can allow the user to interrogate the vessel over the entire length.

Image Interpretation and Diagnostic Capabilities

Two-dimensional images produced by IVUS catheters not only outline the luminal and adventitial surfaces of vessel segments but also can discriminate between normal and diseased components within the wall. In muscular arteries, distinct sonographic layers are visible, with the media appearing as an echolucent (dark)

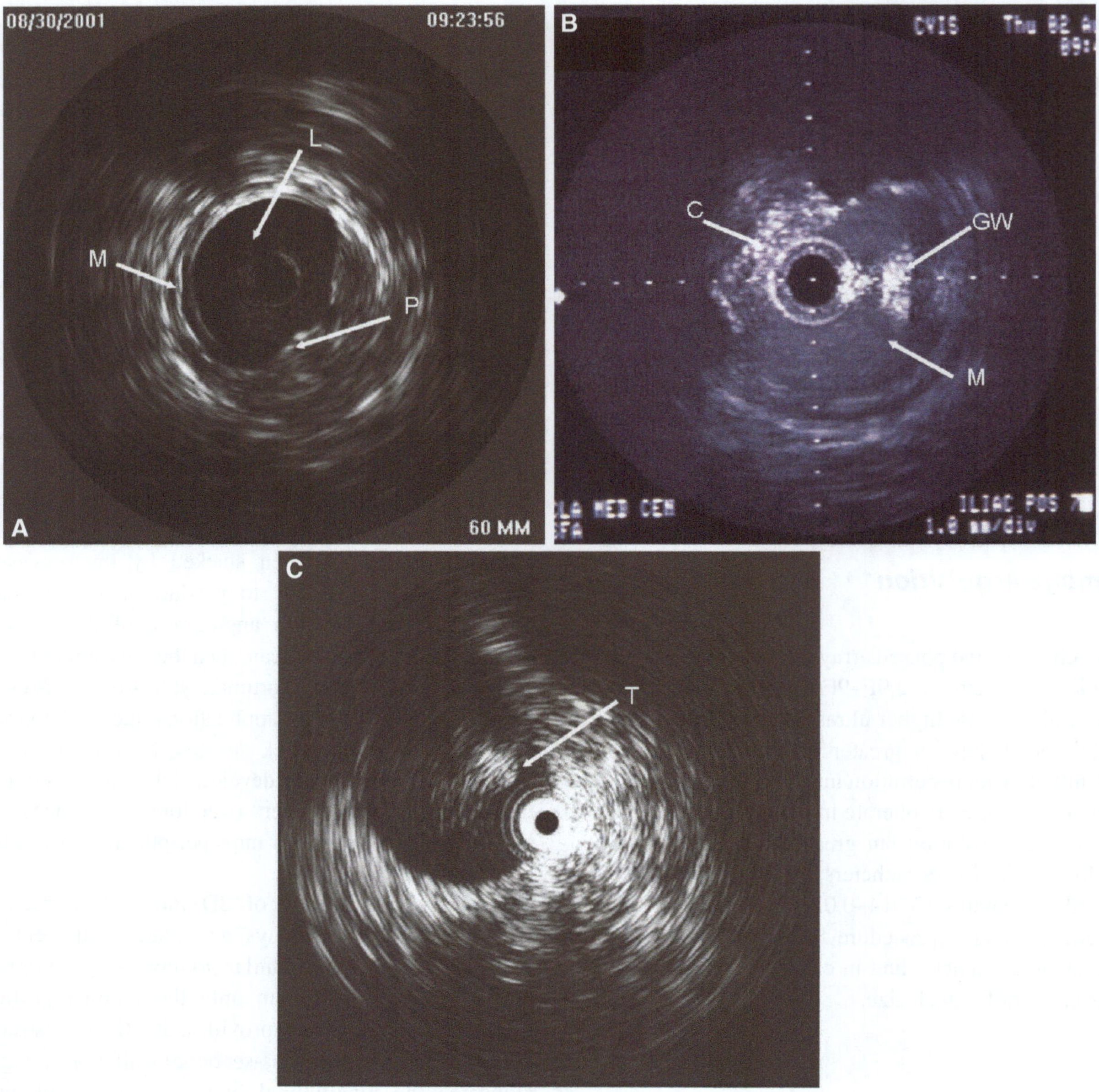

Fig. 11.3 **A**, Phase array IVUS image of diseased human iliac artery demonstrating flow through the lumen (L) and the intima, media (M, dark band), and adventitial arterial layers from 7:00 to 1:00. Areas of soft atheromatous type plaque are seen from 1:00 to 7:00 region. **B**, Mechanical rotating image of a diseased iliac artery demonstrating the highly echogenic image produced by calcified lesions. Note there in no signal penetration beyond the calcium. Also note the intima, media (M), and adventitial layers, from 1:00 to 6:00, as well as the guidewire (GW) artifact. **C**, Phase array image of soft echogenic appearance of thrombus (T) in the vena cava

layer sandwiched between the more echodense intima and adventitia (Fig. 11.3). The precise correlation between the ultrasound image and the histology of the muscular artery wall is still uncertain. The internal and external elastic laminae and adventitia are considered to be the backscatter substrates for the inner and outer echodense zones [9, 10]. Precise measurements of adventitial thickness may be difficult to obtain unless the vessel is surrounded by tissues of differing echogenicity, such as echolucent fat. Even small lesions such as intimal flaps or tears are well visualized because of their high fibrous tissue content and the contrasting echoic properties of surrounding blood. The three-layer appearance of medium-sized muscular arteries is lost in smaller distal vasculature and larger elastic vessels such as aorta because of the increased elastin content in the media. Fresh intraluminal thrombus can be distinguished from underlying vessel wall. It typically appears as a highly echogenic, homogeneous mass with varying image attenuation beyond its location.

IVUS devices are sensitive in differentiating calcified and noncalcified vascular lesions. Because the ultrasound energy is strongly reflected by calcific plaque, it appears as a bright image with dense acoustic shadowing behind it (Fig. 11.3). For this reason, the exact location of the media and adventitia cannot be seen in segments of vessels containing heavily calcific disease, and dimensions must be estimated by interpolation of adjacent size data. Gussenhoven et al. have described four basic plaque components that can be distinguished using 40-MHz IVUS in vitro [10]. Hypoechoic images denote significant lipid deposits. Soft echoes represent fibromuscular tissue or intimal proliferation with varying amounts of dispersed lipid. Bright echoes denote collagen-rich fibrous tissue, whereas bright echoes with acoustic shadowing beyond the lesion represent calcified tissue.

IVUS is capable of identifying intimal flaps and arterial wall dissections and determining the size, location, and extent of these lesions [11, 12]. IVUS has been used in diagnostic assessment of a number of other pathologic vascular scenarios. Accelerated intimal thickening in the coronary arteries of cardiac transplant recipients has been documented by IVUS when angiograms appear normal [13, 14]. Ricou et al. used IVUS to determine candidacy for pulmonary thromboendarterectomy as treatment for pulmonary hypertension in patients with chronic pulmonary thromboembolic disease [15]. Intravascular tumors such as vena caval extensions of renal cell carcinoma can be localized by IVUS to aid in planning resection [16].

Measurements

Luminal dimensions and wall thickness determined by IVUS of normal and minimally diseased arteries both in vitro and in vivo are accurate to within 0.05 mm [9, 17–20]. Determination of outer vessel diameter may be less accurate, with error up to 0.5 mm. Additional studies have compared contrast angiography and IVUS for determining luminal dimensions of normal and moderately atherosclerotic human arteries [21, 22]. The luminal cross-sectional areas calculated from biplanar angiograms and measured from IVUS correlate well for normal or minimally diseased peripheral arteries in vivo. Uniplanar and biplanar angiography and IVUS also correlate well when used to image mildly elliptical lumens. In severely diseased vessels with elliptical lumens, angiography is less accurate in calculating luminal cross-sectional area and tends to underestimate the severity of atherosclerosis in the wall compared with IVUS.

Angulations caused by tortuosity may also cause an elliptical image of the vessel lumen. This is especially true in tortuous aortas and the thoracic arch. When this occurs, the minimal diameter (minor axis) should be used to measure the diameter. Investigators have demonstrated that the minor axis is the most accurate measurement in angled images and/or tortuous anatomy [23]. In another study, investigators found that off-center IVUS measurements may not be as accurate as centerline CT measurements [24]. However, in this study, they included both the long axis and the minor axis measurements. In a study comparing 2D versus 3D CT scans for aortic measurement, investigators found that the minor axis measurement on axial CT scans had a high correlation with the centerline 3D measurements [25]. The conclusion was that the minor axis measurement can substitute for 3D centerline measurements in most situations.

Therapeutic Interventions

Diagnostic

Intravascular ultrasound is an invasive procedure and is normally limited to an adjuvant to other procures such as a contrast angiogram or balloon angioplasty. However, when contrast agents are contraindicated and/or when contrast CT scans are inconclusive, IVUS can serve as a useful tool for pre-diagnostic evaluation. This is especially true for evaluating patient suitability for abdominal or thoracic endoluminal graft (ELG) procedures. Figure 11.5 demonstrates a longitudinal gray-scale image of a patient, with a large abdominal aortic aneurysm, in which contrast was contraindicated. The IVUS pull-through identifies the diameter and length of the proximal (infrarenal aorta) and distal (iliac arteries) landing zones, as well as the overall length between the origin of the renal artery and hypogastric artery. Based on this information, this patient was successfully treated with an aortic endoluminal graft.

Balloon Angioplasty

Adjunctive use of IVUS has allowed description of the mechanism of percutaneous transluminal angioplasty (PTA) in treating coronary and peripheral arterial occlusive disease and helped to define the factors associated with restenosis. Gussenhoven et al. studied 16 patients with superficial femoral artery lesions before and after PTA [26]. IVUS accurately detected the presence of dissections, plaque fractures, and internal elastic lamina ruptures with thinning of the media. This study demonstrated that increased luminal dimensions occurring after PTA are due to overstretching of the arterial wall while the volume of the lesion remained relatively constant. Intravascular ultrasound can provide useful information for both pre-procedural and post-procedural assessment of balloon angioplasty procedures. It provides intraluminal cross-sectional measurements along with precise determination of the arterial morphology and lesion pathology. Post-procedural assessment also provides an accurate assessment of the end result and may determine if a stent may be needed to improve overall result. Studies have shown that post-procedural assessment with IVUS may improve the overall results of percutaneous coronary angioplasty [27]. In this study, it was found that IVUS guidance during coronary interventions improved long-term outcome and cost-effectiveness.

Stent Deployment

Intravascular stents have been used in various applications including post-PTA situations. Common indications for stent deployment after angioplasty are deep arterial wall dissections, elastic recoil, residual stenosis, the presence of a significant residual pressure gradient across the lesion, or plaque ulceration with local thrombus accumulation. Proper stent selection and deployment are critical for salvage of the angioplasty procedure and improving chances of long-term patency. It has been shown that inadequate stent expansion can lead to early thrombosis or stent migration, whereas overexpansion can result in excessive intimal hyperplasia or vessel perforation [28]. IVUS is effective in assessing the result of the primary intervention, establishing the need for stenting and guiding stent deployment and has shown to improve long-term patency rates [29–33].

As with balloon angioplasty, IVUS is useful for determining accurate diameters and exact locations for stent deployment. Arteriography, which is thought to be the gold standard for assessing endovascular therapy, has limitations when evaluating stent-based procedures. Specifically, the uniplanar images produced with arteriography details only the out edges of the artery and stent. This limits the ability to adequately evaluate stent to vessel apposition. In one study it was demonstrated that vessel size and lumen diameter were underestimated 62% of the time by arteriography and that 40% of the stents placed in the iliac arterial system were under deployed, which might lead to related treatment failure [30, 33]. Figure 11.4 demonstrates a femoral artery pre-balloon, post-balloon, and post-stent deployment. Chromaflo was used to observe flow through the lumens, although velocities cannot be measured with this technology.

Endoluminal Grafts for Abdominal Aortic Aneurysm

As with stenting, IVUS can be an important adjuvant in the deployment of endoluminal grafts for the treatment of AAA disease. Although most of the pre-procedural evaluations can be adequately performed using contrast-enhanced spiral CT imaging, IVUS can be used to validate measurements of proximal and distal fixation points, ensure healthy arterial wall and distribution of atherosclerotic lesions, and to determine the optimal device length [34–37]. In our practice, we commonly place radio-opaque scale placed behind the patient and use this to locate the major landmarks such as the aorta just distal to the lowest renal artery, the aortic bifurcation, and the location of the hypogastric arteries (Fig. 11.5). At each given point, the IVUS

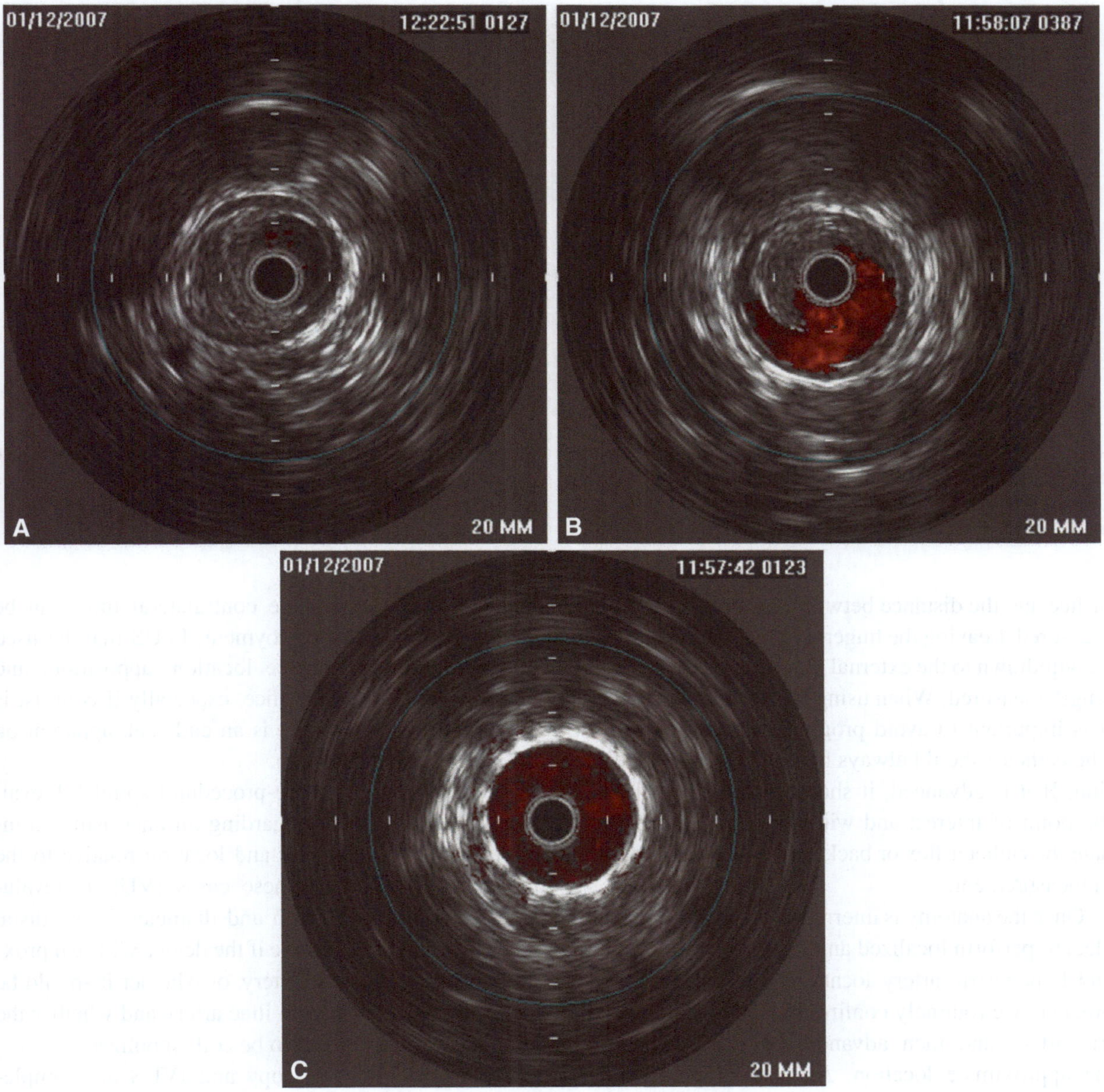

Fig. 11.4 **A**, Femoral artery prior to balloon angioplasty. **B**, Same artery after balloon angioplasty using Chromaflo imaging. Note the plaque fracture created by the angioplasty. **C**, A stent was deployed and appears to be well apposed to the lumen with good flow

catheter is centered on the fluoroscopic screen to eliminate fluoroscopic parallax. That landmark's location is identified and the diameter measured. If the aorta is tortuous, the minor diameter is used as described earlier. The catheter is then advanced or retracted to the next landmark and measurement repeated. This technique allows the interventionalist to interrogate the entire aortailiac system with minimal fluoroscopy time and no contrast. It also verifies the results of the CT scan and enables the physician to further examine the fixation points. Several times in our experience the normal aortic wall seen on the CT scan was aneurysmal or had evidence of a pseudoaneurysm on IVUS evaluation. Once the landmarks are located and measured, the investigator can verify the length from the infrarenal fixation point to the iliac bifurcation and the external iliac orifice. This is accomplished by placing the IVUS catheter at the level of the distal renal orifice and grasping the IVUS catheter as it exits the access sheath. The catheter can then be withdrawn to the level of the iliac

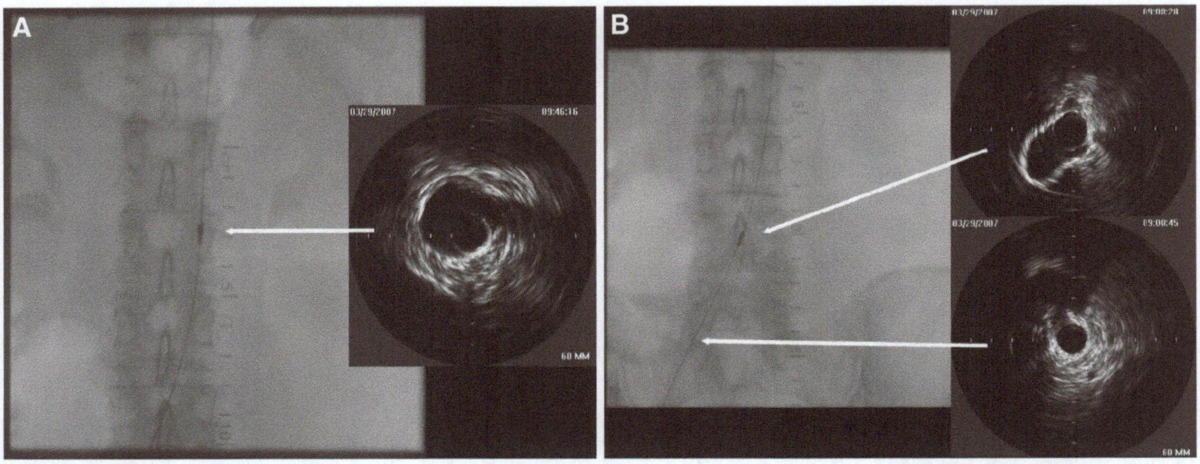

Fig. 11.5 Fluoroscopy and IVUS can be used to map out the aorta (thoracic or abdominal) without the use of contrast. Clinicians can either use radio-opaque rulers, anatomical landmarks, or mark the fluoroscopic screen. **A**, This demonstrates how the IVUS can be used to locate the renal artery orifice located at ~2.5 cm on the screen. **B**, The location of the aortic bifurcation and hypogastric artery can also be identified

orifice and the distance between the sheath and fingers measured. Leaving the fingers in place, the catheter can be withdrawn to the external iliac artery and the overall length measured. When using this technique, however, it is important to avoid prograde catheter movement. The catheter should always be pulled in a distal direction. If it is advanced, it should be advanced beyond the point of interest and withdrawn distally to eliminate the catheter flex or backlash and consequent error in measurement.

Once the anatomy is interrogated, the physician may elect to perform localized angiograms to confirm renal and hypogastric artery locations and patency. In our practice, we routinely confirm the ipsilateral hypogastric artery and then advance the ELG device into the approximate location. An angiographic catheter is positioned alongside the device and a small bolus of contrast injected to confirm the infrarenal fixation point relative to the ELG.

Once the ipsilateral device is deployed, the angiographic catheter is withdrawn into the aneurysmal sac and used with a soft tip guidewire to cannulate the contralateral limb. IVUS is then used to verify proper positioning of the guidewire in the main graft body and to evaluate proximal graft apposition as well as location relative to renal arteries. Several times in our practice, the guidewire was found between the ELG and the aortic wall on IVUS examination. In these cases, it was very easy to withdraw the guidewire and reposition in the correct lumen. Once guidewire location is confirmed, the contralateral limb can be deployed. Following deployment, IVUS may be used to further evaluate device location, apposition, and proximity to the renal orifice, especially if contrast is not being used or if there is an endoleak apparent on the completion angiogram.

In many cases, the pre-procedural spiral CT evaluation is inconclusive regarding an aneurismal common iliac artery diameter and location relative to the hypogastric orifice. In these cases IVUS is invaluable for measuring length and diameter of the distal fixation point, to determine if the device will seal proximal to the hypogastric artery, or whether it should be extended into the external iliac artery and whether the hypogastric artery needs to be coil embolized.

Although cinefluoroscopy and IVUS are complementary in enabling expedient placement of endoluminal grafts, an additional important aspect supporting the use of IVUS in this application is that fluoroscopy time and contrast usage can be reduced significantly during the procedures, minimizing the exposure of both the personnel and the patient. In fact, several investigators have reported deploying both thoracic and abdominal ELGs without the use of contrast agents [7, 37]. Figure 11.6 demonstrates an ELG AAA case performed with IVUS guidance and CO_2 completion angiogram.

One study, which utilized IVUS, digital subtraction angiography and spiral CT scans to evaluate patients preoperatively, found that IVUS may identify patients

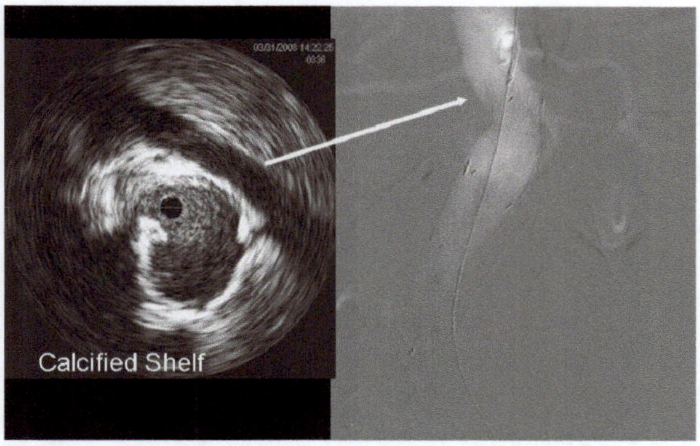

Fig. 11.6 No contrast was used to deploy this infrarenal endoluminal graft. IVUS evaluation noted a calcified shelf just distal to the renal orifice. A CO_2 angiogram demonstrates that the device is not fully apposed at the level of the plaque. A compliant balloon was used to gently confirm the device to the aortic wall without rupturing the calcified plaque

at risk of major adverse complications following endovascular repair [38]. In this study, investigators found that in addition to providing precise measurements, IVUS provided important qualitative information on luminal morphology, including atherosclerotic plaque, calcification, fibrous lesions, and intraluminal thrombus. Investigators found that high-grade atheromatous burden at the level of the aortic neck may lead to increased risk of embolic complications. The presence of thrombus within the neck was associated with increased risk of complications such as immediate and delayed proximal endoleak, graft migration, and distal embolization [39].

Thoracic Aorta

Endovascular treatment of aortic dissection was first described in 1999 [40, 41]. Since then, improvements of the endoluminal graft design and delivery systems have broadened there utility throughout the world. However, many challenges remain in device design [42]. These challenges include the ability to accurately deploy the device around the tortuous curvature of aortic arch and proximal descending aorta and the overall delivery system size. Devices currently range from 20 to 25 Fr. There is also concern over long-term durability of the treatment.

Accurate screening and evaluation are critical to the decision-making process for treatment of the thoracic aorta. Multislice spiral computed tomography (CT) or magnetic resonance imaging (MR) has been proven to provide detailed information of thoracic aneurysms and dissections [42, 43]. However, once the decision has been made to intervene with an endovascular graft, these imaging modalities are limited during the actual deployment.

Thoracic Dissections

Preliminary investigations confirm the utility of intravascular ultrasound in identifying and reconfirming the important parameters required for successful treatment of acute aortic dissection by endoluminal stents [44, 45]. These parameters include (1) site of proximal entry point and distal extent of the dissection, (2) relationship of the false lumen to major aortic branches, (3) measurement of aortic dimensions to allow selection of correct stent size, (4) confirmation that the stent is being deployed in the true lumen, to obliterate the false lumen, and (5) to confirm blood supply to major branch vessels has not been compromised during device deployment. As with AAA intervention, IVUS can be used to identify these landmarks and confirm that the morphology has not changed in the time between initial evaluation and treatment.

Proximal and distal entry points can be readily evaluated with IVUS examination. The use of Chromaflo, in the future, may also enhance the ability to evaluate flow through the false lumen or entry/exit points. If the dissection propagates into the branch vessels, perfusion of end organs must be maintained. Although this can generally be determined pre-intervention, the relationship of major branch vessels to true and false lumens should be reconfirmed prior to exclusion of the proximal entry point. IVUS can be used to evaluate this relationship at the time of the endovascular intervention [42]. Figure 11.7 demonstrates how IVUS can differentiate true and false lumen and evaluate post-deployment changes. In this case, there was a small true lumen (A) just proximal to the celiac artery, with almost no lumen at the celiac and SMA orifices (B & C). The large false lumen was sandwiching the

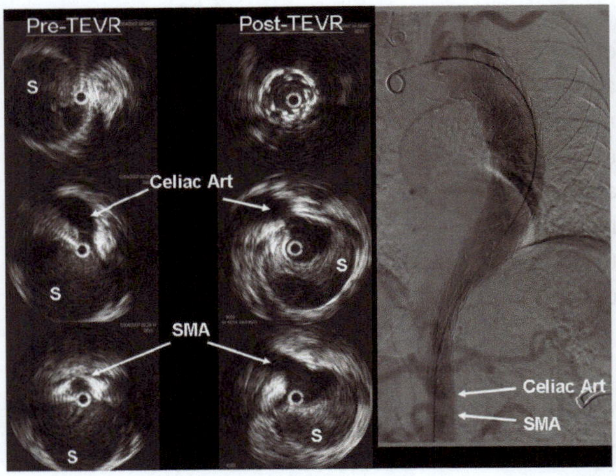

Fig. 11.7 IVUS images demonstrate a small true lumen (*top left*) just proximal to the celiac artery, with almost no lumen at the celiac and SMA orifices (*middle* and *bottom left*). Note the large false lumen is sandwiching the IVUS catheter in the very small true lumen. Also note the stagnant (s) flow in the false lumen at these locations. Immediately after TEVAR deployment the TEVAR device (just proximal to the celiac) is seen partially compressed from the small true lumen (*top middle image*), there is blood flow to the celiac and SMA and the false lumen has no flow. The completion angiogram demonstrates narrowing of the TEVAR due to an intact true lumen and blood flow to the visceral vessels

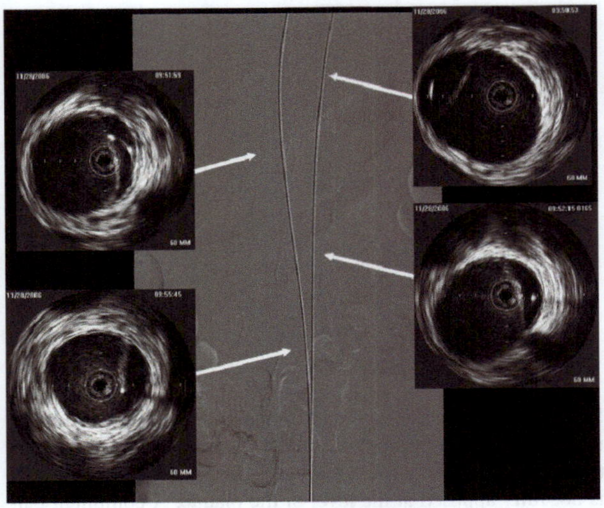

Fig. 11.8 The figure demonstrates a case in which the guidewire continually advanced into the false lumen from the femoral artery. Eventually, investigators place a second guidewire from the right radial artery to gain access to true lumen

IVUS catheter in the very small true lumen. There was also stagnant flow in the false lumen at these locations. Immediately after TEVAR deployment the device became partially compressed along the distal section from the small true lumen. It was also noted that the true lumen dilated at the celiac and SMA and the false lumen compress and has no blood flow. The completion angiogram demonstrated narrowing of the TEVAR due to an intact true lumen and blood flow to the visceral vessels.

Access to the true lumen is essential to the treatment of thoracic dissections. Many times this lumen is compromised and difficult to confirm on fluoroscopy and angiography. IVUS has been useful in our practice to guide the guidewire past the distal entry point, into the true lumen of the proximal aorta. Figure 11.8 demonstrates a case in which the guidewire continually advanced into the false lumen from the femoral artery. Eventually, investigators place a second guidewire from the right radial artery to gain access to the true lumen. All of the clinical thoracic dissection cases described above were performed as part of a single center investigator sponsored, FDA approved, IDE (investigational device exemption).

Thoracic Aneurysms, Ulcerations, and Transections

The treatment of thoracic aneurysms and ulcerations is a little more straightforward and generally associated with favorably primary success rates than aortic dissections [46]. However, given the high flow of the thoracic aorta, IVUS can be very useful for identifying the extent of the aneurysm, to confirm healthy aortic wall for proximal and distal fixation, and to identify the site for endoluminal graft deployment [47]. All of these pre-deployment assessments can readily be performed without the use of contrast. The importance of evaluating aortic wall integrity can be demonstrated in Fig. 11.9. In this case, the preoperative contrast CT scan revealed a small pseudoaneurysm on the mid-descending thoracic aorta (Fig. 11.10). The angiogram would have confirmed the diagnosis and a TEVAR would have been placed in the mid-thoracic aorta. However, IVUS examination revealed a circumferential dissection with intramural thrombus and flow in some areas, extending up to the left subclavian artery. Based on the IVUS findings, the TEVAR was place distal to the left carotid artery.

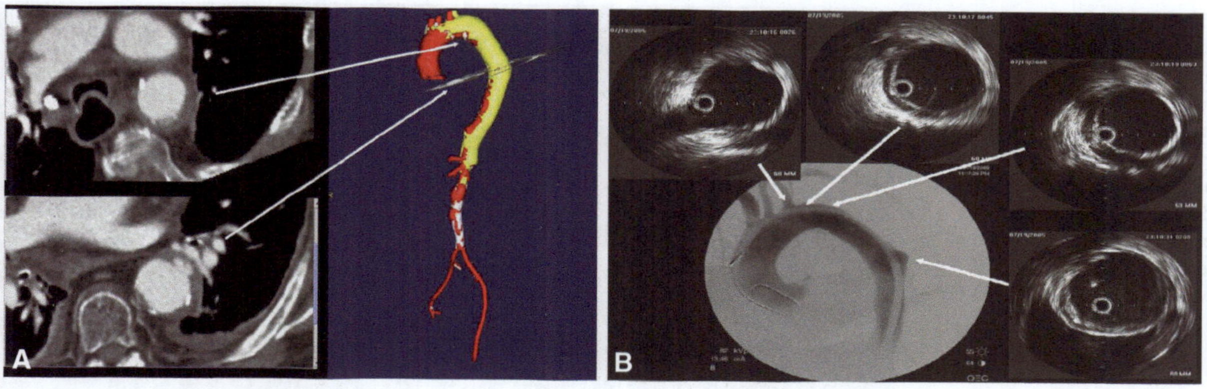

Fig. 11.9 **A**, The preoperative contrast CT scan revealed a small pseudoaneurysm on the *mid-descending thoracic aorta* as seen on this M2S 3D reconstruction. **B**, The angiogram reconfirmed the CT findings. Based on these findings, a TEVAR would have been placed in the *mid-thoracic aorta*. IVUS examination revealed a circumferential dissection with intramural thrombus and flow in some areas, extending up to the *left subclavian artery*. Based on the IVUS findings, the TEVAR was place distal to the *left carotid artery*. Note that IVUS evaluation was performed, and the great branch vessel locations marked on the fluoroscopic screen, prior to advancing the device and taking our first angiogram

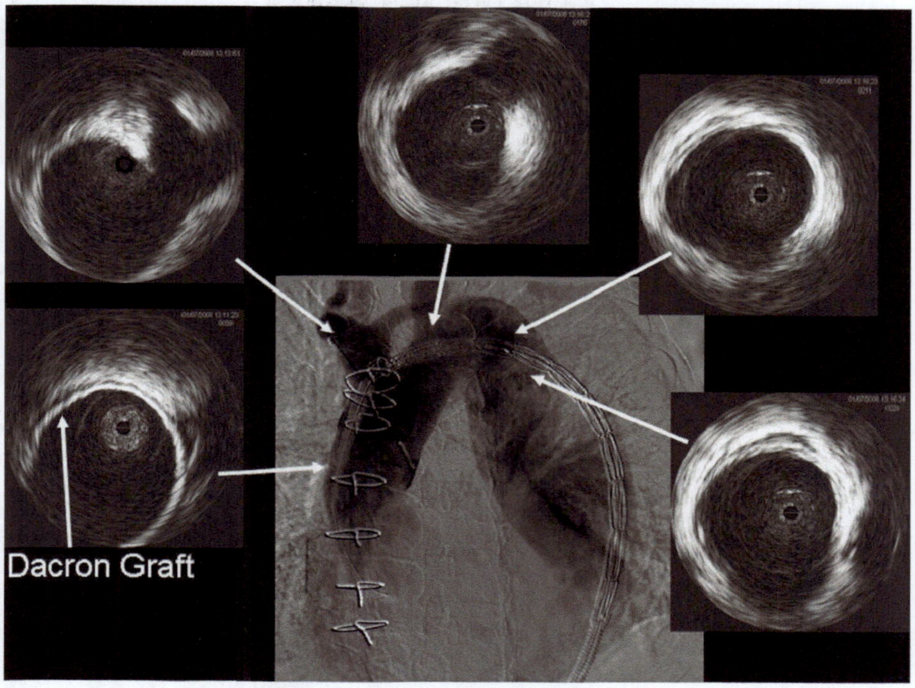

Fig. 11.10 Angiogram and IVUS evaluation of a thoracic pseudoaneurysm of a patient who had a previous ascending arch repair. *Lower left*, Note the echogenic signature of the Dacron prosthetic graft. It appears as a bright ring, with perfect uniformity. Some times there is no signal beyond the prosthesis. *Upper left*, Bovine arch. Upper middle, Left subclavian artery. *Upper right*, Aorta with the beginning of the defect at 6:00. *Lower right*, Aorta with the wall defect at 6:00. Again note that the device is in location prior to our first angiogram

Post-procedural Assessments and Troubleshooting

As noted earlier, IVUS is an invaluable tool in the assessment of ELG apposition following deployment. Although it is usually difficult to image an ELG along its length, due to the air in the pores of the graft material, IVUS can be very useful to assess proximal and distal fixation points. Advancing and retracting the IVUS catheter over the transition area can accomplish this. Any gap between the device and the arterial wall verifies poor apposition and a potential endoleak.

Any time guidewire access through an ELG is compromised, or if there is a re-intervention in a previously deployed device, luminal position should be verified. IVUS is very useful to confirm access through a device and ensure the guidewire is not trapped between the device and the aorta. Figure 11.11 demonstrates the

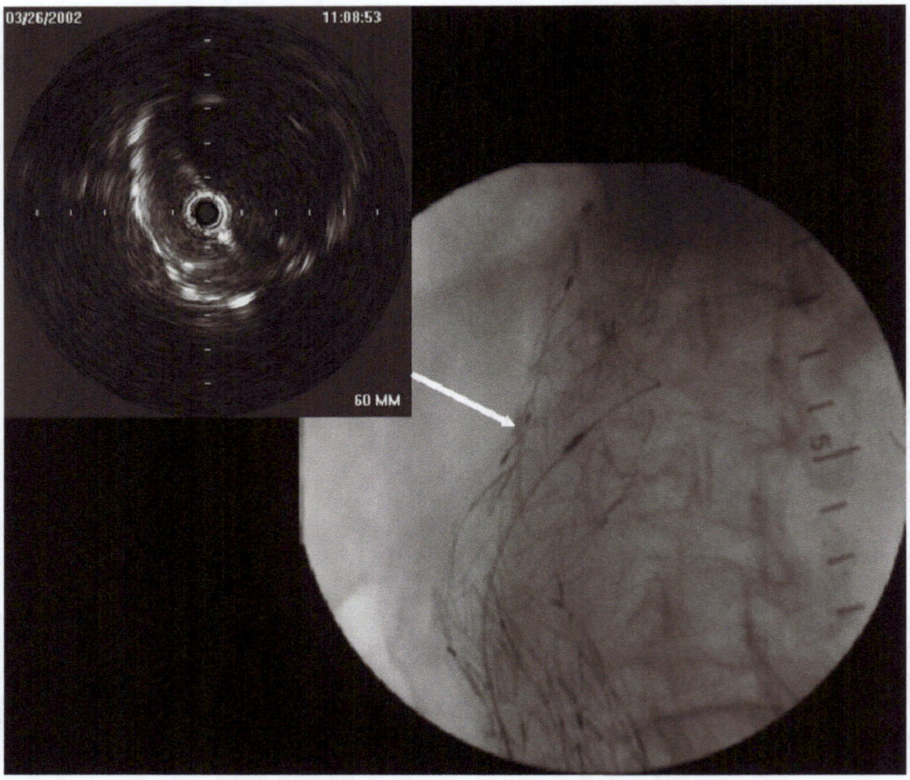

Fig. 11.11 On fluoroscopic examination the guidewire appears to be in the device lumen. However, the IVUS images clearly show that the guidewire and IVUS catheter are positioned between the device and the aorta. In this case, guidewire access was temporarily loss while withdrawing a thoracic ELG

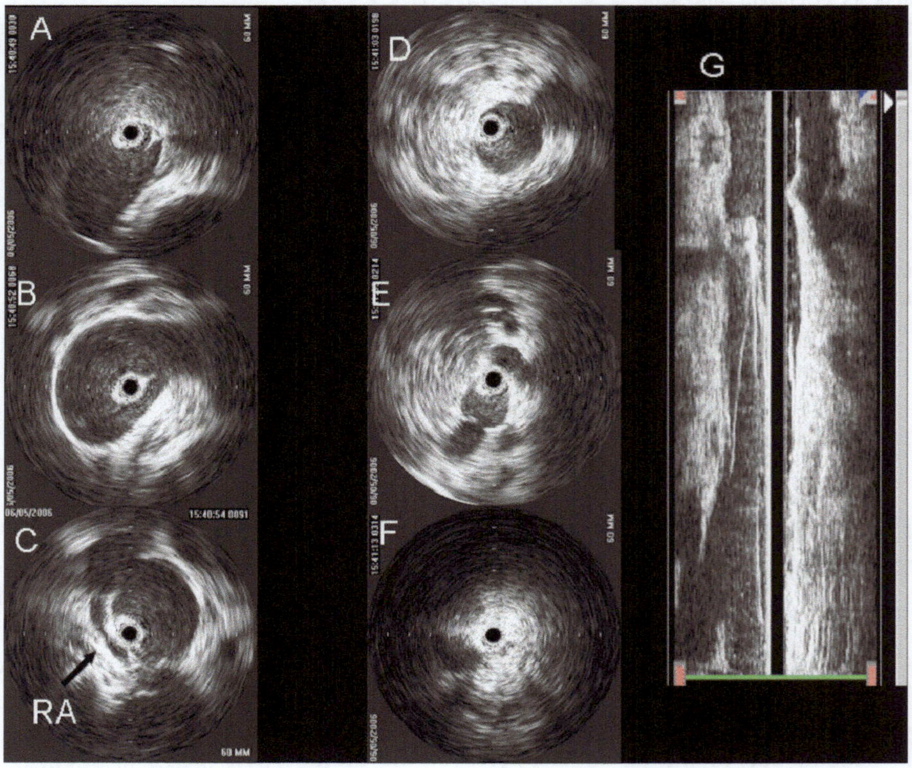

Fig. 11.12 Identifying the venous anatomy is crucial to correct placement of IVUS-guided vena cava filters. **A**, Liver parenchyma. **B**, *Left* renal vein. **C**, *Right* renal vein with crossing renal artery (RA). **D**, Iliac vein bifurcation. **E**, Hypogastric vein. **F**, Access sheath in tissue. **G**, Longitudinal *gray-scale* image of deployed filter

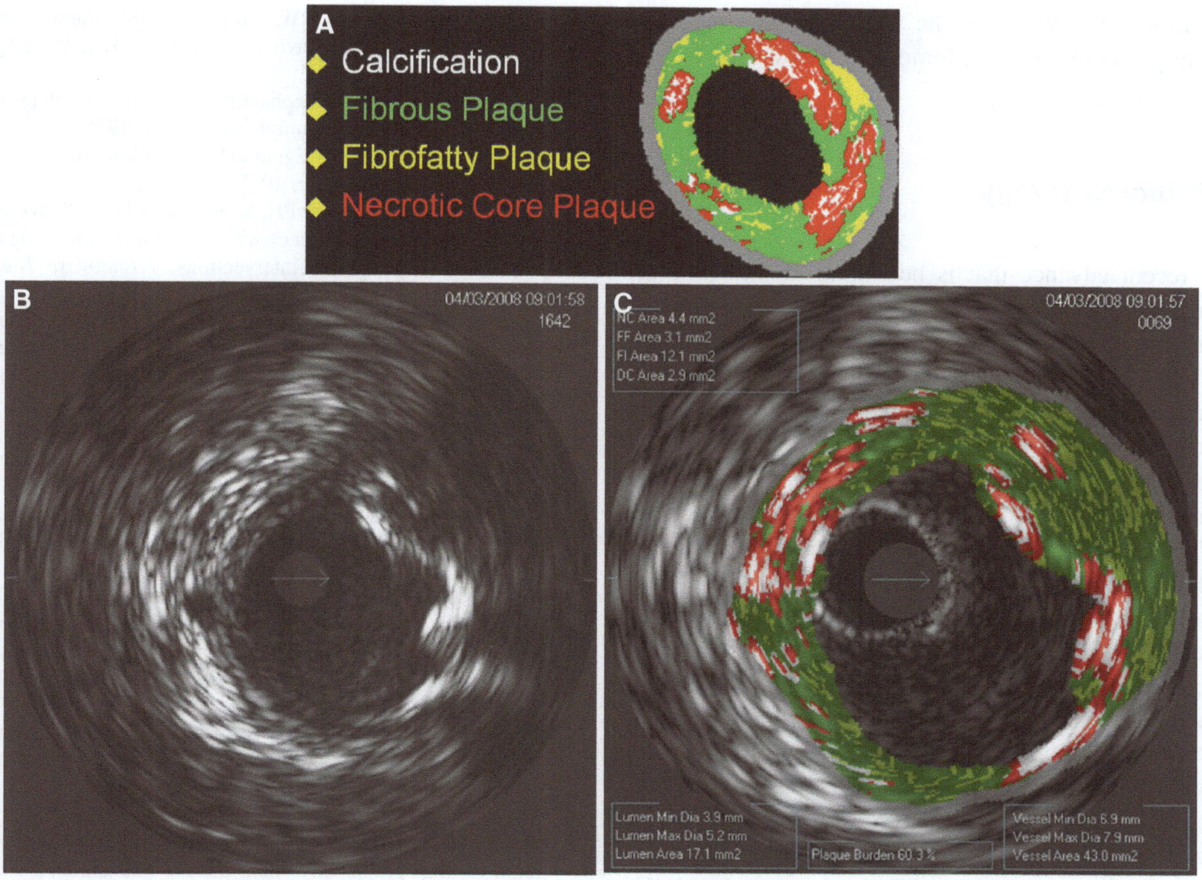

Fig. 11.13 **A**, Virtual histology can differentiate different components of arteriosclerotic plaque and assign them different colors (*dark green*: fibrous, *yellow/green*: fibrofatty, *white*: calcified, and *red*: necrotic lipid core). **B**, *Gray-scale* IVUS image of a diseased iliac artery. **C**, Virtual histology of the same lesion demonstrating a fibrous lesion with area calcified surface

limitation of fluoroscopy for the purpose. On fluoroscopic examination, the guidewire appears to be in the device lumen. However, the IVUS images clearly show that the guidewire and catheter are position between the device and the aorta. In this case, guidewire access was temporarily loss while withdrawing a thoracic ELG.

Bedside Vena Cava Placement

Pulmonary thromboembolism continues to be a major complication in the treatment of critically ill patients [48, 49]. Vena cava filters have been shown to reduce the incidence of pulmonary embolization in patients prone to develop deep venous thrombosis. In this regard, there has been a growing interest in the "bedside" placement of vena cava filters with IVUS guidance. In these cases, IVUS has been used to ensure correct guidewire position and interrogate the inferior vena cava. In these cases, the renal veins can usually be identified by their proximity to the renal artery. The artery appears as a dark structure crossing directly underneath the vena cava. The renal veins are usually located within a few centimeters of the artery. After the anatomy is defined with IVUS, the same guidewire is used to deliver the IVC filter at the appropriate distance from the access sheath. A flat plate abdominal radiograph is used to confirm satisfactory position. This technique allows filter deployments to be performed in the intensive care unit or in morbidly obese patients with minimal radiographic equipment, thus avoiding the complications associated with transporting and imaging these patients. Figure 11.12 demonstrates the anatomical anatomy of the vena cava starting at the liver parenchyma to the femoral access sheath.

Virtual Histology

A recent advance that is beginning to find its place in peripheral vascular interventions is virtual histology intravascular ultrasound (IVUS-Virtual Histology (IVUS-VH), Volcano Therapeutics). Virtual histology images are computer generated using the amplitude, power, and frequency to characterize plaque from the reflected IVUS signals of the artery wall. The images produce a color-coded map of the arterial disease morphology [50, 51]. Different histological constituents of the plaque produce different reflected signals and these are assigned different colors (dark green, fibrous; yellow/green, fibrofatty; white, calcified; red, necrotic lipid core plaque). This color-coded map assists the interventionalist in understanding morphology of the arterial disease. Although currently used for coronary evaluations and therapies, its utility to assist in assessing plaque morphology in carotid disease is proving invaluable. In one study evaluating the diagnostic accuracy, there was a strong correlation between VH IVUS plaque characterization and the true histological examination, particularly in vulnerable plaque types [52]. This feasibility study was done following FDA and Institutional Review Board approval and supports a larger prospective study. In a similar study, investigators found that using VH to assess plaque morphology prior to carotid artery stenting may lead to the selection of appropriate plaque with more favorable outcomes [53]. Figure 11.13 demonstrates the utility of VH compared to the gray-scale image of a diseased iliac artery.

References

1. Born N, ten Hoff H, Lancee CT et al.: Early and recent intraluminal ultrasound devices, *Int J Card Imag* 4:79–88, 1989.
2. Cieszynski T: Intracardiac method for the investigation of structure of the heart with the aid of ultrasonics, *Arch Immunol Ter Dow* 8:551–557, 1960.
3. Kossof G: Diagnostic applications of ultrasound in cardiology, *Australas Radiol* X:101–106, 1966.
4. Carleton RA, Sessions RW, Graettinger JS: Diameter of heart measured by intracavitary ultrasound, *Med Res Eng* 28–32, May 1969.
5. Frazin L, Talano JV, Stephanides L et al.: Esophageal echocardiography, *Circulation* 54:168–171, 1976.
6. Born N, Lancee CT, Van Egmond FC: An ultrasonic intracardiac scanner, *Ultrasonics* 10:72–76, 1972.
7. Irshad K, Reid DB, Miller PH, Velu R, Kopchok GE, White RA: Early clinical experience with color three-dimensional ultrasound in peripheral interventions, *J Endovasc Ther* 8:329–339, 2001.
8. Yock PG, Linker DT, Angelsen BAJ: Two-dimensional intravascular ultrasound: technical development and initial clinical experience, *J Am Soc Echocardiogr* 2(4):296–304, 1989.
9. Gussenhoven WJ, Essed CE, Lancee CT: Arterial wall characteristics determined by intravascular ultrasound imaging: an in-vitro study, *J Am Coll Cardiol* 14:947–952, 1989.
10. Gussenhoven WJ, Essed CE, Frietman P et al.: Intravascular echographic assessment of vessel wall characteristics: a correlation with histology, *Int J Cardiac Imag* 4:105–116, 1989.
11. Tobis JM, Mahon D, Lehmann K et al.: The sensitivity of ultrasound imaging compared to angiography for diagnosing coronary atherosclerosis, *Circulation* 82(suppl III):439, 1990, abstract.
12. Cavaye DM, French WJ, White RA et al.: Intravascular ultrasound imaging of an acute dissecting aortic aneurysm: a case report, *J Vasc Surg* 13:510–512, 1991.
13. St Goar FG, Pinto FJ, Aldermann EL et al.: Intracoronary ultrasound in cardiac transplant recipients: in-vivo evaluation of angiographically silent intimal thickening, *J Am Coll Cardiol* 17:103A, 1994, abstract.
14. Pinto FJ, St. Goar FG, Chaign M et al.: Intracoronary ultrasound evaluation of intimal thickening in cardiac transplant recipients: correlation with clinical characteristics, *J Am Coll Cardiol* 17:103A, 1994, abstract.
15. Ricou FJ, Nicod PH, Moser KM: Intravascular ultrasound imaging of chronic pulmonary thromboembolic disease: correlation with surgical results, *Circulation* 82(suppl 3):441, 1990, abstract.
16. Barone GW, Kahn MB, Cook JM et al.: Recurrent intracaval renal cell carcinoma: the role of intravascular ultrasonography, *J Vasc Surg* 13:506–509, 1991.
17. Kopchok GE, White RA, Guthrie C et al.: Intraluminal vascular ultrasound: preliminary report of dimensional and morphologic accuracy, *Ann Vasc Surg* 4:291–296, 1990.
18. Kopchok GE, White RA, White G: Intravascular ultrasound: a new potential modality for angioplasty guidance, *Angiology* 41:785–792, 1990.
19. Mallery JA, Tobis JM, Griffith J et al.: Assessment of normal and atherosclerotic arterial wall thickness with an intravascular ultrasound imaging catheter, *Am Heart J* 119:1392–1400, 1990.
20. Nissen SE, Grines CL, Gurley JC et al.: Application of new phased-array ultrasound imaging catheter in the assessment of vascular dimensions, *Circulation* 81:660–666, 1990.
21. Nissen SE, Gurley JC, Grines CL et al.: Intravascular ultrasound assessing of lumen size and wall morphology in normal subjects and patients with coronary artery disease, *Circulation* 88:1087–1099, 1993.

22. Tabbara MR, White RA, Cavaye DM et al.: In-vivo human comparison of intravascular ultrasound and angiography, *J Vasc Surg* 14:496–504, 1991.
23. Geselschap JH, Heilbron MJ, Hussain FM, Daskalakis TM, Wilson EP, Kopchok GE, White RA: The effect of angulation on intravascular ultrasound imaging observed in vascular phantoms, *J Endovasc Surg* 5:126–133, 1998.
24. Fernandez JD, Donovan S, Garrett E Jr, Burgar S: Endovascular thoracic aorta aneurysm repair: evaluating the utility of intravascular ultrasound measurements, *J Endovasc Ther* 15(1):68–72, 2008.
25. Dillavou ED, Buck DG, Muluk SC, Makaroun MS: Two-dimensional verse three-dimensional CT scan for Aortic Measurement, *J Endovasc Ther* 10:531–538, 2003.
26. The SHK, Gussenhoven WJ, Zhong Y et al.: Effect of balloon angioplasty on femoral artery evaluated with intravascular ultrasound imaging, *Circulation* 86:483–493, 1992.
27. Gaster AL, Skjoldberg US, Larsen J: Continued improvement of clinical outcome and cost effectiveness following IVUS guided PCI, *Heart* 89(9):1043–1049, September 2003.
28. Busquet J: The current role of vascular stents, *Int Angiol* 12(3):206–213, 1993.
29. Tobis JM, Mahon DJ, Goldberg SL et al.: Lessons from intravascular ultrasonography: observations during interventional angioplasty procedures, *J Clin Ultrasound* 21:589–607, 1993.
30. Lee SD, Arko FR, Buckley CJ: Impact of intravascular ultrasonography in the endovascular management of aortoiliac occlusive disease, *J Vasc Nurs* 16(3):57–61, September 1998.
31. Diethrich EB: Endovascular treatment of abdominal aortic occlusive disease: the impact of stents and intravascular ultrasound imaging, *Eur J Vasc Surg* 7:228–236, 1993.
32. Cavaye DM, Diethrich EB, Santiago OJ et al.: Intravascular ultrasound imaging: an essential component of angioplasty assessment and vascular stent deployment, *Int Angiol* 12:212–220, 1993.
33. Arko F, Mettauer M, McCollough R, Patterson D, Manning L, Buckley CJ: Use of intravascular ultrasound improves long-term clinical outcome in the management of atherosclerotic aortoiliac occlusive disease, *J Vasc Surg* 27(4):614–623, 1998.
34. van Essen JA, van der Lugt A, Gussenhoven EJ, Leertouwer TC, Zondervan P, Sambeek MR: Intravascular ultrasonography allows accurate assessment of abdominal aortic aneurysm: an in vitro validation study, *J Vasc Surg* 27(2):347–353, 1998.
35. van Essen JA, Gussenhoven EJ, Blankensteijn JD, Honkoop J, van Dijk LC, van Sambeek MR, van der Lugt A: Three dimensional intravascular ultrasound assessment of abdominal aortic aneurysm necks, *J Endovasc Ther* 7(5):380–388, 2000.
36. White RA, Donayre C, Kopchok GE: Utility of intravascular ultrasound in peripheral interventions, *Tex Heart Inst J* 24:28–34, 1997.
37. Nishanian G, Kopchok GE, Donayre CE, White RA: The impact of intravascular ultrasound (IVUS) on endovascular interventions, *Seminars Vasc Surg* 12(4):285–299, 1999.
38. Slovut DP, Ofstein LC, Bacharach JM: Endoluminal AAA repair using intravascular ultrasound for graft planning and deployment, *J Endovasc Ther* 10:463–475, 2003.
39. Thompson MM, Smith J, Naylor AR et al.: Microembolization during endovascular and conventional aneurysm repair, *J Vasc Surg* 25:179–186, 1997.
40. Dake MD, Kato N, Mitchell RS et al.: Endovascular stent-graft placement for treatment of acute aortic dissection, *N Engl J Med* 340:1546–1554, 1999.
41. Nienaber CA, Fattori R, Lund G et al.: Nonsurgical reconstruction of thoracic aortic dissection by stent graft placement, *N Engl J Med* 340:1539–1545, 1999.
42. Greenberg RK, Haulon S, Khwaja J, Fulton G, Ouriel K: Contemporary Management of acute aortic dissection, *J Endovasc Ther* 10:476–485, 2003.
43. Quint LE, Platt JF, Sonnad SS, Deep GM, Williams DM: Aortic intimal tears: detection with spiral Computer Tomography, *J Endovasc Ther* 10:505–510, 2003.
44. Waller BF: The eccentric coronary atherosclerotic plaque: morphologic observations and clinical relevance, *Clin Cardiol* 12:14–20, 1989.
45. White RA, Donayre C, Walot I, Lee J, Kopchok GE: Regression of a descending thoracoabdominal aortic dissection following staged deployment of thoracic and abdominal aortic endografts, *J Endovasc Ther* 9(suppl II):84–92, 2002.
46. Chabbert V, Otal P, Bouchard L, Soula P, Van TT, Kos X, Meites G, Claude C, Joffre F, Rousseau H: Midterm outcomes of thoracic aortic stent-grafts: complications and imaging techniques, *J Endovasc Ther* 10:494–504, 2003.
47. Woody JD, Walot I, Donayre CE, Eugene J, Carey JS, White RA: Endovascular exclusion of leaking thoracic aortic aneurysms, *J Endovasc Ther* 9:II-79–II-83, 2002.
48. Oppat WF, Chiou AC, Matsumura J: Intravascular Ultrasound-guided vena cava filter placement, *J Endovasc Surg* 6:285–287, 1999.
49. Matsuura JH, White RA, Kopchok GE, Nishinian G, Woody JD, Rosenthal D, Clark MD: Vena cava filter placement by intravascular ultrasound, *Cardiovascular Surg* 9(6):571–574, 2001.
50. Diethrich EB, Irshad K, Reid DB: Virtual histology and color flow intravascular ultrasound in peripheral interventions, *Semin Vasc Surg* 19:155–162, 2006.
51. Rodriguez-Granillo GA, Mc Fadden E, Ligthart JM, Aoki J, Regar E, de Feyter PJ, Serruys PW: Geometrical validation of intravascular ultrasound radiofrequency data analysis (Virtual Histology) acquired with a 30 M Hz Boston Scientific corporation imaging catheter, *Catheter Cardiovasc Inter* 66(4):514–518, 2005.
52. Diethrich EB, Pauliina Margolis M, Reid DB, Burke A, Ramaiah V, Rodriguez-Lopez JA, Wheatley G, Olsen D, Vermani R: Virtual histology intravascular ultrasound assessment of carotid artery disease: the Carotid Artery Virtual Histology Evaluation (CAPITAL) study, *J Endovasc Ther* 14(5):687–688, 2007.
53. Schiro BJ, Wholey MH: The expanding indications for virtual histology intravascular ultrasound for plaque analysis prior to carotid stenting, *J. Cardiovasc Surg (Torino)* 49(6):729–736, 2008.

Part IV
Endovascular Instrumentation and Devices

Biomaterials: Considerations for Endovascular Devices

12

Martin R. Back

Continued evolution of catheter-based technology has expanded applications of endovascular therapy for the treatment of cardiac and peripheral vascular diseases. Research and development advances have affected metal, textile, and polymer biomaterials and have facilitated refinements in design and construction of endovascular devices. As a result, the performance of these devices has improved, complications have been reduced, and the uses of minimally invasive applications have expanded. This chapter reviews the biomaterial properties and design characteristics of existing guidewires, angioplasty balloons and catheters, and metallic intravascular stents and filters with reference to their implementation and function. Design and biomaterial considerations for newer endoluminal grafts and their applications are also discussed.

Guidewires

Few balloon or other angioplasty catheters are sufficiently steerable and so require advancement through the vascular lumen over guidewires. Guidewires serve to find and secure a pathway through the vascular system from an entrance site and across a target lesion. Proper guidewire selection is as important as the choice of angioplasty device and catheters during endovascular interventions. Ideal guidewire characteristics include strength (to track across lesions and transmit torque), softness at the tip (atraumatic to vessel wall), steerability, and slipperiness (to minimize friction between wire, lesion, and catheter).

Standard larger diameter guidewires are composed of a stiff inner core wire and an outer spring coil (Fig. 12.1). The central core wire usually does not extend to the tip and is tapered distally to allow a gradual decrease in stiffness. Guidewires contain a safety wire anchored to the end of the inner core and welded to the distal end of the outer coil to prevent separation of these components and allow shaping of the tip.

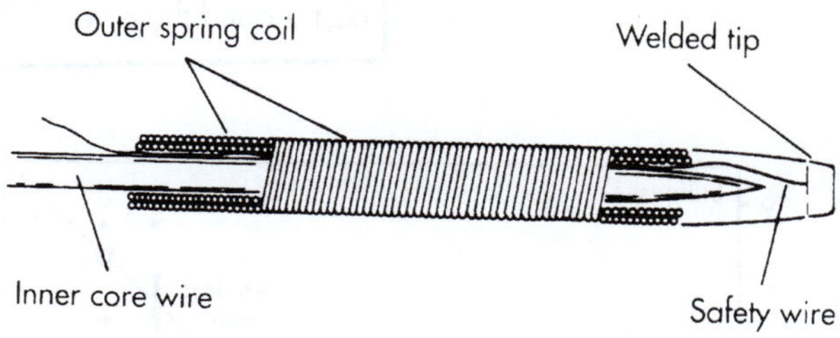

Fig. 12.1 Components of standard stainless steel guidewire

The mechanical properties of guidewires determine their performance. The stiffness of a guidewire in its shaft portion varies directly with the fourth power of the inner core wire diameter [1]. Torsional strength and resistance to kinking are also dependent on the fourth power of the core diameter and the component metal used. The outer spring coil does not provide stiffness or torsional strength along the guidewire shaft but does influence function at the tip. Variation in construction at the guidewire tip affects its distal stiffness, which is generally less than that in the shaft (Fig. 12.2). Guidewires composed of stainless steel for an equivalent diameter are four times stiffer than titanium alloy wires (Fig. 12.3). Steel core wires are also more kink resistant and are the chief component of most available

M.R. Back (✉)
Associate Professor, Division of Vascular and Endovascular Surgery, Department of Surgery, University of South Florida Health, Tampa, FL, USA

T.J. Fogarty, R.A. White (eds.), *Peripheral Endovascular Interventions*,
DOI 10.1007/978-1-4419-1387-6_12,

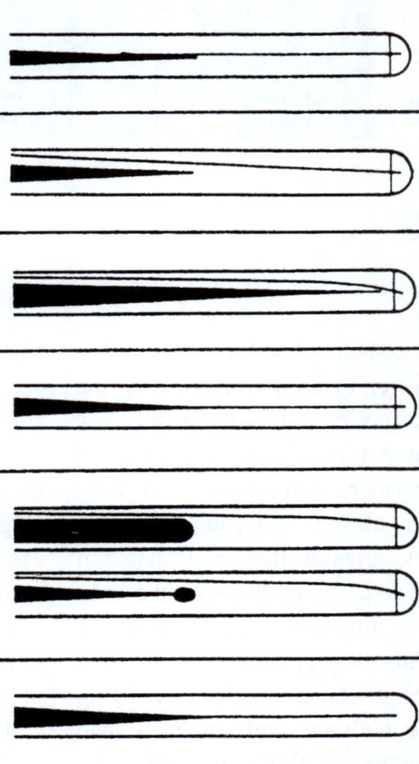

Type of construction of the wire tip	Mean stiffness of the tip.10^{-6}/Nm^2/°
Short safety wire welded onto the core at the front	0.04
Core shorter than safety wire	0.08
Core extends up to the tip (at the side of the safety wire)	0.15
No safety wire, tip fixed on the core	0.26
Moveable core without tapering of the tip / Tapered at the tip	0.07
Titanium wire, hydrophilic plastic cast around the core	0.03

Fig. 12.2 Effect of construction at the guidewire tip on average tip stiffness (Modified from Schroder [1], with permission.)

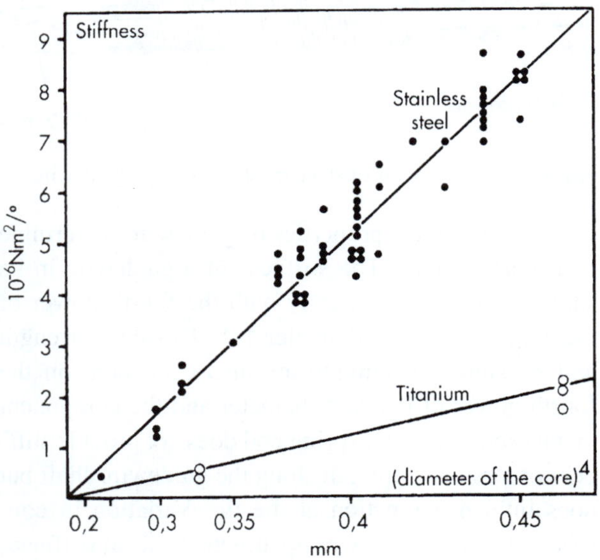

Fig. 12.3 Dependence of guidewire stiffness on the fourth power of the inner core diameter (Modified from Schroder [1], with permission.)

guidewires [2]. Frictional resistance of a guidewire is determined by the stiffness of the wire and a coefficient of friction that depends on the surface characteristics (Fig. 12.4). Tetrafluoroethylene (Teflon) coating reduces the coefficient of friction by 50% for both steel solid wires and guidewires with an outer spring coil [3]. The addition of a hydrophilic polymer (silicone) decreases the coefficient of friction to one-sixth the value for uncoated steel guidewires. Most guidewires have surface coating to facilitate passage through long catheters and across narrow, tortuous vessels.

Most standard steel guidewires have adequate strength and slipperiness for positioning and catheter exchanges yet lack steerability. Straight wires are relatively traumatic and are rarely used. J-shaped guidewires have tapered, softer distal ends that can be straightened or curled by moving the inner core relative to the outer coil. Floppy-tip guidewires have no core wire in their distal 10–15 cm and are maximally flexible. Long exchange wires up to 300 cm in length allow shorter catheters to be withdrawn and new ones

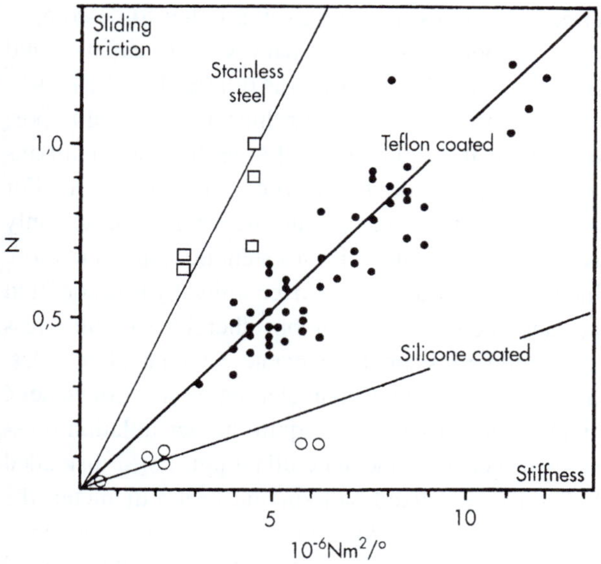

Fig. 12.4 Dependence of sliding friction on guidewire stiffness and material surface (Modified from Schroder [3], with permission.)

to be loaded over the wire without moving the distal tip from its position across a lesion.

Steerable guidewires are required when the diseased vessel lumen is tortuous, is nearly occluded, or has branches that are difficult to cannulate owing to acute angulation. They contain a relatively long, tapered, distal segment with gradual reductions in the stainless steel core wire diameter to provide a maneuverable leading end. The proximal shaft must be relatively stiff to transmit torque and steer the distal tip. The guidewire tip may be steered by bending the proximal shaft and rotating it or applying a torque device over the proximal shaft to facilitate rotation. Steerable guidewires range from 0.014 to 0.035 in. in diameter and have variable distal tip curvatures and degrees of floppiness. In general, smaller diameter guidewires are more fragile and deform easily. Slippery guidewires are frequently coated with layers of silicone, creating a low-friction surface when wetted. A slippery guidewire originally distributed as the Glidewire (Terumo, Somerset, NJ) has several unique features. Its core wire is composed of minimally elastic nickel–titanium alloy, is tapered at its distal end, and has an outer surface of polyurethane rather than spring coil. This wire is pliable yet kink resistant, becomes most slippery when wetted (hydrophilic), and is able to cross occluded arterial segments by virtue of its minimal frictional properties.

Angioplasty Balloons and Catheters

Treatment of symptomatic, focal atherosclerotic lesions in coronary arteries presently relies on percutaneous transluminal angioplasty (PTA) techniques with balloon-tipped catheters. The success of balloon angioplasty in coronary and peripheral arterial applications is related to improved balloon catheter materials and design beginning in 1974 with Gruntzig's development of a more constant volume balloon [4]. A better understanding of how balloon angioplasty dilates a stenotic lesion may also contribute to further catheter refinements. Description of the mechanism of lesion alteration by balloon dilatation has been elucidated [5, 6]. There appears to be little remodeling or compaction of plaque as a result of balloon inflation. Instead, the force exerted by the balloon causes formation of cracks and tears along the luminal surface of the plaque and arterial wall. The intimal plaque is circumferentially separated from underlying media for variable distances, and less diseased arterial wall is radially stretched. The resultant increase in luminal dimensions at both the narrowest stenotic site and along adjacent vessel generally creates noncircular luminal cross sections (Fig. 12.5). Because thin portions of the plaque are more easily cracked than thick atheroma, eccentrically positioned lesions are generally easier to balloon-dilate than concentric stenoses. Eccentric stenoses account for roughly two-thirds of atherosclerotic lesions found in coronary and peripheral arteries [7]. Most cracks and tears occur longitudinally along the vessel. Tears in this orientation are less apt to be lifted and produce local dissections in the wall following restoration of blood flow. This accounts for the relatively infrequent observation of significant intimal

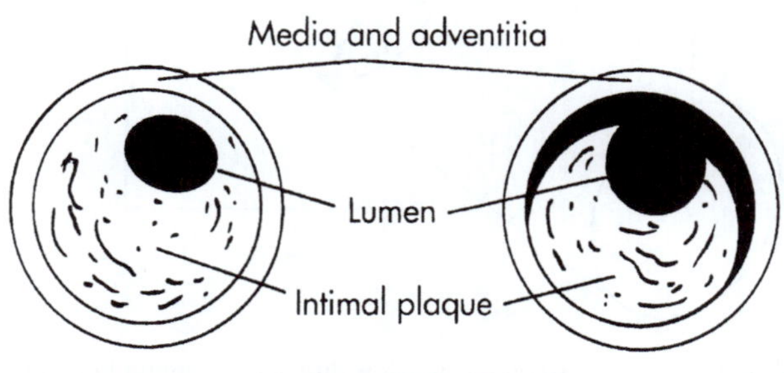

Fig. 12.5 Mechanism of dilatation of an atherosclerotic stenosis by transluminal balloon angioplasty with a resulting noncircular luminal cross section

flap formation and early thrombotic occlusion after balloon angioplasty.

Balloon Mechanics

Adequate luminal enlargement within a stenotic lesion depends on the radial dilating force generated by the inflated angioplasty balloon. This dilating force is influenced by a number of factors including balloon diameter and length, inflation pressure, compliance of the balloon, and the length and degree of stenosis. If the balloon surface is indented by a localized stenosis, the dilating force is the sum of radial forces generated by the hydrostatic pressure of fluid within the balloon and the radial component of tangential stress along the balloon membrane as it expands [8]. According to Laplace's law for cylindrical thin-walled structures, this tangential membrane tension or hoop stress is equal to the product of the internal pressure and the radius (Fig. 12.6). Large-diameter balloons generate more hoop stress at their surface for the same applied internal pressure and thus more dilating force on a stenotic lesion. The radial force component of the hoop stress generated at the balloon membrane is greatest when the balloon is most "hourglass" in shape as occurs with large balloons and in discrete stenotic lesions with steep constriction angles. The "clothesline effect" describes the diminishing radial force component of hoop stress as the balloon fully expands and loses its "waist" as the stenosis dilates (Fig. 12.7) [9].

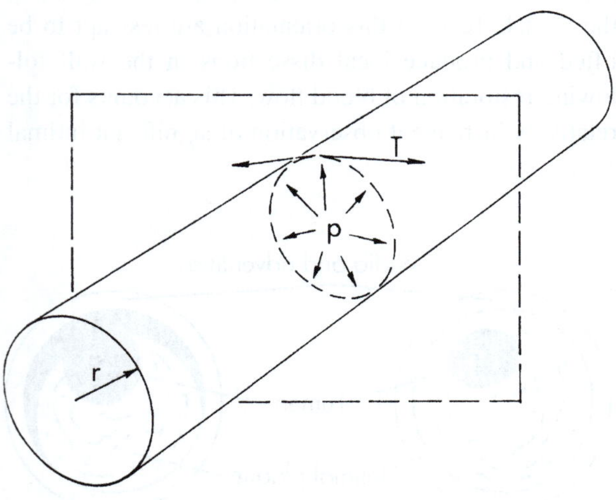

Fig. 12.6 Circumferential tension directed tangentially at the surface is known as hoop stress (*T*) for thin-walled cylindrical structures. According to Laplace's law, hoop stress is equal to the product of internal pressure (*p*) and the radius (*r*)

These mechanical relationships have several important clinical implications. Large-diameter balloons generate greater dilatation force for two reasons. For a given inflation pressure in large balloons, not only is hoop stress greater within a stenotic lesion, but more internal surface area exists over which hydrostatic fluid pressure acts. Large balloons therefore require less distending pressure to generate an equivalent dilating force than small-diameter balloons. Conversely, small-diameter balloons require higher inflation pressures to generate adequate dilatation. For a distended balloon with a fixed balloon and lesion diameter, the dilating force linearly increases with inflation pressure. Applying more pressure to eliminate a small dent in the balloon produces little additional dilating force owing to the "clothesline" effect and is more likely to rupture the balloon. Hoop stress exists in the vessel wall as well. In general, large-diameter vessels require less pressure to dilate and potentially to rupture. In addition to the dilating force generated by the balloon, the composition of the stenotic lesion influences the degree of luminal enlargement. Diffusely calcified plaques may resist displacement despite use of large-diameter balloons and high inflation pressures. However, because wall stresses tend to concentrate within calcific regions, balloon angioplasty more effectively cracks plaque adjacent to focal calcifications.

The relation between balloon stretch and inflation pressure (i.e., compliance) determines how effective the balloon is in terms of generating dilating force. If yield strength (i.e., the force causing permanent deformation) of the material approximates its ultimate tensile strength (i.e., the force required for material breakage), the diameter changes little with increasing inflation pressure. Inelastic balloons with low compliance provide more dilating force for a given inflation pressure at the stenosis and more predictable diameter and shape, and they resist inefficient overexpansion at the ends of the balloon (Fig. 12.8). With non-stretch balloons the dilating force is not affected by balloon length. In an eccentric lesion, however, where the vessel opposite the lesion is relatively elastic, a longer balloon provides more surface area to anchor the balloon during attempted displacement of the plaque.

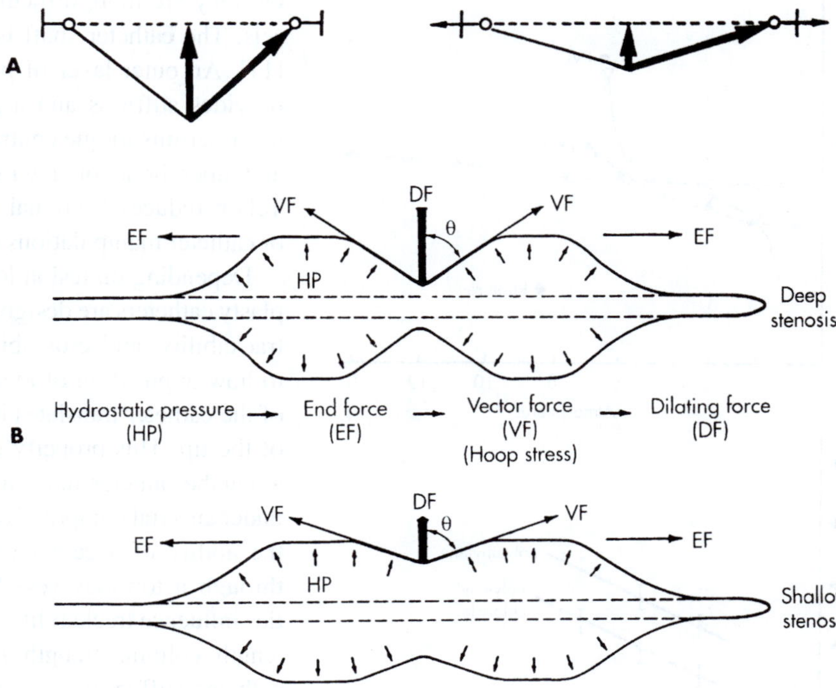

Fig. 12.7 Dilating force and clothesline effect. **a**, When weight hanging at the center of the clothesline is lifted by pulling on each end of the line, the force vector pushing upward decreases as the line straightens. **b**, Same principle applies to balloon dilatation. If the balloon surface is indented by localized stenosis, the radial force component force pushing outward is the dilating force. With progressive balloon expansion or dilatation of the stenosis, the dilating force decreases (From Abele [12], with permission.)

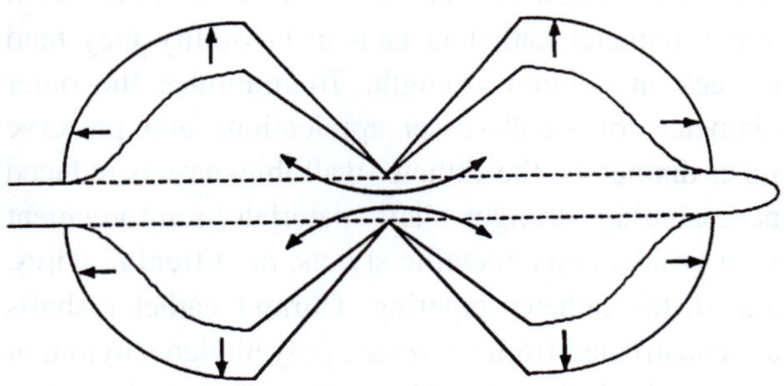

Fig. 12.8 Overdistention of a compliant balloon, which stretches longitudinally and outward around the stenosis (From Abele [8], with permission.)

Balloon Materials

Several polymers have been utilized in constant volume balloons of low compliance [10]. Early balloons and several current designs are constructed of polyvinyl chloride (PVC). Because PVC balloons are more compliant than those made of other available materials, they continue to elongate and are prone to rupture with increasing inflation pressures. Large-diameter PVC balloons are more compliant than small ones. Polyethylene (PE) balloons are generally less compliant, generate greater dilating force, and have higher burst pressure than equivalent-sized PVC balloons (Fig. 12.9). Diameter changes of less than 2% occur with standard PE balloons during working inflation pressures. Thin-walled PE balloons used with low-profile catheters are more compliant with 5–10% increases in diameter at maximum inflation pressures. Polyethylene can be chemically treated to alter its expansile properties, and these balloons are relatively "scratch resistant" within hard calcified lesions.

Newer polyethylene terephthalate (PET) balloons have low compliance and can withstand inflation pressures above 15 atm. The balloons have thin walls and low profiles and are used in small-diameter applications. They are more prone to rupture than PE balloons in calcified lesions. Balloons of composite nylon derivatives (Duralyn, Nydex) have variable compliance characteristics depending on the individual composition. Polyurethane balloons reinforced with nylon mesh (Olbert design, Meadox Medicals, Oakland, NJ) are relatively noncompliant (less than 2.5% diameter change) and have high burst pressures (more than 12 atm).

Angioplasty Catheters

Catheters used during angioplasty procedures have varying function depending on their length, diameter,

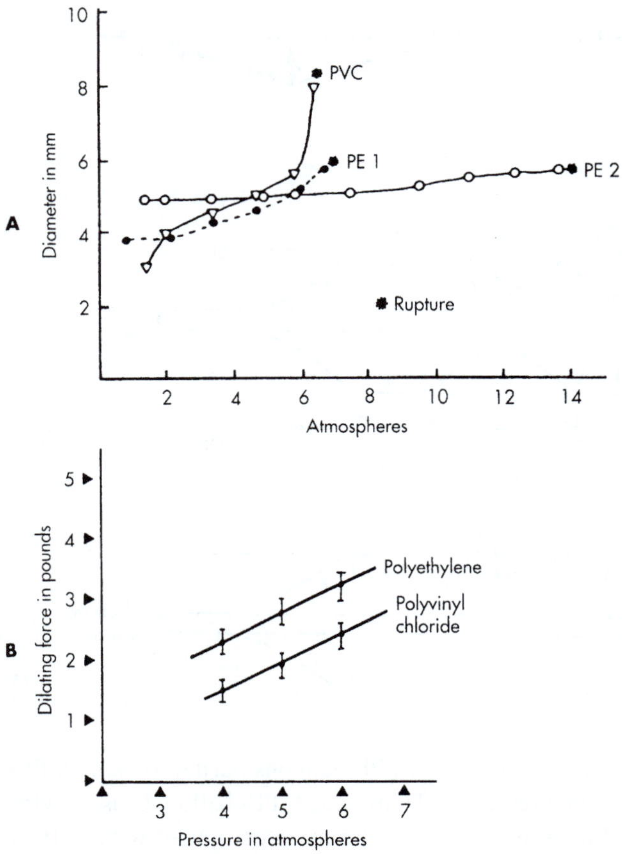

Fig. 12.9 Comparison of balloon materials. **a**, Diameter vs. inflation pressure for polyvinyl chloride (*PVC*) and polyethylene (PE) balloons. *PE1* and *PE2* balloons have been treated differently. PE2 is almost noncompliant compared to the more elastic PVC. **b**, Dilating force for a given inflation pressure is greater for low compliance PE than for a PVC balloon (From Abele [8], with permission.)

and construction. Guiding catheters provide a low-friction, large-bore channel for delivery of endovascular devices to remote target lesion sites. Although less important for interventions of iliac or femoral arteries from a transfemoral approach, guiding catheters are required for selective cannulation of coronary ostia, intra- and extracranial cerebral arteries, visceral branches, and distal extremity vasculature. In addition, these catheters must deliver contrast agents to visualize the distal vessel bed adequately and measure the pressure accurately while not occluding arterial inflow.

Guiding or introducer (sheath) catheters range from 4F to 24F in internal diameter. The shaft is relatively stiff compared to the tapered, preshaped softer catheter tip. Stiff catheters provide more support for positioning and catheter exchanges and a faster torque response, but they are more difficult to advance into distal vessels. The catheter shaft is constructed in three layers [11]. An outer layer of polyethylene or polyurethane provides stiffness and a preformed shape. A middle layer permits torque control and is composed of epoxy and fiber braid or a wire braid. Inner coating with Teflon reduces frictional resistance during guidewire or catheter manipulations through the guiding catheter.

Depending on lesion location and character, angioplasty catheters are designed with differing pushability, trackability, and crossability [12]. *Pushability* refers to how application of axial force to the proximal end of the catheter translates into advantageous movement of the tip. This property depends on column strength along the catheter and resistance to buckling or kinking under an axial compressive load. *Trackability* describes the ability of a catheter to follow over a guidewire through a tortuous vessel. A number of characteristics influence trackability, including shaft diameter and length, column strength, lateral flexibility (opposite of catheter stiffness), and frictional resistance between the inner guidewire, catheter, and vessel wall. What small-diameter catheters gain in flexibility they tend to lack in column strength. To minimize the outer diameter for small-vessel applications and preserve inner diameters, the catheter wall thickness is reduced necessitating stronger shaft materials, reinforcement with braids, coils, metallic stylets, or stiffening wires, and distal catheter tapering. Current catheter shafts are constructed from polyester, polyethylene, nylon, or polyamide derivatives. *Crossability* defines how easily the distal end of the catheter traverses the lesion to be treated. The development of low-profile angioplasty catheters with small-diameter, tapered distal tips, and deflated balloon segments facilitate placement across high-grade stenoses. Balloons with high expansion ratios (inflated/deflated diameters) are ideal. Polymeric surface coatings on angioplasty balloons reduce frictional forces and improve crossability. Application of silicone or similar materials can reduce friction by 30% in vitro [13]. Balloons are attached to catheter shafts by adhesives or thermal bonding. This region tends to be relatively stiff and can hinder catheter tracking. Gradual transitions in catheter stiffness in the distal balloon segment and "matching" the properties of catheters and guidewires optimize lesion crossing and tracking performance.

There are three basic types of balloon angioplasty catheter: over-the-wire, fixed-wire, and monorail [13].

Most balloon catheters employ an over-the-wire system and have two or more channels in their shaft: one for inflation of the balloon and one for guidewire passage, pressure measurement, or dye injection. Early catheters had coaxial shaft lumens. Current catheters have a separate dual-lumen design and allow independent movement of the balloon and the guidewire, thereby facilitating tracking and positioning in tortuous vessels and across difficult lesions. Fixed-wire catheters use a balloon in a guidewire design that reduces shaft diameter. The lower profile and greater flexibility of these catheters provide access to distal vessel lesions and use of smaller bore guiding catheters. Monorail catheters have an exit port for the guidewire 20–40 cm from the distal balloon. The more proximal catheter shaft has a smaller diameter and allows contrast injection during angioplasty. Rapid balloon catheter exchange and lesion access are provided by monorail systems.

Alteration of surface properties of wires and catheters with silicon, polyurethane, or tetrafluoroethylene coatings or constructs, as mentioned above, represented the first wave of technology to reduce overall friction. However, developments in polymer technology have allowed for marked improvements in vascular catheter and guidewire performance mainly due to alteration of surface hydrophilic lubricity [14]. Ideal handling characteristics for endovascular procedures require catheters and wires to possess minimal surface friction when wetted to optimize traversal of difficult lesions but not to be slippery when dry outside the body to allow pushability during entry/advancement and stability during device exchanges. Initial techniques employed physical attachment of hydrophilic polymer coatings (frequently through dip coating) such as poly-*N*-vinylpyrrolidone, polyethylene oxide, or organosiloxane copolymers. Unfortunately, mechanical ablative loss of the surface coating and its associated lubricious properties typically occurs with repeated device use, catheter passages, and wire exchanges. Attempts at improving adhesion between lubricious coatings and underlying biomaterials led to numerous techniques of "immobilizing"/physically intertwining long-chain hydrophilic polymers within complex networks of polyurea–polyurethane or polyacrylate. While these coatings showed improved abrasion resistance and withstood standard sterilization techniques, concerns for suboptimal bonding of coatings to underlying substrate persist. More permanent chemical attachment of coatings using reactive primer systems has been developed. The underlying substrate (i.e., polyurethane) is primed by polyisocyanate and one of the various nonreactive acetone/acetate solvents. Hydrophilic coatings (i.e., polyvinylpyrrolidone) then are applied in a second step and solvent evaporated. The achieved covalent bonding between coating and substrate may have better durability during longer periods of clinical implantation. However, short-term/single use of sterilized catheters and wires during an endovascular procedure does not mandate such durability for the applied lubricious coatings.

Metallic Intravascular Stents and Caval Filters

Several metallic devices are available for endovascular applications, including stents for treatment of difficult arterial and venous stenoses, inferior vena cava filters employed to prevent pulmonary embolism, and coils used to embolize bleeding vessels, arterial true or false aneurysms, and arteriovenous fistulas. Biocompatibility (corrosion resistance, thrombogenicity, toxicity) and the mechanical and physical properties of the commonly utilized metals affect the function and healing characteristics of various stent and filter designs.

Biocompatibility

Metallic devices should not undergo significant change in their mechanical, physical, or chemical properties during the period of implantation (corrosion and fatigue resistant) and should not induce any untoward clinically significant local or systemic changes in the body (nontoxic). Ideally, cardiovascular implants are thromboresistant, easy to produce, manufactured with consistent dimensional accuracy, of good quality without impurities or contaminants, easy to sterilize, and inexpensive, and they have an appropriate surface finish [15].

Corrosion Resistance

All available metallic endovascular devices (stents, filters, coils) are susceptible to corrosion. Because metals have high surface energy compared to that of their core, they tend to reach stability by absorbing elements from the environment. In contact with air they absorb oxygen, forming a thin layer of oxide on their surface. Such a surface is said to be "passive." It is protective for the metal by acting as a physical barrier that separates the metal core from its corrosive environment and prevents the transport of metal cations into solution. Corrosion takes place when this film is removed. The ideal corrosion-resistant metal has the ability to form a thin (1.0–1.5 nm), self-limiting, uniform oxide layer [16]. Corrosion of a vascular implant occurs in the presence of a saline environment by electrochemical mechanisms where the difference between electrical potential of the metal and blood determines how corrosion resistant the metal is. Metals forming a good protective film are aluminum, titanium, tantalum, and chromium, whereas stainless steel is relatively prone to corrosion [17]. Noble metals such as platinum, gold, and titanium are passive and extremely corrosion resistant but have limited use because of their excessive ductility and low tensile strength [17].

Several additional factors influence the overall corrosion resistance of a metallic device including its bulk state, surface state, and design and processing and its handling at the time of implantation. Stainless steel (SS) in its austenitic and annealed forms is more corrosion resistant than the martensitic and work-hardened structures; electropolished surfaces are more resistant than those mechanically polished. The sterilization method also affects the state of the final surface. Sterilization of SS by steam is superior to that by dry heat, moist ethylene oxide, or 24-h immersion in benzalkonium chloride [16]. Corrosion can be limited by avoiding heterogeneities in the material, eliminating crevices or sharp corners, and abolishing friction between metal struts, which can produce fretting corrosion [17].

Of early stent constructs, Wallstents and Strecker stents (Boston Scientific, Watertown, MA) had woven and knitted configurations that were potentially more susceptible to fretting corrosion than Palmaz stents (Cordis, Miami Lakes, FL), which are made from a single piece of SS tube. Coating the implant with metallic plating (chromium, nickel, cadmium) or with organic or inorganic nonmetallic agents can increase corrosion resistance [18, 19]. Scratching, bending, or surface contamination during handling/deployment may accelerate corrosion and produce mechanical failure [17].

Several types of localized corrosion have been described [16, 17]. Interface corrosion develops between two opposing surfaces owing to incomplete physical contact, creating electrolyte exchange (crevice corrosion), or because of two metals with different corrosion potentials exchanging electrons in a common electrolyte solution (galvanic corrosion). Pitting corrosion is the formation of small holes on the metal surface that tend to grow and can cause fracture and fatigue failure of the device. Pitting corrosion can occur with SS but is rare with titanium. Intergranular corrosion, which occurs with SS, is characterized by carbide precipitation and depletion of chromium; it is usually the result of improper manufacturing. Corrosion fatigue is due to repeated cyclic stress, causing disruption of the protective film, thereby promoting pitting corrosion and eventual fatigue cracks. Fatigue corrosion can occur with SS but not with titanium or cobalt–chromium alloys.

Toxicity

Localized or systemic toxicity can result from metal surface corrosion or by element dissolution in the medium. Local signs of biodegradation are common and are manifested by the presence of intracellular particulate matter or areas of discoloration in the tissues adjacent to the implant. Biodegradation of metals in vivo is typically less than that seen in vitro owing to the protective coating of implants by adsorbed proteins that in some cases (i.e., nickel) are metal specific. Few data are available concerning the systemic toxicity of metals commonly used in human implants. In general, no toxicity has been associated with iron, nitinol, tantalum, or titanium compounds, whereas cobalt, chromium, molybdenum, and nickel are potentially toxic [17]. Copper, mercury, chromium, and vanadium can form biopolymer complexes that cross the cell membranes and interrupt nutrient or respiratory pathways [20]. There are also reports of severe allergic reactions to nickel and cobalt–chromium alloys present in fracture plates, joint prostheses [16, 17, 21, 22], cardiac pacemakers [23], and cardiac valves [24, 25] with such reactions often requiring removal of the implant.

Thromboresistance

The thrombogenic activity of a metal implant depends on its chemical and physical parameters, such as the surface charge, surface energy, and texture. The electrical charge of the surface influences the "wettability" (surface area occupied by a drop of blood) of the metal, with greater wettability increasing thrombogenicity [26]. Surfaces that are highly electronegative and donate electrons to blood (i.e., aluminum) are more thromboresistant, whereas those that absorb electrons (i.e., copper) are relatively thrombogenic [27]. Increased thromboresistance is unfortunately associated with decreased corrosion resistance. DePalma et al. [28] studied type 316 SS, tantalum, nickel, and stellite 21 (Co, Cr, Mo, C) but did not find a correlation between preimplantation surface charge and thrombogenicity. A direct correlation did exist between the degree of passivation of the metal by proteinaceous deposits on its surface and thromboresistance. Surface roughness (inhomogeneities more than 1 μm in height) creates steep electrical potential gradients that hinder surface passivation and contribute to local thrombus formation [29]. This phenomenon can be limited by electropolishing and generation of smooth, homogeneous surfaces with uniform surface potential.

Thrombogenicity in vivo also depends on rheologic and hemodynamic factors (blood coagulability, blood flow patterns, shear stress). All cardiovascular devices should ultimately be evaluated in the configuration in which they are going to be used clinically, as flow abnormalities and blood hypercoagulability can lead to failure of an otherwise satisfactory material or device [30]. Available metallic stents are thrombogenic and perform best in high flow locations with adjuvant administration of antiplatelet agents. The amount of thrombus deposition is proportional to the total metal surface area of the stent [18], thus optimal thrombogenicity is gained with low-profile stents with thin struts and large expansion ratios matched to the vessel diameter and lesion length to be treated. These design considerations must be balanced against the degree of mechanical support required of the expanded stent to maximize the luminal cross-sectional area after angioplasty.

Healing

The early and late events reported during the healing around metallic stents deployed in arteries and vena caval filters are derived mainly from animal investigations [31–35]. Metal composition, surface characteristics, thrombogenicity, and device design may each independently influence healing, but similar luminal and vessel wall responses occur after implantation of different stent types.

Immediately after stent implantation, fibrinogen and other blood proteins adhere to the oxide film and form a thin (5–20 nm) proteinaceous layer over exposed metal struts. This layer passivates the metal surface and creates a substrate for platelet and other blood element deposition [31]. After several minutes, an amorphous heterogeneous clot rich in platelets attaches to the protein layer. The early platelet-rich clot tends to fragment and slough but slowly stabilizes as the underlying protein layer thickens. After 24 h the clot becomes less cellular and consists mainly of fibrin strands oriented in the direction of flow [31] (Fig. 12.10). Within 3–4 weeks this thrombotic layer is replaced by a neointima of fibromuscular cells and extracellular matrix. Endothelial coverage over the neointima occurs, although several histologic and ultrastructural abnormalities suggest phenotypic heterogeneity or a cell origin different from that of native vascular endothelium [32]. Thinning of the neointima after 8 weeks is associated with resorption of cellular elements below the endothelium, leaving residual extracellular matrix and scattered fibrocytes.

Maximal neointimal thickness ranges from 50 to 400 μm and varies with the animal model and the stent used. A direct association has been found between the area of metal exposed to blood flow, the amount of initial thrombus formation, and the resulting thickness of the neointima. Stent-induced thrombosis and intimal thickening may be reduced by periprocedural anticoagulation and proper embedding of the stent struts into the arterial wall. Adequate stent deployment in a noncompliant vessel can usually be accomplished by dilating the stent to 10–15% larger than the native arterial diameter, whereas in compliant vessels a 1:1 stent/artery diameter ratio is appropriate [31].

Periadventitial fibrosis occurs around arterial stents implanted clinically and in animal models [35] and may represent an inflammatory response to a metallic foreign body. Alternatively, altered wall stresses imparted by expanded stents may induce local tissue remodeling and inflammatory changes. Thinning of the media under expanded stent struts has been observed with Palmaz stents [36], Wall stents [33, 35, 37, 38],

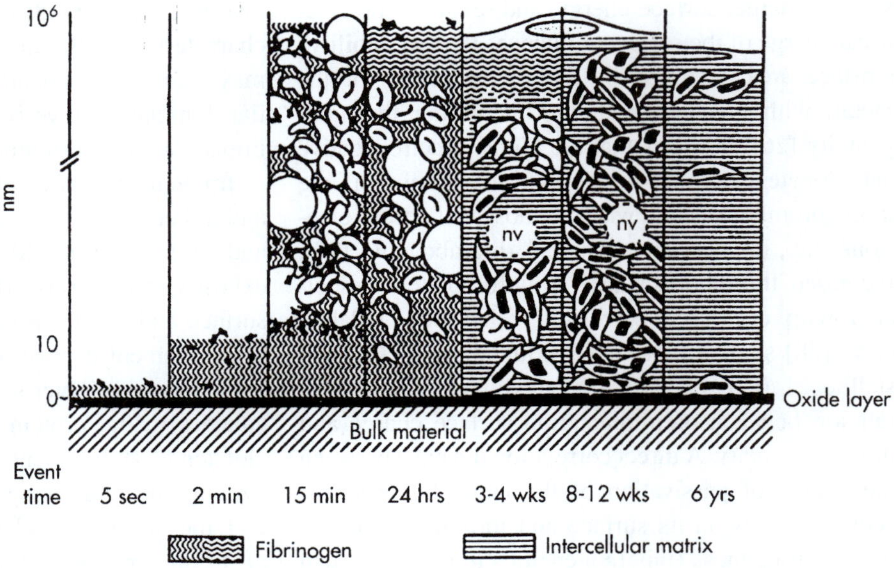

Fig. 12.10 Deposition along the luminal surface of a stent within a vessel. Layer height is in nanometers. *NV*, neovessels. *Vertical undulating lines* represent randomly oriented fibrinogen strands, and *horizontal undulating lines* are fibrinogen oriented in the direction of flow. *Parallel lines* represent extracellular matrix (From Palmaz [31], with permission.)

Strecker stents [39, 40], nitinol stents [41], Gianturco–Roubin "Bookbinder" stents (Cook, Bloomington, IN) [42], and Gianturco Z-stents (Cook) [43]. Medial thinning may be due to mechanical compression of the arterial wall by oversized stents or a result of smooth muscle atrophy caused by diminished pulsatile wall stresses and motion under relatively rigid stents [35].

Mechanical and Physical Properties of Specific Metals

Stainless Steel

Austenitic SS is the most widely used metal in endovascular implants. Type 304 (Fe 70%, Cr 18–20%, Ni 8–12%, Mn < 2%, silicone < 1%, C < 0.08%) is the constituent of Gianturco Z-stents, Gianturco–Roubin "Bookbinder" stents, several vena caval filters, and Gianturco embolization coils. Type 316 (Fe 70%, Cr 16–18%, Ni 10–14%, Mn < 2%, Mo 2–3%, silicone < 1%, C < 0.03%) is the component of Palmaz stents and Greenfield filters (Boston Scientific).

The various elements present in SS provide specific properties. Chromium is a ferrite former and stabilizes iron in a body-centered cube (bcc) crystalline state that is corrosion resistant. Nickel maintains the iron in a fully austenitic crystal structure at room temperature; at concentrations of more than 8% it decreases ferrite production, thereby improving corrosion resistance. Molybdenum is a ferrite stabilizer and at concentrations of 3% confers special resistance against pitting corrosion. Carbon is an austenite former and strengthening agent, but low concentrations are necessary to prevent precipitation in the form of chromium carbide, which decreases the corrosion resistance of the alloy. Silicone favors surface passivation, thereby increasing corrosion resistance [16].

Stainless steel is easy to fabricate and has adequate mechanical properties for use in vascular devices (Table 12.1). High ultimate tensile strength, low-yield stress, and high ductility allow the plastic deformation necessary for construction of balloon-expandable stents. Although 316 SS is less prone to corrosion than other types of SS, its resistance to interface (crevice) corrosion and fatigue is inferior to that of other metals. Stainless steel is generally biocompatible, but several adverse reactions have been reported potentially due to liberation of a nickel derivative or iron deposits [16, 44].

Tantalum

Early Strecker and Viktor stents (Medtronic) were made of tantalum. This metal has a bcc structure and resists corrosion by forming a stable surface film of tantalum pentoxide. In addition to favorable corrosion resistance and biocompatibility [45–47], tantalum is dense and highly radiopaque [15]. Despite its low

Table 12.1 Properties of metals used in endovascular implants

Property	SS (annealed)	Tantalum (annealed)	Beta-titanium (F67)	Nitinol 55–45	Co–Cr alloy (wrought)
Specific gravity (g/cm^3)	7.9	16.6	4.5	4.5	9.2
Elastic modulus (Young's) (MPa)	2.0×10^5	1.0×10^5	1.0×10^5 to 1.2×10^5	0.8×10^5	2.1×10^5 to 2.5×10^5
Yield strength (0.2% strain) (MPa)	2.8×10^2	–	1.6×10^2 to 5.5×10^2	7.6×10^2	4.5×10^2 to 4.9×10^2
Ultimate tensile strength (MPa)	5.5×10^2	0.3×10^2 to 1.3×10^2	4.0×10^2 to 6.2×10^2	1.1×10^3	6.5×10^2 to 6.9×10^2
% Elongation	50	40	30	8	8
Fatigue endurance limit (MPa)	2.3×10^2 to 2.8×10^2	–	–	–	2.4×10^2 to 2.8×10^2

Data were extracted from Keller et al [47]. and Castleman and Motzkin [56].
MPa: megapascals; SS: stainless steel.

tensile strength, tantalum has a relatively high elastic modulus and fatigue resistance, making it a suitable metal for balloon-expandable but not self-expanding stents [37]. Tantalum and SS stents knitted in the same pattern have demonstrated equivalent resistance to compression [45]. Despite in vitro studies showing tantalum's electronegative surface to be more thromboresistant than that of titanium, SS, or copper [48], in vivo evaluation has revealed similar thrombogenicity [49]. Diminished platelet adhesion to tantalum stents has been achieved with polyurethane coating [50], whereas plasma treatment has not decreased the thrombogenicity but has increased the elasticity and flexibility of Strecker stents [19].

Titanium

Titanium has been widely used in orthopedic and oral implants, artificial heart valves, and the newer Greenfield caval filters. Titanium has a crystalline structure that varies with temperature. At low temperatures it has a hexagonal form, but if it is worked above 900°C, beta-titanium in a bcc form is produced [39]. Vanadium added to titanium stabilizes the beta form at lower temperatures. The tensile strength of titanium varies with its oxygen content, and high oxygen concentrations increase strength but compromise ductility. Titanium is flexible, having an elastic modulus roughly one-half that of SS, tantalum, and cobalt–chromium alloy [51]. Titanium's surface readily passivates and is resistant to pitting and crevice and stress corrosion (cracking) [51]. Titanium does have a tendency to gall or seize when in sliding contact with itself or other metals, contributing to relatively poor wear resistance [15]. Greenfield and Savin compared titanium and SS vena caval filters and demonstrated more flexibility, allowing downsizing of titanium devices into 12.5F delivery sheaths from the 19F sheaths required for SS filters [34]. In vitro testing revealed greater resistance to fatigue and less corrosion of titanium filters than for SS devices. Titanium's low specific gravity allows construction of lightweight devices but hinders radiographic visualization of implants. Titanium is relatively biologically inert [52] and thromboresistant.

Nitinol

Devices constructed of nitinol (45–50% titanium and 50–55% nickel) have found increasing endovascular applications beginning with the early Cragg stent (Mintec, Freeport, Bahamas) and Simon caval filter (Nitinol Medical Technologies, Woburn, MA), and more recently in numerous endoluminal stent-graft devices. Nitinol is an acronym for nickel titanium Naval Ordinance Laboratory; the properties of this alloy were discovered by William Buehler [53]. The unique characteristics of this alloy are its shape memory (Marmen) effect and its superelasticity. If plastically deformed at a low temperature, it recovers its original shape when raised to a higher temperature. To possess this shape memory effect, an alloy must have a crystal structure that can shift to a martensitic (ordered, bcc superlattice) configuration when subjected to certain thermal or mechanical stresses and then revert to an austenitic (disordered bcc) structure when the stress is removed. Nitinol wires can be shaped at room temperature and when cooled quickly with saline irrigation they assume straighter, lower profile configurations. Exposure to body temperatures at deployment allows return to its expanded, deformed shape. To achieve full shape recovery, however, the initial deformation must not exceed an internal strain of 3–9%.

Superelasticity is due to the martensitic transformation induced by mechanical stress. The stress–strain relation for nitinol is linear up to a plastic deformation threshold, which is normally an irreversible process where it reverts from the austenitic to the martensitic structure and continues to deform plastically under further stress loading. When the load is removed nitinol can return to its original unstressed dimensions and austenitic structure, as occurs after an elastic deformation. Superelasticity confers to nitinol elasticity approximately 10 times greater than for any other metal alloy [53] and increases the effective expansion ratio of stents by allowing greater initial compression and packaging within smaller introducer catheters. The tensile strength of nitinol is comparable to that of 316 SS, and the Cragg stent has demonstrated a hoop strength double that of the Wallstent [54]. Results of recent fracture testing of thin-walled nitinol tubes (used for stent construction) have differed from initial bulk product nitinol testing (bar and strip) and demonstrated less fracture resistance and greater fatigue-crack growth with cyclic loading [55]. Development of fatigue cracks may affect structural device stability especially if propagation occurs across short distances of thin (0.25 mm) struts commonly used in nitinol stents. These findings may explain the significant incidence of clinical nitinol stent fractures observed after treatment of distal superficial femoral artery occlusive lesions that are typically subjected to repetitive bending, torsional, and compressive forces in the distal thigh/knee region. Refined longer length peripheral stent designs involve helical shapes to reduce circumferential stress concentrations especially at angled strut interfaces. Nitinol also has corrosion resistance comparable to that of titanium [56]. It has been estimated that 0.1% of the population may be allergic to nickel and potentially some of these could develop reaction to nitinol [56]. However, orthopedic devices and endovascular stents implanted in animals were not associated with any local or systemic toxicity [56–59]. Inflammatory responses to implants were not different from those found around other metals despite occasional free nickel and titanium elements released into surrounding tissue.

Cobalt–Chromium Alloys

Several cardiovascular devices are made of cobalt–chromium-based alloys and began with the Vena-Tech (LG Medical, Chasseneuil, France) caval filter (Co 42%, Cr 21.5%, Ni 18%, Fe 8.85%, Mo 7.5%, Mn 2%) and several heart valves and rings. Also, the Boston Scientific Wallstent is constructed of Elgiloy (cobalt–chromium–nickel). These alloys exhibit good wear and corrosion resistance and have a high elastic modulus and ductility. Carbon impurities can lead to the formation of carbides that may induce brittle behavior of the alloy. Cobalt–chromium alloys are biocompatible, but the presence of nickel and chromium has the potential to cause adverse systemic effects [60].

Radiologic Considerations

Endovascular devices ideally are easily visible under fluoroscopy to aid deployment and do not produce artifacts when imaged by computed tomography (CT) or magnetic resonance imaging (MRI). MRI studies may be contraindicated in patients with metallic implants because of concern over potential device displacement generated by the induced electromagnetic field during the procedure. Distortion and artifact on MRI images depends on the magnetic susceptibility of the metal, its specific gravity, its shape, its position and orientation in the body, and the type of image processing [61]. The risk of device displacement is related to the strength of the magnetic field and the length of time since implantation. Endovascular device movement is unlikely after approximately 6 weeks of healing even with ferromagnetic metals.

Few studies have been performed comparing the behavior of endovascular devices when examined by

CT or MRI [46, 61–63]. Because of its high density, tantalum implants are easily visible under fluoroscopy but produce significant artifacts on CT images. Titanium devices are relatively radiolucent but produce little CT artifact owing to their lower specific gravity. MRI imaging artifacts, ferromagnetism, and magnetic torque of several endovascular devices have been investigated by Teitelbaum et al. [62]. Although 304 and 316 SS are both austenitic and therefore nonmagnetic, the type of cold working required to fabricate devices can induce significant ferromagnetism. The 316 SS has higher nickel content than the 304 type, which better stabilizes iron in a nonmagnetic state. However, all SS devices generate marked "black hole" artifacts and MRI image distortion. Elgiloy and nitinol devices create mild MRI artifacts. Titanium devices have little ferromagnetism in fields up to 4.7 T and do not generate MRI artifacts. MRI images of tantalum Strecker stents implanted in dogs showed few luminal artifacts [63], but in general, MRA imaging provides lower clarity in-stent visualization and quantitative assessment than current CTA techniques.

Design Characteristics

Stents

Three general types of intravascular stent have been developed: balloon-expandable, self-expanding, and thermal memory (nitinol) stents (Table 12.2). Available stents are currently made of acceptable biocompatible materials. Performance of a given stent is influenced by the biomaterial properties and the stent design. Characteristics of an ideal intravascular stent have been described by Becker [64].

The in vitro mechanical properties of Palmaz stents [65], Wallstents [38, 66], Gianturco Z-stents [67], and Cragg stents [54] have been reported. Overall stent stiffness is related to the metal used, strut caliber, the length of the stent, and the ratio between the compressed and the expanded diameter [33]. In vitro, the Palmaz stent is three times more rigid and has a higher radial strength than the Wallstent [65]. Cragg et al. reported nitinol spiral stents to have a hoop strength

Table 12.2 Characteristics of early vascular stents

Characteristic	Palmaz	Strecker	Viktor	Gianturco–Roubin	Wallstent	Gianturco Z-Stent	Cragg
Manufacturer	Cordis/J & J	MediTech/ Boston Scientific	Medtronic	Cook	Schneider/ Boston Science	Cook	Mintec
Expansion mode	Balloon exp	Balloon exp	Balloon exp	Balloon exp	Self-exp	Self-exp	Thermal memory
Configuration	Slotted	Knitted mesh	Helical coil	Book-binder coil	Woven mesh	Zigzag pattern	Spiral
Composition	316 SS	Tantalum	Tantalum	304 SS	Elgiloy	304 SS	Nitinol
Strut thickness (mm)	0.12	0.07–0.10	0.13	0.15	0.07–0.17	–	0.27
Delivery sheath (F)	6–9	10	8	–	7–9	–	8–10
Expanded diameter (mm)	3–18	2–14	2.5–3.5	2–4	2.5–15.0	–	8–10
Expansion ratio	High	High	High	Low	High	High	High
Foreshortening	++	++	+	++	+++	0	+
Metal surface	++	+++	+	++	++	+	+
Longitudinal flexibility	0	+++	++	+++	+++	0	++
Radial flexibility	0	+++	+	+	+++	+	+
Retrievable when deployed	No	No	?	No	No	?	Yes
Biocompatibility	+	+	+	+	+	+	+
Radiopacity	+	+++	+++	+	+	+	+
MRI artifacts	++	0	0	+++	++	+++	+

exp: expandable; MRI: magnetic resonance imaging; SS: stainless steel.

twofold that of Wallstents [54]. However, after expansion in vivo, the adequacy of radial stiffness of the stent for optimizing luminal diameter is more dependent on matching stent and artery size, plaque distribution, and morphology than on stent material. Strut thickness of available stents varies with stent diameter but differs among designs. Nitinol's superelastic properties potentially facilitate construction of stents with small struts while maintaining radial strength. Although the surface area occupied by exposed struts in an expanded stent may influence stent thrombogenicity, most early stents had similar metal surface area. Gianturco Z-stents and Viktor and Cragg spiral stents have the least metal surface area, and Strecker stents have the largest area. Palmaz stents have a metal surface area of 31% when collapsed and 12% at 6 mm diameter expansion [36]; expanded Wallstents have 20% exposed metal surface area [33].

Although all early stents had an expansion ratio of approximately 6:1, their degree of foreshortening at full expansion varies. Little foreshortening exists with nitinol spiral stents (about 7%) [54] but increases to between 13 and 25% for Palmaz stents and up to 40% for Wallstents [66]. Significant foreshortening makes precise positioning of the stent difficult, necessitates the use of longer stents for proper lesion treatment, and potentially increases the thrombogenic potential of the stent because of the larger exposed metal surface areas.

Some stent flexibility is required to cross tortuous vessels and is desirable if positioning is required within vessels near flexing joints. Wallstents and Strecker stents have both longitudinal flexibility and radial flexibility [38, 39], whereas Cragg spiral stents have only longitudinal flexibility and Palmaz stents are relatively rigid. Some radial flexibility may decrease the compliance mismatch between the stented and the unstented portions of the vessel and potentially reduce intimal hyperplasia and restenosis phenomena [68]. However, radial flexibility of Wallstents deployed in normal canine arteries is lost within weeks after stenting due to progressive fibrous encapsulation [35]. Recurrent intimal trauma caused by the cyclic motion of flexible stents has been proposed to contribute to a neointimal reaction [31, 33, 37, 64], but no significant differences in neointimal thickness have been found between self-expanding (Wallstent) and balloon-expandable (Palmaz) stents deployed in animals [33, 38]. Strecker stents produce some retraction at the ends of the struts (i.e., flaring), which may protrude into the lumen [39, 49, 69, 70] and potentially contribute to increased intimal thickening, irregular surface contour, and an occasional marked inflammatory reaction around the metal struts [70].

Vena Caval Filters

Several inferior vena cava filters have been developed to prevent PE, and their characteristics have been extensively reviewed [71]. With the exception of the Simon nitinol filter, they are all self-expandable. Greenfield SS filters have been used for more than 12 years and have a filter patency rate of 98%, an inferior vena cava (IVC) patency rate of 95%, and a low incidence of recurrent PE (4%); moreover, only a few cases of migration or perforation have been reported. Hampered by its large delivery system (24F) insertion site, venous thrombosis unfortunately occurs with significant frequency (41%) [71]. Newer models of the Greenfield filter have been constructed of beta-titanium and have modified attachment hooks. The greater elasticity of titanium has facilitated downsizing of the device and delivery through a 12F carrier system (14F sheath), and it has reduced the incidence of insertion site thrombosis to 8% while maintaining comparable efficacy (recurrent PE rate 3.5% and IVC patency rate 99%) [72]. The greater elasticity of titanium may be responsible for the 10% incidence of filter limb asymmetry [72] and potential perforation of the IVC due to excessive limb splaying [73].

The Gianturco–Roehm Bird's Nest filter made of 304 SS can be delivered through a 12F sheath and can expand up to 4 cm, making it ideal for deployment into large IVCs (typically >30 mm diameter). Although its use is associated with an IVC patency rate of 97%, a filter patency rate of 81%, and an incidence of recurrent PE of only 2.7%, cases of filter migration have been reported [71].

Other earlier "permanent" filters included the Vena-Tech/LGM filter composed of a cobalt–chromium alloy, that potentially self-centered when deployed, and was delivered through a 12F sheath. From a multicenter clinical trial in Europe, the incidence of recurrent PE was low (2%) after LGM placements but the complication rate was high (migration 13%, IVC thrombosis 8%, tilting 8%) [74]. The Simon nitinol filter had the lowest profile available (delivered through a 9F sheath) but was associated with a high incidence of

IVC thrombosis (20%) not easily explained by its filter design or new (nitinol) material construct [71, 75].

Temporary and prophylactic uses for IVC filters have been greatly augmented by recent availability of "retrievable" or "optional" filter designs. In theory, these filters could be placed during higher pulmonary embolism risk intervals and be retrieved through a transjugular catheter after clinical improvement, lessening of PE risk, and/or safe administration of anticoagulation. Current retrievable filters are constructed of nitinol (Bard G2, Tempe, AZ and OptEase, Cordis, Miami Lakes, FL) or stainless steel (Cook Gunther Tulip and Celect filters, Bloomington, IN). Unfortunately, many of the recent retrievable filter reports document limited size cohorts with short follow-up periods compared to the more extensive documentation for older permanent filters [76–80]. Surprisingly, only a relatively small fraction (<20–30%) of current filters are actually being retrieved and suggests that current filter designs are being used preferentially over older permanent devices potentially without intention for temporary use. When retrieval has been attempted, it has been successful in generally greater than 80% of cases with filter "tilt"/angulation within the IVC and longer dwell times (>6 months) associated with less successful retrieval and presence of intra-filter/IVC thrombus being an absolute contraindication for removal. There are continuing reports of filter migration, filter strut perforations beyond the IVC wall, and filter/IVC thrombosis but the overall risk of PE after filter deployment remains less than 3%. Based on recent observations, the IVC possesses an elliptical cross-sectional shape that changes significantly with vascular volume fluctuations in the patient (i.e., hydration status) and respiratory variation [81]. These findings will influence further design refinements owing to the need for "soft," flexible struts within an axisymmetric filter able to endure significant shape deformations and maintain capture of thrombus and avoid migration. "Active" fixation, currently provided by barbed struts, appears necessary due to significant IVC shape changes but strut stiffness needed for device anchoring must be countered with diminished perforation potential.

Endoluminal Grafts

Great interest was generated by the early animal and clinical experiences in the 1980s and 1990s with catheter-based delivery of endovascular stent-grafts (endografts) to intraluminally exclude infrarenal abdominal aortic aneurysms (AAA) [82–86]. Various combinations of anchoring stents and stent "scaffolds" attached to prosthetic graft materials have been developed to treat pathological lesions involving the thoracic aorta (aneurysms, dissections, penetrating atherosclerotic "ulcers"), degenerative and pseudoaneurysms (e.g., traumatic, paraanastomotic, mycotic), and atherosclerotic occlusive lesions [87, 88] involving the aortoiliac, femoropopliteal, and supraaortic trunk vessels. Most reports have focused on the relative success of exclusion of these arterial lesions (i.e., prevention of aneurysm rupture, endograft patency) and description of perceived short- and mid-term failure modes. Since limited large animal modeling is available to replicate human pathological arterial diseases being currently treated with endografts, endograft assessment during autopsy procedures is rare and surgical explantation of failing/failed endograft devices is an uncommon event (<1% of implants), little data exist regarding healing characteristics, confirmation of failure modes, and mechanical stability/durability of available devices. Only from such data can optimal design characteristics be discerned.

Prosthetic Graft Materials

Endoluminal prostheses are constructed from currently available graft materials and metallic stents. Both polyester (Dacron) graft materials and polytetrafluoroethylene (PTFE) have been used in thoracic and aortoiliac endograft applications while PTFE has been utilized in most smaller diameter peripheral endografts. Although current endoluminal graft designs vary considerably, the type of prosthetic material has influenced device performance.

Dacron grafts have been the mainstay of aortic reconstruction since the early 1960s, and PTFE found application as an arterial conduit during the 1970s. Dacron grafts are soft and pliable yet relatively inelastic; they demonstrate minimal dilatation after implantation, with a 6–12% increase in cross-sectional area observed during extended in vitro testing [89]. At physiologic arterial pressures Dacron and PTFE vascular grafts have radial compliances much less than that of normal or diseased arteries (Table 12.3) [90–92].

Table 12.3 Radial compliance of human artery and synthetic grafts

Graft	Conduit time after implantation	Species	Compliance (% diameter change/mmHg × 10^{-2})
Thoracic aorta [98]		Human	
		Age 20 years	27
		Age 40 years	20
		Age 60 years	14
Femoral artery [99]		Human (age > 50 years)	6–11
Woven Dacron [100]	0	Human	0.16
Knitted Dacron [99, 100]	0	Human	1.5–1.9
	8 months		0.8
Double velour Dacron [100]	0	Human	3.4
Standard PTFE [99]	0	Human	1.6

PTFE: polytetrafluoroethylene.

Compliance of synthetic grafts tends to decrease further after implantation owing to necessary fibrous tissue ingrowth and encapsulation. Strength in the polyester fabric structure is cumulatively determined by basic polymer, individual fiber, and yarn structure properties (Figs. 12.11, 12.12, and 12.13) [93]. Tensile yield strengths range from nearly 100 times that of native aorta for woven Dacron and standard wall PTFE grafts to 10-fold greater for double velour knits (Table 12.4) [91]. Radial burst strengths are 110–120 pounds per square inch (psi) for double velour knitted Dacron grafts and 30 psi for thin-walled PTFE grafts—considerably more than the maximal arterial pressure (250 mmHg = 4.8 psi) [89, 94]. Small-caliber, thin-walled, nonreinforced PTFE sleeves used for early endoluminal grafts allowed low-profile device delivery and could be balloon-expanded to three to five times their original diameters [94, 95]. Significant microscopic structural deformation occurred in material dilated beyond this elastic limit, thus generating concern over the long-term stability and strength of PTFE endografts used with large expansion ratios. Adequate short-term (less than 1 year) structural integrity of "super-dilated" PTFE endografts within experimental aortic aneurysms was demonstrated by Palmaz

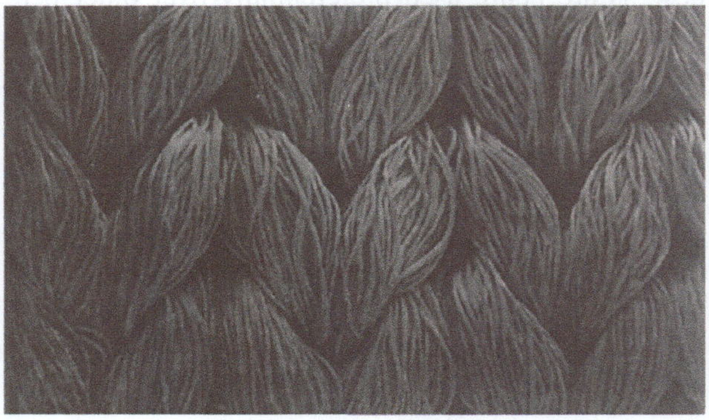

Fig. 12.12 SEM of the outer surface of a DeBakey standard knit Dacron vascular graft. ×37 (From Snyder and Botzko [93], with permission.)

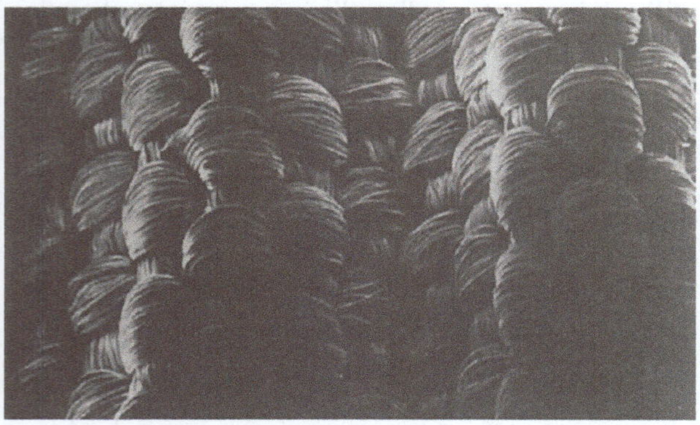

Fig. 12.11 Scanning electron micrography (SEM) of the outer surface of a DeBakey woven Dacron vascular graft. ×37 (From Snyder and Botzko [93], with permission.)

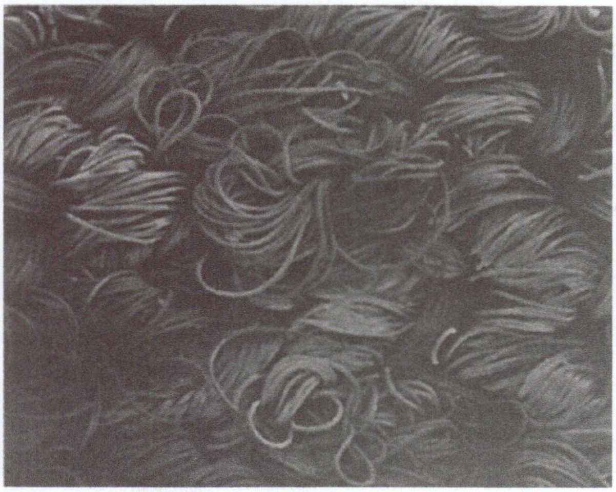

Fig. 12.13 SEM of the inner, luminal surface of a Dacron velour graft. ×37 (From Turner et al. [89], with permission.)

Table 12.4 Tensile yield strength of native artery and synthetic grafts

Material	Yield strength (dynes/cm^2)
Thoracic aorta	3.8×10^7
Woven Dacron	2.2×10^9
Knitted Dacron	0.8×10^9
Double velour knitted Dacron	0.3×10^9
Standard wall reinforced PTFE	3.3×10^9

Modified from Kinley and Marble [91].
PTFE: polytetrafluoroethylene.

et al. [96], but longer term clinical evaluation was lacking.

Porosity is an essential component for the function of synthetic vascular prostheses. For textile grafts this parameter is difficult to describe quantitatively. Wesolowski et al. assessed the porosity of fabric grafts in terms of their permeability by measuring the volumetric flow of water through the material at a pressure differential of 120 mmHg (ml $H_2O/cm^2/min$) [97]. Early studies in pigs and dogs advocated the use of Dacron grafts, with the permeability approaching 5,000 ml/cm^2/min for optimal healing (Gossamer theory) [97]. These porous, ultrathin-wall, knitted grafts were associated with significant dilatation and hemorrhage clinically, however [98]. Current Dacron grafts have lower porosity, thicker walls, greater strength, and improved healing characteristics (Fig. 12.14). Available knitted polyester grafts are currently made impervious (to blood) by gelatin "sealing"/impregnation prior to sterilization and packaging that has not affected healing characteristics. Polyester grafts associated with current endografts are not treated with any "sealing" techniques and remain potentially porous. Connective tissue penetration is not essential for genesis of a pseudointima, but connective tissue support is critical to its long-term existence. This statement is based on the observation that a pseudointima is not formed in areas where tissue incorporation is completely absent, although it is frequently present in areas where adjacent connective tissue is minimal [99]. Extensive proliferation of fibrous tissue as observed in Gossamer grafts in animals may not be desirable but some degree of ingrowth is necessary. Higher porosity (60 μm fibril length) PTFE grafts have shown improved healing and luminal surface endothelialization in animals [100], but clinical evaluation did not demonstrate differences in the healing response compared to standard wall (20–30 μm fibril length) PTFE grafts [101].

In general, more porous, thinner walled polyester grafts have greater distensibility (Fig. 12.15) [93]. Velour Dacron grafts were developed initially to improve healing along luminal and external surfaces (see Fig. 12.13). Early velour grafts (Sauvage Bionit, DeBakey Vasculour) had intermediate porosity compared to woven and knit Dacron but improved handling characteristics. The newer double velour grafts (Microvel and Cooley knit) have permeability similar to that of knit Dacron and are more elastic. The wall thickness of double velour grafts is increased by the inner and outer layers (pile heights 180 and 400 μm, respectively) of perpendicular yarn loops. Thin-walled knitted Dacron (Weavenit) has a wall thickness of 380 μm by comparison. The fine porous surface within the velour pile increases the tissue bond between graft and perigraft tissues and improves the rate of tissue incorporation in Dacron grafts implanted in experimental animals. These studies utilized mechanical peel tests to document more complete and adherent tissue layers along luminal and external surfaces of velour grafts [93]. Lindenauer described enhanced healing of double velour Dacron grafts compared with either internal or external velour surfaces alone [102]. Other studies have noted a more adherent outer fibrous layer with double velour fabrics but no difference in luminal surface healing [93]. Claggett reported reduced platelet survival and less pseudointimal development

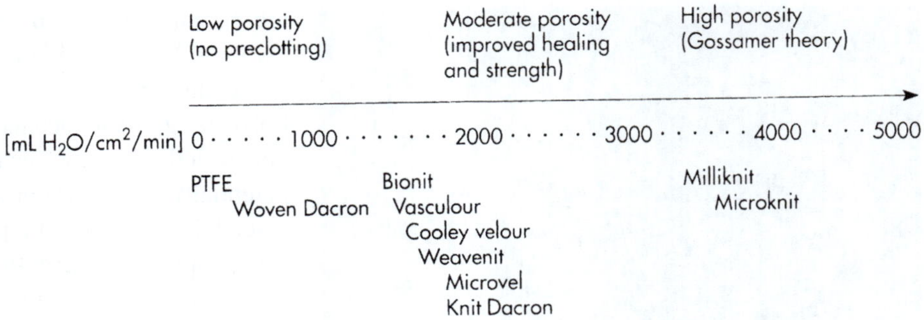

Fig. 12.14 Range of permeabilities and corresponding porosity for available polyester and PTFE vascular prostheses (in milliliters of water per square centimeter per minute) at a 120 mmHg pressure differential (Modified from Snyder and Botzko [93], with permission.)

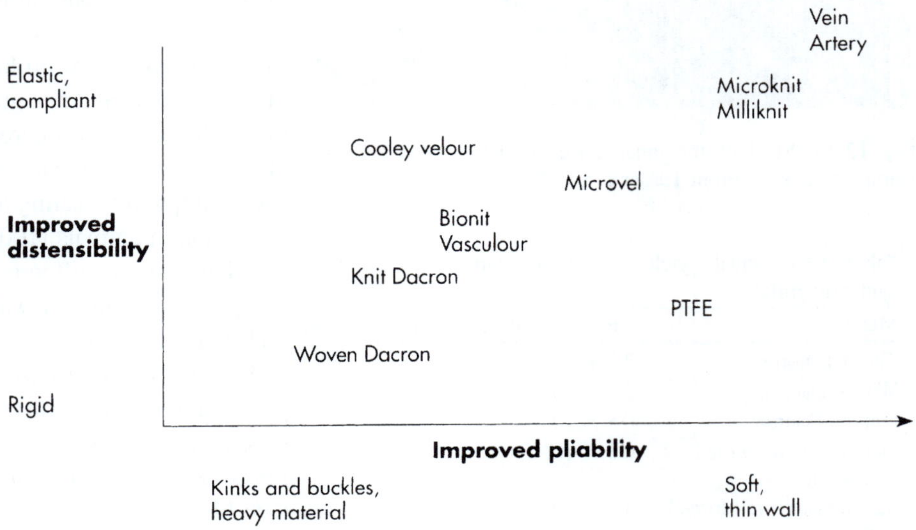

Fig. 12.15 Range of qualitative handling characteristics of available polyester and PTFE vascular graft materials compared to those of native vessels. With a thinner wall, the lighter weight Dacron prostheses tend to be more elastic (From Snyder and Botzko [93], with permission.)

on double velour grafts compared with knitted surfaces for 42 weeks following surgery [103]. At present, improved healing characteristics of velour Dacron fabrics, especially in humans, have not been adequately documented.

Details of healing characteristics of polyester and PTFE coverings of endografts within diseased human arteries remain largely unknown. Prosthetic coating over stents has been proposed to inhibit the neointimal ingrowth that limits long-term patency rates following angioplasty and stenting of occlusive lesions, but evidence of this benefit is lacking. Preliminary studies of endoluminal prostheses constructed from PTFE grafts and Palmaz stents deployed in nondiseased canine iliac arteries showed more neointimal development but a preserved luminal cross-sectional area compared to that of the anastomotic regions of interposition PTFE grafts [104]. Interestingly, more complete endothelial cell coverage of endoluminal PTFE/Palmaz stented grafts has been observed in dogs than occurred on the inner surface of interposition PTFE grafts [104, 105]. Descriptions of clinical endograft healing are limited to several brief reports [106–108]. Detection of endothelial cell coverage up to 7 cm into an endograft (distance from device edge) by factor VIII staining was noted 5 months after device deployment for arterial occlusive disease [106]. In that series, a local inflammatory response to endografting appeared to be related to the presence or absence of a reinforcing wrap on the PTFE used and the depth within the wall in which the device recanalized the occlusion. It remains to be seen whether reendothelialization occurs with intraluminal positioning of stent-graft devices in aneurismal segments compared to the expected pseudointima forming within most prosthetic reconstructions that remains devoid of endothelial cells.

A pronounced, early, systemic inflammatory response to endoluminal grafts has been observed in several small series, manifested by fever and leukocytosis. Elevated levels of various serum markers of inflammation were noted by Hayoz et al. [109] in patients after deployment of Cragg Endopro System

1 devices (Mintec Minimally Invasive Technologies SARL, La Ciotat, France) when compared to nitinol stents implanted for occlusive disease and by Norgren and Swartbol [110] after endografting of AAA compared to conventional open repairs. Despite significant proinflammatory cytokine and leukocyte adhesion molecule responses after endografting, no correlation was found between inflammatory mediator levels and the presence of patient symptoms [109]. Interestingly, in vitro neutrophil activation could be elicited only by exposure to complete endoluminal devices but not to individual biomaterial components of the endografts [109]. The clinical importance of systemic inflammatory responses and their specific cause as related to device construction and deployment remain unknown.

Endograft Design and Structural Stability

Current endografts have substantially evolved from early constructs (Table 12.5). Bifurcated aortoiliac devices assembled in situ from modular components have replaced earlier single, tubular designs for treating AAAs. Current devices are completely or nearly completely supported along the graft material length by self-expanding stent "scaffolding." Earlier devices employed balloon-expandable proximal stents with unsupported polyester graft throughout most of the device body and limbs and were associated with risk of limb kinking/stenosis and thrombosis [111]. Proximal fixation is provided by "passive" frictional forces by self-expanding stent radial expansion (Medtronic AneuRx, Santa Rosa, CA, Endologix Powerlink, Irvine, CA), "active" infrarenal attachment by extraluminal barbs (WL Gore Excluder, Flagstaff, AZ, Guidant EVT/Ancure, Indianapolis, IN), or suprarenal/visceral bare stent expansion with (Cook Zenith, Bloomington, IN) or without (Medtronic Talent, Santa Rosa, CA) barbs. Some bifurcated devices utilize a shorter body/longer iliac limb design (AneuRx, Talent, Excluder) while others use long body/short limbs (Zenith, Powerlink, EVT/Ancure). Graft materials used are PTFE (Excluder, Powerlink) or polyester (AneuRx, Talent, Zenith, EVT/Ancure) and stent metals are stainless steel (Zenith), Elgiloy (EVT/Ancure), or nitinol (AneuRx, Talent, Excluder, Powerlink).

Associated with early attempts to minimize delivery catheter profile, ultrathin endograft materials were used (woven polyester for AneuRx, thin-walled PTFE for Excluder and thoracic TAG devices). Early clinical evaluations of these devices revealed persistent transgraft microleaks after AneuRx implantation [112], infrequent development of AAA sac hygromas requiring device explantation, and AAA diameter growth by more than 5 mm (without rupture) in 38% of patients in the Excluder's 5-year follow-up report [113]. Blood or serum transgraft leak and continued sac pressurization without identifiable endoleak (endotension) were attributed to persistent permeability/porosity of the ultrathin graft materials used. Both companies altered

Table 12.5 Aortic endograft designs

Device	Application	Configuration	Graft material	Support
Parodi [83]	AAA	Aortomonoiliac	Dacron (ultrathin, knit)	Palmaz stent (prox, distal)
Chuter [84]	AAA	Singular, bifurcated	Dacron (thin, woven)	Gianturco Z (prox, distal, barbed)
EVT/Ancure [85]	AAA	Tubular, aortoaortic	Dacron (thin, woven)	Elgiloy stents (prox & distal, barbed)
Vanguard (Meadox) Boston Scientific)	AAA	Modular, bifurcated	Dacron (ultrathin, woven)	Nitinol scaffold (self-exp)
AneuRx (Medtronic)	AAA	Modular, bifurcated	Dacron (ultrathin, woven)	Nitinol scaffold (self-exp)
Talent (Medtronic)	AAA	Modular, bifurcated	Dacron	Nitinol Z-stent scaffold (self-exp)
Excluder (WL Gore)	AAA	Modular bifurcated	PTFE, reinforced	Nitinol scaffold (self-exp)
TAG (WL Gore)	thoracic	Tubular	PTFE	Nitinol scaffold (self-exp)
Zenith (Cook)	AAA	Modular bifurcated	Dacron	Stainless steel Z-stents (self-exp)
Powerlink (Endologix)	AAA	Singular, bifurcated	PTFE	Nitinol scaffold (self-exp)

AAA: Aortic Endograft Designs; AAA: abdominal aortic aneurysm; prox: proximal; exp: expandable.

their graft materials to reduce permeability in 2004 without having to increase delivery catheter diameter. Medtronic tightened the weave pattern of the AneuRx polyester to create a denser material with 50% lowering of permeability (Resilient Graft Material). WL Gore added a thin, non-porous expanded PTFE reinforcing film to the outer surface of Excluder and TAG components (low-permeability endoprostheses). For the modified Gore devices, greater fractions of aneurysm sac regression and reduction of sac expansions to <3% of patients were documented in subsequent reports [114, 115].

Owing to a rigorous surveillance follow-up regimen that included multiview plain film radiographs in addition to CT scans, the extensive aortic endograft experience of Michael Marin offers the most complete documentation of mechanical device failure [116]. Sixty patients were identified (15%) with device fatigue from 696 thoracic and abdominal/aortoiliac aneurysm cases treated with a variety of first- and second-generation stent-grafts. Endoleaks associated with device fatigue were found in 40% of cases with five patients requiring open conversion and endograft explantation. Most (43) device failures were related to stent strut fractures involving nitinol, stainless steel, and Elgiloy constructs. Stent fractures involved the nitinol longitudinal connecting bar of Talent and Gore TAG devices and typically angled regions of the Z-shaped stent scaffolding within proximal endograft locations. During the initial development of larger diameter thoracic endografts and over early concern for the increased deformation forces expected in the thoracic aorta, WL Gore subsequently modified the original TAG device in 2004 to remove the "at risk" longitudinal connecting bar. Fabric fatigue and perforation of endograft covering material was noted in all five explantation cases [116]. These appear to occur at contact regions of repetitive motion/friction between the adjacent stent scaffolding and the endograft material. There was minimal evidence of stent metal corrosion detected by electron microscopy of explanted devices. Fine permanent sutures are used in most devices to secure endograft prosthetic coverings to the adjacent stent scaffolding during construction. Numerous suture disruptions and long length separations of stent "rows" within the early Vanguard device were documented by Jacobs et al. [116] and were reported as part of a clinical trial [117]. The high incidence of mechanical failures halted any further modification or clinical development of the Vanguard device. Mechanical device failure has been an infrequent event for most current aortic endografts but longer term observations are required.

References

1. Schroder J: The mechanical properties of guidewires. Part I. Stiffness and torsional strength, *Cardiovasc Intervent Radiol* 16:43–46, 1993.
2. Schroder J: The mechanical properties of guidewires. Part II. Kinking resistance, *Cardiovasc Intervent Radiol* 16:47–48, 1993.
3. Schroder J: The mechanical properties of guidewires. Part III. Sliding friction, *Cardiovasc Intervent Radiol* 16:93–97, 1993.
4. Gruntzig A, Hopff H: Percutane Rekanalisation chronischer arterieller Verschlusse mit einem neuen Dilatationskatheter: Modification der Dotter-Technik, *Dtsch Med Wochenschr* 99:2502–2505, 1974.
5. Castaneda-Zuniga WR, Formanek A, Tadaverthy M et al.: The mechanism of balloon angioplasty, *Radiology* 135:565–571, 1980.
6. Chin AK, Kinney TB, Rurik GW et al.: A physical measurement of the mechanisms of transluminal angioplasty, *Surgery* 95:196–200, 1983.
7. Waller BF: The eccentric coronary atherosclerotic plaque: morphologic observations and clinical relevance, *Clin Cardiol* 12:14–20, 1989.
8. Abele JE: Balloon catheters and transluminal dilatation: technical considerations, *Am J Radiol* 135:901–906, 1980.
9. Abele JE: Balloon catheter technology. In Castaneda-Zuniga WR, Tadavarthy SM, editors: *Interventional radiology*, Baltimore, 1992, Williams & Wilkins, pp. 345–350.
10. Matsumoto AH, Barth KH, Selby JB, Tegtmeyer CJ: Peripheral angioplasty balloon technology, *Cardiovasc Intervent Radiol* 16:135–143, 1993.
11. Jacobs AK: Selection of guiding catheters. In Faxon DP, editor: *Practical angioplasty*, New York, 1993, Raven Press, pp. 43–52.
12. Abele JE: Balloon engineering and materials. In Vlietstra RE, Holmes DR, editors: *Coronary balloon angioplasty*, Boston, 1994, Blackwell Scientific, pp. 292–304.
13. Faxon DP: Selection of balloon catheters and guidewires. In Faxon DP, editor: *Practical angioplasty*, New York, 1993, Raven Press, pp. 53–70.
14. Fan YL:: Hydrophilic polymers. In Salamone JC, editor: *Polymeric materials encyclopedia*, Boca Raton, FL, 1996, CRC Press, pp. 3107–3114.
15. Williams DF: The selection of implant materials. In Williams DF, Roaf R, editors: *Implants in surgery*, London, 1973, Saunders.
16. Sutow EJ, Pollack SR: The biocompatibility of certain stainless steels. In Williams DF, editor: *Biocompatibility of clinical implants materials*, vol. 1, Boca Raton, 1981, CRC Press.
17. Williams DF: The deterioration of materials in use. In Williams DF, Roaf R, editors: *Implants in surgery*, London, 1973, Saunders.

18. Palmaz JC: Balloon expandable intravascular stent, *AJR* 150:1263–1269, 1988.
19. Crochet D et al.: Plasma treatment effects on the tantalum Strecker stent implanted in femoral arteries of sheep, *Cardiovasc Intervent Radiol* 17:285–291, 1994.
20. Lemons JE: Corrosion and biodegradation. In von Recum A, editor: *Handbook of biomaterials evaluation*, New York, 1986, Macmillan.
21. Fisher AA: Safety of stainless steel in nickel sensitivity, *JAMA* 221:1282, 1972.
22. Fisher AA: Allergic dermatitis presumably due to metallic bodies containing nickel or cobalt, *Cutis* 19:285, 1977.
23. Samitz MH, Katz SA: Nickel dermatitis hazards from prostheses: in vivo and in vitro solubility studies, *Br J Dermatol* 92:287, 1975.
24. Lyell A, Bain WH: Nickel allergy and valve replacement, *Lancet* 1:408, 1974.
25. Pegum JS:: Nickel allergy, *Lancet* 1:674, 1974.
26. Williams DF: The response of the body environment to implants. In Williams DF, Roaf R, editors: *Implants in surgery*, London, 1973, Saunders.
27. Sawyer PN et al.: Electrochemical precipitation of blood cells on metal electrodes: an aid in the selection of vascular prostheses, *Natl Acad Sci* 53:294, 1965.
28. De Palma VA et al.: Investigation of three-surface properties of several metals and their relation to blood compatibility, *J Biomed Mater Res Symp* 3:37, 1972.
29. Sawyer PN et al.: Electron microscopy and physical chemistry of healing in prosthetic heart valves, skirts and struts, *J Thorac Cardiovasc Surg* 67(1):24, 1974.
30. Sawyer PN, Sophie Z, O'Shaughnessy AM: Hemocompatibility assessment. In von Recum A, editor: *Handbook of biomaterials evaluation*, New York, 1986, Macmillan.
31. Palmaz JC: Intravascular stents: tissue–stent interactions and design considerations, *AJR* 160:613, 1993.
32. Robinson KA et al.: Correlated microscopic observations of arterial responses to intravascular stenting, *Scanning Microsc* 3:665, 1989.
33. Rousseau H et al.: Self-expanding endovascular prosthesis: an experimental study, *Radiology* 164:709, 1987.
34. Greenfield LJ, Savin MA: Comparison of titanium and stainless steel Greenfield vena caval filters, *Surgery* 106:820, 1989.
35. Back M, Kopchok G, Mueller M et al.: Changes in arterial wall compliance after endovascular stenting, *J Vasc Surg* 19:905–911, 1994.
36. Palmaz JC et al.: Normal and stenotic renal arteries: experimental balloon-expandable intraluminal stenting, *Radiology* 164:705, 1987.
37. Schatz RA: A view of vascular stents, *Circulation* 79:445, 1989.
38. Vorwerk D et al.: Neointima formation following arterial placement of self-expanding stents of different radial force: experimental results, *Cardiovasc Intervent Radiol* 17:27, 1994.
39. Barth KH et al.: Flexible tantalum stents implanted in aortas and iliac arteries: effects in normal canines, *Radiology* 175:91, 1990.
40. White CJ et al.: A new balloon-expandable tantalum coil stent: angiographic patency and histologic findings in an atherogenic swine model, *J Am Coll Cardiol* 19:870, 1992.
41. Sutton CS et al.: Titanium-nickel intravascular endoprosthesis: a 2-year study in dogs, *AJR* 151:597, 1988.
42. Roubin G et al.: Early and late results of intracoronary arterial stenting after coronary angioplasty in the dog, *Circulation* 76:891, 1987.
43. Rollins N et al.: Self-expanding metallic stents: preliminary evaluation in an atherosclerotic model, *Radiology* 163:739, 1987.
44. Den Otter G: Total prosthetic replacement of atrioventricular valves in the dog, *Thorax* 27:105, 1972.
45. Strecker EP et al.: Expandable tubular stents for treatment of arterial occlusive diseases: experimental and clinical results, *Radiology* 175:97, 1990.
46. Von Holst H, Collins P, Steiner L: Titanium, silver and tantalum clips in brain tissue, *Acta Neurochir (Wien)* 56:239, 1981.
47. Keller JC, Lautenschlager EP: Metal and alloys. In von Recum A, editor: *Handbook of biomaterials evaluation*, New York, 1986, Macmillan.
48. Hearn JA, Robinson KA, Roubin GS: In vitro thrombus formation of stent wires: role of metallic composition and heparin coating [abstract], *J Am Coll Cardiol* 17:302A, 1991.
49. Ribeiro PA et al.: A new expandable intracoronary tantalum (Strecker) stent: early experimental results and follow-up to twelve months, *Am Heart J* 125:501, 1993.
50. Fontaine AB et al.: Decreased platelets adherence of polymer-coated tantalum stents, *J Vasc Intervent Radiol* 5:567, 1994.
51. Williams DF: Titanium and titanium alloys. In Williams DF, editor: *Biocompatibility of clinical implant materials*, vol. 1, Boca Raton, 1981, CRC Press.
52. Williams DF: Titanium as a metal for implantation. Part 2. Biological properties and clinical applications, *J Med Eng Technol* 1:266–270, September 1977.
53. Schetky LM: Shape-memory alloys, *Sci Am* 241:74, 1979.
54. Cragg AH et al.: Nitinol intravascular stents: results of preclinical evaluation, *Radiology* 189:775, 1993.
55. Stankiewicz JM, Robertson SW, Ritchie RO: Fatigue-crack growth properties of thin walled superelastic austenitic Nitinol tube for endovascular stents, *J Biomech Mater Res A* 81:685, 2007.
56. Castleman LS, Motzkin SM: The biocompatibility of nitinol. In Williams DF, editor: *Biocompatibility of clinical implant materials*, vol. 1, Boca Raton, 1981, CRC Press.
57. Haasters J, Bensmann G, Baumgart F: Memory alloys: a new material for implantation in orthopedic surgery. Part II. In Uhthoff HK, editor: *Current concepts of internal fixation of fractures*, New York, 1980, Springer-Verlag.
58. Castleman LS et al.: Biocompatibility of nitinol alloy as an implant material, *J Biomed Mater Res* 10:695, 1976.
59. Oonishi H et al.: Biological reaction of Ni in TiNi shape memory alloy, *Trans Soc Biomater* 7:183, 1984.
60. Williams DF: The properties and clinical uses of cobalt-chromium alloys. In Williams DF, editor: *Biocompatibility of clinical implant materials*, vol. I, Boca Raton, 1981, CRC Press.
61. Shellock FG, Kanal E: MR procedures and patients with biomedical implants, materials, and devices. In Shellock

FG, Kanal E, editors: *Magnetic resonance: bioeffects, safety and patient management*, New York, 1994, Raven Press.
62. Teitelbaum GP, Bradley WG, Klein BD: MR imaging artifacts, ferromagnetism and magnetic torque of intravascular filters, stents and coils, *Radiology* 166:657, 1988.
63. Matsumoto AH et al.: Tantalum vascular stents: in vivo evaluation with MR imaging, *Radiology* 170:753, 1989.
64. Becker GJ: Intravascular stents, general principles and status of lower extremity arterial applications, *Circulation* 83(suppl I):122, 1991.
65. Fluckiger F et al.: Firmness, elasticity and deformation characteristics of metal stents [abstract], *Cardiovasc Intervent Radiol* 16(suppl):19, 1993.
66. Jedwab MR, Clerc CO: A study of the geometrical and mechanical properties of a self-expanding metallic stent—theory and experiment, *J Appl Biomater* 4:77, 1993.
67. Fallone BG, Wallace S, Gianturco C: Elastic characteristics of self-expanding metallic stents, *Invest Radiol* 23:370, 1988.
68. Abbott WM et al.: Effect of compliance mismatch on vascular graft patency, *J Vasc Surg* 5:376, 1987.
69. Laird JR et al.: Placement and angiographic patency of the Strecker coronary stent, *Cathet Cardiovasc Diagn* 31:322, 1994.
70. Santoian EC, King S: Intravascular stents, intimal proliferation and restenosis [editorial comment], *J Am Coll Cardiol* 19:877, 1992.
71. Greenfield LJ, DeLucia A: Endovascular therapy of venous thromboembolic disease, *Surg Clin North Am* 72:969, 1992.
72. Greenfield LJ et al.: Extended evaluation of the titanium Greenfield vena caval filter, *J Vasc Surg* 20:458, 1994.
73. Teitelbaum GP et al.: Vena caval filter splaying: potential complication of use of the titanium Greenfield filter, *Radiology* 173:809, 1989.
74. Ricco JB et al.: Percutaneous transvenous caval interruption with the "LGM" filter: early results of a multicenter trial, *Ann Vasc Surg* 3:242, 1988.
75. Dorfman GS: Percutaneous inferior vena cava filters, *Radiology* 174:987, 1990.
76. Proctor MC, Greenfield LJ: Form and function of vena cava filters: how do optional filters measure up? *Vascular* 16:10, 2008.
77. Rosenthal D, Wellons ED, Hancock SM, Burkett AB: Retrievability of the Gunther Tulip vena cava filter after dwell times longer than 180 days in patients with multiple trauma, *J Endovasc Ther* 14:406, 2007.
78. Kalva SP, Athanasoulis CA, Fan CM et al.: Recovery vena cava filter: experience in 96 patients, *Cardiovasc Intervent Radiol* 29:559, 2006.
79. Schutzer R, Ascher E, Hingorani A et al.: Preliminary results of the new 6F TrapEase inferior vena cava filter, *Ann Vasc Surg* 17:103, 2003.
80. Van Ha TG, Chien AS, Funaki BS et al.: Use of a retrievable compared to permanent inferior vena cava filters: a single institution experience, *Cardiovasc Intervent Radiol* 31:308, 2008.
81. Murphy EH, Johnson ED, Arko FR: Evaluation of wall motion and dynamic geometry of the IVC using intravascular ultrasound: implications for future design, *J Endovasc* Ther 15:349, 2008.
82. Balko A, Piasecki GJ, Shah DM et al.: Trans-femoral placement of intraluminal polyurethane prosthesis for abdominal aortic aneurysm, *J Surg Res* 40:305–309, 1986.
83. Parodi JC, Palmaz JC, Barone HD: Transfemoral intraluminal graft implantation for abdominal aortic aneurysms, *Ann Vasc Surg* 5:491–499, 1991.
84. Chuter TAM, Green RM, Ouriel K et al.: Transfemoral endovascular aortic graft placement, *J Vasc Surg* 18:185–197, 1993.
85. Moore WS, Rutherford RB: Transluminal endovascular repair of abdominal aortic aneurysm: results of the North American EVT phase I trial, *J Vasc Surg* 23:543–553, 1996.
86. White RA, Fogarty TJ, Kopchok GE et al.: Evaluation of a modular endovascular bifurcation prosthesis in a canine aortic aneurysm model, *J Vasc Surg* 24:1034–1042, 1996.
87. Cragg AH, Dake MD: Percutaneous femoropopliteal graft placement, *Radiology* 187:643–646, 1993.
88. Marin ML, Veith FJ, Sanchez LA et al.: Endovascular aortoiliac grafts in combination with standard infrainguinal arterial bypasses in the management of limb-threatening ischemia: preliminary report, *J Vasc Surg* 22:316–325, 1995.
89. Turner RJ, Hoffman HL, Weinberg SL: Knitted Dacron double velour grafts. In Stanley JC, editor: *Biologic and synthetic vascular prostheses*, Orlando, 1982, Grune & Stratton, pp. 509–522.
90. Gonza ER, Marble AE, Shaw A, Holland JG: Age related changes in mechanics of the aorta and pulmonary artery in man, *J Appl Physiol* 36:407, 1974.
91. Kinley CE, Marble AE: Compliance: a continuing problem with vascular grafts, *J Cardiovasc Surg* 21:163–170, 1980.
92. Walden R, L'Italien GJ, Megerman J, Abbott WM: Matched elastic properties and successful arterial grafting, *Arch Surg* 115:1166–1169, 1980.
93. Snyder RW, Botzko KM: Woven, knitted and externally supported Dacron vascular prostheses. In Stanley JC, editor: *Biologic and synthetic vascular prostheses*, Orlando, 1982, Grune & Stratton, pp. 485–494.
94. Diethrich EB: Initial experience with in vivo expansion of PTFE in the treatment of occlusive and aneurysmal disease [abstract], *J Endovasc Surg* 2:308–309, 1995.
95. Bergeron P, Henric A, Bonnet C, Reim R: Tensile characteristics of expanded PTFE for use in endoluminal grafting [abstract], *J Endovasc Surg* 2:302–303, 1995.
96. Palmaz JC, Tio FO, Laborde JC et al.: Use of stents covered with PTFE in experimental abdominal aortic aneurysm, *J Vasc Intervent Radiol* 6:879–885, 1995.
97. Wesolowski SA, Fries CC, Karlson KE et al.: Porosity, primary determinant of ultimate fate of synthetic grafts, *Surgery* 50:91–101, 1961.
98. Ottinger LW, Darling RC, Werthlin LS et al.: Failure of ultra light weight knitted Dacron grafts in arterial reconstruction, *Arch Surg* 111:146–149, 1976.
99. Szilagyi E, Pfeifer JR, DeRusso FJ: Long-term evaluation of plastic arterial substitutes: an experimental study, *Surgery* 55:165–183, 1964.

100. Golden MA, Hanson SR, Kirkman TR et al.: Healing of PTFE arterial grafts is influenced by graft porosity, *J Vasc Surg* 11:838–845, 1990.
101. Kohler TR, Stratton JR, Kirkman TR et al.: Conventional versus high-porosity PTFE grafts: clinical evaluation, *Surgery* 112:901–907, 1992.
102. Lindenauer SM, Weber TR, Miller TA et al.: Velour vascular prostheses, *Trans Am Soc Artif Intern Organs* 20:314–319, 1974.
103. Claggett PC: In vivo evaluation of platelet reactivity with vascular prostheses. In Stanley JC, editor: *Biologic and synthetic vascular prostheses*, Orlando, 1982, Grune & Stratton, pp. 131–152.
104. Ohki T, Marin ML, Veith FJ et al.: Anastomotic intimal hyperplasia: a comparison between conventional and endovascular stent graft techniques, *J Surg Res* 69:255–267, 1997.
105. Ombrellaro MP, Stevens SL, Freeman MB, Goldman MH: Reendothelialization and platelet derived growth factor activity associated with intraarterial stented grafts, *Vasc Surg* 31:631–637, 1997.
106. Marin ML, Veith FJ, Cynamon J et al.: Human transluminally placed endovascular stented grafts: preliminary histopathologic analysis of healing grafts in aortoiliac and femoral artery occlusive disease, *J Vasc Surg* 21:595–604, 1995.
107. White RA, Donayre CE, deVirgilio C et al.: Deployment technique and histopathological evaluation of an endoluminal vascular prosthesis used to repair an iliac artery aneurysm, *J Endovasc Surg* 3:262–269, 1996.
108. McGahan TJ, Barry GA, McGahan SL et al.: Results of autopsy 7 months after successful endoluminal treatment of an infrarenal abdominal aortic aneurysm, *J Endovasc Surg* 2:348–355, 1995.
109. Hayoz D, Do-Dai D, Mahler F et al.: Aortic inflammatory reaction associated with endoluminal bypass grafts, *J Endovasc* Surg 4:354–360, 1997.
110. Norgren L, Swartbol P: Biological responses to endovascular treatment of abdominal aortic aneurysms, *J Endovasc* Surg 4:169–173, 1997.
111. Parent FN, Godziachvili V, Meier GH et al.: Endograft limb occlusion and stenosis after Ancure endovascular AAA repair, *J Vasc Surg* 35:686, 2002.
112. Matsumura JS, Ryu RK, Ouriel K: Identification and implication of transgraft microleaks after EVAR, *J Vasc Surg* 34:190, 2001.
113. Peterson BG, Matsumura JS, Brewster DC et al.: Five-year report of a multicenter controlled clinical trial of open versus endovascular treatment of AAA, *J Vasc Surg* 45:885, 2007.
114. Tanski W, Fillinger M: Outcomes of original and low-permeability Gore Excluder endoprosthesis for endovascular AAA repair, *J Vasc Surg* 45:243, 2007.
115. Makaroun MS, Dillavou ED, Wheatley GH et al.: Five-year results of endovascular treatment with Gore TAG device compared with open repair of thoracic aortic aneurysms, *J Vasc Surg* 47:912, 2008.
116. Jacobs TS, Won J, Gravereaux EC et al.: Mechanical failure of prosthetic human implants: a 10-year experience with aortic stent-graft devices, *J Vasc Surg* 37:16, 2003.
117. Beebe HG, Cronenwett JL, Katzen BT et al.: Results of an aortic endograft trial: impact of device failure beyond 12 months, *J Vasc Surg* 33:S55, 2001.

Ancillary Endovascular Equipment: Catheters, Guidewires, and Procedural Considerations

13

Tony D. Fang

The concept of treating peripheral arterial diseases using catheter and wires is no longer a novel. For instance, a typical vascular surgeon will perform more than 50% of his/her cases using endovascular techniques. Vascular surgery started having endovascular credentialing and defining endovascular procedures as part of fellowship training since 1993 [1–5]. Vascular surgery fellowships today thrive by training practitioners skilled in both open and endovascular interventions. Some programs have taken one step further, using stimulation modules to train their fellows with good results [6]. For the interventional cardiologist training, it is required that fellows spending one full year learning skill sets for peripheral endovascular interventions [7]. The centerpiece of peripheral endovascular training is to be facile in various guidewire and catheter skills. With the excitement of constant evolution of the field, it becomes apparent that no one can master every guidewire and catheter. However, the basic concept of guidewire and catheter skills remains unchanged. It is essential to be familiar with these skills and build upon them in practice.

In this chapter, we will summarize the basics of guidewires and catheters, review some of their unique features, various access techniques, several classic interventions examples, and complications related to guidewires and catheters.

T.D. Fang (✉)
Attending Physician,Division of Vascular Surgery, Southern California Permanente Medical Group, Irvine, CA, USA

Special Terminology of Guidewire and Catheters

Steerability

The tips of the catheters or guidewires change direction in response to the operator's maneuvers at the hub. Catheters and guidewires having angles or curves are steerable. This term applies to both guidewires and catheters. In many situations, a combination of steerable wire and catheter is the only means to pass through stenotic lesions and torturous arteries.

Trackability

This term is specific for catheters. It refers to the ability of a catheter to follow the guidewire in the artery. Catheters having good trackability means they can easily pass through a torturous portion of the arteries over the wires. A good example is that a glide catheter can track over a Glidewire (Terumo Medical Corporation, Somerset, NJ) very easily through the stenosis.

Pushability

This term is also specific to catheters. It stands for the relationship of the operator pushing the catheter at the hub and the forward movement of the tip of the catheter.

T.J. Fogarty, R.A. White (eds.), *Peripheral Endovascular Interventions*,
DOI 10.1007/978-1-4419-1387-6_13, © Springer Science+Business Media, LLC 1998, 2010

Units for Wires and Catheters

Wires are measured in inches (in.). A 0.035 wire is, in fact, a 0.035-in. wire. The diameters of catheters or sheaths are in French size (F). One F ≈ 1/3 mm. The F size for a sheath (access sheath, guiding sheath) represents its inner diameter (ID), while the F size for a catheter or a dilator refers to its outer diameter (OD). Therefore, a 5F catheter should pass through a 5F access sheath. A 5F access sheath actually creates a 6F hole at the arterial wall. A 6F dilator will not pass through a 6F sheath, but actually fits a 7F sheath.

Guidewires

Manipulation of a guidewire is a fundamental skill for peripheral endovascular interventions. Since there is a broad array of products available today, we cannot be familiar with every one. However, the basics of the guidewires remain the same: their coating, diameter, tip property, stiffness, and length. By knowing those components, one should be able to match the guidewire to the appropriate scenario.

Coating

In order to decrease friction, many wires are coated with a layer of either Teflon or silicone. In addition, some guidewires have a layer of hydrophilic coating as the final finish. Guidewires having a hydrophilic coating are particularly valuable in crossing stenosed portions of the arteries and navigating through tortuous vessels. Combined with an angle tipped guide catheter, it becomes a basic technique in peripheral interventions. A classic example of this kind of wire is the Glidewire. However, almost every company today has their version of the "Glidewire" and they come in different lengths, tip shapes, and diameters.

Diameter

Guidewires come in a variety of diameters such as 0.014-, 0.018-, 0.025-, 0.035-, and 0.038-in. when used for gaining initial access, a 0.038-in. wire will pass through an 18 gauge needle, while a 0.018-in. wire will pass through a 21 gauge needle. In general, larger diameter wires are for larger vessels. They are also used to support large interventional devices. Not all wires come with full spectrum of diameters. Certain specialty guidewires are limited to specific diameters and are for special applications. Sometimes devices require a certain size wire for support. Therefore, it is essential to know your intervention and your inventory.

Tip Property

This is the core feature of a wire. Many modifications have been made to the tip of the wire to make them more versatile or specific (Fig. 13.1). Guidewires generally have floppy tip with varying lengths. A floppy tip does not have an inner core, thus decreasing the potential of injuring the vessel during wire advancement. Also, an experienced interventionist can manipulate the guidewire based on the interactions between the floppy tip and the lesion. Wires with longer floppy tips have better safety profiles, such as the wires for thoracic stent graft. Wires having shorter floppy tips yield better instant feedback, such as wires for traversing chronic occlusions (CTO). Some tips of the guidewire are intentionally angled or curved (Fig. 13.1). This simple change makes the wire *steerable*. A steerable wire is essential in negotiating through a stenosis or tortuosity of an artery. A curled-up tip allows the wire to be safely positioned at the part of the artery prone to complications, such as the aortic arch or ascending aorta (Fig. 13.1c).

Stiffness

Stiffness relates to the tightly wound inner steel core that confers differing magnitudes of stiffness on the body of the guidewire. A surrounding wrap of a lighter, more flexible wire helps prevent fracture and fragmentation while the guidewire is in use. Stiffer guidewire give more support. Therefore, they are used for larger devices, such as abdominal or thoracic stent grafts. They are also helpful to straighten a torturous artery. However, one should remember the stiffer the guidewire, the more likelihood to cause iatrogenic injury.

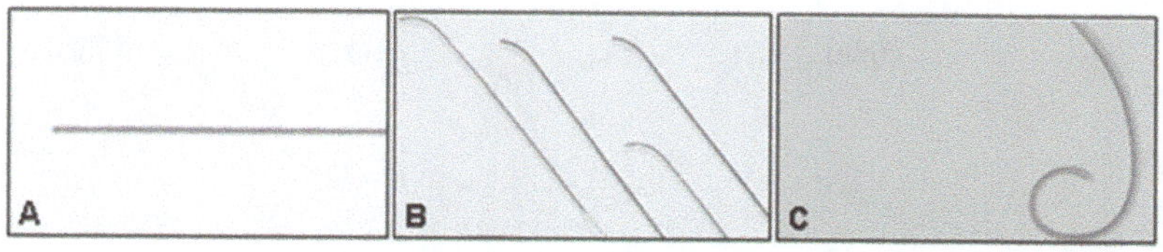

Fig. 13.1 Tip shapes of guidewires. **a**, *straight*, **b**, *angled*, **c**, *curled*

Length

Once gained, the wire access should never be lost until the end of the procedure. Therefore, using the right length of wire is very important. The length of the wire should be estimated based on the distance to the target, and the shaft length of the device being used during the intervention. The following formula will help to estimate the minimal length of the wire needed:

LE (estimated length of the wire) = Lt (access to target lesion) + Ld (shaft length of the device)

Table 13.1 demonstrates the length estimated to the target using femoral retrograde puncture technique. L_E is the minimal length for the particular intervention.

Table 13.1 Estimated distances from femoral artery access

Target location	Estimate distance (cm)
Distal aorta	45–55
Contralateral CFA	65–75
Renal artery and visceral arteries	65–80
Aortic arch	90
Arch vessels	100

CFA: common femoral artery.

Sheathes and Catheters

Just like guidewires, there are ample guide sheaths and catheters available today. Advancements in this technology, alteration of the catheter material, and a variety of head shapes have made the selective catheterization a routine practice. Compared with guidewires, guiding catheters are the main driving force during the cannulation process. Selecting the appropriate catheter will definitely facilitate interventions. Guiding sheaths are conduits for guiding catheter and wires. They essentially shorten the distance between the access sites and the target, especially in torturous arteries. We will go over the basics of catheters and sheath in the following section.

Basic Material

Catheters and sheaths are normally made of materials such as polyethylene, polyurethane, nylon, Teflon, or a combination of these materials. Polyethylene catheters have a low coefficient of friction and are pliable—meaning they have good shape memory. They can be torqued and therefore good for selective catheterization. Catheters made of polyurethane are softer and even more pliable, thus tracking the wires better. Nylon catheters are stiffer and can tolerate a higher flower rate; these are amenable to angiography. Teflon is the stiffest material and is used mainly for dilators and sheaths.

Diameter

Once again, the diameter of a guide catheter relates to its OD, while the diameter of the sheath is the ID. Guiding catheters are normally 4F or 5F for most interventions. The catheter used to cannulate a CTO is only 2.7F.

Length

Catheters are typically between 65 and 100 cm in length. Longer catheters are available for up-and-over interventions. Access sheath is typically 10–15 cm long, but shorter sheaths are available for specific interventions such as dialysis access. Longer sheaths are for arch vessel and up-and-over interventions.

Head Shapes

The configuration of the head shape of the catheter directly determines its application. Certain shape catheters are good for selective arch and cerebral interventions (Fig. 13.2), while others are mainly used for visceral interventions (Fig. 13.3).

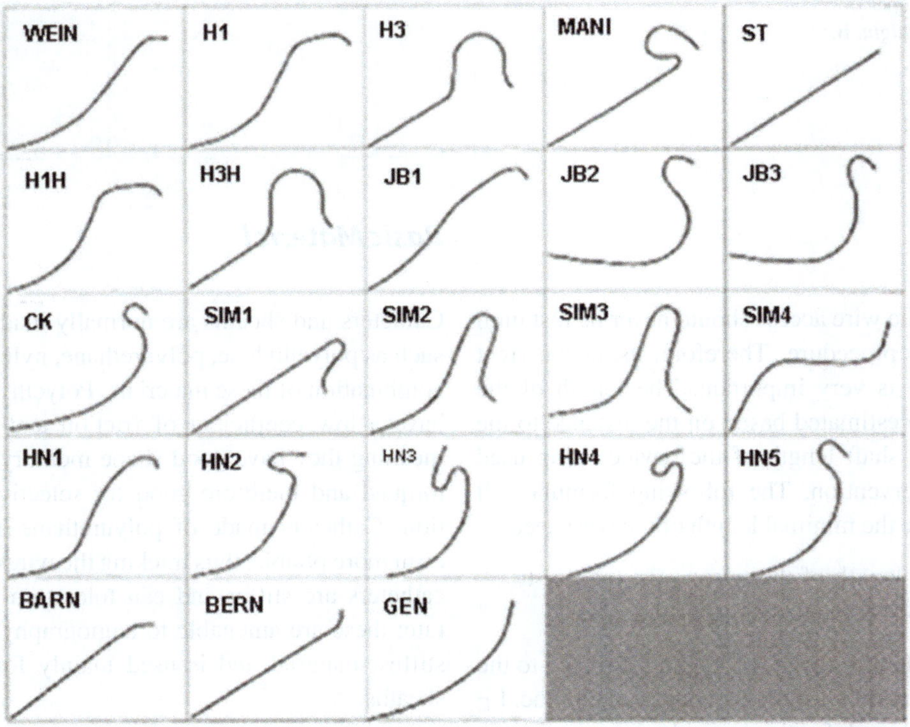

Fig. 13.2 Various catheter head shapes for selective cerebral interventions

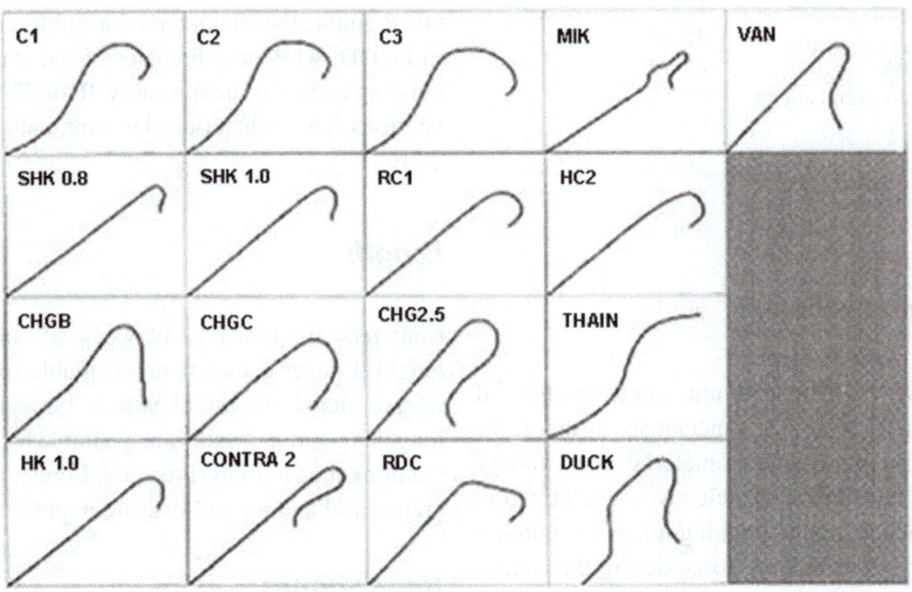

Fig. 13.3 Various catheter head shapes for selective visceral artery interventions

Special Features

Special catheter coatings make them either hydrophilic or not; radiopaque tips make catheters more visible under the fluoroscope. Side holes can divert the pressure, which make them amenable to angiography with power injections, or for therapeutic infusions; marked catheters could help calibrations and measurements.

Guidewire and Lesion Interaction

Always advance the guidewire under fluoroscopy guidance, except during the wire exchange over a catheter. The operator should be very familiar with interpretation between a lesion and a guidewire. Correct interpretation of the wire–lesion relationship will ultimately determine whether the stenotic lesion can be successfully crossed. It also helps to select the appropriate wire and catheter. Fig. 13.4 a–d demonstrates three basic interactions between the wire and lesions:

1. *Floppy portion of the wire moving in a linear fashion* (Fig. 13.4a)—this is what you try to achieve at all times. It means the wire is maneuvering through the stenosis within the flow lumen.
2. *Floppy portion of the wire piles up proximal to the lesion* (Fig. 13.4b)—the wire has no chance to cross the lesion. One should back up, redirect, and advance. If the tip of the wire is straight, change to a steerable one. Also make sure the tip of the wire is still usable and did not bend during the process.
3. *Floppy tip bent with minimal resistance* (Fig. 13.4c)—the wire hits the proximal edge of the lesion and should be able to pass the narrow part of the artery. Cautiously advance the wire. Once passed the lesion, the wire should straighten. This is called advancing a "buckled up" wire. Sometimes it needs to be redirected. Do not force the wire at this point because it may dislodge the plaque and cause distal embolization.
4. *Floppy tip seems "buckled up" with resistance* (Fig. 13.4d)—the guidewire will not pass the lesion. Resistance means the "buckled up" point is at the joint of the floppy and non-floppy parts of the guidewire. Withdraw, redirect, and advance. Forcing ahead will cause dissection, embolization, or damage to the guidewire.

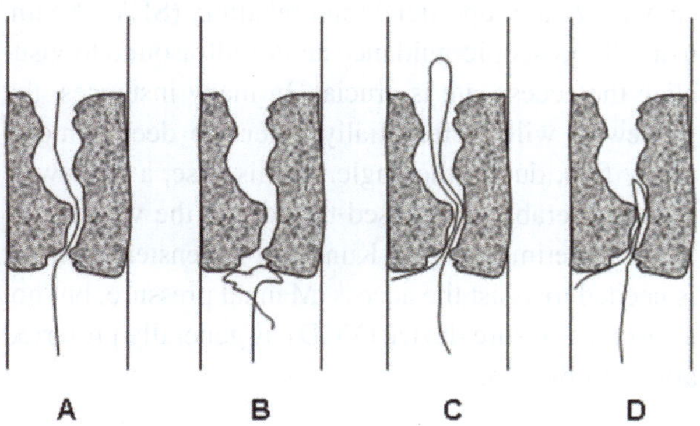

Fig. 13.4 Guidewire and lesion interactions. **a**, Guidewire navigating through the stenosis; **b**, guidewire piled up at the proximal end of the lesion; **c**, tip of the floppy part of the guidewire catches the proximal edge of the lesion, the wire buckled over the lesion with minimal resistance; **d**, tip of the guidewire catches the proximal edge of the lesion, floppy part bent within the lesion with resistance

Vascular Access

Every vascular specialist should familiarize different access options. The general rules for access artery are as follows:

1. Entry site should be relatively disease-free, without significant calcification.
2. Entry site should be over a bony structure, if possible. This will facilitate postprocedural local compression.
3. Angle of the entry needle to skin should be between 30 and 45°.
4. If access vessel is small or potentially diseased, a micropuncture technique is preferred.
5. When in doubt, imaging assistance should be used, such as fluoroscopy or 2-D ultrasound.

Retrograde Femoral Artery Access

The target for the femoral puncture is the infrainguinal portion of the common femoral artery (CFA). Precise entry of this part of the artery allows effective hemostasis by applying local pressure against the femoral head after the procedure (Fig. 13.5a). In most cases, one can

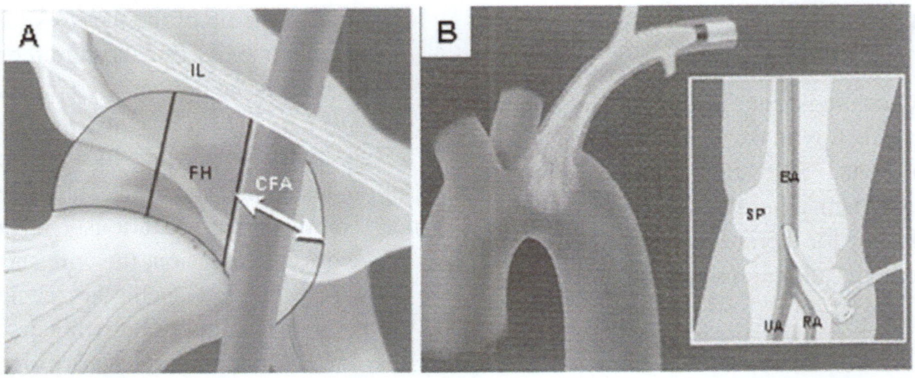

Fig. 13.5 Anatomic landmarks for femoral and brachial artery accesses. **a**, Common femoral artery located at the medial 1/3 of the femoral head. IL: inguinal ligament; CFA: common femoral artery; FH: femoral head; **b**, brachial artery at the antecubital fossa. BA: brachial artery; SP: supracondylar process of the humerus; UA: ulnar artery; RA: radial artery

achieve this by palpating the femoral pulse in the groin region. If the femoral pulse is weak or non-palpable, several techniques can be used to facilitate access.

1. Anatomic reference—The inguinal ligament can be marked prior to the procedure. It extends from the anterior superior iliac spine to the pubic tubercle. A line for the femoral artery can also be marked if there is some femoral pulse. This will provide the operator relative landmarks even after draping.
2. Fluoroscopic-guidance—When placing the femoral head in the center of the imaging, the CFA located at 1 cm lateral to the most medial cortex of the femoral head (Fig. 13.5a). The CFA runs directly over the medial one-third of the femoral head in more than 70% of individuals.
3. Ultrasound-guided access—Even using fluoroscopy cannot guarantee access to the true CFA; high or low femoral bifurcation does occur. The most definitive method is using ultrasound-guidance. However, this technique requires a steep learning curve. Ultrasound can assure the puncture site is within a segment of the CFA and can help to determine whether or not the artery is calcified. This technique is very important. It not only can secure the anatomic puncture site but can also select the most optimal disease-free portion of the CFA. It is especially valuable in percutaneous endovascular abdominal aortic aneurysm (AAA) repair when large sheaths are used.
4. Aortography from the contralateral access serves as a road map for the ipsilateral access.
5. If the femoral vein is inadvertently entered, it can be used as an access guide, either through a venogram or by passing a wire through it.

Antegrade Puncture of the Femoral Artery

Antegrade femoral access is a very useful skill. It allows extra control of the guidewires and catheters for infrainguinal, particularly infragenicular endovascular interventions. In order to access the CFA, the skin entry must be proximal to the inguinal ligament. **A** puncture site that is too high, such as access at the external iliac artery (EIA) will lead to potential retroperitoneal hemorrhage, while access too close to the femoral bifurcation results in inadequate working room to selectively catheterize the superficial femoral artery (SFA). Again, using fluoroscopic-guidance and/or ultrasound to visualize the access site is crucial. In many instances, the guidewire will preferentially enter the deep femoral artery first, due to the angle. In this case, a guidewire with a steerable tip is used to redirect the wire to the SFA. Sometimes, a short Kumpe or Berenstein catheter is needed to assist the access. Manual pressure, but not a vascular closure device (VCD), is generally preferred after completion.

Brachial Artery Access

Although most of the interventions can be performed via femoral accesses, the brachial artery approach is the next best option in some situations. Its advantages include early ambulation and a potentially reduced incidence of bleeding after the procedure. Sometimes it is the preferred access for visceral arterial [celiac artery and superior mesenteric artery (SMA) diseases] interventions. Access can be accomplished via a small cut-down or percutaneously. The patient's arm should be extended and slightly abducted. If choosing percutaneous access, the puncture site should be at, or immediately above, the antecubital fossa. This allows local compression against the supracondylar process of the humerus, after the procedure (Fig. 13.5b). Keep in mind that the percutaneous approach at the brachial artery can lead to a higher complication rate. Upper extremity arteries are generally smaller and more prone to spasm than the arteries of lower extremities. In addition, a small hematoma after the procedure could lead to brachial plexopathy. Therefore, interventions requiring larger than 6F sheaths or in a smaller individual, the open approach is preferred. Left brachial artery access is preferred over the right arm since it can avoid the carotid origin. A micropuncture technique should be used for all percutaneous brachial artery interventions.

Percutaneous Puncture of Prosthetic Grafts

Due to potential scaring and characteristics of the synthetic material, access to the graft requires special attention. Care should be taken to avoid penetrating the back wall of the graft, especially those which are newly implanted. Similarly, access around the anastomosis should be avoided. Once needle access is established, the wire well is introduced into the aorta. The track needs to be dilated before inserting the desired sheath. The dilatation can be accomplished using a dilator set. Typically, it needs a one size up dilator [i.e., using a 6F dilator for a 5F sheath insertion (remember a 5F sheath's OD is 6F)]. Dacron grafts have tightly knitted fabric matrixes which make the accesses particularly challenging.

Micropuncture Technique

A micropuncture introducer set (Cook, Inc, Bloomington, IN) includes a 21 gauge needle (4 cm or 7 cm long), a 0.018-in. guidewire with a floppy tip, and a 4F short catheter with an inner smaller diameter dilator that passes over the 0.018-in. guidewire. When the 21 gauge needle enters the artery, the back bleeding is not pulsatile. The 0.018-in. guidewire should be advanced under fluoroscopic-guidance. The needle is then removed and the 4F short catheter is passed over the guidewire. Remove the guidewire and dilator. Brisk arterial bleeding should occur. A retrograde angiogram can be performed at this time to confirm successful access. A 0.035-in. wire is used to exchange the short catheter for a desired sheath.

Ultrasound-Guided Arterial Access

Ultrasound-guided arterial access is an underutilized technique in peripheral intervention. The success rate of ultrasound-guided arterial puncture in patients having difficult access, such as absent arterial pulse or failed palpation-guided puncture, is quite high [8]. Routine utilization of this technique is still being questioned. Data are not consistent in terms of whether using ultrasound-guidance will decrease postprocedural complications [9, 10]. While some studies have suggested that complications such as pseudoaneurysm formation were significantly decreased in the ultrasound-guided group (2.6%) compared with the palpation-guided (4.5%) group [10], others have shown that ultrasound-guided arterial puncture does not reduce the access time or decrease postprocedural complications; they recommend that this technique should be used only in patients with a weak or absent arterial pulse and in obese patients [9]. With more peripheral interventions performed every year, precise access should be the common goal. A too high or too low access point will lead to a higher complication rate. Precise access will directly decrease the complication rate. Familiarity with ultrasound-guided arterial access is a potential answer to many of the complications.

Vascular Closure Devices

Vascular closure devises (VCD) have been applied to endovascular practice, especially cardiac catheterization, for more than a decade. The purposes of using

Table 13.2 Vascular closure devices overview

Name of the device	Manufacturer	Category	Therapeutic sheath size
AngioSeal	St. Jude Medical St. Paul, MN	Collagen	6–8 F
Prostar	Abbott Vascular Redwood City, CA	Suture × 2 (braided)	10 F
Perclose ProGlide	Abbott Vascular Redwood City, CA	Suture × 1 (monofilament)	5–8 F
StarClose	Abbott Vascular Redwood City, CA	Nitinol clip	5–6 F
Mynx	AccessClosure, Inc Mountain View, CA	Hydrogel Sealant	5–7 F
EVS	AngioLINK Corporation Bloomington, IN	Titanium staples	6–8 F

F: French.

these devices are to prevent postprocedural bleeding complications and to promote early ambulation and early hospital discharge. All VCDs belong to one of the following categories: suture-mediated [11], collagen and procoagulants [12–14], a combination of suture and collagen [15], and, more recently, clip devices (Table 13.2) [16, 17]. Each device is associated with claims that it is at least comparable to manual compression in terms of bleeding complications. Although the utilization of VCDs has steadily increased over the years, they have not yet become standard practice. Of course, the cost-effectiveness is still under debate. In addition, the efficacy of these devices is still raising doubts. Some authors believe that every busy interventionist should become familiar with at least one of these devices, since they can change your practice. Although most of the studies have compared VCDs with manual compressions, the gold standard is ultimately surgical repair. The goal for future VCDs is to be compatible to surgical repair.

The concern related to AngioSeal (St. Jude Medical, St. Paul, MN) (Fig. 13.6f) is its intravascular anchor. Since it is a foreign body, if it fails, the anchor can occlude the atrial lumen and lead to acute vessel occlusion. Mynx (AccessClosure, Inc., Mountain View, CA) (Fig. 13.6d) uses hydrogel sealant to promote active clotting. It accomplishes an initial seal by inflating a temporary balloon at the puncture site; the balloon should be deflated and removed after satisfactory hemostasis is confirmed.

Abbott Vascular (Redwood City, CA) products are either suture or clip based. To date, the Prostar (Fig. 13.6b) can be used to close the largest arterial puncture (Table 13.2). In an off-label application, some practitioners use a single Prostar for percutaneous endovascular AAA repair, where sometimes the access sheaths are 22F. Prostar's magnesium is different from

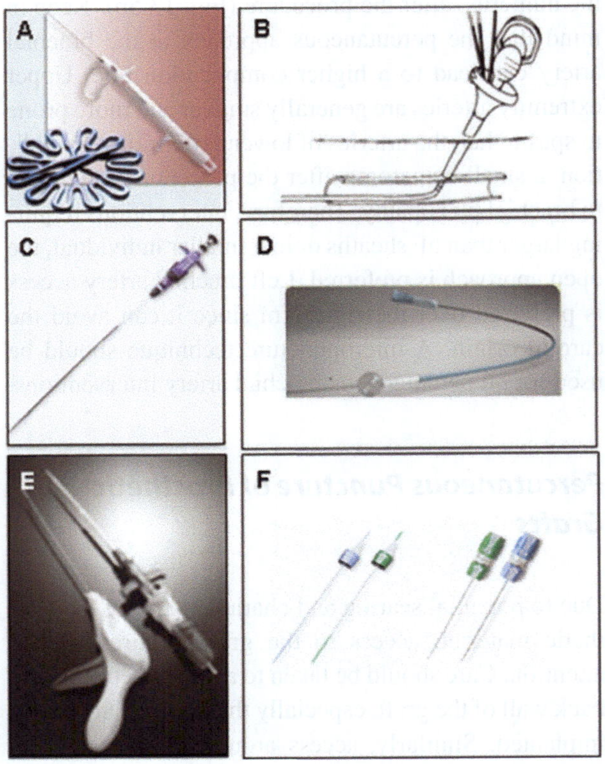

Fig. 13.6 Vascular closure devices. **a**, Starclose, **b**, Prostar, **c**, Perclose ProGlide, **d**, Mynx, **e**, EVS, **f**, AngioSeal

the Perclose ProGlide. The needles of the Prostar are deployed from inside the artery to the outside of the arterial wall. This is particularly helpful in patients with a diseased anterior wall of the femoral artery. This is the best device to prevent arterial dissections during its application. However, it requires operator know-how to tie knots and the learning curve is quite steep. Perclose ProGlide (Fig. 13.6c) is very compact and easy to use. It is pretty much a one handed technique. The pre-knot design will benefit the non-surgeon user. The polypropylene monofilament suture will decrease access site infection. The Starclose (Fig. 13.6a), however, is a new concept compared with Abbott's two other series. It uses a star-shaped titanium clip to close the arterial puncture hole by clipping from the outside; nothing is left inside the artery.

Fairly good at achieving their original goal of decreasing local bleeding complications, VCDs do have some device-related complications, which will be discussed later in this section. Furthermore, they are all relatively expensive compared with manual compression. Whether they are cost-effective still remain controversial.

Examples for Guidewire and Catheter Interventions

In the following sections, we will review several basic interventions in today's practice. We will focus on the wires and catheters, not the exact step-by-step manual.

Catheter and Wire 101

1. Do not insert the sheath if in doubt whether you are intraluminal. When in doubt, a retrograde angiogram should be done to confirm the location of the needles. Micropuncture kits should be used for every case.
2. Advance sheath, catheter over the wire at all times.
3. Never give up the wire access until just prior to completion.
4. Introducing a large sheath requires a stiff wire and should be done under direct fluorovision.
5. Know where your wire is at all times, especially stiff wires.
6. Always mark the pedal arterial sites on both feet prior to the intervention. Re-examine again after the intervention.

Collect Your Thoughts Prior to Percutaneous Interventions

1. Determine the entry site.
2. Evaluate the quality of the desired entry site artery. You can use physical examination, fluoroscopy, or ultrasound mapping.
3. Unless it is a very low-risk patient, do not hesitate to use image guidance, such as fluoroscopy or ultrasound.
4. Rehearse the intervention step-by-step prior to making the puncture. Size of the sheath, length of the target lesion, and the need for heparinization must be determined before the start of the procedure.
5. Consider your closure methods before gaining access, manual compression, or using VCDs.
6. Determine your "plan B" (or even plan C) if something goes wrong with plan A.

Accesses and Selective Guiding Catheters for Some Basic Interventions

Carotid Artery

1. First choice access—either femoral artery
2. Alternative access—left brachial artery
3. Selective catheter—right carotid artery: H1, Simmons, Vick; left carotid artery: angled Clidecath, H1, or Simmons

Subclavian Artery

1. First choice access—either femoral artery
2. Alternative access—ipsilateral brachial artery
3. Selective catheter –angled Glidecath, H1, Simmons or H3

Celiac or SMA

1. First choice access—either femoral artery
2. Alternative access—left brachial artery
3. Selective catheter—RIM, Chuang-C, Chuang-3

Renal Artery

1. First choice access—contralateral femoral artery
2. Alternative access—left brachial artery

3. Selective catheter—C2 cobra, renal double curve, Sos-omni

Infrarenal Aorta

1. First choice of access—either femoral artery
2. Alternative access—left brachial artery
3. Selective catheter—omin-flush, RIM, C2 cobra

Superior Femoral Artery

1. First choice of access—contralateral femoral artery
2. Alternative access—ipsilateral retrograde femoral for run-off; ipsilateral antegrade for intervention
3. Selective catheter—Berenstein, Kumpe, Vertebral

Tibial Arteries

1. First choice of access—contralateral femoral artery
2. Alternative access—ipsilateral retrograde femoral for run-off; ipsilateral antegrade for intervention
3. Selective catheter—Kumpe, Vertebral

Complications and Troubleshootings

Peripheral endovascular intervention has its unique complications compared with other invasive procedures. If endovascular interventions are meant to be less invasive, an effort should also be made to reduce potential morbidities. Knowing possible complications related to guidewire and percutaneous catheterization is essential for today's practice. We will discuss complications during access and the interventions.

Access Site Complications

Access site complications are a major source of morbidity following peripheral endovascular interventions. The incidences vary in the literature. Most common complications are hematoma (6–10%), pseudoaneurysm formation (0.02–9%), and arterial dissection or occlusion (0.3–1.0%) [18–22]. Incidences of other complications, such as arteriovenous fistula, perforation, distal embolization, and infection, are relatively low.

Hematoma and Bleeding

This is the most common complication in endovascular interventions. Most of the series reported in the literature are from investigations of cardiac interventions. Puncture sites too high or too low will lead to postprocedural bleeding. The fundamental reason resides in that only the CFA anatomically lies over the head of the femur (Fig. 13.5a), and the brachial artery immediately above the antecubital crease is over the supracondylar process of the humerus (Fig. 13.5b). These allow effective compression over the bony structures after removing the sheath. Puncture site too high will cause retroperitoneal hematoma or hemorrhage. The consequences are normally significant and likely need transfusion or even surgical interventions. Hematoma can also be the result of a low arterial puncture. If the hematoma is expending, pseudoaneurysm should be carefully ruled out. Other factors contributing to bleeding or hematoma are the presence of anticoagulations, hypertension, and inadequate manual compression. Vascular closure devices are designed to reduce the bleeding complications. However, are they really working? We discuss later in this chapter.

Pseudoaneurysm Formation

Pseudoaneurysm formation after an endovascular intervention is relatively less common than hematoma. The incidence among the series ranges between 0.02 and 9% [20, 22, 23]. High-risk patients identified in these studies include those taking antithrombotic agents, those with hypertension, gender, obesity, type of procedure performed, and the size of the puncture [20, 22–27]. However, some authors believe that the most important risk factor of pseudoaneurysm formation is, again, inaccurate artery access. The best way to prevent this from happening is to puncture the appropriate segment of the artery. In antegrade or retrograde femoral access, the target for the femoral puncture is the infrainguinal portion of the CFA (Fig. 13.5a). Precise entry of this part of the artery allows effective hemostasis by applying local pressure against the femoral head after the procedure. The CFA can be referenced by fluoroscopy. In brachial artery access, the access site should be right at or immediately at the antecubital crease. This allows local compression against the supracondylar process of the humerus after the procedures. One study confirmed that, during femoral artery puncture, access to the CFA significantly decreased the incidence of pseudoaneurysm formation compared with punctures to the EIA, SFA, or deep femoral artery (DFA) [10]. If the goal is to decrease pseudoaneurysm formation, ultrasound-guided puncture or ultrasound mapping of the puncture area should be a routine procedure, especially in high-risk patients. A micropuncture technique should also be used.

Arterial Access Dissection

The incidence of arterial dissection is relatively low (0.06–0.3%) in the English literature. However, only a few studies address this issue [21, 28–30]. It is safe to say that dissection at the access artery is underappreciated and underreported. Clinically significant arterial dissection is rare and sometimes could be mixed with arterial occlusion. One study specifically investigated the incidence of arterial access dissection during percutaneous cardiac interventions (PCIs) [31]. They defined dissection angiographically. That is when there is (1) a persistent intraluminal linear, (2) a spiral-filling defect, or, (3) as a extraluminal dye extension with persistence of contrast after dye clearance from the lumen. The incidence of access artery dissection in their study of more than 3,000 patients was 0.42%. Although the result is higher than any study reported in the literature prior to this, they still suspect that the real incidence could be even higher [31]. The risk factors for arterial site dissection have never been investigated. However, a high or low puncture point, use of a closure device (especially Perclose) [27, 31, 32], and tortuosity of the artery seemed to contribute to the dissections [31]. One can image that if the access arteries are calcified, especially those having circumferential or anterior wall plaques, needle access would lead to dissections. Early recognition is essential to salvage the patient's limb—or even life. Therefore, we propose the following for every peripheral intervention:

1. Evaluate the access artery prior to the puncture. Try to use as much information as possible such as CT scan, MRI, or angiogram.
2. For high-risk patients, ultrasound-guided arterial puncture is recommended. It not only can identify the spot that is relatively disease-free within the target area but also assure that the punctured segment is not too high or too low.
3. Last but not least, be disciplined, perform routine access site angiogram at its completion or at the very beginning, if suspicion is. Angiogram will not avoid dissection, but it may lead to early diagnosis and early intervention.

Complications During the Intervention

Arterial Wall Dissection

Dissection of the artery could happen during wire and catheter crossing of the lesion, during regular balloon angioplasty, or even during primary stent placement with over postdilatation. Recognizing its occurrence during the procedure may prevent early failure. Anatomic locations prone to dissections include the external iliac artery, especially at its origin, SFA, especially at its origin, and with the adductor canal, aortic bifurcation, common carotid artery, and subclavian artery. Lesion morphology that may be associated with dissection includes lesions at the branch point, diffuse longitudinal plaque formation without natural cleavage lanes, and lesions that are heavily calcified. The appropriate precautions should be taken in these situations:

1. Do not force the guidewires.
2. Do not advance the catheter without wire guidance.
3. Do not over balloon angioplasty the lesion.
4. Consider post-PTA stent placement.
5. Primary stent placement for high risk lesions.
6. Consider open bypass rather than endovascular intervention.

Arteriovenous Fistula Formation or Arterial Rupture

Arterial rupture must be ruled out if the following situations occurs

1. Patient complains of pain during the angioplasty and does not resolve after deflation of the balloon.
2. Patient is under heavy sedation or under anesthesia, a sudden drop in blood pressure or any hemodynamic instability.
3. Contrast extravagation during the follow-up angiogram.

Immediate angiogram should be performed in these situations. If rupture does occur, the best immediate maneuver is to advance the balloon back to the spot of rupture and inflate the balloon completely. This will temporarily tamponade the bleeding. If the rupture site is within the aorta or proximal iliac arteries, a covered stent or emergency open surgery should be considered. However, if it occurs at the infrainguinal area, such as the SFA, popliteal artery, or tibial vessels, life-threatening hemorrhage is normally not likely. A simple balloon tamponade may be sufficient to stop the bleeding, especially after reversing the heparin. If repeat angiogram shows marked improved contrast extravasation, there is no expending hematoma, and the arterial lumen is patent, no further intervention is needed. Many of those localized ruptures heal completely. Nevertheless, additional complications may occur such as acute occlusion or pseudoaneurysm formation.

Distal Embolization

Distal embolization during endovascular intervention is probably more common than one would think. However, clinically significant embolization is rare. Lesions that are prone to cause this complication are total occlusion, highly irregular or ulcerated lesions, those containing fresh thrombus, and aneurysmal lesions. Those complex lesions located at the infrarenal abdominal aorta or innominate artery need special attention for distal embolization. Recommended steps to prevent distal embolization are

1. Consider extra anticoagulation. Systemic heparinization and an extra dose of heparin prior to manipulating the lesion is essential. Some advocate keeping the activated clotting time (ACT) between 250 and 300 s at all times during the intervention. Diagnostic angiogram does not need systemic heparinization.
2. Consider distal outflow protection. A filter or distal protection device has been used in some institutions to prevent distal embolization.
3. Primary stent placement or event covered stent placement should be considered for some of the high risk lesions.
4. Always evaluate the outflow vessels after the intervention before withdrawing the wire access.

The following is a management algorism for clinically significant distal embolization:

1. Full systemic heparinization; give an extra dose if not already done. Consider continuous infusion heparin through the access sheath.
2. Quickly stabilize the culprit lesion by placing a stent.
3. Pass a multi-side-hole infusion catheter distal to the affected area. Pulse spray thrombolytic agents. If completion angiogram does not show improvement, continuous thrombolytic agent infusion should be carried on.

Complications Related to Vascular Closure Devices

In the previous section, we discussed VCDs in today's peripheral endovascular practice. Since the main reason for the emergence of VCDs was to reduce the incidence of bleeding complications after endovascular interventions, why are they only being used in 20% of the cardiac catheterization procedures being performed? [33] Aside from the argument of whether using VCDs is cost-effective, do VCDs really decrease the incidence of bleeding complications?

In a review of all the pivotal studies by various device companies, the overall complications rates were between 3 and 5% (Table 13.3) [11, 15, 17, 34].

Table 13.3 Comparisons of complications associated with vascular closure devices [a]

Device	Hematoma (>6 cm) (%)	Pseudoaneurysm (%)	Occlusive (%)	Infection (%)	Nerve injury (%)
AngioSeal	0.2	0.5	1.4	0.2	N/A
Perclose ProGlide	0	0	N/A	1.6	N/A
Prostar	2.4	3.2	N/A	0	N/A
Starclose	0.7	0	0	0	1.5
Mynx	3.2	3.1	0	0	0
EVS	3.7	2	0	0	N/A

[a] Data quoted here are mainly from FDA approved letter. They do not reflect various trials conducted post-market.
N/A: not applicable.

Case reports of various complications, such as puncture site infection, femoral artery compromise, arterial laceration, uncontrolled bleeding, pseudoaneurysm formation, arteriovenous fistula, and distal embolizations, have raised concerns [17, 35–39]. Reviews of published meta-analyses, multicenter registries, and longitudinal registries have led to the following observations:

1. In patients who underwent diagnostic cardiac catheterization, there is 0.5–1.7% rate of vascular complications. Overall, VCD groups did better than manual compression groups [18, 19, 40–42].
2. In patients who underwent PCIs, there is a 0.8–5.5% rate of loosely defined vascular complications. Some VCD groups did better [19, 43–45], while others did worse, in these studies [41, 44].

Summary

The fact is that, overall, VCDs did reduce bleeding complications. Because patients were normally heparinized and were not reversed, when VCDs failed, the bleeding complications tended to be more serious. Therefore, for diagnostic studies, VCDs are recommended; however, for interventional procedures, the data are neutral.

Vascular surgeons should really take the time to learn about the various kinds of VCDs, and select and use those which they feel the most comfortable with and with which they have had the best success. VCDs should be used selectively and, importantly, a protocol should be in place for rescue if and when failure occurs.

References

1. White RA, Hodgson KJ, Ahn SS, Hobson RW 2nd, Veith FJ: Endovascular interventions training and credentialing for vascular surgeons, *J Vasc Surg* 29(1):177–186, January 1999.
2. Credentialing Criteria for Endovascular Surgery. Report from the Executive Board of the International Society for Endovascular Surgery, *J Endovasc Surg* 2(2):131–132, May 1995.
3. White RA: Endovascular credentialing. Endovascular Surgery Credentialing and Training Subcommittee, *J Vasc Interv Radiol* 6(2):287–289, March–April 1995.
4. Diethrich EB: Regarding "Endovascular surgery credentialing and training for vascular surgery", *J Vasc Surg* 18(6):1073–1074, December 1993.
5. White RA, Fogarty TJ, Baker WH, Ahn SS, String ST: Endovascular surgery credentialing and training for vascular surgeons, *J Vasc Surg* 17(6):1095–1102, June 1993.
6. Tedesco MM, Pak JJ, Harris EJ Jr., Krummel TM, Dalman RL, Lee JT: Simulation-based endovascular skills assessment: the future of credentialing? *J Vasc Surg* 47(5):1001–1008, May 2008, discussion 1014.
7. Beller GA, Bonow RO, Fuster V: ACC revised recommendations for training in adult cardiovascular medicine. Core Cardiology Training II (COCATS 2). (Revision of the 1995 COCATS training statement, *J Am Coll Cardiol* 39(7):1242–1246, April 3, 2002.
8. Wacker F, Wolf KJ, Fobbe F: Percutaneous vascular access guided by color duplex sonography, *Eur Radiol* 7(9):1501–1504, 1997.
9. Dudeck O, Teichgraeber U, Podrabsky P, Lopez Haenninen E, Soerensen R, Ricke J: A randomized trial assessing the value of ultrasound-guided puncture of the femoral artery for interventional investigations, *Int J Cardiovasc Imag* 20(5):363–368, October 2004.
10. Gabriel M, Pawlaczyk K, Waliszewski K, Krasinski Z, Majewski W: Location of femoral artery puncture site and the risk of postcatheterization pseudoaneurysm formation, *Int J Cardiol* 120(2):167–171, Auguat 21, 2007.
11. Baim DS, Knopf WD, Hinohara T et al.: Suture-mediated closure of the femoral access site after cardiac catheterization: results of the suture to ambulate aNd discharge (STAND I and STAND II) trials, *Am J Cardiol* 85(7):864–869, April 1, 2000.

12. Silber S, Bjorvik A, Muhling H, Rosch A: Usefulness of collagen plugging with VasoSeal after PTCA as compared to manual compression with identical sheath dwell times, *J Invasive Cardiol* 11(suppl B):19B–24B, September 1999.
13. Silber S, Bjorvik A, Muhling H, Rosch A: Usefulness of collagen plugging with VasoSeal after PTCA as compared to manual compression with identical sheath dwell times, *Cathet Cardiovasc Diagn* 43(4): 421–427, April 1998.
14. Foran JP, Patel D, Brookes J, Wainwright RJ: Early mobilisation after percutaneous cardiac catheterisation using collagen plug (VasoSeal) haemostasis, *Br Heart J* 69(5): 424–429, May 1993.
15. Sanborn TA, Gibbs HH, Brinker JA, Knopf WD, Kosinski EJ, Roubin GS: A multicenter randomized trial comparing a percutaneous collagen hemostasis device with conventional manual compression after diagnostic angiography and angioplasty, *J Am Coll Cardiol* 22(5):1273–1279, November 1, 1993.
16. Ruygrok PN, Chou TM: StarClose femoral arteriotomy closure device: an advance in arterial closure, *Expert Rev Med Devices* 2(3):247–252, May 2005.
17. Hermiller JB, Simonton C, Hinohara T et al.: The StarClose Vascular Closure System: interventional results from the CLIP study, *Catheter Cardiovasc Interv* 68(5):677–683, November 2006.
18. Applegate RJ, Sacrinty MT, Kutcher MA et al.: Propensity score analysis of vascular complications after diagnostic cardiac catheterization and percutaneous coronary intervention 1998-2003, *Catheter Cardiovasc Interv* 67(4): 556–562, April 2006.
19. Arora N, Matheny ME, Sepke C, Resnic FS: A propensity analysis of the risk of vascular complications after cardiac catheterization procedures with the use of vascular closure devices, *Am Heart J* 153(4):606–611, April 2007.
20. Kresowik TF, Khoury MD, Miller BV et al.: A prospective study of the incidence and natural history of femoral vascular complications after percutaneous transluminal coronary angioplasty, *J Vasc Surg* 13(2):328–333, February 1991, discussion 333–325.
21. Muller DW, Shamir KJ, Ellis SG, Topol EJ: Peripheral vascular complications after conventional and complex percutaneous coronary interventional procedures, *Am J Cardiol* 69(1):63–68, January 1, 1992.
22. Waksman R, King SB 3rd, Douglas JS et al.: Predictors of groin complications after balloon and new-device coronary intervention, *Am J Cardiol* 75(14):886–889, May 1, 1995.
23. Thalhammer C, Kirchherr AS, Uhlich F, Waigand J, Gross CM: Postcatheterization pseudoaneurysms and arteriovenous fistulas: repair with percutaneous implantation of endovascular covered stents, *Radiology* 214(1):127–131, January 2000.
24. Perings SM, Kelm M, Jax T, Strauer BE: A prospective study on incidence and risk factors of arteriovenous fistulae following transfemoral cardiac catheterization, *Int J Cardiol* 88(2–3):223–228, April 2003.
25. Seay T, Soares G, Dawson D: Postcatheterization arteriovenous fistula: CT, ultrasound, and arteriographic findings, *Emerg Radiol* 9(5):296–299, November 2002.
26. Ugurluoglu A, Katzenschlager R, Ahmadi R et al.: Ultrasound guided compression therapy in 134 patients with iatrogenic pseudo-aneurysms: advantage of routine duplex ultrasound control of the puncture site following transfemoral catheterization, *Vasa* 26(2):110–116, May 1997.
27. Nehler MR, Lawrence WA, Whitehill TA, Charette SD, Jones DN, Krupski WC: Iatrogenic vascular injuries from percutaneous vascular suturing devices, *J Vasc Surg* 33(5):943–947, May 2001.
28. Agostoni P, Anselmi M, Gasparini G et al.: Safety of percutaneous left heart catheterization directly performed by cardiology fellows: a cohort analysis, *J Invasive Cardiol* 18(6):248–252, June 2006.
29. Messina LM, Brothers TE, Wakefield TW et al.: Clinical characteristics and surgical management of vascular complications in patients undergoing cardiac catheterization: interventional versus diagnostic procedures, *J Vasc Surg* 13(5):593–600, May 1991.
30. Sherev DA, Shaw RE, Brent BN: Angiographic predictors of femoral access site complications: implication for planned percutaneous coronary intervention, *Catheter Cardiovasc Interv* 65(2):196–202, June 2005.
31. Prasad A, Compton PA, Roesle M et al.: Incidence and Treatment of Arterial Access Dissections Occurring during Cardiac Catheterization, *J Interv Cardiol* 21(1):61–66, February 2008.
32. Derham C, Davies JF, Shahbazi R, Homer-Vanniasinkam S: Iatrogenic limb ischemia caused by angiography closure devices, *Vasc Endovascular Surg* 40(6):492–494, December 2006–January 2007.
33. Dauerman HL, Applegate RJ, Cohen DJ: Vascular closure devices: the second decade, *J Am Coll Cardiol* 50(17):1617–1626, October 23, 2007.
34. Ansel G, Yakubov S, Neilsen C et al.: Safety and efficacy of staple-mediated femoral arteriotomy closure: results from a randomized multicenter study, *Catheter Cardiovasc Interv* 67(4):546–553, April 2006.
35. Carey D, Martin JR, Moore CA, Valentine MC, Nygaard TW: Complications of femoral artery closure devices, *Catheter Cardiovasc Interv* 52(1):3–7, January 2001, discussion 8.
36. Jang JJ, Kim M, Gray B, Bacharach JM, Olin JW: Claudication secondary to Perclose use after percutaneous procedures, *Catheter Cardiovasc Interv* 67(5):687–695, May 2006.
37. Gemmete JJ, Dasika N, Forauer AR, Cho K, Williams DM: Successful angioplasty of a superficial femoral artery stenosis caused by a suture-mediated closure device, *Cardiovasc Intervent Radiol* 26(4):410–412, July–August 2003.
38. Warren BS, Warren SG, Miller SD: Predictors of complications and learning curve using the Angio-Seal closure device following interventional and diagnostic catheterization, *Catheter Cardiovasc Interv* 48(2):162–166, October 1999.
39. Stock U, Flach P, Gross M, Meyhofer J, Albes J, Butter C: Intravascular misplacement of an extravascular closure system: StarClose, *J Interv Cardiol* 19(2):170–172, April 2006.
40. Applegate RJ, Sacrinty M, Kutcher MA et al.: Vascular complications with newer generations of angioseal vascular closure devices, *J Interv Cardiol* 19(1):67–74, February 2006.

41. Koreny M, Riedmuller E, Nikfardjam M, Siostrzonek P, Mullner M: Arterial puncture closing devices compared with standard manual compression after cardiac catheterization: systematic review and meta-analysis, *JAMA* 291(3):350–357, January 21, 2004.
42. Tavris DR, Dey S, Albrecht-Gallauresi B et al.: Risk of local adverse events following cardiac catheterization by hemostasis device use – phase II, *J Invasive Cardiol* 17(12):644–650, December 2005.
43. Resnic FS, Blake GJ, Ohno-Machado L, Selwyn AP, Popma JJ, Rogers C: Vascular closure devices and the risk of vascular complications after percutaneous coronary intervention in patients receiving glycoprotein IIb-IIIa inhibitors, *Am J Cardiol* 88(5):493–496, September 1, 2001.
44. Vaitkus PT: A meta-analysis of percutaneous vascular closure devices after diagnostic catheterization and percutaneous coronary intervention, *J Invasive Cardiol* 16(5):243–246, May 2004.
45. Chevalier B, Lancelin B, Koning R et al.: Effect of a closure device on complication rates in high-local-risk patients: results of a randomized multicenter trial, *Catheter Cardiovasc Interv* 58(3):285–291, March 2003.

Balloon Angioplasty

14

John V. White, Constance Ryjewski, and Richard N. Messersmith

Transluminal angioplasty was initially conceived by Dotter and Judkins in 1964 [1]. Unfortunately, the technical limitations of their stiff, coaxial, Teflon catheters prevented widespread acceptance and use of their technique. When Gruntzig and Hopff introduced the flexible, polyvinyl double-lumen balloon catheter in 1974, they revolutionized angioplasty and set the stage for its extensive use to treat coronary and peripheral vascular occlusive disease [2]. Percutaneous transluminal angioplasty (PTA) is undeniably associated with lower morbidity and cost than conventional open bypass surgery. However, the vascular interventionist (i.e., radiologist, cardiologist, or surgeon) must understand the clinical indications, lasting benefit, and complications of PTA to use this therapy appropriately.

Mechanism

Human atherosclerotic plaque is a complex structure that is composed not only of lipid-laden macrophages but also of a calcific skeleton. Early investigators believed that balloon angioplasty dilated stenotic vessels by exerting pressure and compressing the atherosclerotic plaque [3]. Experimental and cadaver studies, however, showed that atherosclerotic plaques are minimally compressible because of the presence of a calcific skeleton [4]. Plaque compression therefore plays only a minor role in vessel dilation. This was confirmed by Demer and colleagues who measured arterial distensibility of atherosclerotic vessels before and after treatment with intraluminal high-intensity ultrasound energy designed to vibrate and disrupt the calcific skeleton [5]. These investigators noted that there was a significant increase in plaque distensibility after vibratory disruption of the calcific portion of the plaque. In studies of arteries from amputated limbs and cadavers, Lyon and colleagues noted the inelasticity and incompressibility of calcified plaque. After angioplasty of plaque in these vessels, there was fracture of the intima along the edges of the plaque rather than through the plaque itself. The arterial wall fracture continued through the media [6]. Balloon angioplasty fractures the atherosclerotic media along with stretching and rupturing the medial muscle fibers [7, 8]. The adventitia of the artery is also stretched irreversibly, thereby expanding the outer diameter of the vessel (Fig. 14.1).

Remodeling of the angioplasty site, or luminal injury, begins immediately and continues indefinitely. The formation of plaque fissures and damage to the internal elastic membrane expose subendothelial collagen to blood elements, resulting in platelet deposition and the release of a variety of platelet and white blood cell mediators. Using dual-radiotracer scintigraphy, Minar and colleagues evaluated immediate platelet accumulation at peripheral angioplasty sites in 92 patients on aspirin therapy [9]. Despite low or high circulating aspirin levels, there was significant platelet aggregation in all patients. The degree of platelet aggregation paralleled the risk of hemodynamically significant restenosis. Vasoactive substances can induce distal spasm and may initiate the process of intimal hyperplasia. The hallmark of this process is

J.V. White (✉)
Clinical Professor, Department of Surgery, Chairman, Department of Surgery, Chicago School of Medicine, University of Illinois, Advocate Lutheran General Hospital, Park Ridge, IL, USA

T.J. Fogarty, R.A. White (eds.), *Peripheral Endovascular Interventions*,
DOI 10.1007/978-1-4419-1387-6_14,

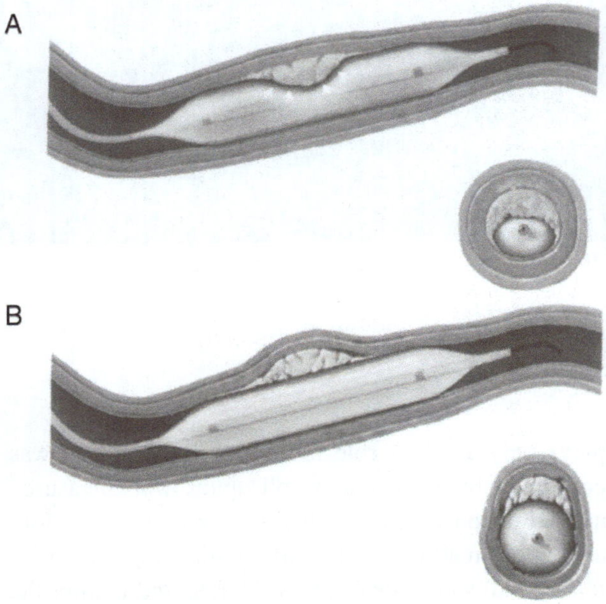

Fig. 14.1 **a**, Once balloon inflation begins, a *waist* forms where the lesion is most resistant. **b**, As inflation progresses, the waist disappears. The media and adventitia are stretched, and the plaque is cracked (Courtesy Medi/tech/Boston Scientific Co., Watertown, MA.)

multiplication and migration of smooth muscle cells. Prevention or control of fibrotic restenosis is currently the target of intense scientific investigation. A recently reported small multicenter trial of local delivery of paclitaxel, a smooth muscle cell inhibitor, at the time of angioplasty of the superficial femoral and/or popliteal arteries significantly reduced restenosis at 6 months [10]. This and similar studies suggest that control of the smooth muscle cell response to the injury of angioplasty may significantly extend the benefits of angioplasty and angioplasty-based procedures.

Indications

Indications for addressing a vascular lesion with balloon angioplasty are frequently controversial, but all agree that patient selection is critical for effective application of this therapeutic modality. The major clinical indications for balloon angioplasty treatment of inflow and outflow lesions of the lower extremity have been well defined in the TransAtlantic Inter Society Consensus on the Management of Peripheral Artery Disease (TASC) I document and updated in the TASC II document [11, 12]. Generally, there should be a clear and compelling reason for the initiation of any form of invasive treatment. For example, invasive treatment should be undertaken when possible for those with limb-threatening ischemia of the lower extremity or for those with intermittent claudication who experience job-threatening or lifestyle limiting symptoms or who are unable to complete cardiac rehabilitation. Generally, asymptomatic stenoses should not be dilated. PTA may also be used as an adjunct to surgery to dilate a stenosis proximal to a planned surgical bypass and save a failing graft.

Arterial balloon angioplasty is ideally suited for patients who have symptomatic short-segment concentric stenoses, rather than occlusions, of a major vessel. Complete occlusions have a higher complication rate and a lower long-term patency rate than stenoses. Acceptable long-term results can be expected when short-segment concentric stenoses are dilated in the presence of good distal runoff and there is an immediate return of distal pulses.

Lesion

The arterial lesion best suited for balloon angioplasty is a concentric plaque located at least 5 mm beyond the origin of a medium to large artery. As a rule of thumb, the length of the stenosis or occlusion is inversely proportional to durability of result. This is in part due to the fact that maintaining contact with normal proximal and distal arterial wall minimizes extension of the fissuring process beyond the stenotic area. Longer lesions have traditionally been dilated by centering the balloon near an end of the lesion and then advancing or withdrawing the balloon after each successive dilation. Such a practice does not limit the extent of the plaque fracture. There are now angioplasty balloons that are 10–20 cm in length that can traverse most long lesions. The treatment of orificial lesions remains challenging and often yields poorer results because of the inability to maintain balloon contact with normal proximal arterial wall. Similarly, dilating an eccentric plaque may lead to differential distribution of lateral wall stress, resulting in subplaque hemorrhage and dissection. PTA of an anatomically or morphologically unfavorable lesion may be considered in a poor-risk patient with limb-threatening ischemia as suggested in recent guidelines [12, 13].

Balloon Angioplasty Equipment

Introducer Sheaths

The introducer sheath provides a hemostatic connection between the surface of the skin and the lumen of the artery. In its simplest form, it is a thin-walled, hollow tube with a hemostatic valve on the external end. There are many types of sheaths with a wide variety of features now available, including those with an internal wire to prevent kinking, a hydrophilic coating to ease introduction, and a variable diameter. Most of them are available with a side arm for the administration of fluids and medications or the monitoring of pressures. The introducer sheath is packaged with a dilator that extends beyond the end of the sheath and is tapered so that the arterial puncture site can be gently expanded to accommodate the introducer. The device is sized by length and internal diameter, and various combinations are available (Fig. 14.2). It is generally best to choose a sheath that is at least 0.5F larger in diameter than the largest catheter to be used. For the performance of angioplasty, a small introducer can be inserted initially to permit contrast angiography with a small catheter, such as one with a 4F diameter. Once the decision is made to perform an angioplasty and the size of the balloon catheter is established, the smaller sheath can be exchanged for a larger one. Though short sheaths are most commonly used for the performance of diagnostic angiography or simple angioplasty, longer sheaths are frequently placed across a difficult lesion to be treated to prevent loss of access to the proximal and distal normal vessel.

Guidewires

Guidewires are the basic tools for crossing stenoses and occlusions and guiding catheters and angioplasty balloons to the treatment area for the performance of angioplasty. They are essential for safe navigation of the arterial tree and for minimizing subintimal dissection and arterial perforation during the introduction and withdrawal of endovascular instruments. The ideal wire is frictionless and atraumatic, resists kinking and fraying, and has good torque response. Wires are available in a variety of lengths and diameters. They are made of a stiff inner core that is wrapped in a more flexible outer layer coated by agents to reduce friction. They are also available in different tip configurations,

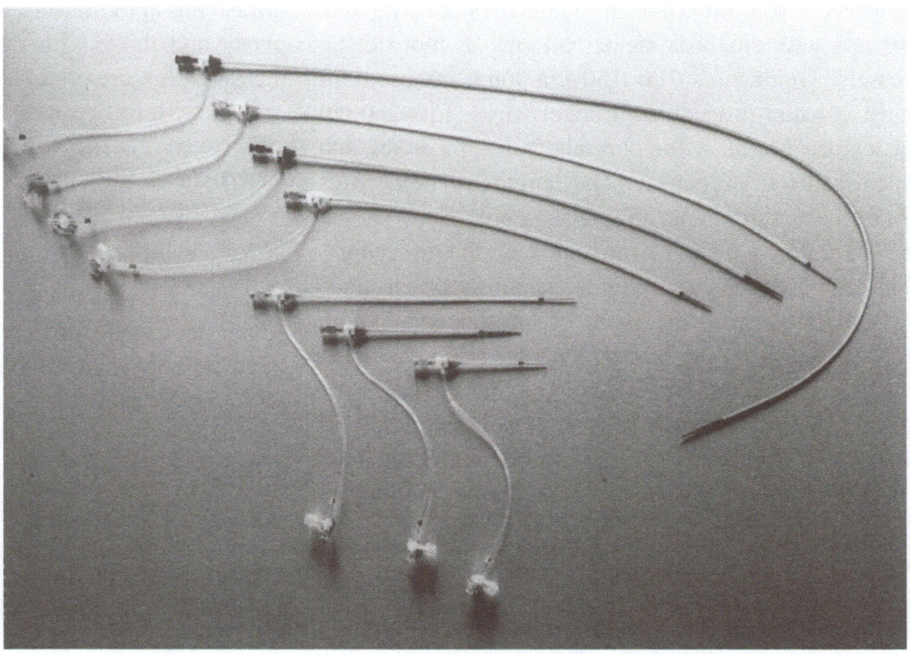

Fig. 14.2 Introducer sheaths come in different sizes and lengths that target different sites (Courtesy of Cordis Corporation.)

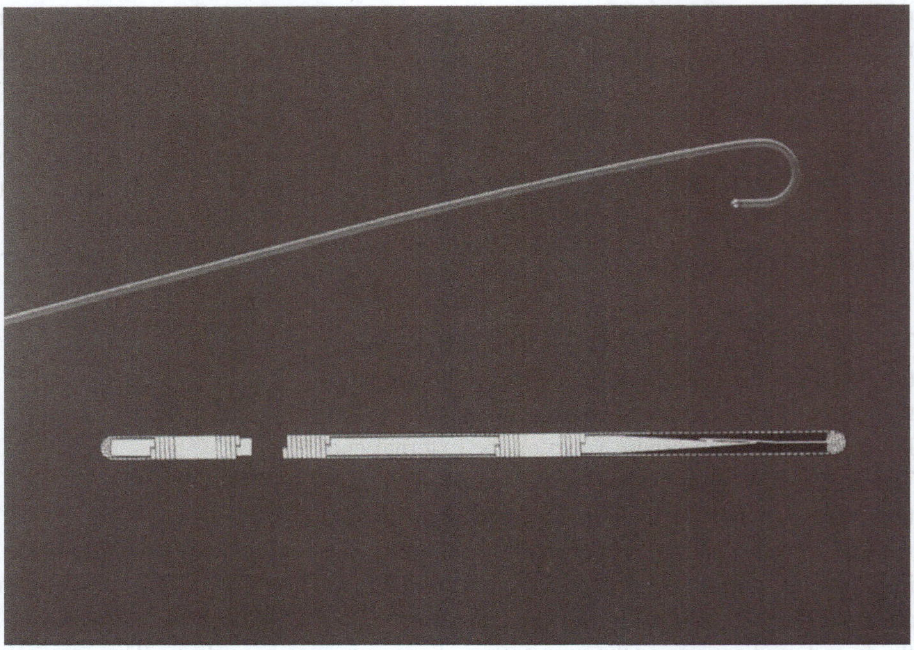

Fig. 14.3 Guidewire configuration and construction schematic (Courtesy of Cook Incorporated, Bloomington, IN.)

including J, angled, straight, or deformable distal tips. Wires with a soft or J tip cause the least trauma to fragile surfaces during manipulation (Fig. 14.3). Stiff wires are used to steer large balloon catheters through tortuous vessels without buckling. Wires coated with hydrophilic materials are the best choice to pass across a long, tortuous channel of disease [14].

Standard 0.038- or 0.035-in. guidewires are useful for guiding most diagnostic and balloon catheters; however, 0.010- to 0.028-in. guidewires are available for use with small-diameter balloons in more distal vessels. Guidewires 100–150 cm long are used for most vascular procedures. Longer wires (150–260 cm in length) are used for contralateral approaches and distal catheter exchanges. The lengths of guidewires to be used during an angioplasty procedure should be determined prior to the onset of the procedure. This can be done simply by determining the distance of the lesion from the point of arterial cannulation and the length of the longest catheter to be used during the procedure. The guidewire length should be greater than the sum of these lengths. For example, if a common iliac artery lesion is to be treated is 10 cm from the point of femoral cannulation and the longest catheter, including the balloon catheter, is 80 cm, a 140 cm guidewire is adequate. If, however, the target is a proximal subclavian artery lesion that is to be approached from the groin, it is likely that a 260 cm wire will be needed. Conversely, surgeons can use shorter (40–80 cm), more maneuverable wires intraoperatively since the distance of the lesion from the point of guidewire introduction is often quite short.

A variety of specialty wires are also available. Some wires contain radiopaque markers and can be used for length and diameter measurements during angioplasty procedures. There are also guidewires containing intravascular Doppler probes for intravascular ultrasonography during the performance of angioplasty and those with pressure sensors in the tip to measure pressure gradients across a lesion [15–17].

Catheters

Catheters are used to perform angiography, direct balloon angioplasty catheters and stents, and help position a wire or a smaller catheter into difficult locations. The large number of available catheters differ in diameter, length, distal shape, and material, and the choice depends on the intended use of the catheter (Fig. 14.4). Catheter length depends on the location of the target area, and the preconfigured distal shape of a catheter is selected based on the specific branch to be cannulated or lesion to be crossed. The material of the catheter determines its behavior during the procedure, but all shaped guide catheters track in a linear manner

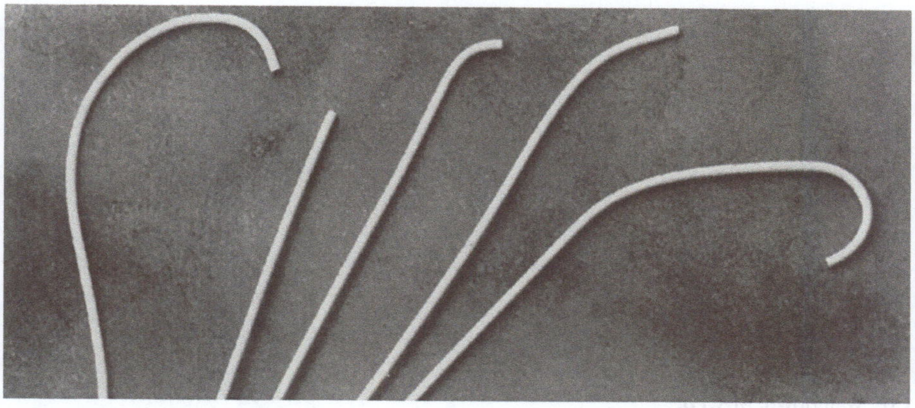

Fig. 14.4 Guiding catheters with variable tip designs provide enhanced torque control when advancing through tortuous lesions (Courtesy of Medi-65 tech/Boston Scientific Co., Watertown, MA.)

over the stiff portion of the guidewire and resume their preformed shapes as they track over the softer end of the wire. To cross difficult arterial lesions, the catheter shape and guidewire should be chosen based upon their interaction. For example, a Berenstein catheter will direct an angled hydrophilic wire in a small arc, whereas a pigtail catheter will direct the wire in a broad arc as the wire is advanced through the preshaped distal tips of these endovascular instruments. Polyethylene catheters have good shape memory and are pliable, which makes them suitable for selective catheterization of branch vessels. Polyurethane catheters have a higher coefficient of friction but are softer and more pliable and thus easier to slide over wires. Nylon catheters are the stiffest and tolerate high flow rates, a characteristic useful during aortography. The most common catheter diameter for routine angiography is a 4F or 5F pigtail or tennis racket catheter that tracks over a 0.035-in. guidewire. This catheter is straightened when tracking over the stiff portion of the wire but resumes its curved head over the softer part of the wire or after the wire is withdrawn. This ability enables it to pass through tortuous vessels, navigate the aortic bifurcation, rapidly deliver contrast, and record pre- and post-angioplasty pressures.

Balloons

The balloon angioplasty catheter has two lumens: The lumen through which the guidewire passes is coaxial, allowing the catheter to track along the wire; the other lumen, which is connected to the balloon, permits inflation. Angioplasty balloons have changed and improved over the years, and it is important for the interventionist to understand the various balloon characteristics and their optimal uses. The most useful catheters have a low profile and high trackability. Low-profile catheters are designed to be as thin as possible in the deflated state, thereby minimizing entry-site complications and optimizing the interventionist's ability to negotiate tight, tortuous stenoses (Fig. 14.5a). Trackability refers to the tendency of the balloon catheter to follow a previously placed wire without pulling the wire out of the desired position. Angioplasty balloons are selected by length, diameter, and bursting pressure. The length is defined as the portion of the balloon that has parallel walls when completely inflated. Bursting pressure is the level of pressure at which the balloon material begins to split and pressure is lost. With the current standards of construction, balloon rupture rarely results in shredding and the loss of material within the blood vessel. The dilating balloons now available are constructed with low-compliance, high-strength materials that are able to exert sufficient dilating force without becoming distorted or rupturing.

Most current balloons are made from polyethylene terephthalate or other low-complaint, strong plastic polymers. These balloons inflate to various preset diameters and pressures. Standard peripheral angioplasty balloons track smoothly over a 0.035-in. guidewire and have a safe operating range of 4–12 atm of dilating pressure. They are available in inflated balloon diameters of 3–10 mm, balloon lengths of 2–10 mm, and hydrophilic coating to enhance performance. Balloons constructed of stiffer materials such as woven nylon have higher burst pressures (more than 17 atm) and are used to cross and dilate tight, calcific

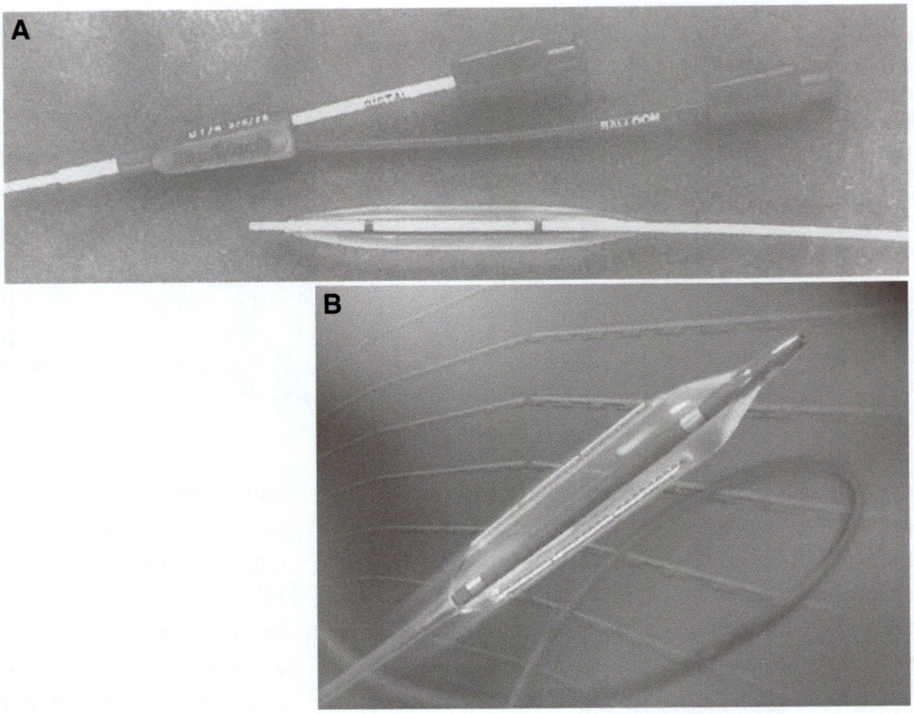

Fig. 14.5 **a**, Typical angioplasty balloon. (Courtesy of Medi-tech/Boston Scientific Co., Watertown, MA.) **b**, Cutting balloon (Courtesy of Boston Scientific Co., Waterman, MA.)

stenoses. To dilate infrapopliteal vessels, balloons are available which accept 0.014- and 0.018-in. guidewires and are mounted on 3.8F catheter shafts. There are also balloons mounted directly on guidewires that can be used in coaxial fashion. These lowest profile balloons are ideal for intraoperative angioplasty and can be placed through a 4F introducer sheath. The balloon should be inflated with a device that monitors pressure inside the balloon.

There are now specialty balloons to assist the interventionalist with specific problems, such as restenosis. Cryoballoons generate very cold temperatures during inflation to defunctionalize the arterial smooth muscle cells in the area of dilation. Since rapid multiplication and migration of smooth muscle cells is an initial step in the formation of restenosis, cryotherapy may reduce the likelihood of restenosis. Once formed, the fibrotic neotintimal hyperplastic lesion is able to stretch and then rapidly contract with balloon inflation and deflation. Therefore, standard balloon angioplasty is only minimally effective in producing a durable reduction in the degree of luminal compromise. To address this problem, a cutting balloon has been developed (Fig. 14.5b). This balloon has four small cutting blades on its surface that cut into the fibrotic material and allow it to be more effectively dilated without shredding it. The balloon is placed across the lesion and inflated. The blades located at 3, 6, 9, and 12 o'clock cut into the wall as it is being dilated. After deflation of the balloon, it is rotated 60° and reinflated to produce more cuts and further expand the lesion. Finally, based upon the success of drug-coated stents, a drug delivery balloon has been the subject of small clinical trials. In a multicenter, prospective trial of 154 patients undergoing balloon angioplasty of the superficial femoral artery and/or popliteal artery, patients were randomized to treatment with either a standard balloon or a balloon coated with paclitaxel [18]. Follow-up angiography was performed at 6 months posttreatment and demonstrated a statistically significant reduction in the rate of restenosis among those who were treated with a paclitaxel-coated balloon. These innovative devices and those in development are likely to greatly improve the durability of balloon angioplasty.

Technique

The patient is placed in the supine position on the imaging table so the arterial segments, from the cannulation point to a few centimeters beyond the region to be dilated, can be easily visualized. The patient is sedated, and a vasodilator such as nifedipine may be given 30 min before the procedure to help prevent vessel spasm. All patients should undergo cardiac rhythm, oxygen saturation, and blood pressure monitoring throughout the procedure.

Once the appropriate site is chosen, the selected groin is prepared and infiltrated with lidocaine. A Seldinger needle is advanced into the artery and when pulsatile backflow is visualized, a standard short 0.035-in. guidewire is advanced through the needle into the common femoral artery. Typically, a 5F introducer sheath is advanced over the guidewire and positioned to protect the insertion site without crossing the lesion. The short guidewire is then replaced by a torquable, soft-tipped guidewire that is advanced with the assistance of fluoroscopy to the level of the stenosis or occlusion and then continued a reasonable distance beyond the lesion. An exchange of guidewires may be necessary to cross the lesion. A specialized adapter with a hemostatic valve such as the Tuohy-Borst Y adapter can be connected to the introducer sheath to facilitate contrast injections through a rotating side port. Additional vasodilators may also be required. When the guidewire is in the correct position, a diagnostic catheter is advanced along the guidewire proximal to the lesion to record arterial pressures above and below the lesion.

A diagnostic angiogram that provides road mapping capabilities is obtained to help select the approach and size of the angioplasty balloon. An arterial puncture site is chosen that is most appropriate for the lesion being treated. In most cases the preferred entry site for balloon angioplasty is the common femoral artery just below the level of the inguinal ligament. Typically, an ipsilateral approach is used to prevent injury to the less diseased extremity. A contralateral route that directs the guidewire and catheter across the aortic bifurcation can be employed, but it makes guidewire manipulation more difficult. An antegrade approach is usually used in patients with superficial femoral artery lesions, and a retrograde approach is used for more proximal stenoses.

After traversing the stenosis, the patient is heparinized. The diagnostic catheter is then removed, and a balloon catheter with a diameter that matches the outflow vessel beyond the lesion as determined by angiogram is inserted. The balloon length should be greater than that of the lesion. The balloon is centered on the lesion and inflated slowly via an inflation device that also measures the intraballoon pressures. The balloon is inflated using dilute contrast so the dilation can be monitored fluoroscopically. When the balloon contacts the lesion, the contrast is pushed to the polar ends of the balloon, creating an hourglass configuration. As the pressure within the balloon increases, the waist of the balloon widens and eventually disappears. Inflation is maintained for 20 s. The balloon is deflated, the vessel is allowed to relax for a few seconds, and the balloon is reinflated. The inflation/deflation cycle is repeated so that the lesion is treated with a total of three inflations of 20 s. The balloon is then withdrawn several centimeters from the lesion site so contrast can be injected and the results evaluated.

Recently, the technique of subintimal angioplasty has been advocated for the treatment of total occlusions when the luminal surface of the plaque cannot be traversed (Fig. 14.6). The initial approach is similar to that of conventional angioplasty for the placement of the sheath and the introduction of the guidewire. If a hydrophilic guidewire will not pass along the flow surface, then it can be carefully advanced into the subintimal plane. If the wire does not spontaneously pass into this plane, the gentle inflation of an angioplasty balloon at the edge of the plaque will frequently separate the plaque from the more normal intima and create a subintimal pathway for the wire. Once the wire has traversed the lesion in the subintimal plane, a hydrophilic catheter or other re-entry device is passed over the wire to guide it back into the lumen. Standard angioplasty of the subintimal plane is performed, with stent placement reserved only if the channel collapses completely.

A technically successful procedure leaves a residual stenosis of 30% or less at the angioplasty site. If a significant stenosis remains or a small dissection is evident after balloon inflation, the process is repeated. Because successful angioplasty does produce small, local wall dissections, postangioplasty injections should not be made within the dilated segment and guidewires should not be advanced across dilated vessels. On completion of the procedure, the arterial pressures above and below the site of the lesion are measured to quantify the new arterial hemodynamic profile. The sheath can be removed and a closure device placed immediately after completion of the procedure. There are a variety of such devices available [19–21]. Though when inappropriately deployed they may be associated with bleeding, thrombosis,

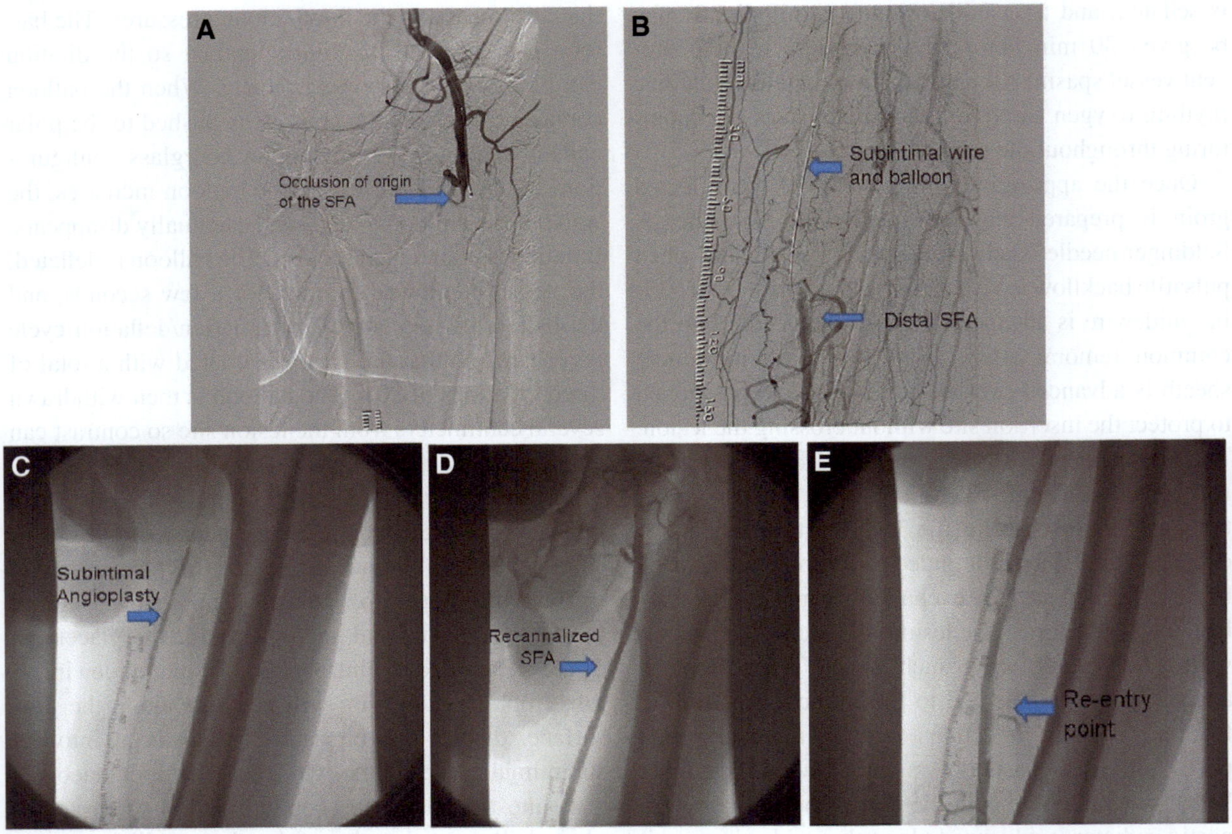

Fig. 14.6 **a**, Subintimal angioplasty may be a useful technique for patients with long-segment occlusions of the superficial femoral artery (SFA). **b**, The subintimal passage of the wire is recognized by its separation from the true lumen. Return to the true lumen often requires a re-entry tool. **c**, Once the guidewire is placed into the distal true lumen, subintimal angioplasty of the entire segment is performed. Stents are used only if there is a severe residual stenosis. **d**, The final result demonstrates a wide open origin of the SFA. **e**, The final result demonstrates a smooth transition to the true lumen with a small distal dissection

embolization, or false aneurysm formation, a closure device when properly placed can seal effectively the cannulation and decrease the likelihood of post-procedure complications [20, 22]. Women are at higher risk than men for arterial complications from closure devices but the rate is still less than 2% [23].

If manual compression is to be used for hemostasis, it is common to defer pulling out the sheath until the activated clotting time falls to a level of 160 s or less. Pressure over the site of arterial puncture rather than skin puncture should be maintained for 20–30 min. Patients are required to remain at bed rest with the cannulated leg straight for a period of time depending upon the size of the sheath and the procedure for achieving hemostasis. The duration of activity restriction is also impacted by the use of arterial closure devices, various anticoagulants and antiplatelet agents, and is maintained for a longer period of time when greater inhibition of coagulation cascade or platelets is present. It is now common to begin antiplatelet agents shortly before or at the time of angioplasty which, in the setting of heparin-induced anticoagulation, raises the risk of bleeding from the puncture site. For example, after removal of a 6F sheath and control of the cannulation site with manual compression, bed rest is generally in the range of 3–4 h. In the presence of an antiplatelet agent, such as clopidogrel, this might be extended to 4–6 h. Baseline noninvasive ankle-brachial pressure measurements are obtained shortly after angioplasty to confirm the hemodynamic improvement and document a new baseline for future evaluations.

Site-Specific Interventions

Aortic Angioplasty

Aortobifemoral bypass grafting is generally indicated for diffuse, multifocal aortoiliac occlusive disease.

Angioplasty can be effectively performed on concentric, focal, distal abdominal aortic stenoses. When the stenosis is proximal to the bifurcation, a single 15–20 mm balloon is used. Stents are placed in most patients. Initial success rates exceed 85% in most studies and approach 100% in many reports [24–26]. The associated mortality of treatment of this large vessel is low. Feugier and associates were able to treat 86 patients with aortic stenosis with angioplasty and stent placement with a technical success rate of 95% and a mortality of 1.2% [27]. The results of infrarenal aortic angioplasty are also durable, with excellent mid- and long-term outcomes. In a study of 17 patients followed for a mean of 27 months after infrarenal aortic angioplasty and stenting, a primary patency of 83% was noted at 3 years [26]. These results are similar to a study of 15 patients who underwent angioplasty of a focal, infrarenal stenosis with primary stent placement. At 3-year follow-up evaluation, primary clinical and technical patency was noted to be 85% with a secondary patency of 100% [28]. Little is lost over time in those successfully treated. In a study of 92 patients with aortic or bifurcation stenoses treated with angioplasty and stent placement, the technical success rate was 85% and the 10-year stent patency was 72%. There were 15 episodes of aortic stent restenosis during the mean follow-up interval of 51 months and 11 were successfully treated with endovascular techniques [29]. Similarly, during treatment of 69 patients with isolated infrarenal aortic stenosis, de Vries and associates achieved a 98% technical success rate, a 5-year primary patency rate of 75%, and a 5-year secondary patency of 97%. Over the period of observation, 12 patients (17%) developed a recurrence of their symptoms due to restenosis and eight were successfully treated with angioplasty [30]. At a mean follow-up of 86 months, 10 patients treated with angioplasty and stent placement for treatment of a focal distal aortic stenosis were evaluated with duplex sonography and ankle-brachial index calculation. The mean ABI was 0.90 + 0.20 and Duplex imaging detected no hemodynamically significant restenosis [31]. Experience is limited and most reported series are small, not because of the technical difficulty of this procedure but because isolated infrarenal aortic flow-restricting lesions are uncommon. Disease that involves both the distal aorta and the iliac arteries is more common. Stenotic lesions associated with aortic aneurysms should not be dilated unless part of a predetermined aneurysm treatment plan to reduce the likelihood of disruption of the intraluminal thrombus and distal embolization or breach of the aneurysm wall.

Atherosclerosis of the aortic bifurcation involves both iliac arteries and requires a bilateral femoral artery approach using the “kissing balloon” technique described by Tegtmeyer et al. [32]. With this technique, two 8–12 mm balloons can be simultaneously inflated within the aortoiliac region without the risk of iliac rupture. Once dilated, kissing stents can be placed with a small segment of the proximal stents anchored in the distal aorta to fully support the bifurcation (Fig. 14.7). This technique has become well established with a technical success rate of greater than 90% and a low complication rate [33–36]. Successful endovascular treatment of aortic bifurcation disease is also durable. The primary patency at 10-year follow-up in a clinical series of 43 patients treated with kissing balloon angioplasty and stent placement for bifurcation disease was noted to be 68% with a secondary patency of 86% [37]. As with all sites treated with angioplasty and stent placement, in-stent restenosis does occur. In a study of 66 patients with distal aortic and/or proximal iliac disease, technical success was achieved in

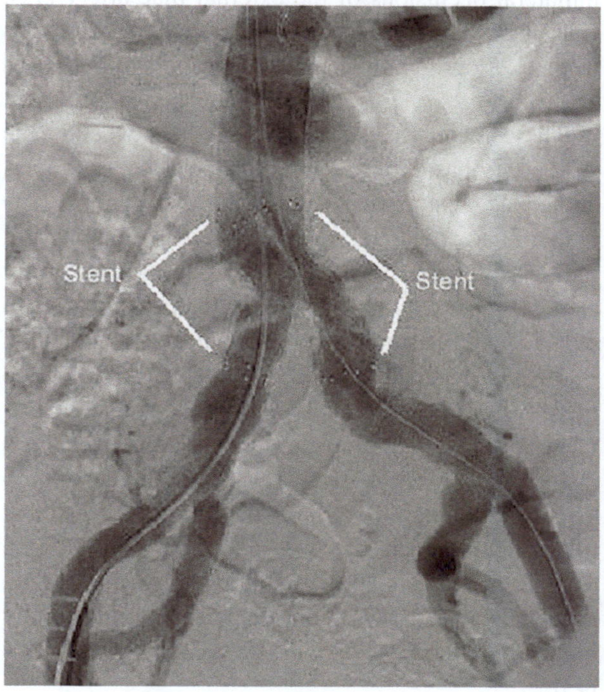

Fig. 14.7 Angiographic image of bilateral iliac arteries after kissing balloon angioplasty and placement of stents

94%. At 3-year follow-up, primary patency was noted in 86% with restenosis documented in 14%. Univariate analysis indicated that restenosis was most significantly associated with stent-lumen mismatch where stents failed to fill the distal aortic lumen [38]. In a similar study of 68 patients who underwent kissing balloon angioplasty and stent placement, patient age <50 years, iliac artery occlusion, and a crossed configuration of stents in the distal aorta were risk factors for reduced primary patency [39].

Iliac Artery Angioplasty

The common iliac artery is ideally suited for balloon angioplasty. It is a large, high-flow vessel that responds well to dilation and offers the highest initial and long-term success rates. The TASC II guidelines suggest that balloon angioplasty is indicated as the preferred intervention for TASC A and B lesions of the iliac arterial tree including unilateral or bilateral stenoses of the common iliac artery, unilateral or bilateral single short stenosis <3 cm in length of the external iliac artery, unilateral common iliac artery occlusions, multiple short stenoses of the external iliac artery, and unilateral occlusions of the external iliac artery [12]. Iliac angioplasty with primary or selective stenting has become a low-risk procedure with excellent outcomes [40].

These recommendations indicate that whether the iliac artery has a long stenosis or total occlusion, percutaneous treatment provides effective therapy. The Dutch Iliac Stent Trial, a prospective, randomized, multi-institutional study of patients with iliac artery stenoses up to 10 cm in length or occlusions up to 5 cm in length, demonstrated a technical success rate of >80% and stent patency of 83% with a mean follow-up of 6.3 years [41]. A French trial of percutaneous treatment of common and/or external iliac artery occlusions in 105 patients reported a technical success rate of 88% and stent patency of 61% at 6 years after treatment [42]. Technical success was independent of location (common iliac versus external iliac) and lesion length, though those with occlusions <6 cm had a significantly higher long-term patency (72% vs. 44%, $p < 0.004$) [43].

PTA of the iliac artery has also been effective in increasing inflow in patients for whom distal bypass grafting is being considered [44]. Noted more than 20 years ago, endovascular treatment of iliac artery stenoses prior to the construction of a femorofemoral or femorodistal bypass is effective for improving inflow sufficiently to support graft flow [45]. Initially performed as a staged procedure, there have been follow-up reports indicating similar success of a single-stage approach to combined iliac angioplasty and bypass. Comparing the results of combined iliac angioplasty and distal bypass to surgical correction of iliac stenoses or occlusions and distal bypass, Alimi and colleagues noted a trend toward a lower mortality among those treated with a combined procedure with equivalent patency rates [44].

Femoral and Popliteal Artery Angioplasty

Dilation of distal extremity lesions has become technically possible and relatively safe with the development of lower profile angioplasty balloons and steerable, hydrophilic guidewires. An ipsilateral approach provides the interventionist with the greatest wire and catheter maneuverability. The contralateral femoral artery approach is effective and necessary in proximal common femoral artery lesions. Because distal vessels are prone to spasm, the use of vasodilators is more important than with balloon angioplasty of aortoiliac disease.

Regardless of the technical feasibility of femoral and popliteal angioplasty, there is still some controversy about which patients should undergo PTA and which should proceed directly to surgical bypass. The indications for percutaneous intervention are similar to those for open surgery. Treatment is indicated for those who have intermittent claudication that interferes significantly with work or home life, who cannot walk adequately for cardiac rehabilitation, or who have limb-threatening ischemia. The TASC guidelines strongly recommend an initial attempt at treatment with angioplasty for stenosis or occlusion of the superficial femoral artery up to 15 cm in length, multiple stenoses or occlusions each less than 5 cm, heavily calcified occlusions up to 5 cm in length, or a single popliteal stenosis [12].

More important than patency rate is the lasting clinical benefit. A study of 117 patients with critical limb ischemia who underwent femoropopliteal angioplasty as their primary form of treatment reported primary technical success rates of 92% for stenoses and 80% for occlusions, with 1-, 2-, and 3-year limb salvage rates of only 56, 49, and 49%, respectively. Becquemin and colleagues compared 4-year patency rates of angioplasty and surgery for the treatment of femoropopliteal disease and found 44% of those treated with angioplasty still patent but 65% of those treated with bypass grafting patent [46]. The routine use of stents for angioplasty of the superficial femoral artery stenosis or occlusion continues to be debated, but there are increasing data that for small lesions stenting may enhance patency. In a randomized, prospective study of selective versus routine stenting after angioplasty of superficial femoral artery lesions up to 5 cm in length, the technical success rates were equivalent (100% for selective stent and 98% for primary stent placement). The 2-year primary patency rates were better with routine stenting (55% for selective stent and 73% for routine) [47]. Bare metal stents are clearly helpful in the setting of an inadequate angioplasty result or with longer lesions. Drug-eluting stents do not yield better results. The Sirolimus-Coated Cordis Self-expandable Stent (SIROCCO) II trial was a randomized, prospective, double-blind study that compared the treatment of long superficial femoral artery stenoses or occlusions (mean length 8.15 + 4.12 cm) with sirolimus-eluting stents to bare metal stents. The technical success rate was 100% for both groups. The 6-month patency was 95% in the drug-eluting stent group compared to 100% in the bare metal stent group [48]. This was followed by another randomized, prospective study comparing angioplasty and selective stenting to angioplasty and primary stenting for treatment of long superficial femoral artery lesions. The mean length of the lesions was greater than 12 cm. At 1-year follow-up, those patients treated with primary stent placement had a higher patency rate (63% vs. 37%) [49]. Though very long lesions may also be treated with a high technical success rate, the result is less durable. In a study of the results of angioplasty of 55 SFA lesions with a mean length of 16.5 cm, Gray and colleagues noted a primary patency at 1 year of only 22% [50]. Treatment of these very long lesions remains one of the significant challenges of the vascular interventionalist. Comparing 193 femoropopliteal angioplasties (116 stenoses and 77 occlusions), Murray et al. described a 4.5-year patency rate of 54.4% for 116 stenoses and 72.9% for 77 occlusions. Stenotic lesions larger than 7 cm demonstrated the worst patency rate: only 23.1% at 6 months [51].

Infrapopliteal Angioplasty

With the application of coronary angioplasty techniques, there has been increased enthusiasm for PTA of the infrapopliteal vessels (Fig. 14.8). Balloon

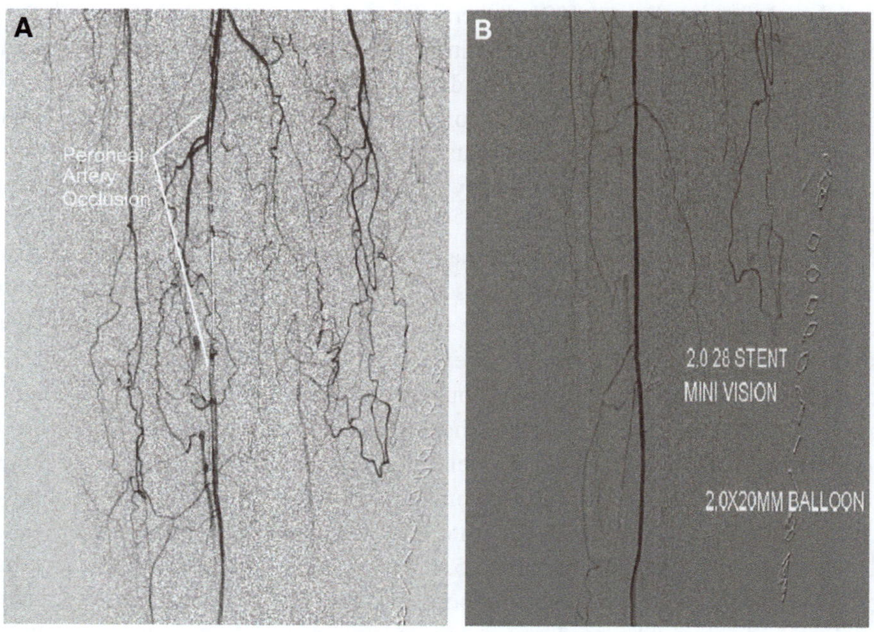

Fig. 14.8 **a**, Angiographic image of peroneal artery occlusion. **b**, Patent peroneal artery after angioplasty and stent placement

angioplasty of the tibioperoneal vessels is usually performed in poor-risk patients for limb salvage. The most common indications at this time are acute ischemia, rest pain, and tissue loss in patients whose vessels are otherwise unreconstructible by surgery. The procedure requires an antegrade common femoral artery puncture and insertion of a 5.5–6F vascular sheath. Generally, a steerable platinum-tipped guidewire along with a small-vessel (4F) angioplasty balloon is advanced across the lesion. Because there is very limited distensibility of the tibial arteries, a balloon diameter that is equal to or slightly smaller than the outflow vessel is used. Over-expansion of the tibial artery as is done in other, more elastic vessels will frequently result in dissection or rupture. Spasm and thrombosis must be treated aggressively with intraarterial vasodilators, thrombolytic agents, and intravenous heparin. Systemic heparinization is often continued for 48–72 h.

The best results for infrapopliteal angioplasty are achieved in short-segment focal stenoses (less than 2 cm). Technical success rates of 75–100% have been reported. In an analysis of 176 extremities with limb-threatening ischemia treated with balloon angioplasty, Giles and colleagues noted a technical success of 93%. At 2-year post-procedure, primary patency of the target site was 51% and freedom from restenosis, reintervention, or amputation was 35%. Nonetheless, limb salvage was 84% during this interval. The 30-day mortality was 5% and the 2-year mortality was 35%, consistent with the end-stage nature of this form of peripheral arterial disease [52]. Several factors have been implicated as adversely influencing the outcome, including the presence of diabetes, distal gangrene, more than six stenoses, occlusions more than 5 cm in length, and significant proximal or distal disease.

Because of the difficulties of elderly patients recovering their ability to independently ambulate after tibial artery bypass grafting, there has been continued efforts to improve the outcomes and durability of infrapopliteal angioplasty. The use of drug-eluting stents has recently been explored to extend the durability of tibial artery angioplasty. Though most series are small and non-randomized, the short-term results appear promising. Using 102 drug-eluting stents to treat lesions in 62 tibial arteries, Commeau and associates reported a technical success rate of 100% and 100% limb salvage at 7 months [53]. In a study of 24 patients with isolated infrapopliteal arterial occlusive disease who underwent angioplasty and placement of a drug-eluting stent, technical success was 96%. Limb preservation and healing of ulcers was achieved in 20 of 24 patients (83%) and angiographic confirmation of target site patency was obtained in 18 of 19 patients (95%) [54]. The continued development of lower profile catheters and balloons and the refinement of subintimal techniques may further enhance both the short- and the long-term outcomes of tibial artery angioplasty.

Renal and Mesenteric Angioplasty

Compared with peripheral vascular procedures, angioplasty of the branches of the abdominal aorta is technically more demanding. Stenoses of these vessels should be treated only by skilled interventionists. These lesions are usually caused by atherosclerosis, fibromuscular dysplasia, extrinsic compression, or vasculitis. Generally, a femoral artery approach is used, although a left brachial or axillary artery approach is recommended when there is an abdominal aortic aneurysm or an acute angle between the diseased artery and aorta. Most renal and mesenteric arteries can be cannulated with a cobra-shaped catheter. Torquable and hydrophilic guidewires used to cross tight stenoses may need to be exchanged for stiffer wires before advancing the balloon across the lesion. Heparin and nitroglycerin should be used before balloon inflation. When dilating renal arteries, it is important to use balloon catheters with the shortest length of catheter distal to the balloon to minimize trauma to the branch vessels. The procedural complication rate ranges from 5 to 18% [55, 56]. Technical success is generally high.

Angioplasty of non-orificial lesions has an immediate technical success rate of 80% to greater than 95% in recent reports [55, 57, 58]. The technical success rate is significantly improved with stents, especially if there is ostial involvement (Fig. 14.9) [59–61]. Stents provide a higher technical success and a longer primary patency [62]. A recent meta-analysis identified a statistically significant improvement in technical result associated with stent placement compared to balloon angioplasty alone (98 vs. 77%, $p < 0.001$) [57]. The addition of drug-eluting stents does not significantly improve either technical success or patency [63, 64]. In a direct comparison of bare metal and drug-eluting stents for renal artery stenosis in 105 patients, there was no statistically significant difference in

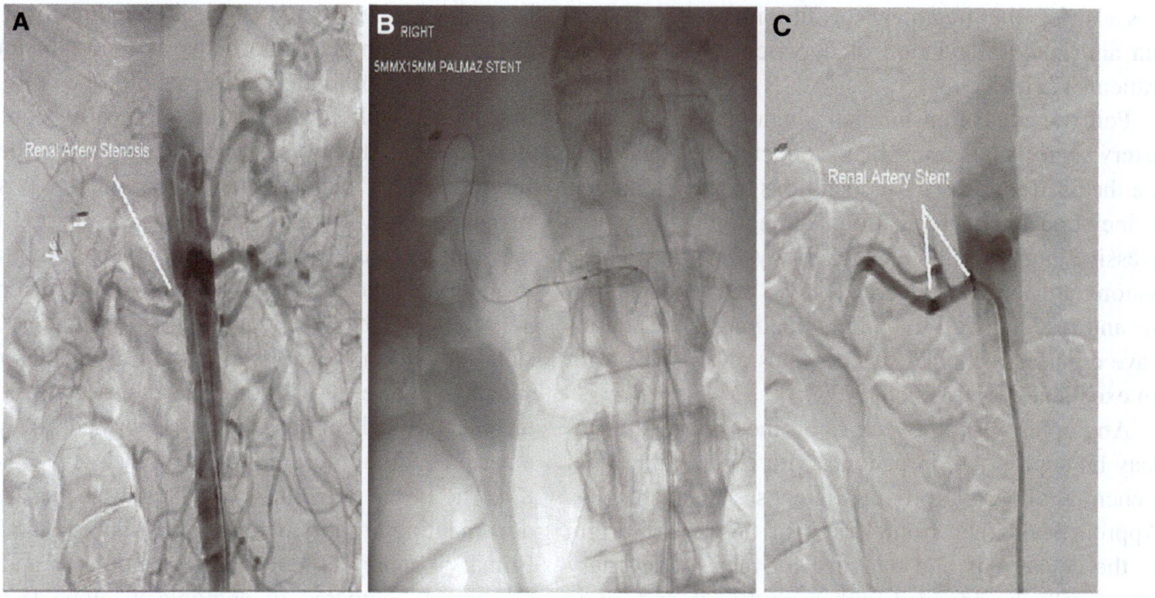

Fig. 14.9 **a**, Right renal artery stenosis. **b**, Balloon expandable stent placed through a well-positioned guide catheter. **c**, Completed angioplasty and stent in place with excellent flow through the renal artery

either technical success or angiographic appearance at 6-month post-procedure. Therefore, the use of drug-eluting stents is not indicated for the treatment of renal artery stenosis at this time.

Percutaneous transluminal renal angioplasty is most commonly indicated for the treatment of poorly controlled hypertension or progressive ischemic nephropathy resulting from renal artery stenosis. The clinical success rates for improvement in blood pressure are somewhat less than the high technical success rates. In a meta-analysis, the technical success rate for renal artery angioplasty was estimated at 98% with a major complication rate of 11% [57]. Though hypertension is uncommonly cured by angioplasty and stent placement (<10%), it is significantly improved in 40–60%, permitting better blood pressure control with fewer medications [55, 56, 60]. A mean arterial pressure >110 mmHg despite medications and bilateral hemodynamically significant renal artery stenoses appear to be predictive of those who will have the best blood pressure response to renal artery angioplasty [65].

Overall, hypertension is initially cured in 10–20% and improved in 40–60%, renal function improved in only 30% and is stabilized in 38% [57]. Of note in that analysis, stent placement was associated with a better response in hypertension control but a lower incidence of improvement in renal function. A subsequent meta-analysis confirmed this discrepant result [66]. Some investigators have postulated that the reason for failure in improvement of renal function after angioplasty is embolization of the kidney during angioplasty and stent placement. To prevent this, several investigators have begun to use embolic protection devices. In a study of 28 patients treated with renal artery angioplasty and stent placement performed with an embolic protection device in place, Edwards and colleagues noted a significant embolic burden in the embolic protection devices at the conclusion of the procedure. There was a negative association between the glomerular filtration rate and the entrapment of particles >60 μm in diameter [67]. Other investigators have noted a synergistic benefit of embolic protection devices and abciximab on renal function after renal artery angioplasty and stent placement [68, 69].

Angioplasty is more effective treatment for stenoses caused by fibromuscular dysplasia than those secondary to atherosclerosis. In a series of 55 renal angioplasty patients, Beebe et al. documented a 33% total cure rate and 50% improvement rate in patients with fibromuscular dysplasia but showed only a 10% cure rate and 42% improvement rate in patients with atherosclerotic plaques [70]. More recently, Davies and colleagues reported an initial improvement in hypertension in 72% of the 28 patients treated for renal artery fibromuscular dysplasia with angioplasty. Of those who responded, 75% retained their reduction in blood pressure at 5 years [71]. Cluzel and colleagues aggressively pursued angioplasty of renal branch vessels for the treatment of fibromuscular dysplasia and noted alleviation of hypertension in 92% of patients [72].

Percutaneous transluminal angioplasty of renal artery stenosis in a transplant is effective and can obviate the need for difficult reoperations to salvage failing kidney transplants. Indications for angioplasty are progressive hypertension and graft dysfunction. These lesions are most frequently located at the anastomosis and respond well to balloon dilation. Some studies have reported technical success rates of 75–93%, with an excellent 2-year benefit [73, 74].

Angioplasty of the celiac or mesenteric arteries may be appropriate in patients with chronic intestinal ischemia who have proximal stenoses or occlusions. Approached either from below or above the origin of the celiac axis and the superior mesenteric artery can usually be engaged with a guidewire and guide catheter. Angioplasty and selective stent placement is the most common form of endovascular treatment. The technical success rate for the treatment of stenoses ranges from 97 to 100% but is 85–100% for the treatment of occlusions. The associated morbidity is 10–15% in most reports. No procedural 30-day mortality was reported in recent series [75–79].

The immediate clinical success rate is 90–100% [75, 76, 78]. Restenosis had been a significant problem, however. The 1-year primary patency ranges from 47 to 70% and reintervention is required frequently. Compared to open surgery, patients treated with angioplasty and stent placement are 15 times more likely to require reintervention [76]. Nonetheless, angioplasty with selective stenting is appropriate for those patients with proximal mesenteric stenosis or occlusion who will reliably participate in a lifelong surveillance program and consent to retreatment when needed. Patients with aortic aneurysms, celiac axis syndrome, or other causes of extrinsic vascular compression should not be treated by PTA.

Brachiocephalic Vessels

Subclavian and Innominate Arteries

Balloon dilation of the subclavian and innominate arteries is effective in treating some patients with subclavian steal syndrome and upper extremity ischemia. Because open surgical techniques are associated with significant morbidity and mortality, angioplasty of the aortic arch vessels should be considered in patients with focal, hemodynamically significant stenoses that do not involve the origin of the vessel. Indications include upper limb ischemia, posterior fossa ischemia, or reduced flow to an internal mammary artery used for coronary artery bypass grafting [80]. Immediate technical success has been reported in 94–98%. The technical success is 99–100% for stenoses but only 69–90% for total occlusions of the subclavian artery [81–86]. These procedures while technically challenging may be performed safely with a periprocedural mortality of 1.5% or less [83, 84, 86, 87]. The 1-year outcome is excellent, with most reports documenting primary patency of 87–93% [82–85, 88]. Primary patency is better with angioplasty and stent placement compared to angioplasty alone [82, 88]. These results are generally sustained with a 10-year patency of 78% reported on long-term follow-up [85]. Although few neurologic complications have been reported, the risk of cerebral embolization must be considered when manipulating these vessels [86]. The risk of this procedure is minimized if the vertebral artery is also occluded.

Carotid Artery

Both tools and techniques of carotid angioplasty and stent placement have evolved significantly over the past several years. Initially performed without embolic protection, there is now substantial evidence that, when an embolic protection device is used, carotid angioplasty can be performed in selected patients with a low morbidity and mortality [89–91]. Few continue to debate the benefit of embolic protection [92]. The procedure is generally performed by cannulating the common femoral artery. After heparinization to an ACT greater than 300 s, a long 6F sheath that extends from the common femoral artery to the mid-cervical common carotid artery is placed over a stiff guidewire, such as a Rosen wire, to establish direct access to the carotid bifurcation and the internal carotid artery. An embolic protection device is carefully advanced across the lesion into the distal internal carotid artery and deployed to provide protection from emboli during angioplasty, stent placement, and post-stent dilation.

The lesion is pre-dilated with a 3 or 4 mm angioplasty balloon. The appropriately sized stent, usually tapered, such as 10–7 mm, is deployed across the stenosis to extend from the common carotid artery proximal to the lesion to the internal carotid artery beyond the lesion. An angiogram is performed. If a residual stenosis of greater than 30% remains then a post-deployment angioplasty is performed to eliminate that narrowing. A completion angiogram that includes intracranial views is obtained before removal of the sheath and placement of a closure.

Carotid angioplasty has been approved by the Centers for Medicare and Medicaid Services (CMS) for patients who have a symptomatic extracranial carotid artery stenosis that is 70% or greater and are at high risk for complications or death from carotid endarterectomy (Fig. 14.10). Risk factors include a high bifurcation that is surgically inaccessible, a hostile neck from either radiation, prior significant neck surgery, such as a radical neck dissection, or the presence of a tracheostomy, or cardiac dysfunction as defined by an ejection factor less than 30%. Pre-angioplasty angiography must document a stenosis of 70% or greater. If a lesser grade of stenosis is identified, then an open carotid endarterectomy must be performed. The hospital where the procedure is performed must be approved by the CMS by submitting an affidavit that confirms the institution has the facilities, support services, and outcomes required for performing carotid angioplasty [93]. Currently, there is no approval by CMS for carotid angioplasty and stent placement for patients with an asymptomatic lesion unless as part of an Food and Drug Administration (FDA)-approved clinical trial.

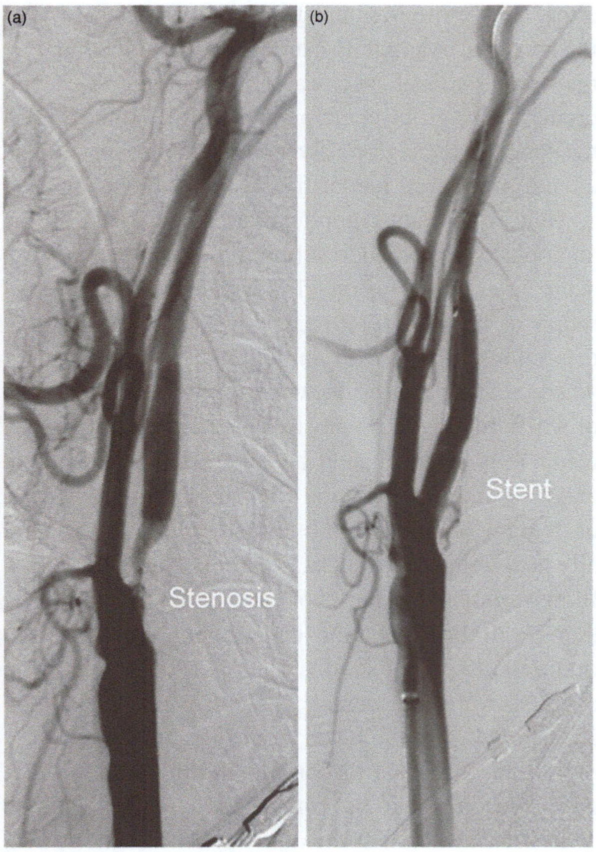

Fig. 14.10 **a**, Origin of internal carotid artery with critical stenosis. **b**, Widely patent internal carotid artery after angioplasty and stent placement

Overall the results have been acceptable in selected patients. The trials through which carotid angioplasty and stent placement was granted approval by the FDA were non-inferiority trials designed to determine whether endovascular treatment was inferior to carotid endarterectomy. The Carotid Revascularization using Endarterectomy or Stenting Systems (CARESS) Trial randomized 254 patients to carotid endarterectomy and 153 to carotid angioplasty and stent placement [94]. No significant difference was found between the two treatment modalities when analyzed for all-cause mortality and stroke [93]. The Stenting and Angioplasty with Protection of Patients with High Risk for Endarterectomy (SAPPHIRE) trial of 334 patients deemed to be at high risk for carotid intervention because of co-morbid conditions, such as cardiac dysfunction. Using a composite endpoint of ipsilateral stroke, death, or myocardial infarction, the trialists found no significant difference between carotid angioplasty and stent placement and carotid endarterectomy when evaluated for non-inferiority [89]. Similar findings were reported by the Carotid Artery Revascularization Using the Boston Scientific EPI FilterWire EX/EZ and the EndoTex NexStent (CABERNET) trial which treated symptomatic patients with a stenosis of 50% or greater and asymptomatic patients with a stenosis of 60% or greater. Using a weighted objective performance criterion, these investigators demonstrated non-inferiority of carotid angioplasty [95]. Several subsequent studies, however, have failed to document superiority or equivalence of carotid angioplasty and stent placement to carotid endarterectomy for the treatment of carotid bifurcation disease. The Endarterectomy

Versus Angioplasty in Patients with Symptomatic Severe Carotid Stenosis (EVA 3S) trial, a European multicenter randomized prospective trial comparing the two treatment modalities in symptomatic patients with at least 60% stenosis of the cervical carotid artery. The trial was halted after 527 patients were enrolled because of concerns of patient safety. The 30-day incidence of stroke and death was 3.9% after carotid endarterectomy but 9.6% after carotid angioplasty and stent placement. The 30-day incidence of disabling stroke was higher after angioplasty at 3.4% compared to 1.5% for those who had endarterectomy [96]. Similarly, the Stent Protected Angioplasty versus Carotid Endarterectomy (SPACE) trial compared carotid angioplasty to endarterectomy in 1,200 patients with symptomatic cervical carotid artery stenosis. This trial also failed to establish non-inferiority of angioplasty [97]. Numerous other studies have been reported leading to several meta-analyses to more clearly determine the role of angioplasty for the treatment of cervical carotid artery disease. These meta-analyses of carotid angioplasty versus carotid endarterectomy trial document an advantage of reduced cranial nerve injury [98–100]. In comparisons of death and stroke, however, nearly all of the meta-analyses conclude that carotid angioplasty has a higher stroke and death rate compared to endarterectomy. Therefore, at this time, carotid endarterectomy remains the treatment of choice for most patients undergoing treatment for symptomatic or asymptomatic carotid stenosis [98, 99, 101–104].

Complications

Although less invasive than surgery, angioplasty is an invasive procedure with well-recognized complications (Table 18.3). A review of the literature reveals an overall complication rate of 7.9–26.0% [105–109]. Most of these complications are minor and resolve without additional therapy, but surgical management is required in 2–3% [110]. The most common complications occur at the puncture site. Other problems can occur at or distal to the angioplasty site. Still other adverse effects have systemic sequelae.

Fruhwirth and colleagues reviewed 15,460 femoral punctures and identified 81 vascular complications [111]. They noted 65 pseudoaneurysms, eight acute arterial occlusions, seven profusely bleeding arteries, and one arteriovenous fistula. Hematoma is the most common puncture site complication. Significant bleeding at the arterial entrance site occurs in 0.2–4.6% of patients. Risk factors include obesity, hypertension, large balloon size, overly aggressive anticoagulation, severe atherosclerosis at the puncture site, and inadequate postprocedural groin compression. Although these groin hematomas rarely require surgical evacuation, they do increase the possibility of infection. Pseudoaneurysm at the cannulation site occurs in 0.1–1.5% of patients [105]. Duplex imaging can quickly confirm this diagnosis. The false aneurysm cavity of small pseudoaneurysms (less than 1.5 cm in greatest diameter) can be thrombosed by ultrasound-guided compression [112]. Large pseudoaneurysms should be treated surgically. A more disastrous puncture-site complication is retroperitoneal hemorrhage or hematoma, occurring in fewer than 0.1% of patients [105]. This complication is usually caused by attempting to puncture the common femoral artery above the inguinal ligament but instead entering the distal external iliac artery. Profuse bleeding into the retroperitoneal space can ensue without the development of a groin hematoma. Careful monitoring of the patient after angioplasty along with prompt surgical attention can avert hemorrhagic shock and death.

Other important complications associated with the angioplasty site include subintimal dissection (4.4%), acute arterial occlusion (1–7%), and arterial perforation or rupture (0.1%) [105–109, 113]. Subintimal dissections, along with intimal flaps, usually occur when crossing the lesion with a guidewire or catheter or when dilating the stenosis. This intimal trauma may result in acute occlusion and the need for emergent endovascular manipulation (i.e., angioscopy, stenting) or bypass surgery. Small dissections or flaps usually heal within 4–6 weeks. Vessel occlusion resulting from thrombosis can be treated with thrombolytic therapy. Balloon dilation occasionally causes vessel rupture [113]. This serious complication results from overdistending the vessel with an oversized balloon and should be anticipated if the patient experiences more than the usual discomfort during balloon inflation. Bleeding can be controlled by reinflating the angioplasty balloon at the injury site while the patient is prepared for surgery.

Clinically significant distal embolization is seen in fewer than 1% of patients, although clinically silent microemboli occur more frequently [108]. Longstanding occlusions or lesions associated with fresh thrombus are prone to showering debris and should not be dilated before first receiving a trial of lytic therapy. If the embolic debris leads to significant distal vessel occlusion, surgical embolectomy or bypass may be required. Distal vessel spasm can be treated pharmacologically.

Renal insufficiency is the most significant systemic complication after angioplasty, occurring in 1.5% of all patients [105, 109]. Worsening renal function occurs most often in the subset of patients undergoing renal angioplasty (6% of patients) and can be minimized by keeping patients well hydrated [114]. Other systemic complications include stroke (0.1%), myocardial infarction (0.1–0.8%), and congestive heart failure (1.9%). The direct mortality associated with angioplasty is between 0.2 and 2.2% [105, 108].

Summary

As technologic advances continue, more patients suffering from peripheral vascular disease are treated with balloon angioplasty. Medications to prevent myointimal hyperplasia, which causes restenosis, are being developed. Stenting devices are currently available to help prevent dissection, elastic recoil, and rapid reocclusion after balloon dilation. Techniques such as thermal, radiofrequency, and laser balloons are also being used in investigational settings to "weld" acute dissections and reduce elastic recoil. The endovascular industry has created a multitude of devices such as atherectomy catheters, intravascular ultrasound instruments, and angioscopes, which can be used as adjuncts to balloon angioplasty. As in all medical procedures, long-term patient benefit from balloon angioplasty depends on proper patient selection and close surveillance.

References

1. Dotter CT, Judkins MP: Transluminal treatment of arteriosclerotic obstruction: description of a new technique and a preliminary report of its application, *Circulation* 30:654–670, 1964.
2. Gruntzig A, Hopff H: Perkutane Rekanalisation chronischer arterieller Verschlusse mit einem neuen Dilatationskather: Modification der Dotter-Technik, *Dtsch Med Wochenschr* 99:2502–2505, 1974.
3. Dotter CT, Judkins MP, Rosch J: Nonoperative treatment of arterial occlusive disease: a radio-logically facilitated technique, *Radiol Clin North Am* 5:531–542, 1967.
4. Chin AK, Kinney TB, Rurik GW et al.: A physical measurement of the mechanisms of transluminal angioplasty, *Surgery* 95:196–200, 1984.
5. Demer LL, Ariani M, Siegel RJ: High intensity ultrasound increases distensibility of calcific atherosclerotic arteries, *J Am Coll Cardiol* 18(5):1259–1262, November 1, 1991.
6. Lyon RT, Zarins CK, Lu CT, Yang CF, Glagov S: Wessel, plaque, and lumen morphology after transluminal balloon angioplasty. Quantitative study in distended human arteries, *Arteriosclerosis* 7:306–314, 1987.
7. Block PC, Baughman KL, Pasternak RC et al.: Transluminal angioplasty: correlation of morphologic and angiographic findings in an experimental model, *Circulation* 61:778, 1980.
8. Zarins CK, Lu CT, Gewertz BL et al.: Arterial disruption and remodeling following balloon dilatation, *Surgery* 92:1086–1095, 1982.
9. Minar E, Ehringer H, Ahmadi R et al.: Platelet deposition at angioplasty sites and its relation to restenosis in human iliac and femoropopliteal arteries, *Radiology* 170:767–772, 1989.
10. Tepe G, Zeller T, Albrecht T, Heller S, Schwarzwalder U, Beregi J-P, Claussen CD, Oldenburg A, Scheller B, Speck U: Local delivery of paclitaxel to inhibit restenosis during angioplasty of the leg, *N Engl J Med* 358:689–699, 2008.
11. Rutherford RB, Dormandy JA: The TransAtlantic Inter-Society consensus on the management of peripheral arterial disease, *J Vasc Surg* 31(Part 2):S1–S296, 2000.
12. Norgren L, Hiatt WR, Dormandy JA, Nehler MR, Harris KA, Fowkes FGR: Inter-society consensus for the management of peripheral arterial disease (TASC II), *J Vasc Surg* 45(suppl S):S49–50, 2007.
13. Hirsch AT, Haskal ZJ, Hertzer NR, Bakal CW, Creager MA, Halperin JL et al.: ACC/AHA guidelines for the management of patients with peripheral arterial disease (Lower extremity, renal, mesenteric, and abdominal aortic): A collaborative report from the American associations for vascular surgery/society for vascular surgery, society for cardiovascular angiography and interventions, society for vascular medicine and biology, society of interventional radiology, and the American college of cardiology/American heart association task force on practice guidelines (Writing committee to develop guidelines for the management of patients with peripheral arterial disease) – Summary of recommendations, *J Vasc Interv Radiol* 17(9):1383–1397, September 2006.
14. Schneider PA:: Guidewire-catheter skills. In Schneider PA, editor: *Endovascular skills*, St. Louis, 1998, Quality Medical Publishing, pp. 3–21.
15. Hoppe M, Wagner HJ, Klose KJ: Assessment of the hemodynamic result of PTA with a Doppler guide wire: initial experience, *J Vasc Intervent Radiol* 7: 89–93, 1996.
16. Garcia LA, Carrozza JP Jr.: Physiologic evaluation of translesion pressure gradients in peripheral arteries: comparison of pressure wire and catheter-derived measurements, *J Interv Cardiol* 20(1):63–65, 2007.

17. Cavendish JJ, Carter LI, Tsimikas S: Recent advances in hemodynamics: noncoronary applications of a pressure sensor angioplasty guidewire, *Catheter Cardiovasc Interv* 71(6):748–758, 2008.
18. Tepe G, Zeller T, Albrecht T, Heller S, Schwarzwalder U, Beregi J-P, Claussen CD, Oldenburg A, Scheller B, Speck U: Local delivery of paclitaxel to inhibit restenosis during angioplasty of the leg, *New Engl J Med* 358:689–699, 2008.
19. Lewis-Carey MB, Kee ST: Complications of arterial closure devices, *Tech Vasc Interv Radiol* 6:103–106, 2003.
20. Applegate RJ, Sacrinty M, Kutcher MA, Gandhi SK, Baki TT, Santos RM, Little WC: Vascular complications with newer generations of angioseal vascular closure devices, *J Interv Cardiol* 19(1):67–74, February 2006.
21. Hermiller JB, Simonton C, Hinohara T, Lee D, Cannon L, Mooney M, O'Shaughnessy C, Carlson H, Fortuna R, Zapien M, Fletcher DR, DiDonato K, Chou TM: The StarClose vascular closure system: interventional results from the CLIP study, *Catheter Cardiovasc Interv* 68(5):677–683, November 2006.
22. Meyerson SL, Feldman T, Desai TR, Leef J, Schwartz LB, McKinsey JF: Angiographic access site complications in the era of arterial closure devices, *Vasc Endovascular Surg* 36(2):137–144, March–April 2002.
23. Eggebrecht H, von Birgelen C, Naber C, Kröger K, Schmermund A, Wieneke H, Bartel T, Wörtgen U, Baumgart D, Haude M, Erbel R: Impact of gender on femoral access complications secondary to application of a collagen-based vascular closure device, *J Invasive Cardiol* 16(5):251, May 2004.
24. Schedel H, Wissgott C, Rademaker J, Steinkamp HJ: Primary stent placement for infrarenal aortic stenosis: immediate and midterm results, *J Vasc Interv Radiol* 15(4):353–359, April 2004.
25. Stoeckelhuber BM, Stoeckelhuber M, Gellissen J, Kueffer G: Primary endovascular stent placement for focal infrarenal aortic stenosis: long-term results, *J Vasc Interv Radiol* 17:1105–1109, 2006.
26. Simons PC, Nawijn AA, Bruijninckx CM, Knippenberg B, deVries EH, van Overhagen H: Long-term results of primary stent placement to treat infrarenal aortic stenosis, *Eur J Vasc Endovasc Surg* 32:627–633, 2006.
27. Feugier P, Toursarkissian B, Chevalier JM, Favre P: Endovascular treatment of isolated atherosclerotic stenosis of the infrarenal abdominal aorta: long-term outcome, *Ann Vasc Surg* 17:375–385, 2003.
28. Schedel H, Wissgott C, Rademaker J, Steinkamp HJ: Primary stent placement for infrarenal aortic stenosis: immediate and midterm results, *J Vasc Interv Radiol* 15(4):353–359, April 2004.
29. Audet P, Therasse E, Oliva VL et al.: Infrarenal aortic stenosis: long-term clinical and hemodynamic results of percutaneous transluminal angioplasty, *Radiology* 209:357–363, 1998.
30. de Vries JP, van Den Heuval DA, Vos JA, van Den Berg JC, Moll FI: Freedom from secondary interventions to treat stenotic disease after percutaneous transluminal angioplasty of the infrarenal aorta: long-term results, *J Vasc Surg* 39:427–431, 2004.
31. Ruppert V, Wirth S, Rieger J, Kueffer G, Steckmeier B, Stoeckelhuber BM: Long-term results after primary stenting of distal aortic stenosis, *J Endovasc Ther* 13(2):229–236, April 2006.
32. Tegtmeyer CJ, Kellum CD, Kron IL, Mentzer RM, Jr: Percutaneous transluminal angioplasty in the region of the aortic bifurcation, *Radiology* 157:661–665, 1985.
33. Silva MB Jr, Hobson RW II, Jamil Z et al.: A program of operative angioplasty: endovascular intervention and the vascular surgeon, *J Vasc Surg* 24:963–971, 1996.
34. Bosch JL, Hunink MGM: Meta-analysis of the results of percutaneous transluminal angioplasty and stent placement for aortoiliac disease, *Radiology* 204:87–96, 1997.
35. Piffaretti G, Tozzi M, Lomazzi C, Rivolta N, Laganà D, Carrafiello G, Caronno R, Castelli P: Mid-term results of endovascular reconstruction for aorto-iliac obstructive disease, *Int Angiol* 26(1):18–25, March 2007.
36. van't Riet M, Spronk S, Jonkman J, Den Hoed T: Endovascular treatment of atherosclerosis at the aortoiliac bifurcation with kissing stents or distal aortic stents: a temporary solution or durable improvement?, *J Vasc Nurs* 26(3):82–85, September 2008.
37. Houston JG, Bhat R, Ross R, Stonebridge PA: Long-term results after placement of aortic bifurcation self-expanding stents: 10 year mortality, stent restenosis, and distal disease progression, *Cardiovasc Intervent Radiol* 30(1):42–47, January–February 2007.
38. Sharafuddin MJ, Hoballah JJ, Kresowik TF, Sharp WJ, Golzarian J, Sun S, Corson JD: Long-term outcome following stent reconstruction of the aortic bifurcation and the role of geometric determinants, *Ann Vasc Surg* 22(3):346–357, May–June 2008.
39. Yilmaz S, Sindel T, Golbasi I, Turkay C, Mete A, Lüleci E: Aortoiliac kissing stents: long-term results and analysis of risk factors affecting patency, *J Endovasc Ther* 13(3):291–301, June 2006.
40. Sullivan TM, Childs MB, Bacharach JM et al.: Percutaneous transluminal angioplasty and primary stenting of the iliac arteries in 288 patients, *J Vasc Surg* 25:829–838, 1997.
41. Klein WM, van der Graaf Y, Seegers J et al.: Dutch iliac stent trial: long-term results in patients randomized for primary or selective stent placement, *Radiology* 238:734–744, 2006.
42. Henry M, Amor M, Ethevenot G, Henry I, Mentre B, Tzvetanov K: Percutaneous endoluminal treatment of iliac occlusions: long-term follow-up in 105 patients, *J Endovasc Surg* 5:228–235, 1998.
43. Reyes R, Maynar M, Lopera J et al.: Treatment of chronic iliac artery occlusions with guide wire recanalization and primary stent placement, *J Vasc Intervent Radiol* 8:1049–1055, 1997.
44. Alimi Y, Di Mauro P, Barthèlemy P, Juhan C: Iliac transluminal angioplasty and distal surgical revascularisation can be performed in a one-step technique, *Int Angiol* 16(2):83–87, June 1997.
45. Brewster DC, Cambria RP, Darling RC, Athanasoulis CA, Waltman AC, Geller SC, Moncure AC, Lamuraglia GM, Freehan M, Abbott WM: Long-term results of combined iliac balloon angioplasty and distal surgical revascularization, *Ann Surg* 210(3):324–330, September 1989.

46. Becquemin JP, Cavillon A, Allaire E et al.: Iliac and femoropopliteal lesions: evaluation of balloon angioplasty and classical surgery, *J Endovasc Surg* 2:42–50, 1995.
47. Cejna M, Thurnher S, Illiasch H et al.: PTA versus Palmaz stent placement in femoropopliteal obstructions: a multicenter prospective randomized study, *J Interve Radiol* 12:23–31, 2001.
48. Duda SH, Bosiers M, Lammer J et al.: Sirolimus-eluting versus bare nitinol stent for obstructive superficial femoral artery disease: the SIROCCO II trial, *J Vasc Interv Radiol* 16:331–338, 2005.
49. Schillinger M, Sabeti S, Loewe C et al.: Balloon angioplasty versus implantation of nitinol stents in the superficial femoral artery, *N Engl J Med* 354:1879–1888, 2006.
50. Gray BH, Sullivan TM, Childs MB, Young JR, Olin JW: High incidence of restenosis/reocclusion of stents in the percutaneous treatment of long-segment superficial femoral artery disease after suboptimal angioplasty, *J Vasc Surg* 25:74–83, 1997.
51. Murray RR Jr, Hewes RC White RI Jr et al.: Long-segment femoropopliteal stenoses: is angioplasty a boon or bust? *Radiology* 162:473–476, 1987.
52. Giles KA, Pomposelli FB, Hamdan AD, Blattman SB, Panossian H, Schermerhorn ML: Infrapopliteal angioplasty for critical limb ischemia: relation of TransAtlantic InterSociety Consensus class to outcome in 176 limbs, *J Vasc Surg* 48(1):128–136, July 2008, Epub 2008 May 23.
53. Commeau P, Barragan P, Roquebert PO: Sirolimus for below the knee lesions: mid-term results of SiroBTK study, *Catheter Cardiovasc Interv* 68(5):793–798, November 2006.
54. Rosales OR, Mathewkutty S, Gnaim C: Drug eluting stents for below the knee lesions in patients with critical limb ischemia : long-term follow-up, *Catheter Cardiovasc Interv* 72(1):112–115, July 1, 2008.
55. Yutan E, Glickerman DJ, Caps MT, Hatsukami T, Harley JD, Kohler TR, Davies MG: Percutaneous transluminal revascularization for renal artery stenosis: veterans affairs puget sound health care system experience, *J Vasc Surg* 34:685–693, 2001.
56. Sivamurthy N, Surowiec SM, Culakova E, Rhodes JM, Lee D, Sternbach Y, Waldman DL, Green RM, Davies MG: Divergent outcomes after percutaneous therapy for symptomatic renal artery stenosis, *J Vasc Surg* 39:565–574, 2004.
57. Leertouwer TC, Gussenhoven EJ, Bosch JL, van Jaarsveld BC, van Dijk LC, Deinum J, Man In't Veld AJ: Stent placement for renal arterial stenosis: where do we stand? *Radiology* 216:78–85, 2000.
58. White CJ, Olin JW: Diagnosis and management of atherosclerotic renal artery stenosis: improving patient selection and outcomes, *Nat Clin Pract Cardiovasc Med* 6(3):176–190, March 2009.
59. Tuttle KR, Chouinard RF, Webber JT, Dahlstrom LR, Short RA, Henneberry KJ, Dunham LA, Raabe RD: Treatment of atherosclerotic ostial renal artery stenosis with the intravascular stent, *Am J Kidney Dis* 32:611–622, 1999.
60. Lim ST, Rosenfield K: Renal artery stent placement: indications and results, *Curr Interv Cardiol Rep* 2:130–139, 2000.
61. Rocha-Singh K, Jaff MR, Rosenfield K: Aspire-2 trial investigators. Evaluation of the safety and effectiveness of renal artery stenting after unsuccessful angioplasty: the ASPIRE-2 study, *J Am Coll Cardiol* 46:776–783, 2005.
62. Gill KS, Fowler RC: Atherosclerotic renal arterial stenosis: clinical outcomes of stent placement for hypertension and renal failure, *Radiology* 226:821–826, 2003.
63. Zeller T, Rastan A, Rothenpieler U, Muller C: Restenosis after stenting of atherosclerotic renal artery stenosis: is there a rationale for the use of drug-eluting stents? *Catheter Cardiovasc Interv* 68:125–130, 2006.
64. Zahringer M, Sapoval M, Pattynama PM, Rabbia C, Vignali C, Maleux G, Boyer L, Szczerbo-Trojanowska M, Jaschke W, Hafsahl G, Downes M, Beregi JP, Veeger NJ, Stoll HP, Talen A: Sirolimus-eluting versus bare metal low-profile stent for renal artery treatment (GREAT Trial): angiographic follow-up after 6 months and clinical outcome up to 2 years, *J Endovasc Ther* 14:460–468, 2007.
65. Rocha-Singh KJ, Mishkel GJ, Katholi RE, Ligon RA, Armbruster JA, McShane KJ, Zeck KJ: Clinical predictors of improved long-term blood pressure control after successful stenting of hypertensive patients with obstructive renal artery atherosclerosis, *Catheter Cardiovasc Interv* 47:167–172, 1999.
66. Nordmann AJ, Woo K, Parkes R, Logan AG: Balloon angioplasty or medical therapy for hypertensive patients with atherosclerotic renal artery stenosis? A meta-analysis of randomized controlled trials, *Am J Med* 114:44–50, 2003.
67. Edwards MS, Corriere MA, Craven TE, Pan XM, Rapp JH, Pearce JD, Mertaugh NB, Hansen KJ: Atheroembolism during percutaneous renal artery revascularization, *J Vasc Surg* 46:55–61, 2007.
68. Cooper CJ, Haller St, Colyer W et al.: Embolic protection and platelet inhibition during renal artery stenting, *Circulation* 117:2752–2760, 2008.
69. Kanjwal K, Haller S, Steffes M, Virmani R, Shapiro JI, Burket MW, Cooper CJ, Colyer WR Jr: Complete versus partial distal embolic protection during renal artery stenting, *Catheter Cardiovasc Interv* 73(6):731–736, 2009.
70. Beebe HG, Chesebro K, Merchant F, Bush W: Results of renal artery balloon angioplasty limits its indications, *J Vasc Surg* 8(3):300–306, 1988.
71. Davies MG, Saad WE, Peden EK, Mohiuddin IT, Naoum JJ, Lumsden AB: The long-term outcomes of percutaneous therapy for renal artery fibromuscular dysplasia, *J Vasc Surg* 48(4):865–871, October 2008.
72. Cluzel P, Raynaud A, Beyssen B et al.: Stenoses of renal branch arteries in fibromuscular dysplasia: results of percutaneous transluminal angioplasty, *Radiology* 193:227–232, 1994.
73. Hagen G, Wadström J, Magnusson M, Magnusson A: Outcome after percutaneous transluminal angioplasty of arterial stenosis in renal transplant patients, *Acta Radiol* 50(3):270–275, April 2009.
74. Valpreda S, Messina M, Rabbia C: Stenting of transplant renal artery stenosis: outcome in a single center study, *J Cardiovasc Surg (Torino)* 49(5):565–570, October 2008.
75. Chahid T, Alfidja AT, Biard M, Ravel A, Garcier JM, Boyer L: Endovascular treatment of chronic mesenteric

ischemia: results in 14 patients, *Cardiovasc Intervent Radiol* 27:637–642, 2004.

76. Brown DJ, Schermerhorn ML, Powell RJ, Fillinger MF, Rzucidlo EM, Walsh DB, Wyers MC, Zwolak RM, Cronenwett JL: Mesenteric stenting for chronic mesenteric ischemia, *J Vasc Surg* 42:268–274, 2005.
77. Landis MS, Rajan DK, Simons ME, Hayeems EB, Kachura JR, Sniderman KW: Percutaneous management of chronic mesenteric ischemia: outcomes after intervention, *J Vasc Interv Radiol* 16:1319–1325, 2005.
78. WyPiffaretti G, Tozzi M, Lomazzi C, Rivolta N, Riva F, Caronno R, Lagana D, Carrafiello G, Castelli P: Endovascular therapy for chronic mesenteric ischemia, *World J Surg* 31:2416–2421, 2007.
79. Sarac TP, Altinel O, Kashyap V, Bena J, Lyden S, Sruvastava S, Eagleton M, Clair D: Endovascular treatment of stenotic and occluded visceral arteries for chronic mesenteric ischemia, *J Vasc Surg* 47:485–491, 2008.
80. Westerband A, Rodriguez JA, Ramaiah VG, Diethrich EB: Endovascular therapy in prevention and management of coronary steal syndrome, *J Vasc Surg* 38:699–703, 2003.
81. Motarjeme A: Percutaneous transluminal angioplasty of supraaortic vessels, *J Endovasc Surg* 3:171–181, 1996.
82. Sixt S, Rastan A, Schwarzwalder U et al.: Results after balloon angioplasty or stenting of atherosclerotic subclavian artery obstructions, *Catheter Cardiovasc Interv* 73:395–403, 2009.
83. Henry M, Henry I, Polydorou A, Polydorou A, Hugel M: Percutaneous transluminal angioplasty of the subclavian arteries, *Int Angiol* 26:324–340, 2007.
84. Van Noord BA, Lin AH, Cavendish JJ: Rates of symptom reoccurrence after endovascular therapy in subclavian artery stenosis and prevalence of subclavian artery restenosis prior to coronary artery bypass grafting, *Vasc Health Risk Manag* 3:759–762, 2007.
85. AbuRahma AF, Bates MC, Stone PA, Dyer B, Armistead L, Scott Dean L, Scott Lavigne P: Angioplasty and stenting versus carotid-subclavian bypass for the treatment of isolated subclavian artery disease, *J Endovasc Ther* 14:698–704, 2007.
86. Patel SN, White CJ, Collins TJ, Daniel GA, Jenkins JS, Reilly JP, Morris RF, Ramee SR: Catheter-based treatment of the subclavian and innominate arteries, *Catheter Cardiovasc Interv* 71:969–971, 2008.
87. Palchik E, Bakken AM, Wolford HY, Saad WE, Davies MG: Subclavian artery revascularization: an outcome analysis based on mode of therapy and presenting symptoms, *Ann Vasc Surg* 22:70–78, 2008.
88. Sixt S, Rastan A, Schwarzwalder U, Schwarz T, Norry E, Frank U, Muller C, Beschorner U, Burgelin K, Nazary T, Hauswald K, Hauk M, Neumann FJ, Zeller T: Long term outcome after balloon angioplasty and stenting of subclavian artery obstruction: a single centre experience, *Vasa* 37:174–182, 2008.
89. Yadav JS, Wholey MH, Kuntz RE, Fayad P, Katzen BT, Mishkel GJ, Bajwa TK, Whitlow P, Strickman NE, Jaff MR, Popma JJ, Snead DB, Cutlip DE, Firth BG, Ouriel K: Stenting and angioplasty with protection in patients at high risk for endarterectomy investigators protected carotid stenting in high-surgical-risk patients: the ARCHeR results, *J Vasc Surg* 44(2):258–268, August 2006.
90. CARESS Steering Committee Carotid Revascularization Using Endarterectomy or Stenting Systems (CaRESS) phase I clinical trial: 1-year results *J Vasc Surg* 42(2):213–219, August 2005.
91. Gray WA, Hopkins LN, Yadav S, Davis T, Wholey M, Atkinson R, Cremonesi A, Fairman R, Walker G, Verta P, Popma J, Virmani R, Cohen DJ: ARCHeR trial collaborators. Protected carotid stenting in high-surgical-risk patients: the ARCHeR results, *J Vasc Surg* 44(2):258–268, August 2006.
92. Jansen O, Fiehler J, Hartmann M, Bruckmann H: Protection or nonprotection in carotid stent angioplasty: the influence of interventional techniques on outcome data from the SPACE Trial, *Stroke* 40:841–846, 2009.
93. Medlearn Matters CMS # MM3811
94. CaRESS Steering Committee: Carotid revascularization using endarterectomy or stenting systems (CARESS): phase I clinical trial, *J Endovasc Ther* 10:1021–1030, 2003.
95. Hopkins LN, Myla S, Grube E, Wehman JC, Levy EI, Bersin RM, Joye JD, Allocco DJ, Kelley L, Baim DS: Carotid artery revascularization in high-surgical risk patients with the NexStent and the Filterwire EX/EZ: 1-year results in the CABERNET Trial, *Catheter Cardiovasc Interv* 71:950–960, 2008.
96. Mas JL, Chatellier G, Beyssen B, Branchereau A, Moulin T, Becquemin JP et al.: Endarterectomy versus stenting in patients with symptomatic severe carotid stenosis, *New Engl J Med* 355:1660–1671, 2006.
97. Collaborative Group SPACE, Ringleb PA, Allenberg J, Bruckmann H et al.: 30-day results from the SPACE trial: Stent-protected angioplasty versus carotid endarterectomy in symptomatic patients: a randomized non-inferiority trial, *Lancet* 368:1239–1247, 2006.
98. Coward LJ, Featherstone RL, Brown MM: Percutaneous transluminal angioplasty and stenting for carotid artery stenosis, *Cochrane Database Syst Rev* 2:CD000515, 2004.
99. Coward LJ, Featherstone RL, Brown MM: Safety and efficacy of endovascular treatment of carotid artery stenosis compared with carotid endarterectomy: a Cochrane systematic review of randomized evidence, *Stroke* 36:905–911, 2005.
100. Qureshi AI, Kirmani JF, Divani AA, Hobson RW 2nd: Carotid angioplasty with or without stent placement versus carotid endarterectomy for treatment of carotid stenosis: a meta-analysis, *Neurosurgery* 56:1171–1181, 2005.
101. Luebke T, Aleksic M, Brunkwall J: Meta-analysis of randomized trials comparing carotid endarterectomy and endovascular treatment, *Eur J Vasc Endovasc Surg* 34:470–479, 2007.
102. Ringleb PA, Chatellier G, Hacke W, Favre JP, Bartoli JM, Eckstein HH, Mas JL: Safety of endovascular treatment of carotid artery stenosis compared with surgical treatment: a meta-analysis, *J Vasc Surg* 47:350–355, 2008.
103. Brahmanandam S, Ding EL, Conte MS, Belkin M, Nguyen LL: Clinical results of carotid artery stenting compared with carotid endarterectomy, *J Vasc Surg* 47:343–349, 2008.

104. Jeng JS, Liu HM, Tu YK: Carotid angioplasty with or without stenting versus carotid endarterectomy for carotid artery stenosis: a meta-analysis, *J Neurol Sci* 270:40–47, 2008.
105. Belli AM, Cumberland DC, Knox AM et al.: The complication rate of percutaneous peripheral balloon angioplasty, *Clin Radiol* 41:380, 1990.
106. Johnston KW, Rae M, Hogg-Johnston SA et al.: Five-year results of a prospective study of percutaneous transluminal angioplasty, *Ann Surg* 206:403, 1987.
107. O'Keeffe ST, Woods BO, Beckmann CF: Percutaneous transluminal angioplasty of the peripheral arteries, *Cardiol Clin* 9:515, 1991.
108. Samson RH, Sprayregen S, Veith FJ et al.: Management of angioplasty complications, unsuccessful procedures, and early and late failures, *Ann Surg* 199:234, 1984.
109. Weibull II, Bergqvist D, Jonsson K et al.: Complications after percutaneous transluminal angioplasty in the iliac, femoral, and popliteal arteries, *J Vasc Surg* 5:681, 1987.
110. Tegtmeyer CJ: Percutaneous transluminal angioplasty, *Curr Probl Diagn Radiol* 16:75–139, 1987.
111. Fruhwirth J, Pascher O, Hauser H et al.: Locale Gefasskomplikationen nach iatrogener femoralarterienpunktion, *Wien Klin Wochenschr* 108:196–200, 1996.
112. Feld R, Patton GM, Carabasi A et al.: Treatment of iatrogenic femoral artery injuries with ultrasound-guided compression, *J Vasc Surg* 16:832–840, 1992.
113. Chong WK, Cross FW, Rapheal MJ: Case report: iliac artery rupture during percutaneous angioplasty, *Clin Radiol* 41:358–359, 1990.
114. Cope C, Burke DR, Meranze S: *Atlas of interventional radiology*, Philadelphia, 1990, Lippincott.

Endovascular Intervention for Lower Extremity Deep Venous Thrombosis

15

Erin H. Murphy, Thomas J. Fogarty, and Frank R. Arko

DVT is the third most common cardiovascular disease in the United States with 600,000 cases reported annually, resulting in more than 100,000 deaths [1, 2]. Clinical sequelae of DVT are significant in both the acute and chronic settings. Initial consequences include acute lower extremity symptoms, risk of pulmonary emboli, and death. Long-term consequences include recurrent DVT, lower extremity venous hypertension, claudication, pain, swelling, and ulceration which can result in significant post-thrombotic morbidity [3–7].

Traditionally, anticoagulation has been the mainstay for DVT therapy [8–12]. While effective in preventing clot propagation and pulmonary emboli (PE), clot resolution is slow, relying on the intrinsic fibrinolytic system [13, 14]. The prolonged venous obstruction prior to complete clot resolution may lead to permanent valvular damage, believed to be responsible for post-thrombotic symptoms and long-term morbidity after DVT treatment [13–16].

Multiple studies have now confirmed that early clot removal can preserve valve function and prevent much of the long-term morbidity associated with DVT. While multiple approaches have been proposed, focus has shifted toward endovascular interventions for DVT. Thus far, results are encouraging and far exceed those obtained with anticoagulation alone when used in the appropriate patient population.

This chapter focuses on the proper management of DVT which requires prompt diagnosis, identification of patients who may benefit from more aggressive endovascular thrombus removal strategies, and early implementation of appropriate treatment.

E.H. Murphy (✉)
Postdoctoral Fellow, Department of Vascular Surgery, Stanford University Medical Center, Dallas, TX, USA

Diagnosis

Clinical Manifestations

Clinical consequences of DVT differ in the acute and chronic settings. Acutely, patients present with symptoms of impaired venous return including unilateral lower extremity pain, erythema, and swelling. Physical examination may reveal tenderness, warmth, and increased calf circumference of the affected limb when compared to the contralateral extremity. Patients may have palpable cords or evidence of superficial venous dilation which could represent underlying obstruction in the venous system [3–7].

Alternatively, patients with lower extremity DVT may present with symptomatic pulmonary emboli manifested as dyspnea, cough, pleuritic chest pain, shock, and even sudden death. Clinical signs include tachycardia, tachypnea, hypoxia, hypotension, and cardiac arrest secondary to cardiac arrhythmia, most commonly pulseless electrical activity. Despite a common origin from DVT of the lower extremities, less than one-third of patients presenting with PE will have any clinical evidence of DVT at the time of presentation [4–8].

In the chronic setting, patients with DVT may progress to develop symptoms of post-thrombotic syndrome. This syndrome may present months to years after initial diagnosis with lower extremity venous hypertension, venous claudication, swelling, pain, discoloration, and ulceration [13–16].

T.J. Fogarty, R.A. White (eds.), *Peripheral Endovascular Interventions*,
DOI 10.1007/978-1-4419-1387-6_15,

Diagnostic Imaging and Hypercoagulable Evaluation

While venography remains the gold-standard DVT diagnosis, this is both invasive and impractical as a standard diagnostic tool. Alternatively, lower extremity duplex ultrasound can accurately diagnose DVT and is minimally invasive, low risk, convenient, and more cost-effective. Ultrasonographic evidence of DVT includes non-compressible or partially compressible venous segments, continuous venous flow patterns, and the absence of normally phasic flow variation. The sensitivity and specificity of duplex ultrasonography in diagnosing proximal lower extremity DVT is 95–97% [17, 18]. While the sensitivity and specificity drops to only 75% when used for the diagnosis of distal calf DVT, these patients may be screened with a repeat ultrasound in 5–7 days if clinical suspicion is high [12, 17, 18].

Workup with a hypercoagulable panel has been suggested in patients less than 50 years old, an absence of additional risk factors for DVT, a family history of thromboembolic disorders, unusual thrombus location, or recurrence of DVT. These patients should be screened for protein C or S deficiency, antithrombin deficiency, factor V Leiden, protein C resistance, prothrombin gene mutation 2021A, and antiphospholipid antibody syndrome [12]. Further, it may be prudent to screen patients less than 50 years old presenting with left lower extremity DVT for May–Thurner syndrome, a condition caused by compression of the left common iliac vein by the right common iliac artery against the fifth lumbar vertebra, which can predispose to DVT. Diagnosis of these conditions is important as these patients may require additional treatment [19].

Conventional Treatment

Anticoagulation remains the gold standard for treatment of lower extremity DVT. This therapy is well suited for patients with isolated calf DVT who are at low risk of short- and long-term complications. Anticoagulation prevents clot propagation, pulmonary embolism, and DVT recurrence thereby reducing post-thrombotic morbidity and mortality. When contraindications to anticoagulation exist, patients with isolated calf DVT may also be managed with serial duplex ultrasounds. Patients who continue to have DVT isolated to the calf at 1-week will have less than a 1% risk of embolization, a 2% chance of recurrence, and a low incidence of post-thrombotic syndrome [7–9].

However, while anticoagulation also continues to be the most common treatment for patients for proximal DVT, this may be inadequate in a large number of patients. Clot resolution during anticoagulation therapy relies on the endogenous fibrinolytic pathways. This process is slow, particularly in patients with proximal DVT. When patients with proximal DVT underwent repeat venography 6 months after initiation of anticoagulation, complete clot lysis was seen in only 21%, incomplete lysis >50% in 41%, incomplete lysis <50% in 28%, and extension of DVT in 7% of patients [13]. Additionally, up to 50% of patients with proximal DVT treated with anticoagulation alone still have incompressible veins on follow-up duplex ultrasound completed 1-year after initiation of treatment [14].

Prolonged time from initial DVT development to venous recanalization may result in permanent valvular damage. As a direct consequence, patients may develop symptoms of post-thrombotic syndrome. Akesson demonstrated that during a 5-year follow-up of patients with iliofemoral DVT treated with anticoagulation alone, 95% developed venous hypertension, 90% had venous reflux, 15% had venous claudication, and another 15% developed venous ulceration [15]. Delis and colleagues confirmed these findings demonstrating 50% incidence of venous claudication and 15% with limited ambulation during a 5-year follow-up of patients with iliofemoral DVT treated with anticoagulation. This study further noted a poor quality of life reported by these patients following treatment [16].

Early Thrombus Removal: Initial Strategies

Early clot removal strategies have been proposed for patients with proximal DVT to prevent valvular damage and symptoms of post-thrombotic syndrome. The first attempts at thrombus removal were reported by Fogarty and colleagues in 1966 by means of surgical embolectomy [20]. This technique involved operative exposure of the femoral vein and balloon embolectomy of the proximal and distal veins. Improved venographic and clinical outcomes after surgical thrombectomy for proximal DVT have been reported compared to patients receiving anticoagulation alone. Plate and colleagues demonstrated normal venograms in 76, 78, and 84% of patients post-thrombectomy at 6 months, 5-years, and 10 years, compared to only 35, 50, and 41% of patients who received anticoagulation alone at the same time intervals [21–23]. Further, a reduced incidence of post-thrombotic symptoms was observed in the surgical thrombectomy cohort.

The administration of systemic intravenous thrombolytic drugs demonstrated similar promising results without the need for operative exposure. When thrombus removal with lytic therapy was successful, valvular function was preserved and a reduced incidence of post-thrombotic syndrome was observed [24].

While the results of surgical thrombectomy and systemic thrombolytic therapy illustrated the benefits of early thrombus removal in patients with proximal DVT, these therapies have not been widely utilized. Surgical thrombectomy is invasive requiring operative exposure and risks damage to the venous endothelium and valves during embolectomy. The administration of systemic thrombolytics is associated with an unacceptably high rate of bleeding complications including retroperitoneal hemorrhage and intracranial hemorrhage. Further, complete clot resolution is not always achievable with either intervention. In fact, complete clot resolution after systemic thrombolytic administration was only achievable in 50% of patients with non-occlusive thrombi and 10% of patients with occlusive thrombus [24].

Nonetheless, these initial strategies have paved the route for the development of safer, more effective endovascular treatment strategies for thrombus removal in patients with proximal DVT.

Endovascular Management of DVT

Endovascular intervention for DVT should be considered in all patients with proximal lower extremity DVT and a reasonable life expectancy. While multiple techniques and devices are available for endovascular DVT intervention, the majority of available treatment options may be separated by mechanism of action and include catheter-directed thrombolysis, ultrasound accelerated thrombolysis, and percutaneous mechanical thrombectomy.

Percutaneous access for endovascular interventions is most often achieved in the vein distal to the occluded segment. For isolated iliac DVT, an ipsilateral common femoral puncture is most appropriate. Alternatively, a retrograde approach from the contralateral femoral vein may be used for isolated iliac and femoral vein DVT. More commonly, however, patients present with more extensive iliofemoral or iliofemoral popliteal thrombosis, in which case access is best obtained from the ipsilateral popliteal vein while the patient is positioned prone. Figure 15.1 demonstrates a pre- and post-venogram of a DVT following single treatment of the iliofemoral segment.

Ultrasound guidance should be considered for access of the popliteal or tibial veins and for any access obtained while the patient is fully anticoagulated. Further, a micropuncture technique with a 22 gauge needle and 0.014-in. guidewire may minimize bleeding complications and vessel wall trauma. Following initial access, the thrombus is crossed with a guidewire to facilitate catheter or device positioning.

The use of retrievable inferior vena caval filters during catheter-directed thrombolysis (CDT) or percutaneous mechanical thrombectomy (PMT) may be prudent for prevention of peri-procedural pulmonary embolization as clot is disrupted [25–43]. In an animal model, IVC filters were shown to decrease the incidence of angiographically diagnosed pulmonary emboli after mechanical thrombolysis of DVT [26]. Further, Thery et al. have demonstrated that 31% of patients (41/132) undergoing thrombolysis for lower extremity DVT after placement of retrievable IVC filters had significant thrombus in the filter at the end of the procedure. More importantly, no patients in this study suffered a PE [27]. Subsequent study confirmed these results demonstrating a 40% incidence of thrombus debris in implanted filters following mechanical thrombectomy [28].

It is our standard practice, and recommendation, to use retrievable IVC filters prior to thrombolysis or mechanical thrombectomy [29]. In over 30 patients treated at our institution with IVC filters, mechanical thrombectomy and catheter-directed thrombolysis, there have been no occurrences of symptomatic pulmonary emboli, no filter-related complications and all IVC filters have been successfully removed [29]. Other authors have reported similar success with IVC filters in this setting [30].

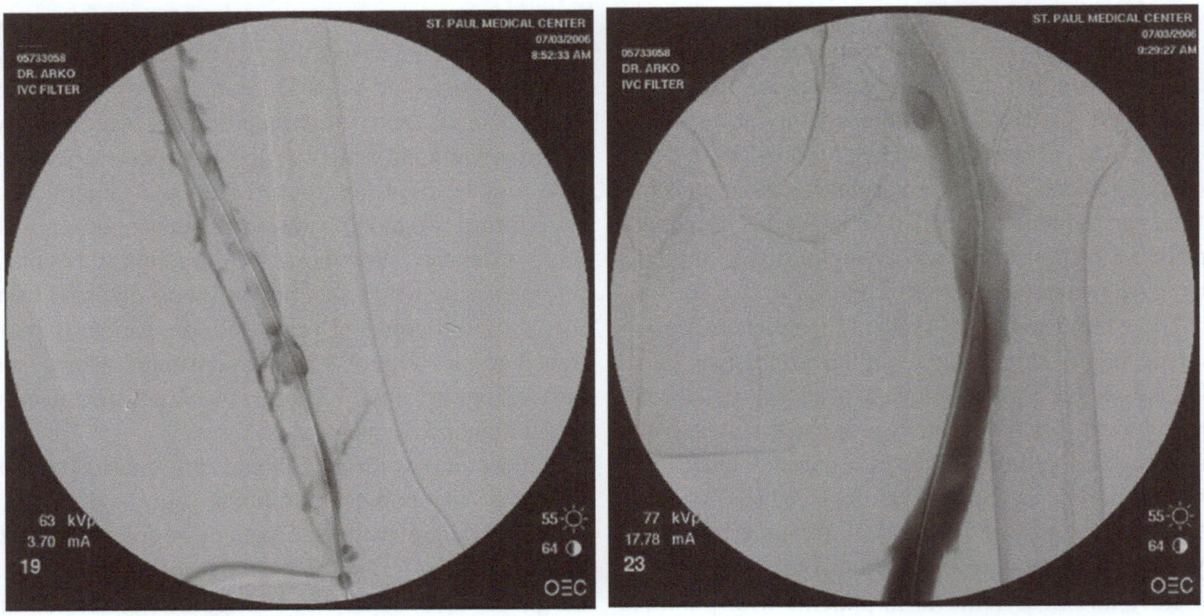

Fig. 15.1 Pre- (**a**) and Post-venogram (**b**) of patient being treated with isolated pharmcomechanical thrombolyis. All thrombus has been removed in this patient who was treated 3 days after developing his DVT

Filters placed prior to CDT or PMT should be placed in standard fashion below the renal veins. In addition, access for filter deployment should be planned such that the endovenous delivery route is free of thrombus. Often, filters may be placed from the contralateral femoral vein in a percutaneous fashion. Extension of DVT into the IVC, however, may require filter placement from the internal jugular vein to avoid thrombus disruption during placement.

Timing of filter retrieval is largely surgeon preference. It is generally accepted that filters may be removed at the end of the procedure if completion venogram reveals no substantial clot burden. However, filter thrombus or persistent post-procedural contraindications to anticoagulation mandate longer filter indwell times [19, 29, 30]. In our experience, these filters may be removed without complications at a later date.

Endovascular Treatment Options

Catheter-Directed Thrombolysis

Catheter-directed thrombolysis (CDT) allows infusion of thrombolytics directly into the venous thrombosis, limiting systemic drug exposure. Thrombolytic agents used with CDT include Urokinase (ImaRx Therapeutics, Tucson, AZ), tissue plasminogen activator (Activase, Genentech, South San Francisco, CA), recombinant tissue plasminogen activator (Retavase, PDL BioPharma, Fremont, CA), or tenecteplase (Genentech).

Most commonly, patients treated with CDT undergo percutaneous access in the operating room and initial venogram to determine extent of thrombus. A small infusion catheter is placed just proximal to the location of thrombus and secured in place externally. Patients are monitored in the in the intensive care unit and thrombolytics are slowly administered through the catheter. The patient undergoes repeat venography in the operating room to assess clot lysis once every 24 h until complete lysis is achieved.

This option has proven effective in proximal DVT resulting in early clot resolution, prevention of PE, prevention of recurrent DVT, preservation of valve function, and improved quality of life over treatment with isolated anticoagulation. Results have demonstrated 60–90% clot resolution in proximal DVT [31–34] with degree of clot removal correlating directly with improvements in long-term patency and reduced incidence of post-thrombotic syndrome [34].

Unfortunately, this therapy is still associated with significant bleeding complications in 11–43% of patients [31–37]. Ouriel et al. demonstrated insertion site bleeding in 22–44%, transfusion requirements in 12–22%, and intracranial hemorrhage in 0.6–3% of patients undergoing CDT with Urokinase and recombinant tissue plasminogen activator, respectively [37]. Further limitations to the widespread use of this technique include prolonged lytic infusion times of 36–72 h, prolonged ICU stay, and expensive drug costs [31–37].

Ultrasound Accelerated Thrombolysis: Ekos EndoWave

The EndoWave (EKOS Corp., Bothell, WA) uses low-power, high-frequency ultrasound (2 MHz) in combination with catheter-directed thrombolysis to achieve clot disruption (Fig. 15.2). Ultrasound waves generated by the unit do not directly macerate the clot but rather create microstreams which increase thrombus permeability via alteration of fibrin composition. Increased permeability results in augmented lytic dispersion within the thrombus [38–40]. In fact, a 65% increase in the number of fibrin strands exposed to thrombolytic drugs has been demonstrated to occur with a 44% ultrasound-mediated reduction in the diameter of fibrin strands [39]. This translates to increased

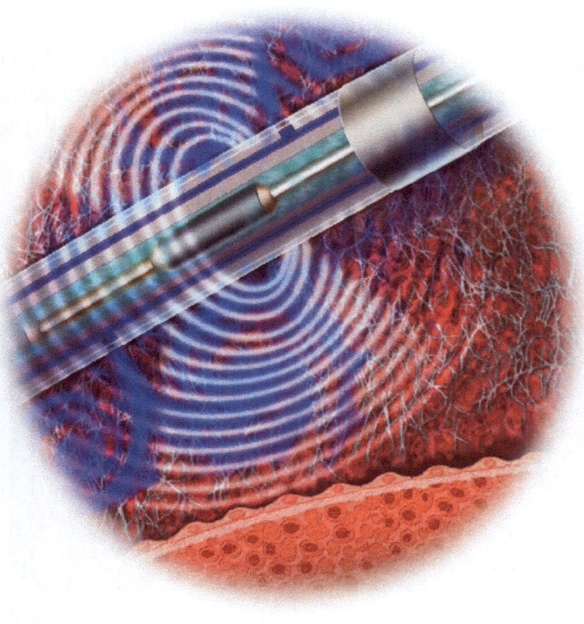

Fig. 15.2 Example and principle of the EKOS ultrasound facilitated thrombolysis (Courtesy of EKOS Corp., Bothell, WA.)

thrombus uptake of recombinant tissue plasminogen activator by 48, 84, and 89% at 1, 2, and 4 h, respectively [40]. Further, the ultrasound waves penetrate past valves, allowing for thrombus removal behind the valves which may be inaccessible with other PMT devices.

The device consists of an infusion/aspiration catheter, an ultrasound core wire, and a drive unit. The catheter, available in treatment lengths of 6–50 cm, contains a central lumen which accommodates the 0.035 ultrasound core wire and normal saline infusate used for central cooling. In a triangular distribution around the central lumen are three separate infusion channels containing microinfusion pores for drug delivery and thermocouples to monitor changes in temperature and flow patterns. The ultrasound core wire has transducers (2.2 MHz) located at 1 cm intervals. When the drive unit is activated, ultrasound waves are delivered to the core wire and transmitted through the catheter, penetrating thrombus and allowing lytic dispersion.

Access is obtained with a 6Fr introducer sheath and the lesion is crossed with a 0.35-in. guidewire. The catheter is positioned such that the treatment zone extends through the length of the thrombosed venous segment. After positioning, the guidewire is exchanged for the ultrasound core wire. The three separate drug infusion lumens are primed with unfractionated heparin. The control unit is activated and delivers ultrasound energy via the core wire, while the thrombolytic agent of choice is administered through micropores located throughout the length of the treatment zone on each of the three catheters. Normal saline is infused through the central lumen continuously during the procedure to dissipate heat production. The drive unit automatically adjusts power according to changing vessel conditions, reducing power as flow is restored. The procedure is continued until complete lysis is achieved.

Early evaluation of the EndoWave system in 53 patients, including 32 patients with lower extremity DVT, demonstrated greater than 90% clot lysis in 70% of patients and at least partial thrombus resolution in 91%. Importantly, at least partial lysis was achieved in 96% of acute DVT (<14 days), 100% of subacute DVT (15–28 days), and 77.8% of chronic (>28 days) and acute DVT. Median lytic infusion time was 22 h and bleeding complications were low (3.8%). Further, median infusion times and median total drug dosages administered were lower with ultrasound mediated thrombolysis compared to standard CDT when using UK, tPA, or rtPA. The median dosages and infusion times were similar for CDT and US-mediated thrombolysis when tenecteplase was used [41]. The Ekos EndoWave system is used and functions in the same manner as the EndoWave system; however, the company is promoting faster clot lysis with this newer device.

Percutaneous Mechanical Thrombectomy

Percutaneous mechanical thrombectomy offers the benefit of early thrombus removal while limiting thrombolytic dosages and bleeding complications. PMT additionally offers a treatment option for patients with absolute contraindications for lytic therapy as the AngioJet, a PMT device discussed below, is the only device that can be used without the addition of lytics. PMT has further been shown to be more cost-effective than alternative treatment regimens when considering the lower thrombolytic dosages administered and decreased length of ICU stay compared to CDT [42] and the decreased long-term morbidity from post-thrombotic syndrome compared to traditional anticoagulation.

AngioJet Rheolytic Thrombectomy System—Pulse-Power Spray Technique

The AngioJet catheter system (Possis Medical, Inc., Minneapolis, MN) is comprised of a single-use catheter, a single-use pump set, and a drive unit. The catheter, which is available in working lengths of 60, 100, and 120 cm, contains a central lumen for infusate and a larger lumen encompassing the central channel, the guidewire, and aspirate from the thrombus. The drive unit generates 10,000 psi of pulsatile infusion flow which is released from the catheter in retrograde-directed high-velocity saline jets. These jets create a localized low-pressure zone (Bernoulli's principle) at the catheter tip macerating thrombus and redirecting flow and debris into outflow channels directed behind the catheter tip for aspiration and removal.

Access for the AngioJet system requires a 6F introducer sheath. The AngioJet catheter is then advanced over a 0.035-in. guidewire through the thrombus load (Fig. 15.3). While this system was originally intended for use without adjunctive thrombolytics, it has been demonstrated that the addition of lytics to the infusion solution results in decreased treatment time and improved results. We recommend that thrombolytics be routinely used except when contraindicated, as is our practice. While thrombolytic choice and dose will vary dependent on surgeon preference we have experienced good results using 10 mg of tenecteplase in 50 ml of sodium chloride infusing solution [29].

With the aspiration port clamped, infusate is released into the thrombosed venous segment during a slow pullback of the catheter, effectively lacing the clot with thrombolytic drug. After 10 min the aspiration function of the catheter is turned on. The catheter is then advanced through the thrombosed segment a second time removing macerated thrombus through the

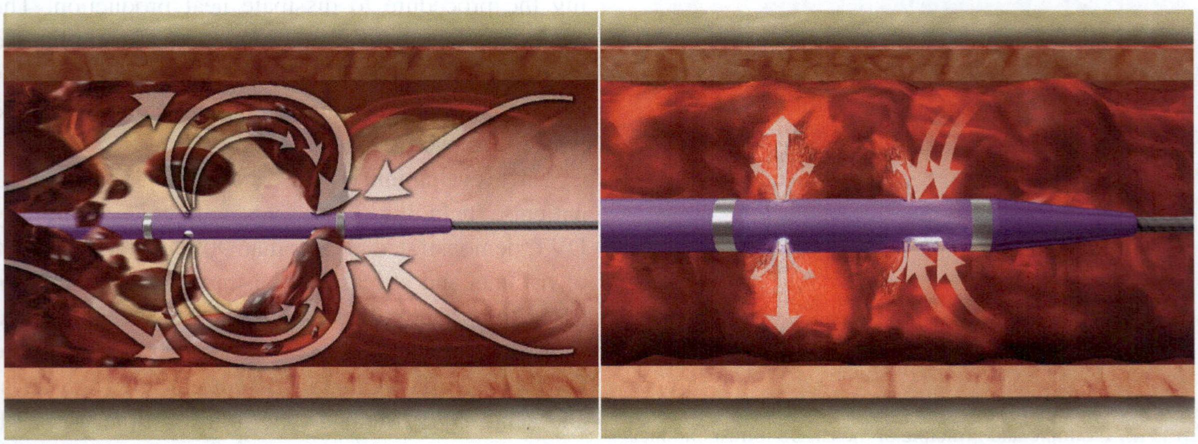

Fig. 15.3 (**a** and **b**) Example and principle of AngioJet Power-Pulse spray for DVT (Courtesy of Possis Medical, Inc., Minneapolis, MN.)

aspiration ports as the catheter is advanced. This process may be repeated if there is remaining thrombus burden at the end of the first-pass. Alternatively, as is often our preference, the patient may then undergo catheter-directed thrombolysis in the intensive care unit (ICU) overnight and return to the operative room the following day for re-evaluation with venography and possible repeat thrombectomy or venous stenting if indicated.

Success in thrombus removal, restoration of venous patency, and preservation of valvular function have been demonstrated with the use of the AngioJet pulse-power spray technique. While Kasirajan reported only 24% of patients had >90% clot resolution, 35% had 50–90% resolution, and 41% had less than 50% resolution [43], improved results have been demonstrated with the addition of lytics to the infusate as discussed above. Bush et al. reported complete thrombus resolution in 65% of patients with at least partial resolution seen in all of the remaining patients [30]. Lin et al. demonstrated that PMT with the AngioJet system was at least as effective as CDT in treating lower extremity DVT. They showed complete clot lysis in 75% of patients treated with AngioJet versus 70% in patients treated with CDT (p = NS) with similar patency at 1-year follow-up of 64 and 68%, respectively. Additionally, they demonstrated a reduced ICU stay, hospital length of stay, and reduced costs in the PMT cohort [42]. In our series we demonstrated a 90% venous patency restoration and maintenance of venous valvular function in 88% at a mean follow-up of 6 months [29].

This therapy is associated with a low incidence of hemorrhagic complications. Isolated case reports of pancreatitis resulting from massive hemolysis with use of the AngioJet system have been reported but appear to be rare occurrences [44].

Trellis-8 Infusion System—Pharmacomechanical Thrombectomy

The Trellis-8 infusion system (Bacchus Vascular, Inc., Santa Clara, CA) incorporates the use of both chemical thrombolysis and mechanical thrombectomy (Fig. 15.4). The Trellis device consists of a single-use catheter, a dispersion wire, and an integral drive unit. The catheter contains proximal and distal occlusion balloons which allow infusion of thrombolytics

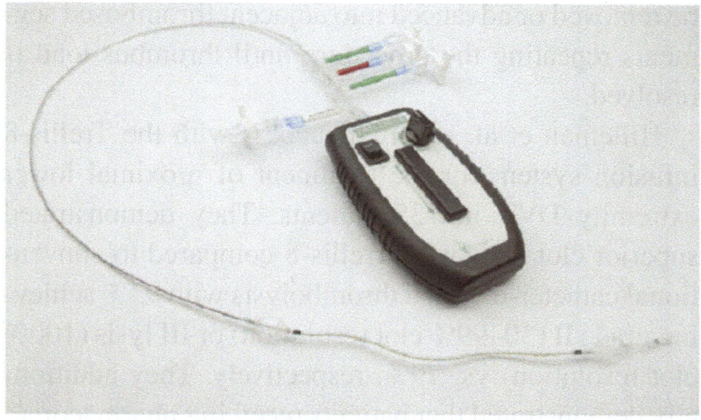

Fig. 15.4 Example of Trellis-8 infusion catheter for DVT. Thrombolytics are isolated between the two balloons and thrombus macerated with the dispersion wire connected to the motor unit (Courtesy of Bacchus Vascular, Inc., Santa Clara, CA.)

to an isolated segment of thrombosed vein. Catheters are available in lengths of 80 or 120 cm with varied distances between occlusion balloons allowing treatment of 10, 15, or 30 cm venous segments. Selection of which catheter to use will depend on the location and length of the thrombosed segment determined on initial venogram, with the goal of minimizing treatment length of non-thrombosed vein. The drive unit is attached to the sinusoidal dispersion wire which creates catheter oscillatation at 500–3,500 rpm causing dispersion of lytics within the thrombus load and mechanical clot disruption. Aspiration of thrombus debris and lytic remaining in the isolated segment completes treatment of the isolated venous segment.

Access for the Trellis-8 infusion system requires 8F introducer sheath. A 0.35 glidewire is used to cross the thrombosed venous segment and the Trellis-8 catheter is advanced over the glidewire. With proximal and distal balloons inflated, 5–10 mg of lytics is infused within the thrombus. After 10 min, the dispersion wire is inserted into the catheter. Catheter vibration between the occlusion balloons aids in clot maceration and increases the thrombus surface area exposed to the lytics. The dispersion wire may further be advanced and retracted once a minute during the treatment interval to further assure mixing of the lytics with the thrombus. After 5–15 min, the distal balloon is deflated and the catheter aspirated via a side-port to remove macerated thrombus and a substantial portion of the remaining lytics. The proximal balloon is left inflated during aspiration to prevent embolization of clot. After aspiration, with both balloons deflated, the system may be removed or advanced into adjacent thrombosed segments repeating the procedure until thrombus load is resolved.

Hilleman et al. reported success with the Trellis-8 infusion system for the treatment of proximal lower extremity DVT in 135 patients. They demonstrated superior clot lysis with Trellis-8 compared to conventional catheter-directed thrombolysis with 93% achieving grade II (50–99% clot resolution) or III lysis (100% clot resolution) vs. 79%, respectively. They additionally demonstrated that patients receiving pharmacomechanical lysis required lower lytic dose, was more cost-effective and associated with significantly lower rates of hemorrhage (0% vs. 8.5%, $p < 0.001$) [45]. Arko et al., further demonstrated 80% of patients experienced complete clot resolution with this technique in a single setting with venous patency maintained in 88% of patients treated with this device at a mean follow-up of 6-months [29]. O'Sullivan demonstrated grade II or III lysis in 96% of patients in a single setting with 100% assisted primary patency at 30 days [46].

Adjunctive Endovascular Procedures

Use of Multiple PMT Devices or Adjunctive CDT

Recalcitrant thrombus after initial treatment with PMT may require further therapy. While small residual thrombus may respond to venous angioplasty and stenting discussed in the text to follow, larger amounts of residual thrombus may require use of a second PMT device or overnight catheter-directed thrombolysis [19, 29, 30, 38]. Use of an adjunctive device or CDT should not be regarded as a failure of the first device but rather as complementary procedures [38]. The initial device achieves significant clot burden reduction paving an easier path for the second intervention. Use of a second PMT device can be performed in the same setting, often with lower doses of thrombolytics [19, 29]. Alternatively, overnight CDT therapy may be sufficient to eliminate residual thrombus after debulking of clot with PMT [19, 29, 30]. This significantly reduces the time required for effective CDT and thereby reduces the associated bleeding risks with this treatment modality [19, 29, 30]. Patients should then undergo a second evaluation with intravascular ultrasound and/or completion venography to evaluate vessel conditions.

Adjunctive Venoplasty and Stenting

Post-treatment evaluation of the venous segment may reveal areas of venous compression, stenosis, or recalcitrant thrombus in greater than 90% of patients [19, 29, 30]. May–Thurner anatomy is the most common anatomic variant found on completion of imaging during the treatment of proximal DVT (Fig. 15.5). This syndrome is characterized by compression of the left common iliac vein by the right common iliac artery against the fifth lumbar vertebrae resulting in venous compression, development of venous scar tissue, and eventually venous stenosis. This condition then predisposes to left iliofemoral DVT [47, 48]. With anticoagulation alone, untreated iliac vein obstruction prevents vessel recanalization in 70–80% of patients and clot propagation may continue in up to 40% [49, 50]. Further, patients with iliofemoral DVT and untreated May–Thurner anatomy experience increased risk of recurrent DVT and universally experience symptoms of post-thrombotic syndrome during follow-up [5, 51].

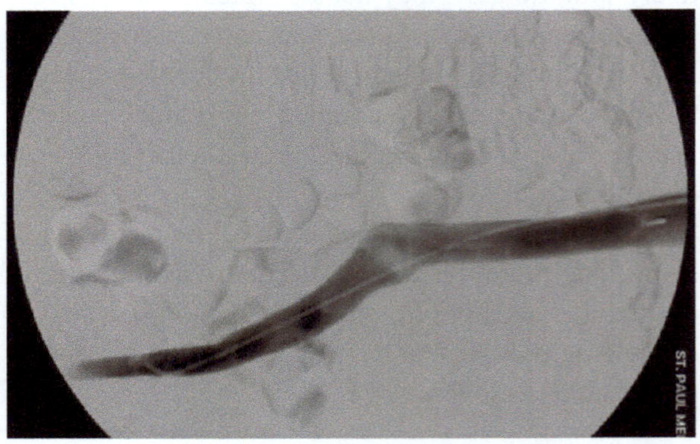

Fig. 15.5 Venogram 6 weeks following EKOS and AngioJet with stent in *left* common iliac vein. Vein is widely patent without thrombus in filter which was removed

Adequate treatment of anatomic compression, stenosis, or persistent small thrombus after CDT or PMT requires angioplasty and stenting [52–60]. Patel et al. demonstrated 100% symptom resolution in May–Thurner syndrome and acute DVT treated with early thrombus removal and venous stenting. They further demonstrated preservation of valvular function in all

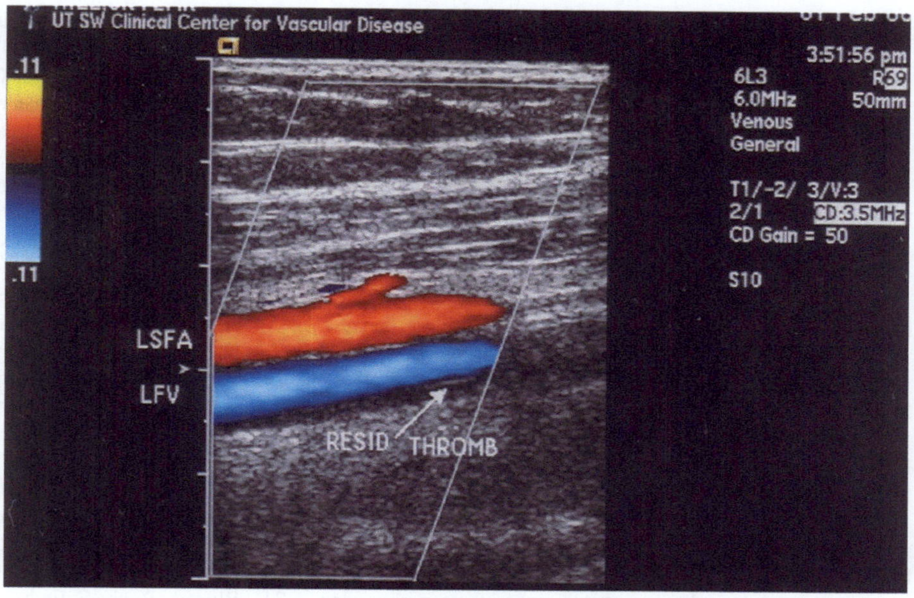

Fig. 15.6 Follow-up 6 month DUS with vein widely patent with mild amount of chronic residual thrombus with phasic flow and no evidence of venous insufficiency

patients on follow-up ultrasound [56]. Additionally, we have reported on the use of PMT and iliac vein stenting in 12 women, with May–Thurner syndrome demonstrating a 100% intraoperative clot resolution and 100% primary stent patency with follow-up up to 45 months. All patients have had complete symptom resolution and there were no occurrences of post-thrombotic syndrome [19].

Follow-Up After Endovascular DVT Management

Patients should be anticoagulated post-procedure with unfractionated heparin or low-molecular weight heparin and transitioned to oral warfarin for 6-months (goal international normalized ratio 2.0–3.0). Patients with recurrent DVT or hypercoagulable disorders may require a longer duration of anticoagulation and consultation with primary care physicians is recommended. Patients with venous stents require lifelong aspirin therapy. Follow-up with duplex ultrasound is also recommended at 1 and 6 month intervals and yearly thereafter (Fig. 15.6).

Conclusions

Endovascular options are more effective in reducing long-term morbidity after proximal DVT when compared to anticoagulation alone. These options should be considered for all patients with proximal lower extremity DVT and a reasonable life expectancy. Percutaneous mechanical thrombectomy is at least as effective as catheter-directed thrombolysis with reduced ICU and hospital stays and decreased overall costs. Further, use of a second PMT device or adjunctive CDT may allow optimal results. Venous angioplasty and stenting may be required to treat recalcitrant thrombus or anatomic causes of DVT. With widespread implementation of these advanced treatment options for DVT we can achieve a significant reduction in long-term morbidity after proximal DVT.

References

1. Wells PS, Forster AJ: Thrombolysis in deep vein thrombosis: is there still an indication? *Thromb Haemost* 86:499–508, 2001.
2. Strandness DE Jr, Langois Y, Cramer M, Randlett A, Thiele BL: Long-term sequelae of acute venous thrombosis, *JAMA* 250:1289–1292, 1983.
3. Blann AD, Lip GYH: Clinical review: venous thromboembolism, *BMJ* 332(28):215–219, 2006.
4. White RH: The epidemiology of venous thromboembolism, *Circulation* 107(suppl 1):14–18, 2003.
5. O'Donnell TFJR, Browse NL, Burnand KG, Thomas ML: The socioeconomic effects of an iliofemoral venous thrombosis, *J Surg Res* 22:483–488, 1977.
6. Kraaijenhagen RA, Lensing AW, Wallace JW, van Beek EJ, ten Cate JW, Buller HR: Diagnostic management of venous thromboembolism, *Baillieres Clin Haematol* 11:541–586, 1998.

7. Kearon C: Natural history of venous thromboembolism, *Circulation* 107:I22–I30, 2003.
8. Buller HR, Sohne M, Middledorp S: Treatment of venous thromboembolism, *J Thromb Haemost* 3:1554–1560, 2005.
9. Fifth ACCP consensus conference on antithrombotic therapy. *Chest* 114(suppl):439S–769S, 1998.
10. Kearon C, Gent M, Hirsh J et al.: A comparison of 3 months of anticoagulation with extended anticoagulation for a first episode of idiopathic venous thromboembolism, *N Engl J Med* 341:801–806, 1999.
11. Ofri D: Best practice: evidence-based case review. Diagnosis and treatment of deep vein thrombosis, *WJM* 173:194–197, 2000.
12. Tovey C, Wyatt S: Diagnosis, investigation and management of deep vein thrombosis, *BMJ* 326:1184–1190, 2003.
13. Holmstrom M, Lindmarker P, Granqvist S, Johnson H, Lockner DA: 6-month venographic follow-up in 164 patients with acute deep vein thrombosis, *Thromb Haemost* 78:803–807, 1997.
14. Piovella F, Crippa L, Barone E: Normalization rates of compression ultrasonography in patients with a first episode of deep vein thrombosis of the lower limbs: association with recurrence and new thrombosis, *Haematologica* 87:515–522, 2002.
15. Akesson H, Brudin L, Dahlstom JA, Eklof B, Ohlin P, Plate G: Venous function assessed during a 5 year period after ilio-femoral venous thrombosis treated with anticoagulation, *Eur J Vasc Surg* 4:43–48, 1990.
16. Delis KT, Bountouroglou D, Mansfield AO: Venous claudication in iliofemoral thrombosis: long-term effects on venous hemodynamics, clinical status, and quality of life, *Ann Surg* 239:118–126, 2004.
17. Kraaijenhagen RA, Lensing AW, Wallace JW, van Beek EJ, ten Cate JW, Buller HR: Diagnostic management of venous thromboembolism, *Baillieres Clin Haematol* 11:541–586, 1998.
18. Kearon C, Ginsberg JS, Hirsh J: The role of venous ultrasonography in the diagnosis of suspected deep venous thrombosis and pulmonary embolism, *Ann Intern Med* 128:1044–1049, 1998.
19. Murphy EH, Davis CM, Journeycake JM, Demuth RP, Arko FR: Symptomatic ileofemoral DVT after onset of oral contraceptive use in women with previously undiagnosed May-Thurner syndrome, *J Vasc Surg*, 30:460–65, 2009.
20. Fogarty TJ, Dennis D, Krippaehne WW: Surgical management of iliofemoral venous thrombosis, *Am J Surg* 112:211–217, 1966.
21. Plate G, Einarsson E, Ohlin P et al.: Thrombectomy with temporary arteriovenous fistula: the treatment of choice in acute iliofemoral venous thrombosis, *J Vasc Surg* 1:867–876, 1984.
22. Plate G, Akesson H, Einarsson E et al.: Long-term results of venous thrombectomy combined with a temporary arterio-venous fistula, *Eur J Vasc Sur* 4:483–489, 1990.
23. Plate G, Eklof B, Norgren L et al.: Venous thrombectomy for iliofemoral vein thrombosis—10-year results of a prospective randomized study, *Eur J Vasc Endovasc Surg* 14:367–374, 1997.
24. Comerota AJ, Aldridge SA: Thrombolytic therapy for acute deep vein thrombosis, *Semin Vasc Surg* 5(2):76–84, 1992.
25. Kinney TB: Update on inferior vena cava filters, *J Vasc Interv Radiol* 14:425–440, 2003.
26. Trerotola SO, McLennan G, Eclavea AC, Salis A, Davidson D, Dreesen RG, Tennery J: Mechanical thrombolysis of venous thrombosis in an animal model with use of temporary caval filtration, *JVIR* 12:1075–1085, 2001.
27. Thery C, Bauchart J, Lesenne M, Asseman P, Flajollet JG, Legghe R, Marache P: Predictive factors of effectiveness of streptokinase in deep venous thrombosis, *Am J Cardiol* 69:117–122, 1992.
28. Lam R, Bush RL, Lin PH, Lumsden AB: Early technical and clinical results with retrievable inferior vena caval filters, *Vasc Endovasc Surg* 38:658–665, 2005.
29. Arko Fr, Davis CM, Murphy EH et al.: Aggressive percutaneous mechanical thrombosis: early clinical results, *Arch Surg* 142:513–518, 2007.
30. Bush RL, Lin PH, Bates JT, Mureebe L, Zhou W, Lumsden AB: Pharmacomechanical thrombectomy for treatment of symptomatic lower extremity deep venous thrombosis: safety and feasibility study, *J Vasc Surg* 40:965–970, 2004.
31. Blum A, Roche E: Endovascular management of acute deep vein thrombosis, *Am J Med* 118(suppl):31S–36S, 2005.
32. Comerota AJ, Throm RC, Mathias SD, Haughton S, Meiwissen M: Catheter-directed thrombolysis for iliofemoral deep venous thrombosis improves health-related quality of life, *J Vasc Surg* 32:130–137, 2000.
33. Semba CP, Razavi MK, Kee ST, Sze DY, Dake MD: Thrombolysis for lower extremity deep venous thrombosis, *Tech Vasc Interv Radiol* 7:68–78, 2004.
34. Mewissen MW, Seabrook GR, Meissner MH, Cynamon J, Labropoulos N, Haughton SH: Catheter-directed thrombolysis for lower extremity deep venous thrombosis: report of a national multicenter registry, *Radiology* 211:39–49, 1999.
35. Lieberman S, Safadi R, Aner H, Verstandig A, Sasson T, Bloom AI: Local thrombolysis for the treatment of patients with proximal deep vein thrombosis of the leg, *Harefuah* 141:424–429, 2002.
36. AbuRahma AF, Pekins SE, Wulu JT, Ng HK: Iliofemoral deep vein thrombosis: conventional therapy versus lysis and percutaneous transluminal angioplasty and stenting, *Ann Surg* 233:752–760, 2001.
37. Ouiel K, Grey B, Clair DG, Olin J: Complications associated with the use of urokinase and recombinant tissue plasminogen activator for catheter directed peripheral aterial and venous thrombolysis, *J Vasc Interven Radiol* 11:295–298, 2000.
38. McLafferty RB: Endovascular management of deep venous thrombosis, *Perspect Vasc Surg Endovasc Ther* 20:87–91, 2008.
39. Braaten JV, Goss RA, Francis CW: Ultrasound reversibly disaggregates fibrin fibers, *Thromb Haemost* 78:1063–1068, 1997.
40. Francis CW, Blinc A, Lee S, Cox C: Ultrasound accelerates transport of recombinant tissue plasminogen activator into clots, *Ultrasound Med Biol* 21:419–424, 1995.
41. Parikh S, Motarjeme A, McNamara T, Raabe R, Hagspiel K, Benenati JF, Sterling K, Comerota A: Ultrasound-accelerated thrombolysis for the treatment of deep vein thrombosis: initial clinical experience, *J Vasc Interv Radiol* 19:521–528, 2008.

42. Lin PH, Zhou W, Dardick A, Mussa F, Kougias P, Hedayati N, Naoum JJ, Sayed HE, Peden EK, Huynh TT: Catheter-direct thrombolysis versus pharmacomechanical thrombectomy for treatment of symptomatic lower extremity deep venous thrombosis, *Am J Surg* 192:782–788, 2006.
43. Kasirajan K, Grey B, Ouriel K: Percutaneous AngioJet thrombectomy in the management of extensive deep venous thrombosis, *JVIR* 12(2):179–185, 2001.
44. Piercy KT, Ayerdi J, Geary RL, Hansen KJ, Edwards MS: Acute pancreatitis: a complication associated with rheolytic mechanical thrombectomy of deep venous thrombosis, *J Vasc Surg* 44(5):1110–1113, 2006.
45. Hillman DE, Pharm D, Razavi MK: Clinical and economic evaluation of the Trellis-8 infusion catheter for deep vein thrombosis, *J Vasc Interv Radiol* 19:377–383, 2008.
46. O'Sullivan GJ, Lohan DG, Gough N, Cronin CG, Kee ST: Pharmacomechanical thrombectomy of acute deep vein thrombosis with the Trellis-8 isolated thrombolysis catheter, *J Vasc Interv Radiol* 18(6):715–724, 2007.
47. May R, Thurner J: The cause of predominately sinistral occurrence of thrombosis of the pelvic veins, *Angiology* 8:419–427, 1957.
48. Kim D, Orron DE, Porter DH: *Venographic anatomy, technique and interpretation. Peripheral Vascular Imaging and Intervention*, St. Louis, MO, 1992, Mosby-Year Book, pp. 269–349.
49. Krupski WC, Bass A,, Dilley RB,, Bernstein EF,, Otis SM: Propagation of deep venous thrombosis identified by duplex ultrasonography, *J Vasc Surg* 12:467–475, 1990.
50. Cockett FB, Thomas ML, Negus D: Iliac vein compression. Its relation to iliofemoral thrombosis and the post-thrombotic syndrome, *Br Med J* 2:14–19, 1967.
51. Calnan J, Kountz S, Pentecost B, Shillingford JP, Steiner RE: Venous obstruction in the aetiology of lymphoedema praecox, *Br Med J* 2:221–226, 1964.
52. O'Sullivan GJ, Semba CP, Bittner CA, Kee ST, Razavi MK, Sze DY et al.: Endovascular management of iliac vein compression (May Thurner) syndrome, *J Vasc Interv Radiol* 11:823–836, 2000.
53. Kwak HS, Han YM, Lee YS, Jin GY, Chung GH: Stents in common iliac vein obstruction with acute ipsilateral deep venous thrombosis: early and late results, *J Vasc Interv Radiol* 16:815–822, 2005.
54. AbuRahma AF, Perkins SE, Wulu JT, Ng HK: Iliofemoral deep vein thrombosis: conventional therapy versus lysis and percutaneous transluminal angioplasty and stenting, *Ann Surg* 233:752–760, 2001.
55. Nazarian GK, Bjarnarson H, Dietz CA, Bernadas CA, Hunter DW: Iliofemoral venous stenosis: effectiveness of treatment with metallic endovascular stents, *Radiology* 200:193–199, 1996.
56. Patel NH, Stookey KR, Ketcham DB, Cragg AH: Endovascular management of acute extensive iliofemoral deep venous thrombosis caused by May-Thurner syndrome, *JVIR* 11:1297–1302, 2000.
57. Hollis K, Olivier J, Raju S: Stenting of the venous outflow in chronic venous disease: long-term stent-related outcome, clinical, and hemodynamic result, *J Vasc Surg* 46(5):979–990, 2007.
58. Hartung O, Benmiloud F, Barthelemy P, Dubuc M, Boufi M, Alimi YS: Late results of surgical venous thrombectomy with iliocaval stenting, *J Vasc Surg* 47(2):381–387, 2008.
59. Schwarzbach MH, Schumacher H, Bockler D, Furstenberger S, Thomas F, Seelos R et al.: Surgical thrombectomy followed by intraoperative endovascular reconstruction for symptomatic ilio-femoral venous thrombosis, *Eur J Vasc Surg* 29(1):58–66, 2005.
60. Husmann MJ, Heller G, Kalka C, Savolainen H, Schmidli J, Baumgartner I: Stenting of common iliac vein obstructions combined with regional thrombolysis and thrombectomy in acute deep venous thrombosis, *Eur J Vasc Endovasc Surg* 34(1):87–91, 2007.

Remote Femoral and Iliac Artery Endarterectomy

16

Wouter J.M. Derksen, Jean-Paul P.M. de Vries, Gerard Pasterkamp, and Frans L. Moll

Atherosclerosis is still the leading cause of death in Western countries. Ischemic heart disease and cerebrovascular disease (stroke) are responsible for more than a fifth of all deaths worldwide [1]. Total disease prevalence is 3–10%, increasing to 20% in persons older than 70 years. The first symptom caused by atherosclerotic obstruction in the peripheral arteries is intermittent claudication, with a total prevalence of up to 10% in patients older than 60 years [2]. Atherosclerosis in the peripheral arteries develops slower compared with atherosclerosis in the coronary and carotid arteries. However, the occurrence of atherosclerotic plaques in the superficial femoral artery (SFA) is usually associated with atherosclerotic coronary arteries, and in younger patients, the presence of plaques in the SFA is associated with cardiovascular vulnerability and adverse events [3].

Only a quarter of patients with intermittent claudication will ever significantly deteriorate. Clinical stabilization or improvement is due to the development of collaterals, metabolic adaptation of ischemic muscles, or the patient alters his or her gait to favor non-ischemic muscle groups [2]. Major amputation is a relatively rare consequence of peripheral arterial disease (PAD), with an incidence of 1–3.3% in claudicant patients during a 5-year period [2].

All risk factors for atherosclerosis contribute to the progression of PAD; however, predicting the risk of deterioration to Fontaine classes III and IV remains difficult. A decreasing ankle-brachial index (ABI) over time is probably the best individual predictor. Intermittent claudication patients with an ABI <0.50 face a two-times higher risk of deterioration (i.e., need for arterial surgery or major amputation) compared with patients with an ABI >0.50 [2].

In 70% of patients with PAD, the SFA is affected. Location of the distal SFA between the tight adductor muscles, the S-shaped configuration of the artery at this level, and the high incidence of arterial branching causing unfavorable hemodynamic circumstances are possible explanations of the high incidence of SFA obstructions [4].

Primary treatment of PAD is supervised exercise treatment combined with medical and lifestyle management to decrease the risk for future cardiovascular adverse events [2]. When primary treatment is not sufficient, a wide variety of interventions are possible as a result of rapidly evolving endovascular techniques. The low morbidity and mortality of endovascular techniques makes it the preferred choice of treatment in limited disease such as stenoses or occlusions up to 10 cm in length, defined as types A and B according to TransAtlantic InterSociety Consensus (TASC) classification [2]. However, patency rates for percutaneous interventions of long-segmental occlusions (>10 cm in length) are still disappointing. For such long lesions, designated as types C and D according to the TASC classification, surgical intervention is recommended [2]. Remote endarterectomy is a combination of surgical debulking and endovascular treatment of the occluded peripheral artery without the need for bypass grafting and with at least the same patency rates as prosthetic supragenicular bypass grafts [5].

W.J.M. Derksen (✉)
Surgical Resident, Experimental Cardiology Laboratory, Department of Vascular Surgery, University Medical Center Utrecht, Utrecht, The Netherlands

T.J. Fogarty, R.A. White (eds.), *Peripheral Endovascular Interventions*,
DOI 10.1007/978-1-4419-1387-6_16, © Springer Science+Business Media, LLC 1998, 2010

Remote Endarterectomy

Remote endarterectomy can be performed for long-segment occlusions of the SFA as well as the external and common iliac arteries. The technique of remote endarterectomy has been described previously in detail [5–7]. Remote endarterectomy will be discussed in summary.

Remote Superficial Artery Endarterectomy

A single vertical groin incision is used to expose the common femoral artery (CFA), the profunda femoral artery, and the SFA, and 5,000 IU of heparin is administered systemically. The proximal SFA is clamped to leave the flow in the profunda femoral artery uninterrupted during the procedure (Fig. 16.1). A longitudinal arteriotomy is then made in the occluded proximal SFA. The right cleavage plane is defined by a meticulous dissection of the intimal core between the lamina elastica interna and the circular fibers of the media or, preferably, between the media and the smooth lamina elastica externa of the adventitia (Figs. 16.2 and 16.3).

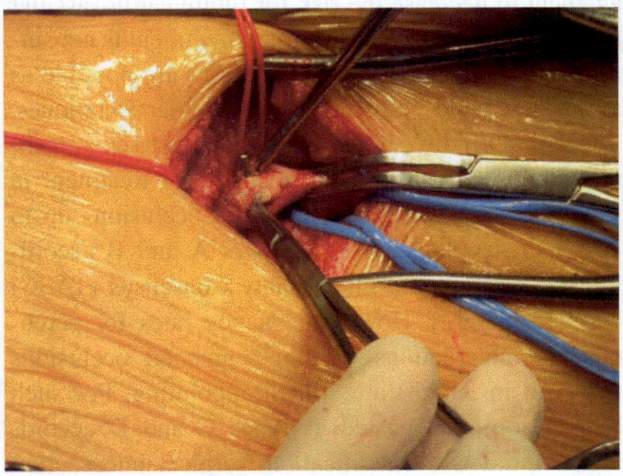

Fig. 16.1 The superficial femoral artery (SFA) is clamped and a longitudinal arteriotomy is made in the occluded proximal SFA

The intimal core is dissected using the Vollmar ring stripper (Vollmar Dissector, Aesculap, San Francisco, CA, USA) until it reaches the distal limit of the atheroma in the SFA, which is done under fluoroscopic guidance. Next the Vollmar dissector is exchanged for a Mollring cutter (Mollring Cutter, LeMaître Vascutek, San Jose, CA). The Mollring cutter is a modification of the Vollmar ring stripper. The metal shaft has a double-ring construction at the distal end. Both rings have sharpened inner edges, thereby mimicking scissors as the lower ring shears along the upper ring when a trigger is pulled (Fig. 16.4). This allows transection of the distal intimal core.

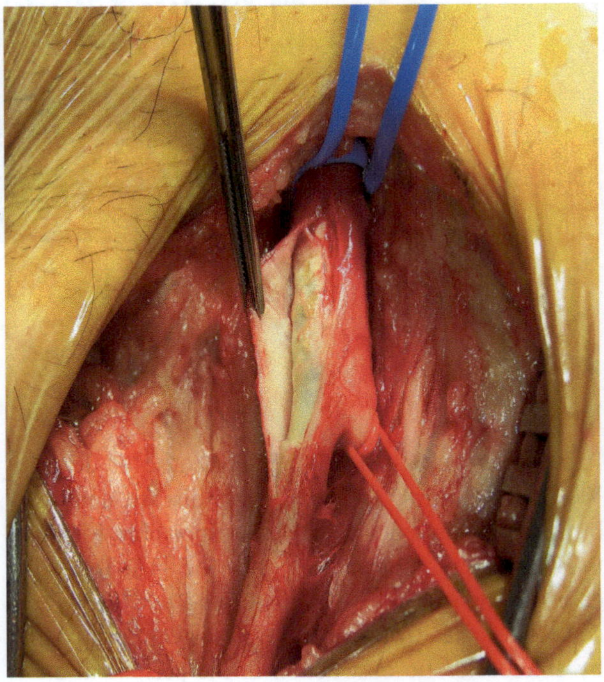

Fig. 16.2 Cleavage plane of the intimal core is made (during remote iliac artery endarterectomy)

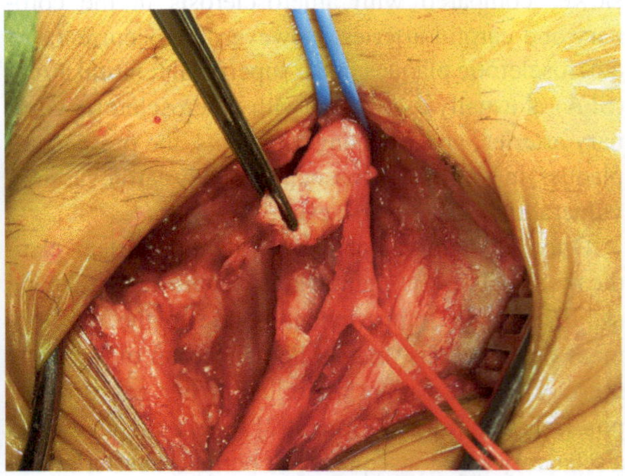

Fig. 16.3 Intimal core is cut and Vollmar device now can be used

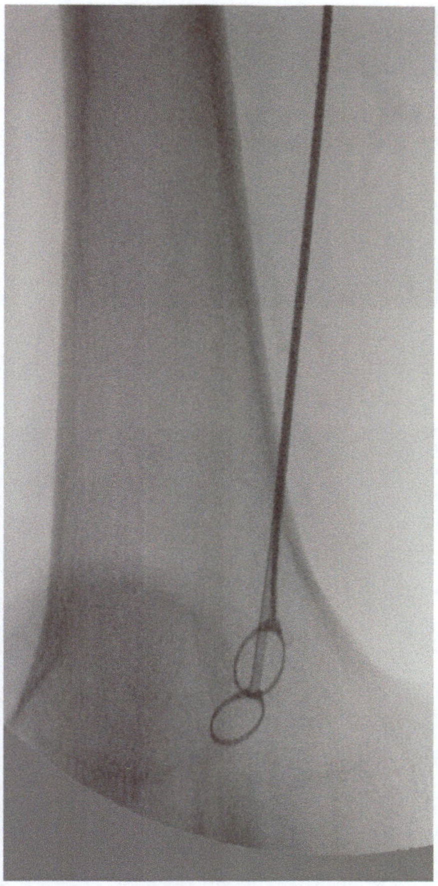

Fig. 16.4 Mollring cutter, with clearly double-ring construction, which cuts the distal intimal core

The Mollring cutter is advanced along the same cleavage plane as the Vollmar ring. After the atheroma is transected at its distal end, the intimal core and Mollring cutter are removed, all under fluoroscopic guidance (Fig. 16.5). The distal transection zone is secured by percutaneous transluminal angioplasty (PTA) with additional stent placement. A commonly used stent is the aSpire stent (aSpire stent, LeMaître Vascutek, San Jose, CA), an expandable polytetrafluoroethylene (ePTFE), covered, double-spiral nitinol stent that is flexible and yet has sufficient high radial strength to withstand torsional stresses proximal to the knee joint (Fig. 16.6). The open helical design of the aSpire stent offers the possibility of preserving the major genicular collateral vessels. It is recommended to use a small angioplasty balloon to unfold the aSpire stent and to start in the middle of the stent with unfolding (Figs. 16.7 and 16.8).

A completion arteriography must be performed after stent placement to check that no distal thromboembolic complications have occurred and to verify the patency of the desobstructed SFA; additional embolectomy must be performed when necessary. If required, a CFA and profunda artery deobstruction can be performed, and the arteriotomy may be closed with or without patch.

Remote Iliac Artery Endarterectomy

The technique is similar to the RSFAE using an arteriotomy at the origin of the CFA. However, the ring stripper is advanced proximally up to the patent common iliac artery. It is important not to pass the aortoiliac bifurcation to prevent thromboembolic load to the contralateral limb. A bony landmark can be useful for orientation. The recommendation is to cannulate the contralateral femoral artery percutaneously, to allow digital subtraction angiography of the aortoiliac arteries during the procedure, and to facilitate additional PTA eventually with additional stent placement [8].

The goal is to debulk the total external iliac artery as well as the common iliac artery. After removal of the intimal core, a PTA, with or without additional stent placement, can be executed. In contrast with RSFAE, a stent is not always necessary. In case of heavily calcified iliac arteries it can be difficult to advance the Vollmar ring beyond the origin of the internal iliac artery. In these patients debulking of the external iliac artery and the CFA may be combined with catheter-based recanalization and stenting of the common iliac artery.

Benefits of Remote Endarterectomy

Remote endarterectomy offers the surgeon a less invasive alternative to treat long-segment atherosclerotic lesions of the SFA through a single groin incision, with almost the same benefits as percutaneous interventions. The hospital length of stay is shorter and fewer wound complications, such as hematomas, edema, lymphoceles, and wound and graft infections, will occur compared with traditional bypass graft surgery. More than 50% of patients can be discharged from the hospital

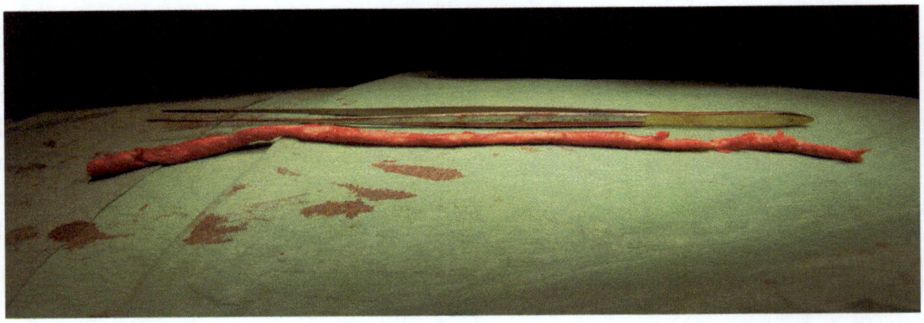

Fig. 16.5 Dissected intimal core

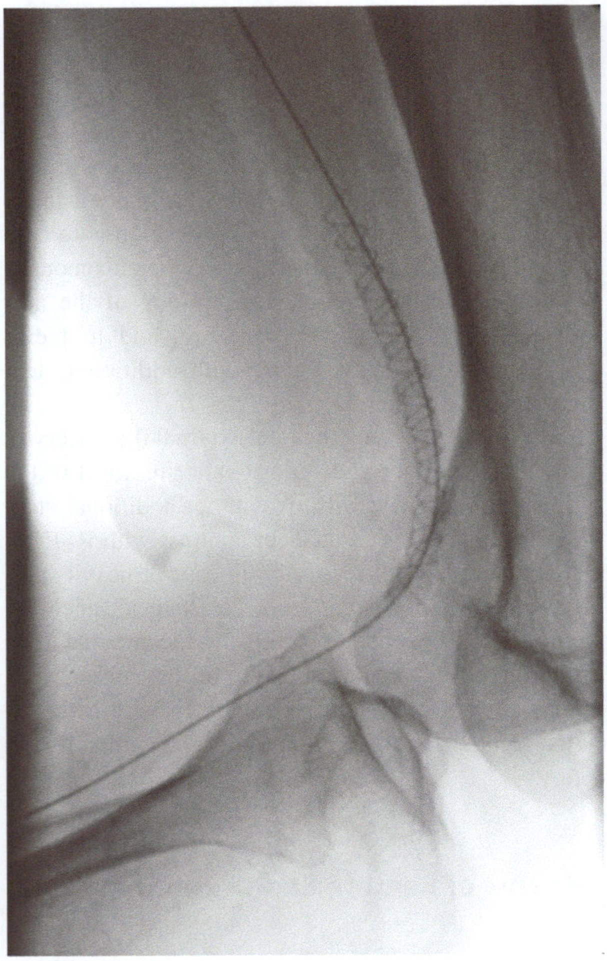

Fig. 16.6 aSpire stent that has sufficient high radial strength to withstand torsional stresses proximal to the knee joint

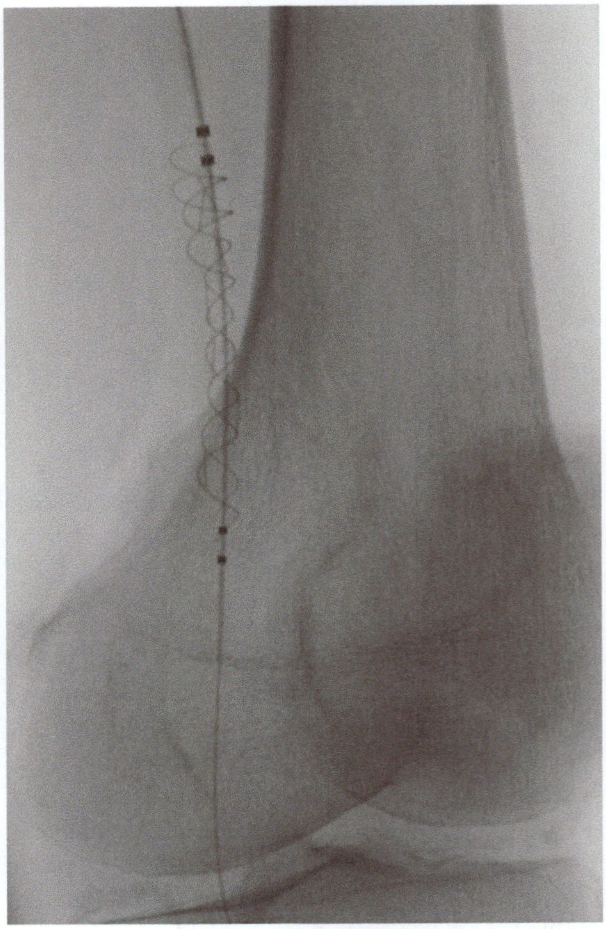

Fig. 16.7 Unfolded aSpire stent in the distal superficial femoral artery

on the second postoperative day, which will result in lower hospital costs [6].

The advantage of remote endarterectomy compared with bypass surgery is the avoidance of synthetic and venous materials, with no need for a second distal incision, resulting in fewer postoperative complications, as previously mentioned. Thereby, the ipsilateral saphenous vein, which is the preferred choice for a distal bypass graft, has been reported to be of poor quality or has been previously stripped or harvested for

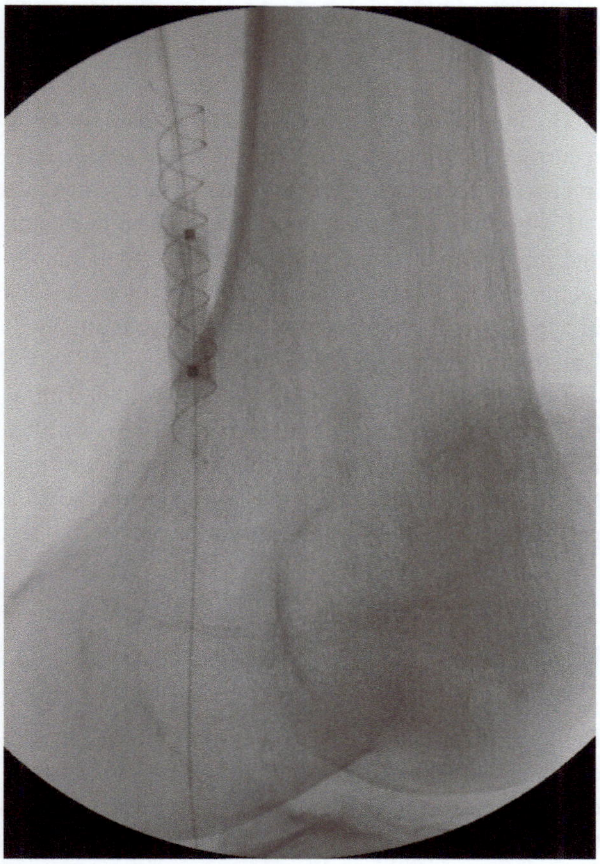

Fig. 16.8 A small angioplasty balloon unfolding the stent, starting in the middle of the stent

coronary bypass grafts in up to 40% of patients who require a distal bypass operation [9, 10].

The saphenous vein is the preferred choice for infragenicular bypass grafts, especially in patients with Rutherford classes V and VI [11]. If the great or small saphenous vein is only partially available or suitable, RSFAE in combination with distal venous bypass grafting seems to be a safe and moderately durable procedure in case of limb salvage. In such combined revascularization procedures, the proximal anastomosis of the venous graft is made at the level of the transaction zone in the distal SFA or proximal popliteal artery [9].

In addition to procedurally related complications, it is also important to determine the clinical consequences of failure of revascularization procedures, because 5–10% of failed femoropopliteal bypass grafts in claudicant patients result in amputation; this increases up to 50% in patients with critical limb ischemia [12–14]. Smeets and coworkers reported that the clinical consequences of re-occlusion after 239 initially successful RSFAEs with long-term follow-up were mild, with only two major amputations (2.5%) in a population with 27% critical limb ischemia patients [15].

The explanation for this remarkable difference compared with bypass graft surgery is the preservation of the collaterals during RSFAE. Because the aSpire stent provides for preservation of the collateral arteries, the genicular side branches are still patent if the SFA re-occludes. This is in contrast with occlusion of supragenicular bypass grafts, which often results in worsening of symptoms compared with the original complaints before surgery because of thrombosis of collaterals and runoff vessels [7, 15, 16]. The attendant benefit of RSFAE is the fact that the saphenous vein is spared for possible secondary bypass graft surgery when the SFA is re-occluded.

Another advantage of remote endarterectomy is the possibility of a relatively simple additional open endarterectomy of the CFA and profunda femoral artery. The CFA is not an optimal site for percutaneous intervention, but an advantage of both RSFAE and iliac artery endarterectomy is that this additional intervention can be performed through the same single groin incision. Fifty percent of the remote endarterectomies are extended with an additional endarterectomy of the CFA, with or without profunda plasty, and thereby improving inflow and patency rate (unpublished data).

Patency Rates

Sole endovascular treatment, both PTA and percutaneous recanalization of infrainguinal atherosclerotic disease, is an established treatment modality due to the low morbidity, low mortality, and high technical success rate [17–20]. However, patency rates for the treatment of more extensive disease (TASC C and D lesions) with percutaneous intervention remain disappointing [2]. Wolf and colleagues showed 1-year primary patency rates for extensive SFA lesions of 43% after PTA and 82% after bypass surgery [21]. Five-year primary patency and secondary patency rates of 25 and 41%, respectively, are published for PTA of long-segment lesions [22], demonstrating that surgery is the preferred treatment modality for long-segment SFA stenoses or occlusions and endovascular interventions are reserved for type A and B lesions [2, 21–24].

Multiple studies have been published that have proved the superiority of venous bypass grafts over synthetic bypass grafts for supragenicular obstructions. A review article showed 2-year primary patency rates of 81% for venous above-knee bypass grafts and 67% for synthetic above-knee bypasses, and the rates after 5 years were 69 and 49%, respectively [25]. A recent meta-analysis showed a pooled primary graft patency of 57% for supragenicular synthetic bypass grafts and 77.2% for supragenicular vein grafts. Pooled secondary patency rates were 73.2 and 80.1%, respectively. Patency rates for patients with critical limb ischemia are approximately 10% lower compared with claudicants [26]. No statistically significant differences between Dacron and PTFE for above-knee synthetic bypass grafts were determined [27].

Patency rates for RSFAE have been studied by various authors. Rosenthal and colleagues published an 18-month primary cumulative patency rate of 68.6% and primary-assisted patency rate of 88.5% [28]. Furthermore, the 3-year cumulative primary patency rate was 60.6% and the assisted primary patency rate was 70.2% [7]. Martin and coworkers published 3-year primary and assisted primary patency rates of 70 and 76%, respectively [6]. The only prospective study (non-randomized) was published by Knight and colleagues, with short-term (18 months) cumulative patency rates of 60% and assisted primary patency rates of 70% [16]. However, there is a strong need for a prospective, randomized controlled study that compares RSFAE with above-knee bypass surgery. At the end of 2005, a randomized, controlled multicenter trial was started that included more than 100 patients. Short-term results, which have not been published, showed that venous supragenicular bypass grafts are superior to remote superficial artery endarterectomy (RSFAE) and synthetic supragenicular bypass grafts. Besides, RSFAE has at least comparable patency rates with synthetic grafts and shorter hospital stay, with primary patency rates of 63% for synthetic bypass graft and 61% for RSFAE. At 1-year of follow-up, assisted primary patency rates were 63 and 73% and secondary patency rates were 63 and 79%, respectively.

The Achilles heel of RSFAE is the restenosis rate in the first year postoperatively, which is when more than 80% of all restenoses after RSFAE will occur. Restenosis of more than 50% within the first year has been associated with a higher risk for occlusion. Furthermore, the restenotic lesions are equally distributed in the endarterectomized SFA, including the distal part of the SFA with stented transaction zone [14].

Ho and colleagues discovered that revision of early recurrent stenoses (<1 year) after RSFAE significantly improved the primary patency rates. Late restenoses (>1 year) do not seem to progress to re-occlusion and may be treated conservatively. This phenomenon seems identical to graft failure. Early restenotic lesions in bypass grafts in the first postoperative year often will lead to graft failure unless treated [29].

Because of this, a program of intensive duplex ultrasound imaging is needed at 3, 6, and 12 months after RSFAE. In case of early restenotic lesions (asymptomatic lesions >70% and symptomatic lesions >50%), percutaneous re-intervention is strongly advised.

Remote Iliac Artery Endarterectomy

Remote endarterectomy of the iliac artery (RIAE) offers the advantage of a single groin incision instead of the need for an abdominal approach or retroperitoneal dissection with graft-related complications. The procedure can be performed with regional or local anesthesia and is therefore particularly useful in patients with chronic obstructive pulmonary disease or previous abdominal surgery [8].

Midterm results of RIAE (primary patency rate of 60.2% and primary-assisted patency rate of 85.7%) are comparable with semi-closed endarterectomy. Repeat endovascular interventions are usually possible in the event of restenosis [8]. According to the literature, possible initial conversion of RIAE to more extensive surgical procedures has no significant adverse clinical effect on early and 5-year clinical outcome and follow-up [30].

Preferred surgical revascularization method for unilateral iliac occlusive disease is, according to the literature, the retroperitoneal unilateral iliac artery bypass, with long-term patency rates between 90 and 100% [31–33]. However, this operation required more extensive surgery and the use of synthetic material, subsequently resulting in a higher rate of morbidity compared to RIAE.

RIAE has equal patency rates compared with conventional treatment of iliac occlusive disease and offers the advantages of a less invasive surgical procedure.

For this reason, RIAE is worth considering as a treatment option for long-segmental iliac occlusive disease. However, prospective studies that compare RIAE with open unilateral iliac artery (bypass) surgery are lacking. These studies will need to be done in the near future to validate RIAE.

Improving Treatment Outcome and Future Perspectives

Despite all of the new developments to treat long atherosclerotic lesions of the SFA, long-term patency remains disappointing. New medicines or techniques will need to be discovered in the near future.

Lifestyle modification can reduce the substantial and increasing burden of PAD and its local and systemic complications. Smoking cessation reduces the severity of claudication and the risk that rest pain will develop [34]. In patients with intermittent claudication, exercise significantly improves the maximal walking time and overall walking ability. Exercise is more effective than angioplasty and antiplatelet therapy for improving walking time and statin drugs improve pain-free walking time [35–37].

PAD patients also require treatment for systemic complications of coronary and cerebral atherosclerotic arterial disease because they are at increased risk of vascular events. Prolonged treatment with a statin and at least one agent to lower blood pressure should be considered in every PAD patient, independent of the baseline cholesterol level and blood pressure. Antiplatelet therapy with aspirin should be used in every PAD patient, when not contraindicated, because it is effective in reducing the risk of myocardial infarction, stroke, or cardiovascular death by 25%, and is also relatively inexpensive [34].

The Achilles heel of RSFAE is the high percentage of restenosis during the first postoperative year due to neointimal hyperplasia, which causes significant lower primary patency rates compared with venous bypass grafts. New insights to improve first-year postoperative patency rates need to be discovered.

Recent published data showed promising results for restenosis reduction in the SFA. The use of paclitaxel-coated angioplasty balloons (e.g., balloons with a chemotaxis substance) or drug-eluting stents during percutaneous intervention of femoropopliteal lesions (7.4 ± 6.5 cm) is associated with significantly less restenosis. The effect of paclitaxel is attributed to inhibition of vascular smooth muscle cell proliferation after exposure to the chemotaxis substance, which subsequently results in less neointimal hyperplasia [38].

However, we want to minimize the use of synthetic material as much as possible during RSFAE. Ideally, it is better to perform the RSFAE without additional stent placement. Cryo-balloon angioplasty of the distal transaction zone might be a solution to replace the stent. A cryoplasty balloon with a comparable diameter to the desobstructed SFA is positioned centrally at the transaction zone, a standard cryo-balloon angioplasty procedure is performed, and the distal intimal flap is tacked without a stent.

The functioning mechanism of cryo-balloon angioplasty combines mechanical force and localized supercooling of the arterial wall to induce apoptosis and lower cell proliferation, in endothelial cells of the intima and mainly in the smooth muscle cells of the medial layer [39]. However, this mechanism has only been proven in in vitro studies. Although there is a lack of evidence and a lack of prospective studies proving the working mechanism of cryo-balloon angioplasty as an addition to single PTA [40], it could be an interesting combination with RSFAE because the intimal core has been removed and cryo-balloon angioplasty can be applied directly on the medial and adventitial layer. First results of additional cryo-balloon angioplasty at the end of the RSFAE procedure are promising with a 100% success rate in tacking the distal intimal core and omitting the distal stent (not published data); patency data will be published in the near future.

There is an urgent need to determine variables that can predict restenosis or systemic cardiovascular events in the individual patient. Traditional risk factors can predict outcome for groups of patients but lack discriminative power to predict which individuals are at risk for local restenosis or systemic adverse cardiovascular event. Many studies have shown that local atherosclerotic plaque characteristics are associated with plaque rupture, resulting in arterial thrombosis [41, 42]. However, it is unknown if the local plaque characteristics hide a positive-predictive value to identify plaques that are prone to rupture. Prospective evidence is lacking, because these are all cross-sectional or retrospective studies.

One recently published article showed that the dissection of an inflammatory and lipid-rich carotid plaque is associated with reduced restenosis, due to the retained inflammatory cells into the backward vessel wall [43]. Thanks to the inflammation in the media and adventitia, matrix metalloproteinase will rise which will cause a decline in collagen, resulting in expansive remodeling, thereby increasing the vessel area during follow-up. Whether atherosclerotic plaque of the peripheral arteries hides predictive value for restenosis is not yet known.

Furthermore, there is increasing evidence that local plaque characteristics could also be predictive for future cardiovascular adverse events. Several studies have shown that the instability of the vascular wall is a systemic process rather than only local inflammation and that the molecular structure of the atherosclerotic vascular wall at one side could hold information about the stability of the entire system [44–46]. Thus, atherosclerotic lesions harvested during surgical endarterectomy may hide predictive biomarkers for adverse systemic cardiovascular events.

This approach is investigated in the Athero-Express study, which includes atherosclerotic specimens harvested with endarterectomy (RSFAE, RIAE, and carotid endarterectomy) and combines the histologic features with 3-year clinical follow-up from each patient [47]. Recently, extensive SFA plaque analyses were completed, and the first results will be published soon. Plaque characteristics of the peripheral artery will help to define the patient cohort that will benefit from RSFAE and which patient group will probably not because of increased risk of restenosis. Gender differences and time interval between SFA occlusion and surgical therapy seem to influence long-term patency. Furthermore, femoral plaque characteristics will help to define the patient who is likely to suffer from restenosis or a future systemic cardiovascular event such as myocardial infarction, stroke, or cardiovascular death.

Summary

Patency rates for the sole endovascular treatment of long-segment (>10 cm) atherosclerotic occlusions of the SFA remain disappointing. Therefore, surgical treatment is still advised for TASC C and D lesions of the SFA. RSFAE seems to be a reliable and safe method to treat these lesions with at least equal patency rates compared with synthetic above-knee bypass grafts. Benefits of RSFAE include its minimal invasiveness, avoidance of synthetic grafts, sparing of the veins, and reduced need for amputation in case of re-occlusion of the desobstructed SFA compared to occluded grafts. Furthermore, remote endarterectomy is a reliable treatment modality for long-segment iliac occlusive disease. At the moment, studies are executed to reduce the short-time restenosis rate of remote endarterectomy which is the Achilles heel of this technique. Atherosclerotic plaques harvested during endarterectomy provide important histological and biochemical information to determine patients who will benefit most from endarterectomy and to determine biomarkers that will predict the individual risk for restenosis or future adverse cardiovascular events.

References

1. Lopez AD, Mathers CD, Ezzati M, Jamison DT, Murray CJ: Global and regional burden of disease and risk factors, 2001: systematic analysis of population health data, *Lancet* 367(9524):1747–1757, May 27, 2006.
2. Norgren L, Hiatt WR, Dormandy JA et al.: Inter-society consensus for the management of peripheral arterial disease (TASC II), *Eur J Vasc Endovasc Surg* 33(Suppl 1):S1–S75, 2007.
3. Dalager S, Falk E, Kristensen IB, Paaske WP: Plaque in superficial femoral arteries indicates generalized atherosclerosis and vulnerability to coronary death: an autopsy study, *J Vasc Surg* 47(2):296–302, February 2008.
4. Scholten FG, Warnars GA, Mali WP, van Leeuwen MS: Femoropopliteal occlusions and the adductor canal hiatus, Duplex study, *Eur J Vasc Surg* 7(6):680–683, November 1993.
5. Ho GH, Moll FL, Joosten PP, van de Pavoordt ED, Overtoom TT: The Mollring Cutter remote endarterectomy: preliminary experience with a new endovascular technique for treatment of occlusive superficial femoral artery disease, *J Endovasc Surg* 2(3):278–287, August 1995.
6. Martin JD, Hupp JA, Peeler MO, Warble PB: Remote endarterectomy: lessons learned after more than 100 cases, *J Vasc Surg* 43(2):320–326, February 2006.
7. Rosenthal D, Martin JD, Smeets L et al.: Remote superficial femoral artery endarterectomy and distal aSpire stenting: results of a multinational study at three-year follow-up, *J Cardiovasc* Surg (Torino) 47(4):385–391, August 2006.
8. Smeets L, de Borst GJ, De Vries JP, van den Berg JC, Ho GH, Moll FL: Remote iliac artery endarterectomy: seven-year results of a less invasive technique for iliac artery occlusive disease, *J Vasc Surg* 38(6):1297–1304, December 2003.
9. Rosenthal D, Wellons ED, Matsuura JH, Ghegan M, Shuler FW, Laszlo PL: Remote superficial femoral artery endarterectomy and distal vein bypass for limb salvage: initial experience, *J Endovasc Ther* 10(1):121–125, February 2003.

10. Battaglia G, Tringale R, Monaca V: Retrospective comparison of a heparin bonded ePTFE graft and saphenous vein for infragenicular bypass: implications for standard treatment protocol, *J Cardiovasc Surg (Torino)* 47(1):41–47, February 2006.
11. Taylor LM Jr, Edwards JM, Porter JM: Present status of reversed vein bypass grafting: five-year results of a modern series, *J Vasc Surg* 11(2):193–205, February 1990.
12. Brewster DC, LaSalle AJ, Robison JG, Strayhorn EC, Darling RC: Femoropopliteal graft failures. Clinical consequences and success of secondary reconstructions, *Arch Surg* 118(9):1043–1047, September 1983.
13. Schouten O, Hoedt MT, Wittens CH, Hop WC, van Sambeek MR, van UH: End-to-end versus end-to-side distal anastomosis in femoropopliteal bypasses; results of a randomized multicenter trial, *Eur J Vasc Endovasc Surg* 29(5):457–462, May 2005.
14. Ho GH, van Buren PA, Moll FL, van der Bom JG, Eikelboom BC: Incidence, time-of-onset, and anatomical distribution of recurrent stenoses after remote endarterectomy in superficial femoral artery occlusive disease, *J Vasc Surg* 30(1):106–113, July 1999.
15. Smeets L, Huijbregts HJ, Ho GH, De Vries JP, Moll FL: Clinical outcome after re-occlusion of initially successful remote endarterectomy of the superficial femoral artery, *J Cardiovasc* Surg (Torino) 48(3):309–314, June 2007.
16. Knight JS, Smeets L, Morris GE, Moll FL: Multi centre study to assess the feasibility of a new covered stent and delivery system in combination with remote superficial femoral artery endarterectomy (RSFAE), *Eur J Vasc Endovasc Surg* 29(3):287–294, March 2005.
17. Cejna M, Thurnher S, Illiasch H et al.: PTA versus Palmaz stent placement in femoropopliteal artery obstructions: a multicenter prospective randomized study, *J Vasc Interv Radiol* 12(1):23–31, January 2001.
18. Grimm J, Muller-Hulsbeck S, Jahnke T, Hilbert C, Brossmann J, Heller M: Randomized study to compare PTA alone versus PTA with Palmaz stent placement for femoropopliteal lesions, *J Vasc Interv Radiol* 12(8):935–942, August 2001.
19. Muradin GS, Bosch JL, Stijnen T, Hunink MG: Balloon dilation and stent implantation for treatment of femoropopliteal arterial disease: meta-analysis, *Radiology* 221(1):137–145, October 2001.
20. Vroegindeweij D, Vos LD, Tielbeek AV, Buth J, vd Bosch HC: Balloon angioplasty combined with primary stenting versus balloon angioplasty alone in femoropopliteal obstructions: a comparative randomized study, *Cardiovasc Intervent Radiol* 20(6):420–425, November 1997.
21. Wolf GL, Wilson SE, Cross AP, Deupree RH, Stason WB: Surgery or balloon angioplasty for peripheral vascular disease: a randomized clinical trial. Principal investigators and their associates of veterans administration cooperative study number 199, *J Vasc Interv Radiol* 4(5):639–648, September 1993.
22. Jamsen TS, Manninen HI, Jaakkola PA, Matsi PJ: Long-term outcome of patients with claudication after balloon angioplasty of the femoropopliteal arteries, *Radiology* 225(2):345–352, November 2002.
23. Ihnat DM, Duong ST, Taylor ZC et al.: Contemporary outcomes after superficial femoral artery angioplasty and stenting: the influence of TASC classification and runoff score, *J Vasc Surg* 47(5):967–974, May 2008.
24. Surowiec SM, Davies MG, Eberly SW et al.: Percutaneous angioplasty and stenting of the superficial femoral artery, *J Vasc* Surg 41(2):269–278, February 2005.
25. Klinkert P, Post PN, Breslau PJ, van Bockel JH: Saphenous vein versus PTFE for above-knee femoropopliteal bypass. A review of the literature, *Eur J Vasc Endovasc Surg* 27(4):357–362, April 2004.
26. Pereira CE, Albers M, Romiti M, Brochado-Neto FC, Pereira CA: Meta-analysis of femoropopliteal bypass grafts for lower extremity arterial insufficiency, *J Vasc Surg* 44(3):510–517, September 2006.
27. Jensen LP, Lepantalo M, Fossdal JE et al.: Dacron or PTFE for above-knee femoropopliteal bypass. A multicenter randomised study, *Eur J Vasc Endovasc Surg* 34(1):44–49, July 2007.
28. Rosenthal D, Martin JD, Schubart PJ, Wellons ED, Shuler FW, Levitt AB: Remote superficial femoral artery endarterectomy and distal aSpire stenting: multicenter medium-term results, *J Vasc Surg* 40(1):67–72, July 2004.
29. Ho GH, van Buren PA, Moll FL, van der Bom JG, Eikelboom BC: The importance of revision of early restenosis after endovascular remote endarterectomy in SFA occlusive disease, *Eur J Vasc Endovasc Surg* 19(1):35–42, January 2000.
30. Smeets L, van der HG, Gisbertz SS, Ho G, Moll F: Does conversion of intended remote iliac artery endarterectomy alter the early and long-term outcome? *Vascular* 13(6):336–342, November 2005.
31. Cham C, Myers KA, Scott DF, Devine TJ, Denton MJ: Extraperitoneal unilateral iliac artery bypass for chronic lower limb ischaemia, *Aust N Z J Surg* 58(11):859–863, November 1988.
32. Rutherford RB: Options in the surgical management of aorto-iliac occlusive disease: a changing perspective, *Cardiovasc Surg* 7(1):5–12, January 1999.
33. Tetik O, Emrecan B, Bayatli K et al.: Surgical treatment of unilateral iliac artery occlusive disease using a retroperitoneal approach, *Acta Chir Belg* 107(4):382–385, July 2007.
34. Hankey GJ, Norman PE, Eikelboom JW: Medical treatment of peripheral arterial disease, *JAMA* 295(5):547–553, February 1, 2006.
35. Gardner AW, Poehlman ET: Exercise rehabilitation programs for the treatment of claudication pain. A meta-analysis, *JAMA* 274(12):975–980, September 27, 1995.
36. Aronow WS, Nayak D, Woodworth S, Ahn C: Effect of simvastatin versus placebo on treadmill exercise time until the onset of intermittent claudication in older patients with peripheral arterial disease at six months and at one year after treatment, *Am J Cardiol* 92(6):711–2, September 15, 2003.
37. Mohler ER III, Hiatt WR, Creager MA: Cholesterol reduction with atorvastatin improves walking distance in patients with peripheral arterial disease, *Circulation* 108(12):1481–1486, September 23, 2003.
38. Tepe G, Zeller T, Albrecht T et al.: Local delivery of paclitaxel to inhibit restenosis during angioplasty of the leg, *N Engl J Med* 358(7):689–699, February 14, 2008.

39. Yiu WK, Cheng SW, Sumpio BE: Vascular smooth muscle cell apoptosis induced by "supercooling" and rewarming, *J Vasc* Interv Radiol 17(12):1971–1977, December 2006.
40. Kessel DO, Samson RH: What is the evidence for the efficacy of cryoplasty? *J Cardiovasc Surg (Torino)* 49(2):179–185, April 2008.
41. Schaar JA, Muller JE, Falk E et al.: Terminology for high-risk and vulnerable coronary artery plaques. Report of a meeting on the vulnerable plaque, June 17 and 18, 2003, Santorini, Greece, *Eur Heart J* 25(12):1077–1082, June 2004.
42. Davies MJ, Richardson PD, Woolf N, Katz DR, Mann J: Risk of thrombosis in human atherosclerotic plaques: role of extracellular lipid, macrophage, and smooth muscle cell content, *Br Heart J* 69(5):377–381, May 1993.
43. Hellings WE, Moll FL, De Vries JP et al.: Atherosclerotic plaque composition and occurrence of restenosis after carotid endarterectomy, *JAMA* 299(5):547–554, February 6, 2008.
44. Lombardo A, Biasucci LM, Lanza GA et al.: Inflammation as a possible link between coronary and carotid plaque instability, *Circulation* 109(25):3158–3163, June 29, 2004.
45. Mauriello A, Sangiorgi G, Fratoni S et al.: Diffuse and active inflammation occurs in both vulnerable and stable plaques of the entire coronary tree: a histopathologic study of patients dying of acute myocardial infarction, *J Am Coll Cardiol* 45(10):1585–1593, May 17, 2005.
46. Rothwell PM, Villagra R, Gibson R, Donders RC, Warlow CP: Evidence of a chronic systemic cause of instability of atherosclerotic plaques, *Lancet* 355(9197):19–24, January 1, 2000.
47. Verhoeven BA, Velema E, Schoneveld AH et al.: Athero-express: differential atherosclerotic plaque expression of mRNA and protein in relation to cardiovascular events and patient characteristics. Rationale and design, *Eur J Epidemiol* 19(12):1127–1133, 2004.

Intravascular Stents

17

Kevin M. Sheridan, Shoaib Shafique, Alan P. Sawchuk, and Michael C. Dalsing

Percutaneous transluminal angioplasty (PTA) has become an accepted treatment for atherosclerotic arterial occlusive disease in properly selected patients. Delivery systems and balloon designs have matured over the last three decades, resulting in improved PTA results and fewer procedural complications [1]. However, this technique does have its limitations. Our personal experience with early technical failures and postprocedural restenosis forced a reevaluation of the technique and a consideration of methods that might improve results in areas of difficulty [2, 3]. The use of supportive endoskeletons (stents), although suggested by Dotter during the late 1960s, was not pursued until the limitations of PTA were widely recognized [4]. Since the mid-1980s, various stent designs have been studied and clinical trials undertaken. Recently, there has been a dramatic increase in the available types and manufacturers of stents. Many are approved for use in other areas of the body but are increasingly used in an off-label capacity.

Indications for Stent Use

There were initially two situations where stent use was theoretically appealing. The primary indication was the potential salvage of an unacceptable angioplasty result. Among PTA attempts, 10–15% are early technical failures, with 25–50% of these involving cases in which a guidewire could be manipulated past the lesion, but PTA could not maintain a functional channel [2, 3, 5]. Such cases might benefit from a device that could mechanically support the lumen until healing could take place. The underlying causes of early balloon failure are many [1, 2, 5, 6]. The desired effect of an arterial balloon dilatation, a controlled dissection, can go awry resulting in a *spiral dissection* that narrows or occludes the lumen. The PTA may expose sufficient subintimal collagen causing an *acute thrombosis* or *spasm* (or both) that, if sufficiently severe, predisposes the vessel to occlusion. One portion of the wall may be essentially normal, whereas the opposite wall is a hard atherosclerotic plaque. When PTA is attempted in such a case, the normal wall may easily expand but then quickly recoil as the intraluminal pressure exerted by the balloon is removed. This is called *elastic recoil*. Furthermore, any or all of these potential events may combine to result in an early technical failure. As long as the guidewire remains across the arterial narrowing, the procedure might be salvaged with an endovascular support (stent) to tack the dissection down and maintain an intraluminal radial force sufficient to prevent elastic recoil, constrictive spasm, or constrictive thrombosis. In practice, a PTA failure is documented by a residual stenosis on angiography of 30% or more or a systolic pressure gradient at rest of 5 mmHg or higher.

The other situation considered potentially amenable to stent use was an early PTA restenosis. Several factors, including site of stenosis, degree of narrowing, length of stenosis, and other patient factors, affect the incidence of PTA restenosis and generally occur within 6 months to 1 year of follow-up with a more gradual failure rate thereafter [2, 3, 5, 7–9]. Restenosis can and does occur at the original site of PTA [2, 5, 7]. It can be caused by fibromuscular hyperplasia or rapid

M.C. Dalsing (✉)
E. Dale and Susan E. Habegger Professor of Surgery, Director of Vascular Surgery, Section of Vascular Surgery, Department of Surgery, Indiana University School of Medicine, Indianapolis, IN, USA

T.J. Fogarty, R.A. White (eds.), *Peripheral Endovascular Interventions*,
DOI 10.1007/978-1-4419-1387-6_17,

progression of the atherosclerotic process [10]. If a stent can prevent such rapid restenosis, its use would be ideal for this particular patient problem.

The primary use of stenting, rather than an attempt at PTA alone, has more recently been considered an option for the treatment of certain difficult clinical situations. It may be especially appropriate in the totally occluded artery where PTA results have been less than optimal owing to distal embolization and poor long-term patency rates [5, 7, 9, 11]. Localized ulcerative plaques, thought to be a source of emboli, may also be appropriate lesions for primary stent placement to prevent dislodgment of plaque debris during PTA. Furthermore, when used intraoperatively in conjunction with a planned distal bypass, it might provide the hemodynamic support thought beneficial for maintaining inflow patency while outflow is being reconstructed [12]. Others have considered primary stent use as a plausible option for all PTA attempts if it can be proven to improve long-term patency rates without increased risk.

Stent Designs

A number of stent designs have been proposed; some have been studied only experimentally, but others have made their way into clinical trials [13–15]. A few have made a significant clinical impact in the peripheral arterial system. Still others proposed mainly for coronary use are currently under investigation for peripheral use. These designs have included the use of absorbable construction materials, antiproliferative coatings, removable designs, and other inventive concepts that may ultimately materialize into usable stents [16–19]. Currently there are two types of stent suitable for clinical use that are distinguished by the method of deployment: balloon-expandable and self-expanding (Tables 17.1 and 17.2). Both the balloon-expandable Palmaz stent and the self-expanding Wallstent are approved by the US Food and Drug Administration (FDA) for intra-arterial use. The Palmaz stent is indicated for use in both the iliac and the renal arterial systems, while the Wallstent has an indication for use in the central venous system as well as the iliac arterial system. However, their clinical use in many other areas of the arterial tree is well accepted and has become standard practice.

The Palmaz-type balloon-expandable stent is a simple stainless steel tube that is available in various diameters and lengths (Fig. 17.1). The walls are etched into multiple rows of staggered rectangles that, like a split-thickness skin graft, allow expansion to a larger area or, in this case, diameter when dilated (Fig. 17.1) (Johnson and Johnson, Interventional Systems, Warren, NJ). Its wall thickness is in the 0.12 mm range. It can be

Table 17.1 Examples of balloon-expandable stents

Stent	Manufacturer	Material	Approved use	Wire compatibility (in.)
Palmaz	Cordis J & J	Stainless steel	Iliac	0.035
Palmaz Genesis	Cordis J & J	Stainless steel	Iliac, renal	0.035
Express LD	Boston Scientific	Stainless steel	Biliary	0.035
Express SD	Boston Scientific	Stainless steel	Biliary	0.018
Visi-Pro	EV3	Stainless steel	Biliary	0.035
Formula 418	Cook Medical	Stainless steel	Biliary	0.018
Racer	Medtronic	Cobalt alloy	Biliary	0.014, 0.018

Table 17.2 Examples of self-expanding stents

Stent	Manufacturer	Material	Cell design	Approved use	Wire compatibility (in.)
Wallstent	Boston Scientific	Elgiloy	Closed	Biliary, tracheal	0.035
S.M.A.R.T. control stent	Cordis J & J	Nitinol	Open	Iliac	0.035
Protégé	EV3	Nitinol	Open	Biliary	0.035
Luminexx	Bard	Nitinol	Open	Biliary	0.035
Zilver 518	Cook Medical	Nitinol	Open	Biliary	0.018
LifeStent FlexStar	Edwards Lifesciences	Nitinol	Open	Biliary	0.035
Supera	IDev	Nitinol	Closed	Biliary	0.018

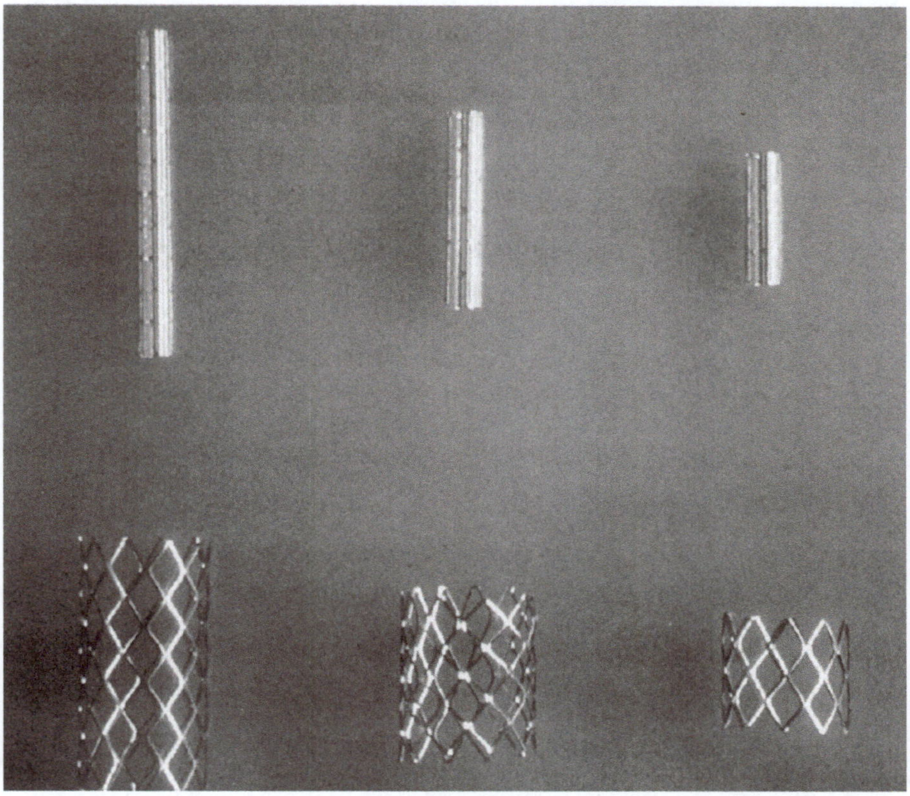

Fig. 17.1 Various diameters and lengths of the commercially available Palmaz stent demonstrating the collapsed and expanded conditions. Note the staggered slits in the collapsed version, which allow expansion when a PTA balloon is dilated within the stent lumen

obtained from the manufacturer premounted on a balloon or alone in a sterile vial, which can then be placed on a variety of balloon catheters. Most stents are available in a wide variety of lengths up to 3 cm and may be dilated to a recommended diameter of 12 mm. The stent may be overdilated if necessary. The small stents can be delivered through a 6F sheath, whereas larger ones require a 10F delivery port. The Palmaz-Schatz long medium stent (available in lengths of 4.2–7.8 cm) has shown promise for eliminating the need to implant multiple overlapping stents for coverage of long lesions. What the Palmaz stent provides in terms of excellent resistance to radial recoil, it relinquishes in overall flexibility. Its biocompatibility, general ease of delivery, and reliable expansion without migration were proven in early experimental studies [20]. Intimal thickening after placement of this stent was observed in this experimental model (approximately 98 μ(mu)m at 6 months) but was a much more gradual process after the initial 2 months of follow-up [20]. Figure 17.2 demonstrates a case with placement of a Palmaz stent in the iliac artery.

The Wallstent (Schneider Peripheral Division, Minneapolis, MN) is made of 16–20 surgical grade stainless steel alloy filaments braided into a flexible tubular structure (Fig. 17.3). The filament's diameter can range from 0.075 to 0.170 mm, providing a thin-walled device. Because the filaments are bound together only at the ends, there is great accommodation for flexibility in all directions. The stent is manufactured in various lengths from 2.0 to 9.4 cm and diameters ranging from 5 to 24 mm. The stents commonly used in the iliac arterial system are deployed through a 6F sheath (Fig. 17.4). What the Wallstent sacrifices in radial strength is compensated for by its flexibility and the ability to accommodate bends in the arterial lumen. Its biocompatibility is similar to that of all stainless steel devices and incites an intimal response with some thickening of the lumen wall [21, 22]. If a Wallstent is deployed in a vessel smaller than the native artery it elongates. The use of the Wallstent in the arterial circulation has gradually declined since the introduction of balloon-expandable and nitinol stents, because they offer better radial

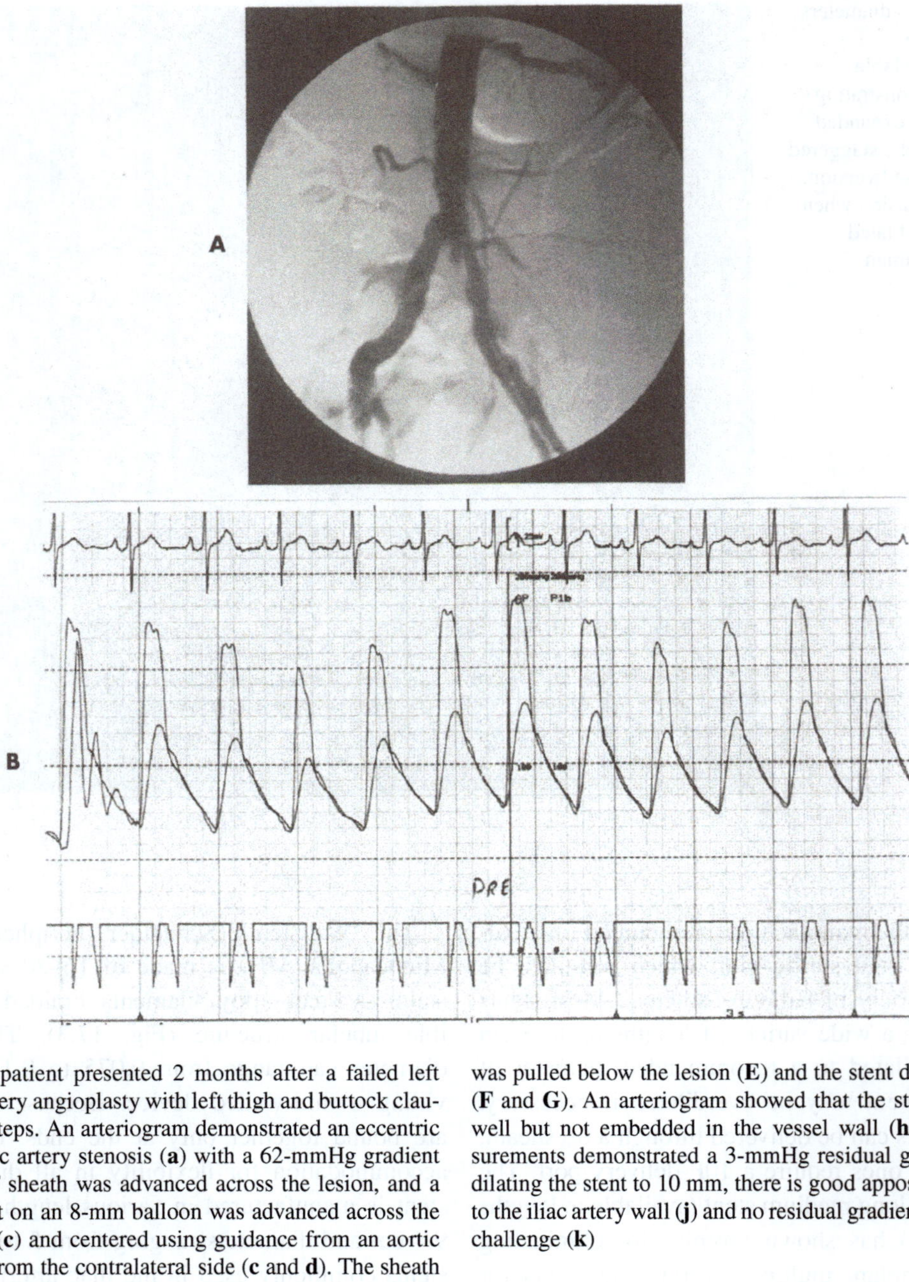

Fig. 17.2 This patient presented 2 months after a failed left common iliac artery angioplasty with left thigh and buttock claudication at 100 steps. An arteriogram demonstrated an eccentric left common iliac artery stenosis (**a**) with a 62-mmHg gradient at rest (**b**). A 9F sheath was advanced across the lesion, and a 308 Palmaz stent on an 8-mm balloon was advanced across the area of stenosis (**c**) and centered using guidance from an aortic catheter placed from the contralateral side (**c** and **d**). The sheath was pulled below the lesion (**E**) and the stent deployed to 8 mm (**F** and **G**). An arteriogram showed that the stent was centered well but not embedded in the vessel wall (**h**). Pressure measurements demonstrated a 3-mmHg residual gradient (**i**). After dilating the stent to 10 mm, there is good apposition of the stent to the iliac artery wall (**j**) and no residual gradient after Priscoline challenge (**k**)

strength. The Wallstent is recapturable even when up to 87% deployed. Since it comes in diameters up to 24 mm, it is also useful for venous interventions such as May–Thurner syndrome or interventions of the vena cava. Figure 17.5 demonstrates the use of a Wallstent to treat an iliac artery lesion.

Another balloon-expandable device (Strecker; Meditech, Watertown, MA) made of a radiopaque material called tantalum has more flexibility than the Palmaz stent but less radial strength. Therefore, it is more like the Wallstent in that aspect of its design. A third type of balloon-expandable stent is too small in diameter for practical use in the large artery peripheral vascular system (e.g., Gianturco Roubin Stent; Cook, Bloomington, IN) [23]. The Gianturco (Z-stent) (Cook), a unique zigzag configuration of bent stainless steel wire (Fig. 17.6), is approved for tracheobronchial use. However, it has been used off-label for inferior vena cava interventions. The new nitinol Symphony Stent (Boston Scientific, Natick,

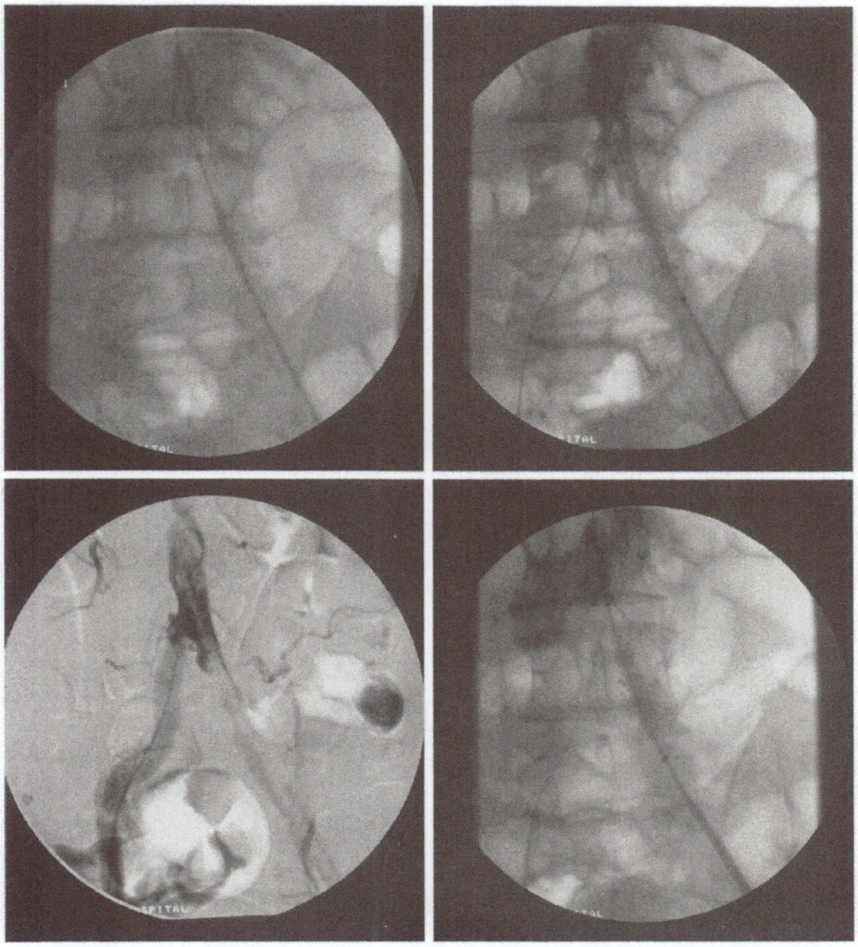

C D E F

Fig. 17.2 (continued)

MA) is flexible and easy to deploy but has yet to be approved for clinical use in the arterial system. Nitinol stents made of a nickel–titanium alloy with thermal memory have been approved for biliary but not arterial use (e.g., Memotherm; Bard Radiology, Covington, GA). Both the Zilver stent (Cook, Bloomington, IN) and the S.M.A.R.T. stent (Cordis, Warren, NJ), which are nitinol self-expanding stents, have gained FDA approval for iliac stenting. Covered stents are also available, which incorporate a polytetrafluoroethylene (PTFE) covering to the stent, the majority of which are really only approved for use in the tracheobronchial system. The Viabahn Endoprosthesis (W. L. Gore, Inc., Flagstaff, AZ) has gained FDA approval in the United States for treatment of superficial femoral artery (SFA) occlusive disease, and more recently has been approved for iliac use.

The Supera stent, developed by IDev Technologies, Inc. (Houston, TX), is a new self-expanding stent made of wire-interwoven nitinol which has been approved for biliary use. The Supera stent has a closed cell design, comes in diameters ranging from 4 to 9 mm, and stent lengths ranging from 40 to 120 mm. Its wire compatibility is 0.018 and it requires at least a 7F sheath. It should be sized 1:1 with respect to native vessel diameter. Bench testing of the Supera stent shows increased radial force, increased flexibility, and ex vivo fracture resistance. The compression fatigue testing was conducted by cycling a 0–4 lb load over 10,000,000 cycles of 120° flexion/bending bench tests and 180° torsion bench tests. The Supera stent had zero fractures and demonstrated exceptional flexibility. Other nitinol stents were subjected to the same testing and they showed fractures before 10,000,000 cycles.

G H I

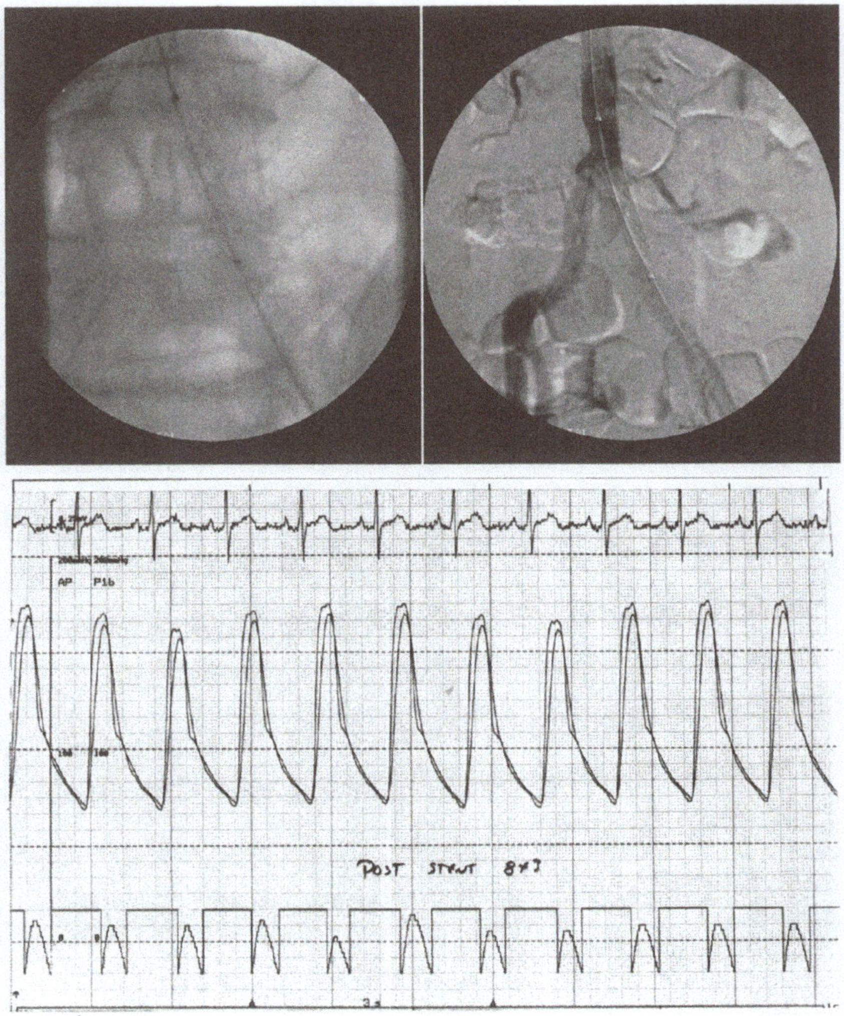

Fig. 17.2 (continued)

The Supera stent has 360% greater radial strength compared to other self-expanding stents. The complexity of motion and variable forces experienced by stents placed in the femoropopliteal arteries have limited the ability to treat many vascular conditions effectively with stents. Ex vivo testing of the Supera stent demonstrates that its unique properties may make it the stent of choice for use in the SFA.

Technical Considerations

Several lesion-related and anatomic factors need to be considered when choosing a stent. If the lesion is located in an area which is not prone to external compression or has an ostial location, balloon-expandable stents are a good choice. Examples of such lesions are renal or mesenteric vessel ostial lesions. Balloon-expandable stents offer better radial strength and more accurate deployment. The sizing needs to be very accurate, since oversizing can lead to edge dissection with flow limitation and undersizing can lead to in-stent restenosis. In case of edge dissection, an overlapping self-expanding stent may need to be placed to cover the dissection starting point. In high-risk interventions, intravascular ultrasound (IVUS) is a very useful modality to make the diagnosis of edge dissection following stent placement. Also, IVUS can confirm complete expansion and apposition of the stent to the wall of the artery. Highly calcified and tight lesions should be predilated, because if the lesion is too tight, the delivery catheter of the stent may not be able to

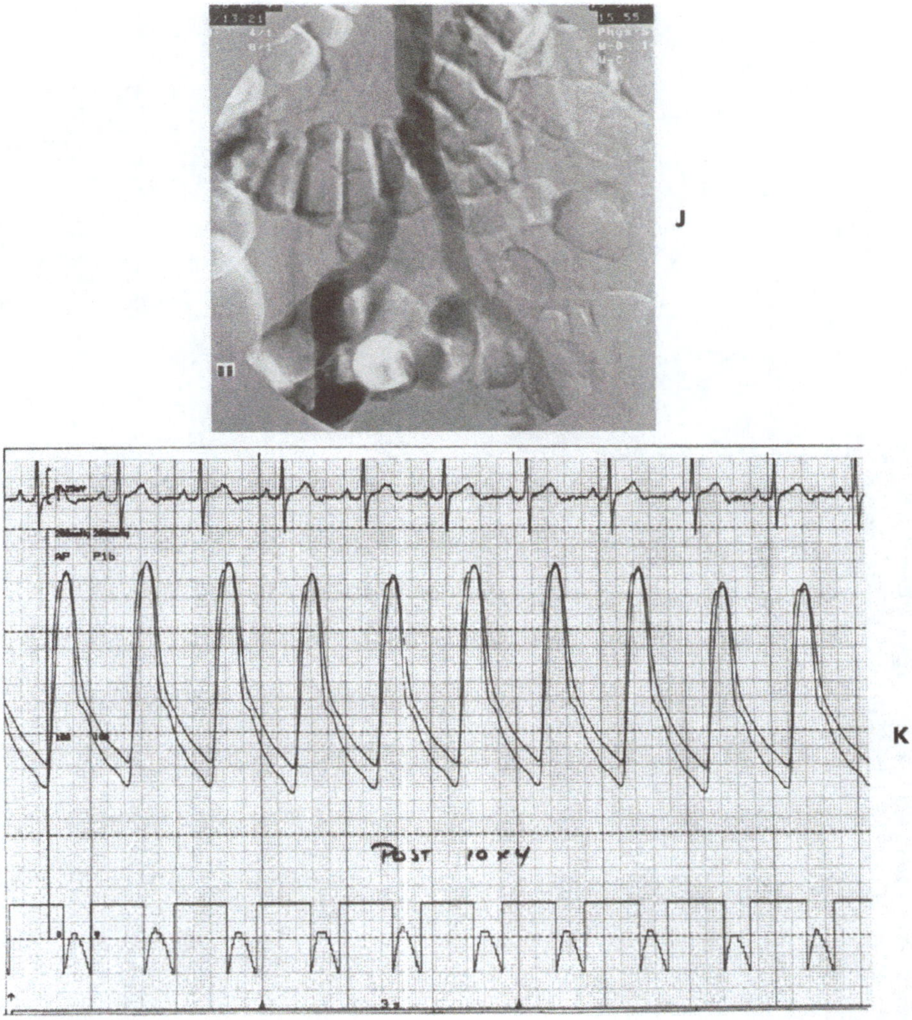

Fig. 17.2 (continued)

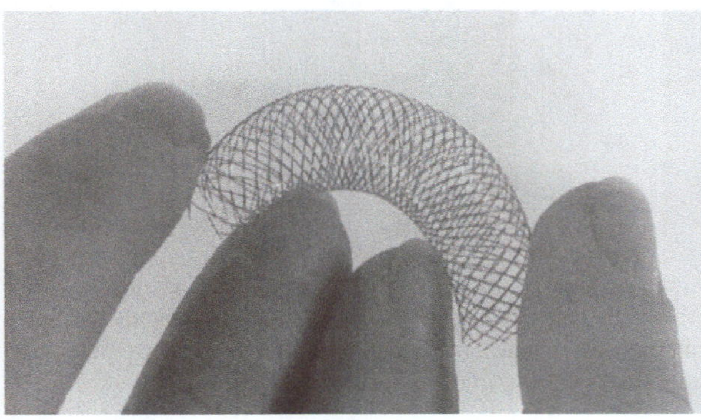

Fig. 17.3 Wallstent demonstrating the braided filament design and flexibility of the stent

cross the lesion. Forcing the delivery catheter through the lesion could dislodge the stent from the balloon.

The self-expanding stents are useful in vascular beds that are subjected to movement and prone to external compression. The newly designed nitinol self-expanding stents offer accurate deployment and good radial strength. If the lesion is too tight it should be predilated, and every attempt should be made to cover the entire lesion with the stent. Self-expanding stent diameters should be oversized about 15–20% greater than the native vessel. Post-stent balloon angioplasty is done to treat any residual stenosis in the vessel and for optimal stent apposition to the arterial wall. Post-stent balloon angioplasty should be done to the profile of the stent/artery, and excessive atmospheres

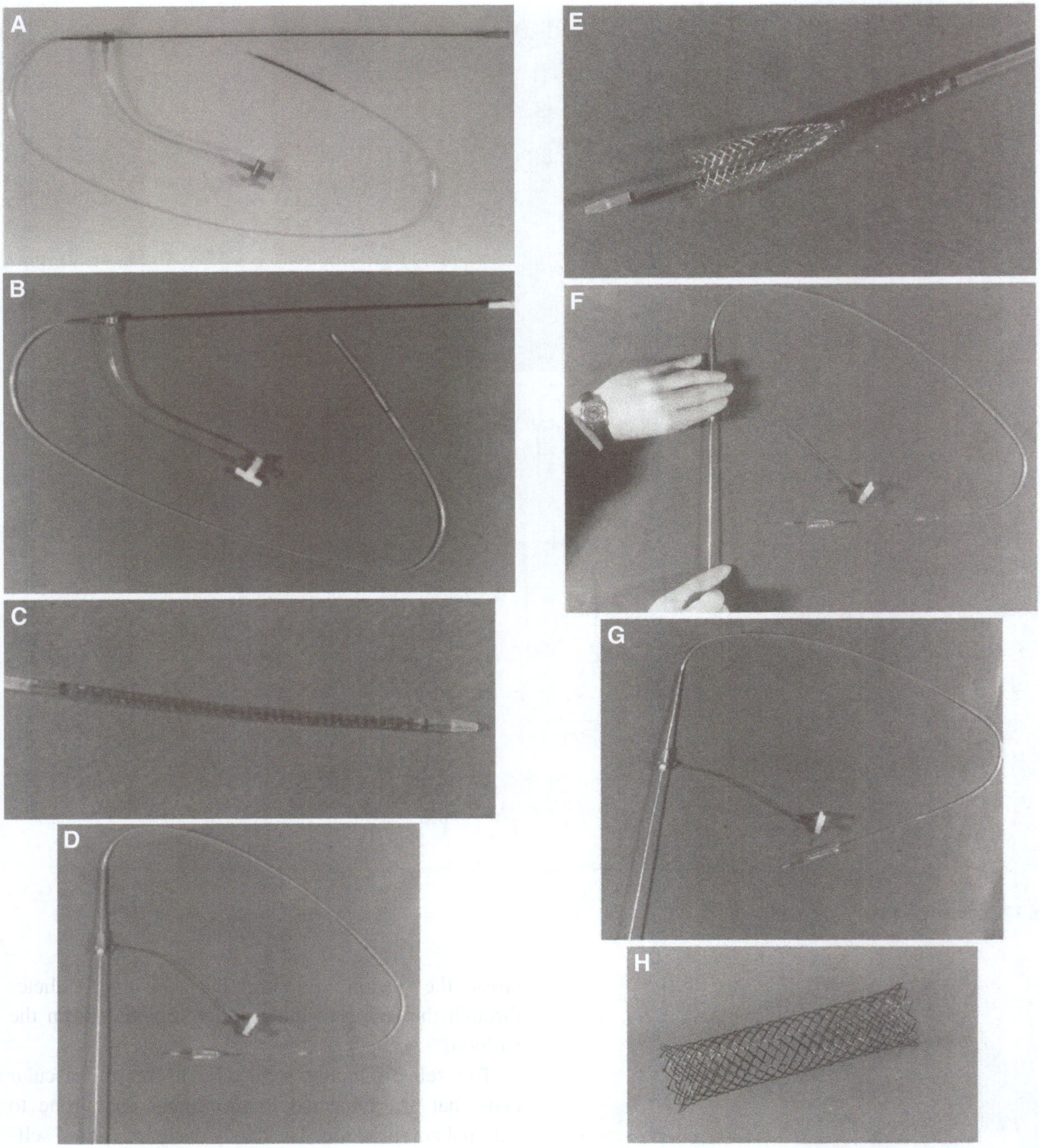

Fig. 17.4 Small (**a**) and large (**b**) Wallstent introducer catheter with stent in place. **c**, Close-up view of the Wallstent within its retractable sheath and mounted on a smaller inner catheter. **d**, Wallstent is partially deployed. **e**, A closer view of (**d**). **f**, Demonstrating how the inner sheath must be held stationary while the outer rolling membrane is pulled back to allow the Wallstent to expand. **g**, Stent is fully deployed with the inner catheter still in place. **h**, Close-up of how the stent would appear fully deployed within the vessel lumen

of pressure should be avoided since the struts of the stent can cut through the plaque causing more disruption of the plaque, leading to distal embolization. During post-stent balloon angioplasty, every attempt should be made to keep the balloon within the stent and avoid the balloon touching the native vessel, since that can cause dissection of the native artery as well. Self-expanding stents have open or closed cell designs. Open cell designs allow various segments of the stent to open up independent of adjacent cells.

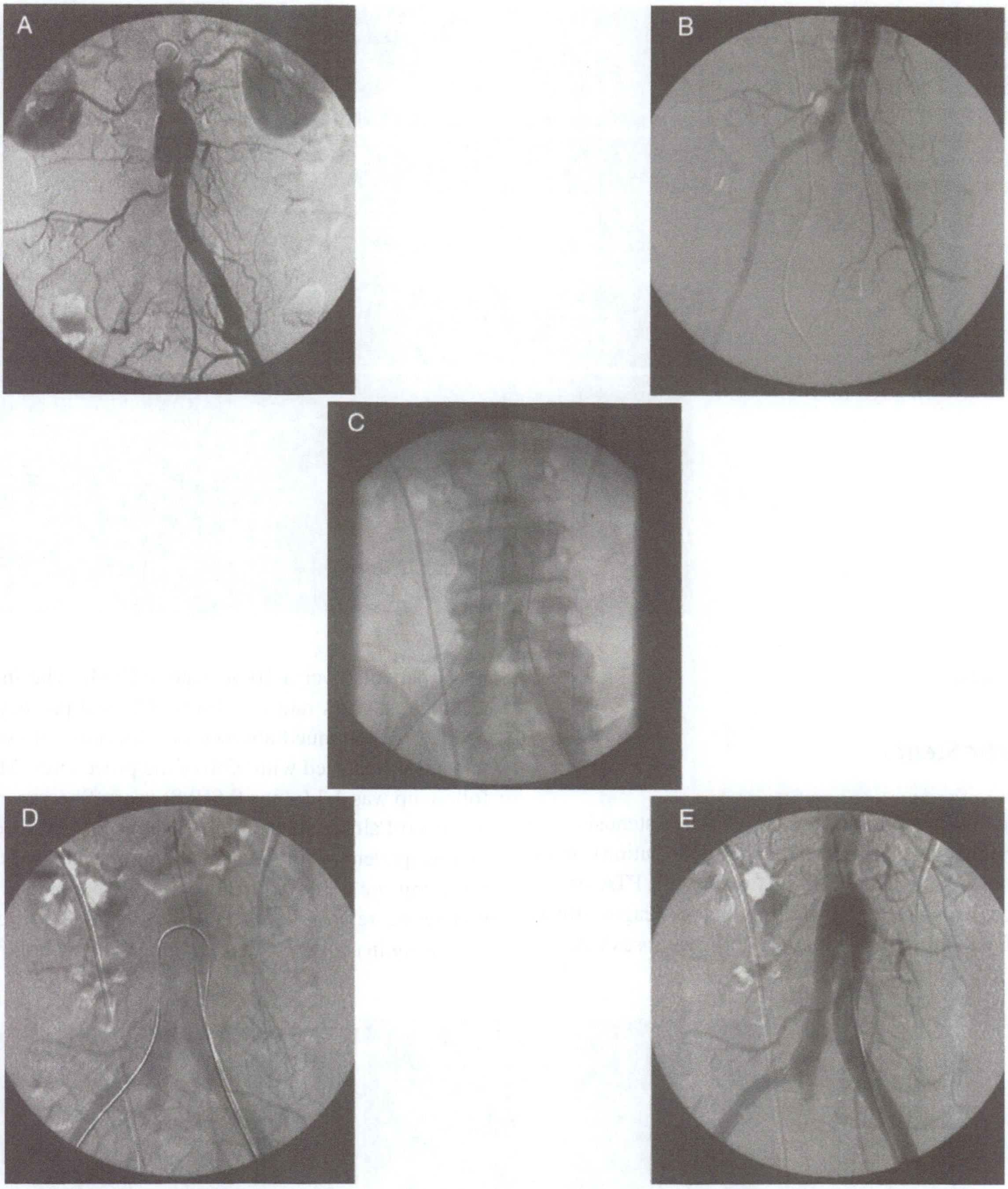

Fig. 17.5 This patient had previously undergone aortobifemoral bypass grafting with subsequent revision of the right limb of the graft. He had acute graft occlusion, **a**. After surgical thrombectomy of the right limb, there was an intimal disruption, **b**. Because there was a fresh incision in the right groin, the retrograde placement of a Palmaz stent in the radiology suite was not deemed appropriate. Therefore, a Wallstent was placed from a contralateral approach. A hydrophilic-coated Simmons catheter and hydrophilic wire were used to negotiate the lesion from a left common femoral artery access, **c**. Next, a 10-mm diameter by 20-mm length Wallstent was deployed across the flap and dilated with a 10-mm balloon. A post-stent arteriogram showed excellent flow through the area without residual stenosis, **d** and **e**

This allows for stent expansion in tortuous vascular anatomy. The closed cell design stents have all of the cells connected to each other. This design helps trap the plaque better with a lower likelihood of distal atheroembolization. The downside of the closed cell design is less flexibility for tortuous vascular anatomy.

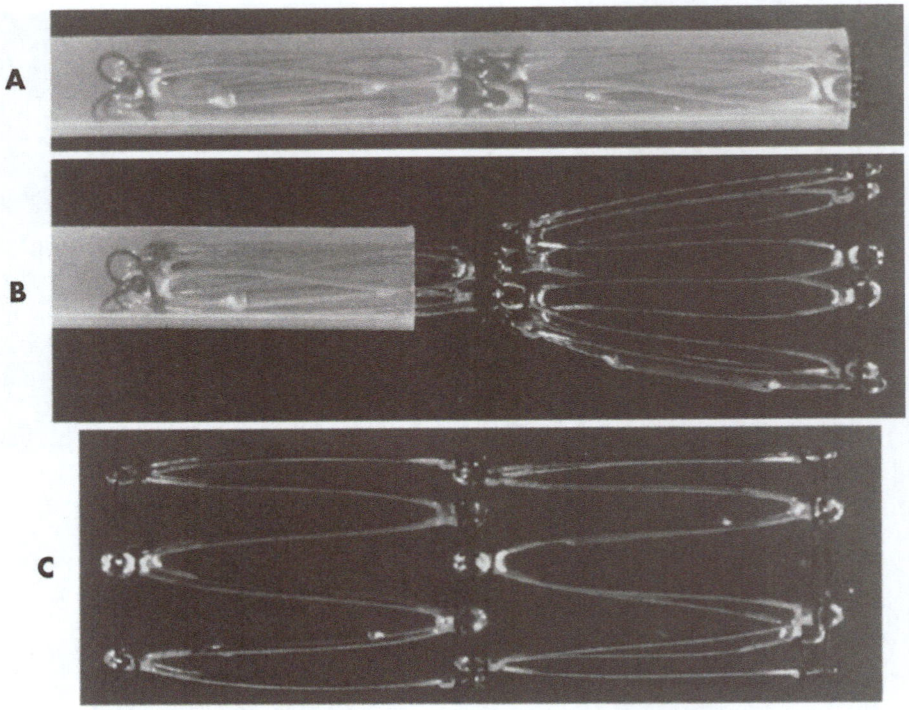

Fig. 17.6 Gianturco stent used in the biliary system presented here to demonstrate the design of the stent, **c** and how it expands from a sheath, **a–c**. A variation on this design has been used clinically in the arterial system in Japan

Results

Aortic Stents

True isolated midabdominal aortic stenosis (i.e., infrarenal lesions sparing the iliac distribution) are rare but may be amenable to treatment with PTA or stent placement (Fig. 17.7). Hallisey and colleagues treated 15 focal infrarenal abdominal aortic stenoses with PTA in 14 patients over a 10-year period [24]. The initial technical success rate was 100%. Clinical patency, as defined by continued absence or alleviation of symptoms, was achieved with 93% of the procedures. Mean follow-up was 4.3 (range 0.6–9.8) years. Sheeran et al. deployed Palmaz stents in six patients and Wallstents in three patients with focal midabdominal stenoses not involving the aortic bifurcation [25]. One patient had undergone remote aortic endarterectomy, and aortic narrowing in another patient developed at the proximal

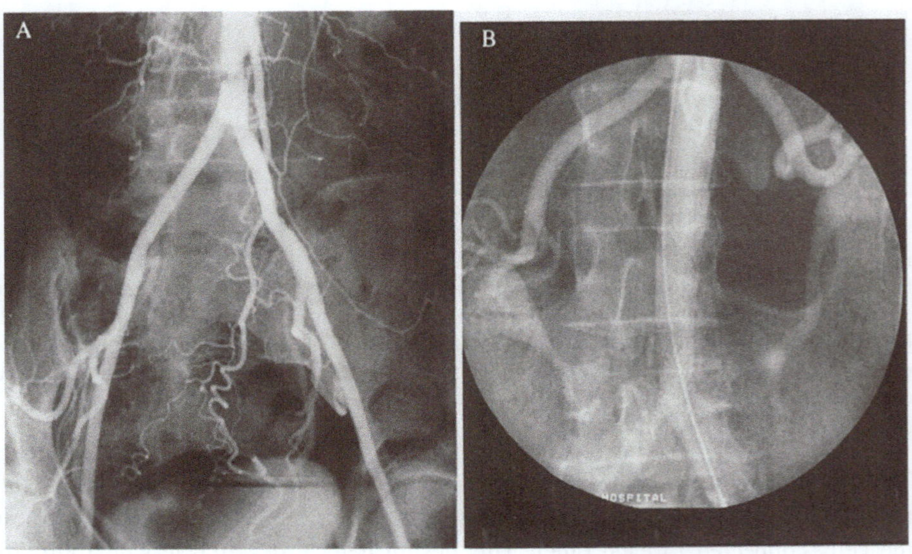

Fig. 17.7 This patient presented with bilateral blue toes and claudication. **a**, Abdominal aortogram demonstrates a severe focal aortic stenosis just above the bifurcation. **b**, After placement of a 16 × 40 mm Wallstent dilated to 14 mm, an arteriogram shows a good cosmetic result

anastomosis of an aortobifemoral graft performed 4 years prior to presentation. Technical success of stent placement was 100%. Follow-up (mean 1.6 years) demonstrated some degree of clinical improvement in all patients treated with Wallstents (100%) and in five patients treated with Palmaz stents (83%); no early or late complications were noted.

Schedel and colleagues reported results of primary aortic stenting in 15 patients [26]. Palmaz stents were used to treat the aortic stenosis in each case. Six patients underwent aortoiliac reconstructions with kissing stents placed in the iliac arteries. Technical success was achieved in 87%, with a primary clinical and hemodynamic patency of 85% observed at the end of a 36-month follow-up period. One case of distal embolization was observed, as well as two minor groin complications. Poncyljusz et al. placed 26 Palmaz stents in 26 patients with infrarenal aortic stenoses [27]. Initial technical and clinical success was 100%, with all stents remaining patent at 24 months by Doppler examination in addition to continued clinical improvement. No major complications were observed. Simons et al. utilized self-expandable nitinol stents in 10 patients (Smart stents) and balloon-expandable stainless steel stents in 7 patients (Palmaz stents in six, a Genesis stent in one) to treat distal aortic stenoses [28]. Technical success (defined as <50% residual stenosis or systolic gradient <10%) was achieved in 82%. During the 86-month follow-up period, primary patency was 55% (83% at 36 months), with a secondary patency of 100%. More recent results have been obtained with similar patency achieved. Klonaris et al. performed primary aortic stenting (without predilation) in 12 patients with immediate technical success achieved in 100% [29]. At the end of a 37-month follow-up period, a primary patency of 91.7% was observed, with no reinterventions performed. One patient died during the follow-up period from complications of chronic renal failure.

Overall, the evidence supports the use of PTA with or without stenting in the infrarenal aorta. While the evidence is largely retrospective, it suggests that this treatment modality is a viable option, especially in patients that would likely not tolerate a large open surgical procedure. It appears that this as a reasonably durable procedure if initial technical success is achieved. It seems unlikely that a prospective, randomized trial with sufficient power would be possible to complete for such a relatively rare condition.

Iliac Artery Stents

Iliac artery occlusive disease treated by PTA is quite successful for localized disease, with 1-year patency rates of 50–93% [3, 5, 7, 8, 30, 31] Five-year results are less well reported but range from approximately 20–76% [7, 8], depending on the indications for angioplasty, run-off, occlusion versus stenosis, and other variables. Initial failure in those cases with guidewire-accessible lesions occurs in about 1.5–7.5% of all iliac PTAs [2, 3, 5], and restenosis (3–17%) [3, 8, 9, 32] or locally progressive disease accounts for most of the chronic failures [2–4, 7–9]. PTA for a totally occluded iliac artery is technically less rewarding than PTA performed for stenosis, and the complication rate appears to be higher [5–7, 9, 11]. Provided optimal patient selection was addressed, these studies suggest that there is room for stent technology to improve the long-term results of iliac PTA.

Palmaz Stent

The Palmaz stent has been studied in the United States via a multicenter trial, with indications for stent placement being an immediate inadequate post-angioplasty response (Fig. 17.8), PTA restenosis, or total iliac occlusion [33–35]. The results were generally not segregated precisely by these categories but were combined to provide an overall success rate. When results were categorized by indication for placement, the findings were consistent with the following generalizations [36]. The findings from this group of patients treated with stents were clinical benefit rates of 90.9% at 1 year and 68.6% at 43 months, the benefit defined as at least a one-stage improvement in the ischemic rating system used [35]. The mean ankle–brachial index (ABI) remained approximately 0.18 above the pretreatment mean of 0.62, corresponding with the fact that approximately 67% of the patients were treated for claudication and only 33% for limb-threatening ischemia. Approximately one-fifth of the participants agreed to a postprocedural angiogram 1–35 months after treatment, and it demonstrated a mean loss of luminal diameter of 15% and a restenosis rate of 2.7% (50% or less of the original stent diameter). Probably more interesting was the approximately 5% per year progression of significant atherosclerotic

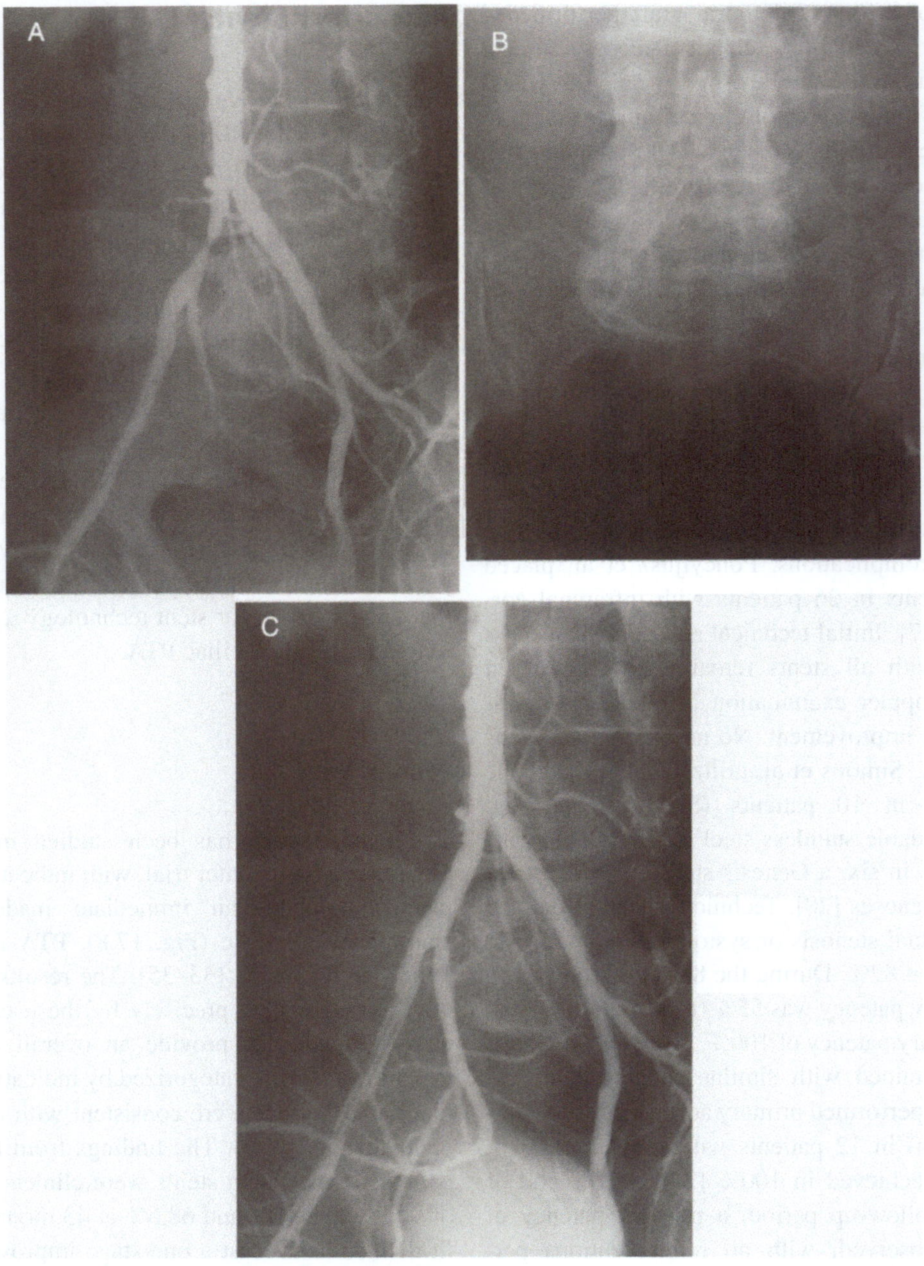

Fig. 17.8 This patient developed recurrent right lower extremity claudication 1 year after a successful right common iliac artery angioplasty. **a**, Arteriogram demonstrates a significant stenosis in the area of prior angioplasty with a 35-mmHg gradient. **b** and **c**, A 308 Palmaz stent was deployed primarily to 10 mm with good cosmetic results and no residual gradient

disease at a site distant from the stent. The 30-day procedural mortality was 1.9%, with a 9.9% rate of complications, of which 1.9% were related to the stent itself. These results suffered from short-term follow-up (only about 20% were more than 2 years) but constitute a dedicated effort to report all aspects of stent placement.

Wolf et al. placed stents in a group of 37 patients (50 stenoses, 6 occlusions, 128 stents) [37]. Resolution of symptoms was noted in 27 patients. One death and four complications (treated nonoperatively) occurred. Follow-up was not lengthy (range 6–21 months). Routine 6-month arteriograms obtained for 19 patients revealed six patients with mild-to-moderate stenoses

(9–43% diameter reduction). Of these six, only two had recurrence of symptoms. These results are comparable to the 17.8% mean stenosis at 6 months reported by Murphy et al. [38], who observed no correlation between outcome and the presence of hypertension, coronary artery disease, obesity, age, or length of stenosis. They did, however, demonstrate a statistically significant difference in maintaining improved symptomatology at 4 years in nondiabetics [38].

Henry et al. stented 230 iliac arteries in 184 patients [39]. The 6-month angiographic restenosis rate was 0.5% with a mean follow-up of 35 months. Life table analysis of their data revealed a 4-year primary patency rate of 86.0 ± 4.1%, with successful treatment of most restenotic lesions by repeat angioplasty resulting in a 4-year secondary patency rate of 94.0 ± 2.8%.

The use of primary stent placement in cases of total iliac artery occlusion may have found a viable application. An early report by Rees et al. demonstrated its success in 12 patients, but the embolic risk was high (16%) [40]. The most recent multicenter study results from this same group found an 87.8% success rate at 40 months in this select group; although it was not statistically different from the stenosis-only group (66.6%), there was a tendency for improved outcome [34]. Surgical exposure to prevent the risk of procedure-induced emboli is a possible solution to a continuing problem of distal embolus [34, 40]. Alternatively, stent grafts (covered stents) to cover embolic sources prior to embolization may help [41].

Scheinert et al. evaluated results of recanalization of chronic iliac artery occlusions with primary stent placement in 212 patients [42]. Recanalization of the arteries was assisted by the Excimer laser system. A total of 527 stents were placed in 196 patients, 346 of those being Palmaz stents and 94 of them being Wallstents. Thirty-one patients had dissections treated with Dacron-covered self-expanding nitinol stents (EndoPro1/Passager). Primary technical success was obtained in 190 patients (90%), and only three patients suffering from major procedure-related complications (two embolizations, one arterial rupture). Clinical improvement measured by the Rutherford claudication scale occurred in 88% of patients. Cumulative patency rates were noted over a 4-year period, with a large amount of patients lost to follow-up (only 15 patients remained at the final analysis). Primary and secondary patency rates at 1 year were 84 and 88%, respectively, and at 4 years were 76 and 85%, respectively. Kaplan–Meier curve analysis comparing those with less than 10 cm stented segments to those with greater than 10 cm stented segments revealed a significantly improved patency. The authors felt the use of the Excimer laser to debulk the occlusions, and the use of a crossover technique may have contributed to their low rate of embolization. They felt that randomized controlled data would be necessary to validate this approach as a first-line treatment for iliac occlusion.

Primary stenting based on the theoretic advantages of a smooth flow surface, optimal resolution of pressure gradients, and reduced subintimal collagen exposure has been an active area of research [43]. Bonn et al. reported a feasibility study and concluded that early stent results were acceptable and did not significantly increase the complication rate of iliac PTA [44]. Williams and colleagues in 1994 confirmed these results but reported a 13% complication rate, but there was also an initial cost saving of 25–66% compared with surgical interventions [45]. Long-term durability could not be confirmed. A randomized trial of PTA versus primary stenting demonstrated a primary patency rate of 93.6% with stents versus a 64.6% rate with PTA alone [46]. The Dutch Iliac Stent Trial recently published its long-term results aimed at determining the validity of primary stenting practices [47]. This was a prospective, randomized trial of PTA and selective stenting versus primary stenting in a total of 279 patients. Patients were randomized to primary stent placement (143 patients) or PTA (136 patients) with selective stent placement (40% of the patients) performed for lesions with a hemodynamically significant residual stenosis (defined as >10 mmHg). Palmaz stents (Johnson and Johnson Interventional Systems, Warren, NY) were used. The investigators found better symptomatic success with PTA and selective stent placement than with primary stent placement (66% of primary stent patients continued to have symptoms versus 51% of the PTA/selective stent group) over a 6- to 8-year follow-up period. Hemodynamic success, patency, and reintervention rate was similar between the two groups. When patients undergoing PTA alone were separated from patients who underwent stent placement, no differences in the above parameters were noted. With the improved symptomatic results and decreased cost associated with selective stent placement, the authors concluded that selective stent placement should be the preferred method of iliac treatment.

Wallstent

The Wallstent has been studied most extensively in Europe as part of the European Wallstent Peripheral Artery Implant Study. Indications for stent placement were a complex lesion, i.e., occlusion (Fig. 17.9), long-segment stenosis with an irregular surface, aneurysm formation, markedly ulcerated plaques, eccentric stenosis, or ostial lesions extending into the aorta—or an acute complication during PTA [48]. The reports generally did not separate the results by indication but did provide an overall estimate of success.

An early report of this experience included 31 iliac lesions (16 occlusions), all but one of which were performed for claudication. Warfarin (Coumadin) was used in 11 early cases but was then deemed unnecessary. At a mean of 5.5 months, one occlusion had occurred and one case of significant restenosis secondary to pseudointimal hyperplasia was reported [49]. In 1991, there were 100 cases available for analysis [50]. Most of the patients (90%) were claudicants, 97% were primary technical stent successes, and thrombosis occurred immediately after stent placement in two patients. In general, the stent dramatically reduced the average degree of residual stenosis by about 30–50% in the patients in whom stents were used. Within the first month, six other stents occluded and were associated with uncorrected inflow disease not completely covered by the original stent in three cases. Two others failed within 3 months, which is a rate of failure similar to that reported by Hausegger et al. [51]. All symptomatic patients and several asymptomatic patients underwent postprocedural angiography. The prevalence of clinically relevant restenosis was 5%. The angiographic prevalence of restenosis was 16% (10 of 62); three of the stenoses were immediately adjacent to the stent. Angiographic restenosis was defined as a more than 20% decrease from the original postintervention luminal diameter, and the results stated were for a mean follow-up of 1 year. In 10 of 14 cases, angiographic restenosis was related to the implant, and in four cases it represented a new lesion. A later report covers a 3-year clinical experience with 125 iliac stents [48]. Eliminating the 22 cases of total iliac occlusion not guidewire-accessible, the 1-year cumulative patency was 94.6% and the 2-year patency

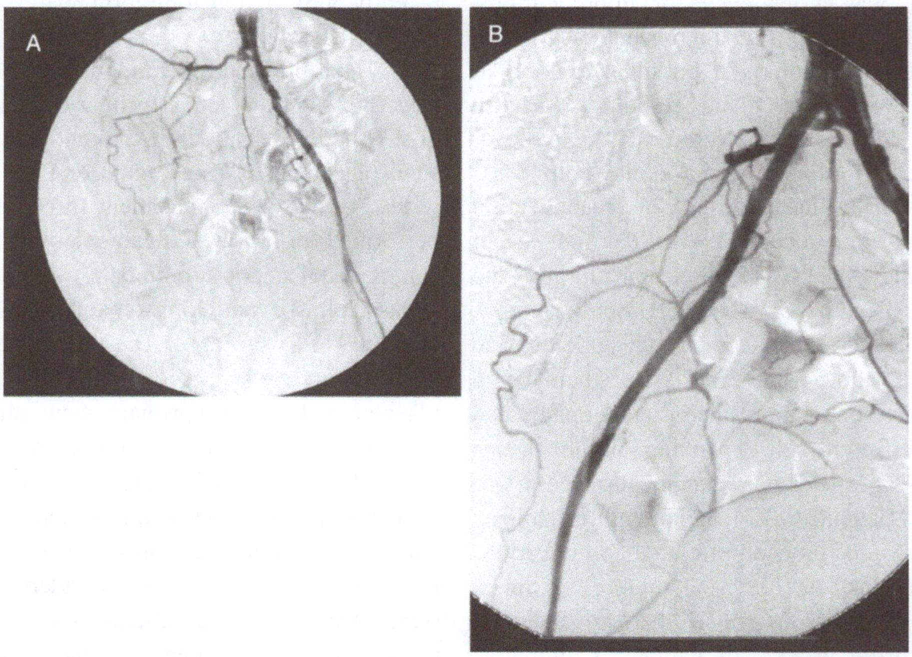

Fig. 17.9 This patient had a history of chronic right lower extremity claudication. **a**, Arteriogram demonstrated occlusion of the right common and external iliac artery. The patient was given 5,000 units of heparin. The right iliac occlusion was then negotiated with a hydrophilic wire from a contralateral approach. Without predilatation, two overlapping 8 × 60 mm Wallstents were deployed and dilated to 8 mm in the common iliac artery and 7 mm in the external iliac artery. **b**, Postprocedural arteriography demonstrated a patent channel through the previously occluded right iliac artery. There was no pressure gradient across the system at the termination of the procedure

86.5%. The procedural mortality was 0%. There was a total complication rate of 4%, but only a 1.6% major complication rate if this was defined as the patient requiring some type of reintervention. Reobstruction (resulting from lesions inside or adjacent to the stented segment) occurred in 6.5% of cases during follow-up, generally more than 6 months after the Wallstent had been placed.

Regarding complex lesions, Vowerk et al. stented 13 ulcerated plaques and 5 aneurysms with a mean length of 3.5 ± 1.0 cm [52]. Follow-up angiography demonstrated lesion ablation in 94% of cases at 3 months and in all cases at 9 months. No embolization occurred. Follow-up revealed a 4-year cumulative patency rate of 82%. Obstruction recurred in two patients. One patient developed a thrombotic occlusion at the site of stent deployment after 17 months but underwent successful percutaneous recanalization that was still patent after 46 months. The other patient underwent successful balloon dilatation for a restenosis within the stent at 26 months, then returned 12 months later with an occlusion of the stent that was also successfully recanalized.

Long et al. reported a 3-year experience of Wallstent use in 47 iliac artery lesions (15 occlusions) in 49 patients; seven Strecker stents were used in the remaining cases [53]. Follow-up averaged 15 months, and postprocedural angiography was undertaken in an impressive 47 cases. The procedural mortality was 2%. Thrombosis occurred in 7.7% of all cases. Significant intrastent hyperplasia was observed in 13.5% of cases (50% or more recurrent luminal narrowing) in addition to a 5.8% incidence of stenosis in adjacent areas where the stent just missed covering an offending lesion. Six of these patients required intervention for symptomatic relief. Long et al. also observed that overlapping the hypogastric artery lumen was not without consequence, as 2 of 18 (11%) occluded and 33% had documented ostial degradation in luminal size over time [53].

Raillat et al., studying 16 symptomatic iliac lesions treated by PTA and stent placement, noted that no stenosis occurred in the stent itself but usually occurred in an area of PTA dissection not covered by the stent, which then resulted in early occlusion [54]. Zollikofer and colleagues treated 24 iliac stenoses in 18 patients; they reported one acute occlusion and two cases of restenosis secondary to intimal hyperplasia at approximately 4 months. At a mean follow-up of 16 months, no clinical or angiographic evidence of restenosis had been observed in any of the other patients [55].

Sapoval et al. stented 101 arteries in 95 patients [56], with a mean follow-up of 29 months. They reported a 4-year primary patency rate of 61% and a secondary rate of 86%, similar to those reported by Murphy et al. [57]. Sapoval et al. identified the following five factors associated with long-term angiographic failure: SFA occlusion, stent diameter less than 8 mm, two or more stents implanted, current tobacco use, and, interestingly enough, the lack of hypertension. They postulated that the presence of hypertension may have caused more frequent visits to the physician and thus better general management [56]. The 1-year patency rates were 95.2 ± 4.8, 88.6 ± 6.2, 78.2 ± 8.7, and 54.9 ± 17.2% for patients with no, one, two, or three risk factors, respectively. No patient with four risk factors had a patent stent at 1 year [56].

Martin and colleagues reported the results of an FDA phase II, multicenter trial [58]. Iliac stents were placed in 140 patients. The 6-month angiographic patency rate was 93%. The 1-year primary patency was 81% and secondary patency 91% and the 2-year primary patency was 71% and secondary patency 86%. The major complication rate was 4.3%. Three patients died during the first 30 days after the procedure, but no death was directly related to stent deployment.

Totally occluded iliac arteries have been treated with the Wallstent. Vorwerk and Gunther reported on the European Wallstent Peripheral Artery Implant Study noting that 48 of 68 total occlusions were successfully recanalized (70.6%) [59]. Once accomplished, there were two early reocclusions (less than 6 months) probably resulting from incomplete stent coverage of a coexisting common iliac artery orificial stenosis. Restenosis developed in two others; one was found at 1 month and corrected by placement of a second stent at a proximal location not previously included in the stenting procedure. The second demonstrated intimal hyperplasia within and proximal to the stent within 6 months. The distal embolus rate was 2.1%, and no thrombolysis had been used in any of these cases. Emboli after treatment of total iliac artery occlusions continued to be a problem during the course of this investigation, as noted by the 4.7% incidence reported during an extended period of follow-up [48]. A more current study by this group noted a 5.1% embolization rate [60]. Long et al. also reported a significant problem with emboli after stent treatment for total occlusions (20%) [53]. Long-term follow-up of the European Wallstent study demonstrated early recurrences from incomplete stenting of the occluded segment in 3.2% of all cases [48]. Clinically relevant late reocclusions occurred 9–30 months (mean 16.4 months) after the procedure and developed in 10 of 123 patients. Interestingly, the rate of late reobstruction was higher for preprocedure iliac stenoses (9.6%) than for iliac occlusions (6.5%) [48]. Another study involving primary Wallstent deployment without thrombolysis involved 61 iliac artery occlusions. The mean length of the occluded segment was 10 cm. The technical success rate was 92%. The 2-year primary and secondary patency rates were 73.0 and 88.0%, respectively. Embolization rates were comparable to those of other studies [61].

More recent long-term results of Wallstent use in iliac arteries were published by Reyes and others [62]. Wallstents were placed in 303 legs of 259 patients over a 10-year period; 141 of these were occluded iliac arteries, with the remaining 162 being angioplasty failures (residual stenosis >50%). At 5 and 7 years, primary patency was 70 and 65%, respectively. Secondary patency was 92 and 87% after 5 and 9 years follow-up, respectively. There were complications in 4% (12 patients) of limbs in the first 24 h, with five patients exhibiting thrombosis of the treated vessel; 42 patients (16%) died during the follow-up interval. Long-term complications were noted in 54 (18%) limbs. The authors concluded that acceptable long-term results can be achieved with the use of Wallstents.

Ten-year results of iliac Wallstents were reported by Schurmann et al. [63]. A total of 110 patients were treated with a total of 167 Wallstents in 123 legs over a 3-year period prior to 1991. During the follow-up period, 46 patients (42%) died, largely due to cardiac causes. Many other patients were lost to follow-up or had arterial bypass surgery, resulting in a significantly decreased number of patients remaining at final follow-up. Five-year primary patency rates were 66%, with secondary patency rates of 79%. Ten-year primary and secondary patency rates were 46 and 55%, respectively. Major complications requiring additional intervention or hospital stay occurred in nine patients. The authors concluded that while long-term results are inferior to surgical intervention, iliac stent placement has a low procedure-related morbidity and mortality rate with a moderate long-term patency rate.

Miscellaneous Iliac Artery Stents

The Gianturco self-expanding metallic stent has been used in Japan for iliac artery stenosis and occlusion [64]. Early animal studies were encouraging [15], but the device never reached clinical trial in the United States for the arterial system. Ten patients were treated in the clinical series; one-half had total occlusions. The technical success rate was 100%. At an average follow-up of 10.3 months no migration or occlusion was noted, and the mean ABI was significantly improved over the preintervention value. Postprocedural angiograms demonstrated mild neointimal thickening. It should be noted that the device used clinically was made of a smaller diameter wire (0.01 in.) than that used in earlier US experimental reports. The authors believed that the small amount of wire present in terms of thickness and overall bulk may help improve endothelial coverage, decrease its thrombogenicity, and allow side-branch interventions if required at a later date. Because of its rigidity, which is similar to that of the Palmaz device, acutely angulated vessels or vessels near bend areas of the body are not candidates for intervention with this device.

The Strecker stent has been used in Europe [51, 64–67]. The number of totally occluding lesions ranged from 22.7 to 47.3%. The indications for stent placement were PTA failures or early restenosis following PTA. Additionally, long iliac occlusions were indications for primary stenting [66]. The patency rates ranged from 98 to 100% after 9 months. Three-year patency rates were significantly higher in short (88%) versus long (63%) lesions (using 4 cm as the line of demarcation) and in stenoses (92%) versus occlusions (63%) [67]. The stent's flexibility, ease of delivery, and ability to be imaged by magnetic resonance imaging (MRI) may be clinically advantageous.

The design of nitinol stents has matured from an early spiral coil used experimentally [13] to a zigzag configuration used in ongoing clinical evaluations following renewed experimental work [68, 69]. Early clinical work involved 14 patients with nine iliac stenoses and five total occlusions after unsuccessful PTA [68]. In the 13 patients available for long-term follow-up (average 12.7 months), the ABI was still more than 0.15 above preinterventional levels and no clinical deterioration had occurred. Eight patients had follow-up angiography; only minimal intimal hyperplasia involving the entire length of the stent(s) was noted. The Zilver stent (Cook, Bloomington, IN), a self-expanding flexible nitinol stent, was recently evaluated for safety and efficacy by Krol and others in a multicenter prospective trial [70]. A total of 204 stents were placed in 177 lesions. Immediate technical success was 98%. At 9 months follow-up, 92.9% of the stents were patent (<50% stenosis) by duplex examination. Slightly lower patency rates were noted in patients requiring multiple overlapping stents versus those with single stents placed (82 versus 95%).

The S.M.A.R.T. stent (Cordis Endovascular, Warren, NJ) has been compared to the Wallstent (Schneider, Minneapolis, MN) in the treatment of arterial stenosis by Ponec and colleagues in the Cardiac Remote Ischemic Preconditioning in Coronary Stenting (CRISP) US trial [71]. This was a multicenter, prospective, randomized trial comparing the two stents in 203 patients with suboptimal PTA of the iliac arteries. Immediate technical success was achieved in 98.2% of the S.M.A.R.T. stent patients and in 87.5% of the Wallstent patients. Duplex ultrasound was used to evaluate patency of the stents in follow-up out to 1 year. Primary and primary-assisted patency for the S.M.A.R.T. stent group was 94.7 and 99.1% versus 91.1 and 95.5% for the Wallstent group, respectively. Repeat procedures were required for patency in 2% of the SMART stent group versus 4% of the Wallstent group. One stent thrombosis was noted in each group. The authors noted that while patency rates were not statistically different, immediate technical success was higher in the S.M.A.R.T. stent group.

The "kissing stents" technique has become a viable treatment option for patients with lesions at the distal aorta and proximal common iliac arteries. Greiner and colleagues published mid-term results of 25 patients treated with "kissing stents" [72]. Balloon-expandable Palmaz stents were used in heavily calcified lesions while self-expanding Wallstents were used in others; eight occlusions were treated. Immediate technical success was achieved in 86%. Primary-assisted patency was reported as 94, 91, and 65% at 6, 12, and 24 months, respectively. Two patients had a distal aortic dissection not requiring treatment, and three patients required surgical treatment for a femoral pseudoaneurysm. The authors concluded that the inferior mid-term results compared to surgery warrant reservation of this technique for patients with high-risk characteristics and a limited life expectancy. Mid-term results from Mohamed et al. evaluated outcomes of 24 patients with "kissing stents" prospectively [73]. Special attention was given to the fate of the non-diseased limb in patients with unilateral proximal disease. Memotherm stents (Bard-Angiomed, Germany) comprised 35 of the stents placed, with a variety of other stents used for the other 20. They noted primary patency rates at 6, 12, and 24 months of 94, 81, and 58%, respectively. A total of 15 reinterventions were necessary in nine patients, three of those in asymptomatic limbs. Four limbs in three patients occluded during the follow-up period, none of which were in asymptomatic limbs. Two occlusions underwent cross-femoral bypass for treatment. The authors felt that the results justified stent placement in non-diseased limbs based on the absence of occlusions in those limbs at mid-term follow-up. Excellent results were reported by Mouanoutoua and others [74]. Fifty patients underwent "kissing stent" placement, 43 of them receiving balloon-expandable stents. Immediate technical success and clinical improvement was achieved in all patients, with 50% asymptomatic after the procedure. The authors reported one dissection (treated with extra stents) and two distal embolizations, along with three minor groin complications. After a mean follow-up of 20 months, primary patency was 92%, with a secondary patency of 100%.

A larger study of "kissing stent" placement has been reported by Bjorses et al. recently [75]. One hundred and seventy-three patients with lesions representing all Transatlantic Intersociety Consensus (TASC) classifications were treated, 50% of them TASC C or D lesions. A wide variety of stents were used, with 63% of cases including self-expanding stents. After a mean follow-up period of 36 months, 25% (43 patients) died, most commonly from cardiovascular disease. Ultimately, only 21 patients (12%) were available for long-term assessment. Primary patency at 36 and 60 months was 83 and 65%, respectively. Primary-assisted patency and secondary patency at 36 months was 90 and 95%, respectively, and decreased to 73 and 83% at 60 months, respectively. Major complications occurred in 3.5% of patients. The authors felt that their findings exhibited good patency at 3 years, regardless of the patient's TASC classification. Longer-term follow-up of this technique has been reported by Houston et al. [76]. A total of 43 patients underwent "kissing stent" placement with self-expanding stents (Memotherm or Wallstent) and follow-up was recorded over a 10-year period. Two-year primary- and secondary-assisted patencies of 89 and 93% were reported. The 5-year primary- and secondary-assisted patencies were 82 and 93%, respectively, while at 10 years they decreased to 68 and 86%, respectively. No limb loss was reported over the 10-year period. The authors again noted the high long-term mortality rate owing to progression of cardiovascular disease.

Femoropopliteal Stents

The need for adjuvants to improve femoropopliteal PTA may be more critical than in the iliac system. The initial success rate for femoropopliteal PTA averaged 80–98%, depending on the type of lesion and the experience and technical skill of the interventionalist [1, 3, 5, 7–9, 32, 77]. The 1-year patency rate was 36–80% [3, 5, 7, 8, 32]. At 5 years the results continued to show a gradual decline, with rates between 13 and 70% [3, 7, 8, 32, 77]. The variety of lesions treated (i.e., length, degree of stenosis) in addition to the variable methods of reporting results account for the wide variation in long-term results observed. Restenosis was a perplexing problem, obviously more common at this site as exemplified by the poorer long-term patency rates than in the larger iliac vessels [78, 79]. Total occlusions initially fared poorly [7, 9, 32]. Stents were considered a possible solution to these problems, especially given the increasing tendency to treat TASC C and D lesions in the femoropopliteal region.

Palmaz Stent

One of the first to evaluate femoropopliteal deployment of the Palmaz stent were Henry et al. [39]. They placed 188 stents in 126 patients. No arteries were primarily stented. In all, 63% of patients had a single stent, and a maximum of five stents was placed in one patient. The lesions were located in the common femoral artery (6 patients), the upper third of the SFA (19 patients), the middle third of the SFA (62 patients), the lower third of the SFA (29 patients), and the popliteal artery (10 patients). Immediate clinical success was achieved in 73 femoral artery stenoses (97%) and 8 popliteal stenoses (80%). Two distal emboli occurred after femoral recanalization and responded to thromboaspiration. Four patients developed stent thromboses within the first 24 h after stent placement, but flow was restored in all by fibrinolytic therapy. The average restenosis rate at 6 months increased as interventional procedures descended within the arterial system: upper femoral artery lesions (4%), middle femoral artery lesions (10%), lower femoral artery lesions (18%), and popliteal artery lesions (20%). The 4-year primary patency rates for femoropopliteal interventions were 80.0 ± 7.4% for stenotic disease and 39.0 ± 11.5% for occlusive disease. Repeat angioplasty improved the secondary patency rates to 94.0 ± 4.3% for stenotic lesions and 86.0 ± 6.7% for occlusive lesions. Henry et al. concluded that for lower SFA and popliteal lesions, and especially for total occlusions, the relative merits of stent placement may not compare favorably with other methods of treatment [39].

Chatelard et al. reviewed a series of 26 cases of stent deployment of SFA stenosis and nine cases of deployment for popliteal artery stenosis [80]. Their initial success rate of insertion was 100%; mean follow-up was 32 months. During the first 6 months after the procedure two patients developed acute thrombosis and five developed restenosis. Of note in this study is that the restenosis rates in the popliteal artery were not significantly greater than in the SFA. The extrapolated 4-year primary patency rate of 75.7 ± 8.0% is comparable to that noted by Henry et al. [39].

Bergeron and colleagues retrospectively analyzed a series of 55 Palmaz stents placed exclusively for SFA lesions in 39 patients. In contrast to other studies, most of the lesions (57%) were occlusions. Two acute thromboses (4.8%) developed within 48 h after the procedure; these particular patients had long segments of occlusion and poor run-off. At 2 years, the primary and secondary patencies were 77 and 89%, respectively [81]. Preprocedure occluded lesions were not statistically more likely to become restenotic when compared to preprocedure stenosis-only lesions.

Cejna and others performed a prospective randomized trial of PTA versus Palmaz stent placement in femoropopliteal lesions [82]. Over a 2-year follow-up period, 154 limbs in 141 patients were evaluated (77 limbs in each group). Immediate technical success was superior in the stent group (99 versus 84% in the PTA alone group). Clinical/hemodynamic success at 1 and 2 years was similar between the two groups (72 and 65%, respectively, in the PTA group versus 77 and

65%, respectively, in the stent group). Likewise, primary and secondary angiographic patency was similar at 1 and 2 years for both groups. Complications were evenly distributed between both groups, with a total of seven peripheral embolizations occurring. The authors did note three early (<24 h) stent thromboses compared to only one in the PTA group. Another more recent randomized study comparing selective stenting to primary stenting echoed these results with similar patency results in both groups [83]. Both groups concluded that routine stenting of the SFA is not justified, and stents should be placed only in patients with suboptimal angioplasty results. Balloon-expandable stents are generally not used in the SFA currently, as forces of external compression can lead to the stent being crushed.

Wallstent

The European Wallstent study analyzed the results of Wallstent placement for atherosclerotic narrowing of the femoral artery. Treatment of 4 stenotic and 10 occlusive femoral arteries were described in an early report from this experience [49]. Most of these patients were anticoagulated for 6 months with sodium warfarin. One acute thrombosis and two cases (14.3%) of distal emboli, which resolved on heparin therapy, were the observed procedural complications. Significant in-stent intimal hyperplasia occurred in three patients (21.4%) in less than 12 months and was most pronounced at the distal end of the stent.

Rousseau and colleagues reported a mid-term analysis of Wallstent deployment for the treatment of femoropopliteal stenosis [84]. Forty implants were performed, and follow-up in all cases was more than 6 months. A 12-month angiogram was performed in 32 cases. Oral anticoagulation (acenocoumarol) was utilized in the last nine cases for a 2-month period. Claudication (78%) was the most common presenting symptom. No stent migration or traumatic dissection during stent deployment was observed, and major collateral vessels crossed by the stent remained open. Nine thromboses occurred within the first month in the subset of patients not undergoing anticoagulation. Four restenoses (10% of cases) of more than 50% narrowing were observed 3–6 months after stent placement and were generally most pronounced at either end of the stent.

A Swiss paper reported on 15 femoropopliteal Wallstent placements; 11 were available for follow-up. Six occlusions occurred within the first month, and only six of the stents were patent at a mean of 20 months [55]. Even in these six, one to three secondary interventions were required for continued patency. Of the six patients available for angiography more than 3 months after stent placement, two had recurrent stenosis outside the stent with moderate in-stent hyperplasia (less than 40% reduction in stent diameter), two demonstrated severe in-stent intimal proliferation, and two others had moderate in-stent hyperplasia.

Sapoval et al. followed 21 patients prospectively who underwent femoropopliteal PTA followed by Wallstent insertion for a mean of 17.6 months with angiography, Doppler ultrasonography, and clinical examinations [85]. Nine occlusions occurred: four during the first 30 days and five during the first 1–5 months after PTA. Three patients developed intrastent intimal hyperplasia requiring additional percutaneous intervention. The 12-month patency rates were 49% (primary) and 67% (secondary). These authors believed that stenting did not decrease the rate of reocclusion after PTA alone and that its use may be indicated only for treatment of acute closure complicating PTA [85]. As part of the FDA phase II multicenter Wallstent trial, Martin et al. placed stents in the femoral systems of 90 patients [58]. The 6-month angiographic patency was 80%. The 1-year clinical patencies were 61% (primary) and 84% (secondary), and the 2-year patencies were 49% (primary) and 72% (secondary). Their results were comparable to those for femoral angioplasty use alone [58].

One investigator compared the results of primary Wallstent placement versus simple balloon angioplasty in the treatment of femoropopliteal artery occlusive disease [86]; there were 26 patients treated in each group. Warfarin therapy was substituted for aspirin (300 mg) and dipyridamole (25 mg b.i.d.) after three early occlusions occurred in the first 11 stent cases. Of 26 stented lesions, 5 (19%) occluded during the first 10 days. Eight others demonstrated severe neointimal hyperplasia within 12 months, and one occlusion at the distal end of a stent was noted. Taking into account 10 successful reinterventions, a secondary patency rate of 69% was reported. In the PTA-only group, there were six stenoses or occlusions within 6 months and four additional ones during the following 6 months.

No reintervention was undertaken, and the primary patency rate was therefore 65%.

Strecker Stent

The Strecker stent was thought sufficiently flexible to be used in this location, and 58 were deployed in one study [65]. At a mean follow-up at 19 months, there were 14 restenoses or reocclusions (29.2%). Within the first 6–9 months after deployment, intimal hyperplasia was generally the cause of arterial narrowing. Redilation was done successfully by PTA, but the problem recurred even more quickly (within 4–6 months). In 10 of the cases, several redilations were required to maintain a stable clinical condition. There were some problems with stent delivery in early cases, but no major complications requiring invasive procedures were reported. Two other studies identified important risks for restenosis: distal SFA or popliteal stent placement and an area of placement longer than 4 cm [66, 87].

Problems with restenosis after the use of the Strecker stent have taken an interesting twist in the treatment of SFA disease. In four early cases, endovascular irradiation with a surface dose of 12 cGy provided encouraging results in that all irradiated stents remained patent at short-term follow-ups [65]. Long-term follow-up (23–30 months) demonstrated no recurrent obstructions in these patients [88, 89]. A larger series ($n = 13$) is showing a similar freedom from restenosis as demonstrated by digital subtraction angiography and magnetic resonance angiography (MRA) with follow-up of 3–27 months [88, 89]. More recently, Schopohl et al. reviewed 6 years of experience with SFA restenosis following stent/intravascular brachytherapy with a 10-Ci ^{192}Ir source [90]. Stent length ranged from 5 to 16 cm. Of the 25 patients available with sufficient follow-up (range 8–71 months), 21 patients (84%) had patent-treated vessel segments [90].

Nitinol Stents

Early nitinol stent results were promising. In one study, SFA lesions (39 stenoses, 6 occlusions) and popliteal lesions (9 stenoses, 7 occlusions) were stented. The stent length was approximately 4 cm, and stent diameter varied from 5 to 8 mm. The respective primary and secondary patency rates at 18 months were 85 and 88%, respectively, for SFA lesions and 87 and 100%, respectively, for popliteal lesions. The 4.1% failure rate within 24 h was comparable to that in other studies [91].

Multiple studies have since validated the improved patency rates of nitinol self-expanding stents in the femoropopliteal segment. Schillinger et al. reported mid-term results of 104 patients randomized to undergo primary stenting in the SFA with nitinol stents (Dynalink or Absolute, Guidant Corp., Santa Clara, CA) or PTA with optional stenting [92]. They noted angiographic restenosis (>50% stenosis) rates of 24% for the nitinol stent group versus 43% for the PTA group at 6 months. Twelve-month follow-up with duplex US yielded restenosis rates of 37% for the stent group and 63% for the PTA group; 32% of patients in the PTA group required secondary stenting due to residual stenosis or dissection. These results were relatively sustained at 2 years in a follow-up study, with 45.7% restenosis noted in the primary stenting group versus 69.2% restenosis in the PTA group [93]. The authors also noted a lower reintervention rate in the primary stenting group. The Femoral Artery Stenting Trial (FAST) evaluated the use of the Bard Luminexx 3 stent (C. R. Bard, Inc., Murray Hill, NJ) in the SFA versus PTA alone with follow-up by duplex ultrasound at 1 year reported [94]. They found no difference between groups in terms of binary restenosis rates. Additionally noted in their study was the 12% rate of stent fractures, although the clinical impact of this was not determined. Ferreira and colleagues evaluated the use of the Zilver stent (Cook, Bloomington, IN) in the recanalized SFA in 74 limbs and carried follow-up out to 5 years with excellent results [95]. Primary patency by duplex ultrasound was 90, 78, 74, 69, and 69% at 1, 2, 3, 4, and 4.8 years, respectively. Assisted primary patency was 96, 90, 90, 90, and 90% at 1, 2, 3, 4, and 5 years, respectively. Ten restenoses (>50% stenosis) and six occlusions occurred, two of which were within the first 30 days; only one stent fracture was noted.

The new Supera stent is a wire-interwoven nitinol self-expanding stent which combines features of increased radial force, more flexibility, and is fracture resistant by ex vivo testing. This stent has not yet undergone clinical testing. However, based on the aforementioned properties, the stent has the potential to fill a need or patients with SFA disease.

The application of drug-eluting stents has been tested in the SFA segment with interesting results. The Sirolimus-Coated Cordis Self-expandable Stent (SIROCCO) I and II trials evaluated a sirolimus-eluting SMART stent (Cordis) versus a bare nitinol stent in the SFA, with a hypothesis that the anti-inflammatory and antiproliferative effects of the sirolimus would improve restenosis rates in the SFA [96–98]. Both trials revealed no statistical difference between the drug-eluting stents and the bare nitinol stents in terms of restenosis rates, though the drug-eluting stents did fare slightly better. Possibly the most interesting finding from these studies was the relatively low rate of restenosis in the bare nitinol stents, with 21.9% restenosis seen at 24 months.

Interest has been generated in the use of a covered stent graft in the femoropopliteal segment based on the potential to minimize myointimal ingrowth at the site of treatment, which was realized by the Viabahn stent graft (W. L. Gore, Inc., Flagstaff, AZ), a flexible nitinol stent with a PTFE covering. Early studies with the Hemobahn stent graft (later changed to Viabahn after a change in the delivery system) showed promising mid-term results, with primary, primary-assisted, and secondary patency rates at 74.1, 80.3, and 83.2%, respectively, at 24 months noted in a study on 52 patients [99]. A small, prospective, randomized comparison trial between the Hemobahn and the PTA alone showed markedly improved patency and clinical outcomes at 2 years [100]. The full multicenter results of this same approval trial were recently released [101]. A total of 244 limbs in 241 patients were randomized to a stent graft group or PTA alone and treated over an 18-month period. Technical success was achieved in 95% of stent graft cases and only 66% of PTA-only cases. Target vessel patency at 1 year by Doppler ultrasound was 65% in the stent graft group versus 40% in the PTA alone group. Additionally, the authors found a patency benefit for lesions 3 cm long or more. Hartung and colleagues published two studies evaluating the patient characteristics that might affect outcomes with Viabahn stent placement. They found no difference in patency of the Viabahn stent in claudicants with good run-off versus chronic limb ischemia patients with bad run-off [102]. TASC D lesions were excluded in this study, and a significant number of outflow treatments were performed in the chronic limb ischemia group. A later publication by the same group expanded the previous study group to include TASC D lesions and showed a significant difference in long-term patency between TASC C and D lesions, with overall primary and secondary patency rates of 71 and 79% at 3 years [103].

Kedora and colleagues performed a randomized, prospective trial comparing the Viabahn stent graft to prosthetic femoral-popliteal bypass grafts [104]. Fifty limbs were treated in each group. During the mean follow-up period of 18 months, 13 stent grafts and 10 prosthetic bypass grafts thrombosed. Six of the thrombosed stent grafts ultimately required surgical bypass. Stent graft primary patency at 3, 6, 9, and 12 months was 84, 82, 75.6, and 73.5%, respectively. Surgical bypass graft primary patency at the same intervals was 90, 81.8, 79.7, and 74.2%, respectively. Secondary patency at 12 months was 83.7% for the stent graft group versus 83.9% for the surgical bypass group. Limb salvage at 12 months was similar between groups at 98% for the stent graft group and 89.6% for the prosthetic bypass group. Wound complication rates were similar between groups as well. The authors concluded that the two treatment methods were comparable in terms of efficacy in treating femoropopliteal disease.

Long-term results of Viabahn stent grafts have even been reported. Saxon and others treated 87 limbs with the Viabahn during 8-year period and reported results of a 4-year follow-up [105]. Three occlusions occurred during the first 30 days, one of which was immediately after placement. Patency of the target vessel was assessed by Doppler examination. The 1-year primary, primary-assisted, and secondary target vessel patency rates were 76, 87, and 93%, respectively. The 4-year respective patency rates were 55, 67, and 79%. Notably, 1-year primary patency rates were actually higher for lesions longer than 12 cm than for those less than 12 cm. The authors also found that device size greater than 6 mm and placement isolated to the SFA-improved primary patency.

Another application for the Viabahn stent graft has been treatment of popliteal aneurysms. Long-term results have not been widely published, but early and mid-term results appear to be promising. Mohan and colleagues published mid-term results of the use of several stent graft devices, including the Hemobahn, to repair 30 popliteal artery aneurysms in 25 patients [106]. Follow-up to 36 months demonstrated primary patency rates by duplex US of 92.9, 84.7, 80, 74.5, and 74.5% at 1, 6, 12, 24, and 36 months, respectively.

Respective secondary patency at the same intervals was 96.5, 88.7, 88.7, 83.2, and 83.2%. Two type II endoleaks (one early, one late) were observed, and one type I endoleak was observed and resolved spontaneously. Antonello et al. compared results with the Hemobahn and open surgery in a prospective randomized trial on asymptomatic popliteal aneurysms [107]. Fifteen patients were enrolled in each group and were followed with duplex ultrasound. They found comparable results between the therapies, with 100% primary patency in the operative group versus 86.7% in the stent graft treatment group at 12 months. Secondary patency of the stent graft was 100% at 36 months versus 90.9% in the operative group. No statistical differences were seen between the two groups in terms of patency, but the operative time was significantly longer and the mean hospital length of stay was significantly shorter in the stent graft group. One endograft thrombosis was noted in the early postoperative period (the day after the procedure). Several other series exist with small numbers of patients treated and reasonable results achieved [108–110]. More data will need to be obtained to determine the durability of this approach, but it appears to be a reasonable alternative to surgery, especially in patient populations with substantial comorbidities prohibitive of an open operative approach. In addition, the new heparin-bonded Viabahn stent graft has been increasingly used for SFA interventions and has the potential for increased patency rates.

Infrapopliteal Stents

Although multiple studies have reported the value of infrapopliteal angioplasty for limb salvage, little data exists to support the use of infrapopliteal stents at this time [111–114]. Small-diameter stents used in the infragenicular arteries were previously coronary balloon-expandable or self-expanding stents placed for balloon angioplasty failure. One such study evaluating the use of coronary stents of multiple types placed empirically in infragenicular lesions yielded initial technical success rates of 94% and limb salvage rates of 96% in treated patients with critical limb ischemia [115]. No major clinical adverse events occurred as a result of the procedures.

A new self-expanding nitinol stent has been developed for use in infrapopliteal arteries (Xpert stent, Abbott Vascular, San Francisco, CA) and a limited amount of data suggests its feasibility. Tepe et al. reported data on a series of 18 patients receiving 24 stents in 21 lesions in infragenicular arteries [116]. The stents were placed for PTA failure in limb salvage patients (most patients had foot ulcerations). The investigators had 100% initial technical success with no adverse events. At 6-month follow-up, two patients had died and five more were lost to follow-up. Overall, 14 stented segments were evaluated at 6 months, with three occluded and one >50% restenosis at that time. The remaining 10 stents were widely patent based on duplex ultrasound or angiogram evaluation. The clinical results (ulcer healing) were not reported in the study.

Kickuth and colleagues evaluated the use of the Xpert stent in the distal popliteal and tibioperoneal arteries [117]. Technical success was 100% in the 35 patients, and primary cumulative patency was 82% at 6 months. Follow-up was largely via noninvasive imaging to determine stent patency. The authors did note 80% sustained clinical benefit and 100% freedom of major amputation at 6 months, though the patient population was comprised of 54% claudicants. There was a major complication rate of 17% reported, with three patient deaths occurring >30 days after the procedure.

Peregrin et al. reported a prospective study of Xpert stent placement in patients with failed PTA of the infrapopliteal arteries and compared the results to patients undergoing successful PTA alone [118]; 23 stents were placed in 16 arteries with 100% immediate technical success. PTA alone was successful in 54 arteries. At 12 months follow-up with Doppler ultrasound, patency in the PTA alone group was 82% while patency in the stent group was 78%. The authors determined that stent placement was a reasonable means of converting a technical failure to success in the treatment of patients with chronic critical limb ischemia.

A report even exists relating the placement of a bare metal coronary stent in the dorsalis pedis artery of two patients with chronic limb ischemia and nonhealing foot ulcers [119]. Both stents were placed for angioplasty failure, and a good angiographic and clinical result was achieved in both patients. The authors reported ulcer healing and symptomatic relief in both patients at the reported follow-up intervals (3 months in one patient and 12 months in the other patient).

In addition to the above studies, evaluation of drug-eluting stents has been performed in the infrapopliteal arteries. Small studies using sirolimus- or paclitaxel-eluting stents have been published, showing reasonable safety and efficacy for both, but with a higher restenosis and reintervention rate for the paclitaxel-eluting stents [120, 121]. The authors noted several differences in the modes of action for the drugs which could contribute to the differences in restenosis patterns, and further data will need to be accumulated on drug-eluting stents in this region to determine their utility [121]. Carbofilm-coated and even absorbable stents have gained some attention in the infrapopliteal arteries as well based on their success in the coronary circulation, with early short-term results suggesting their feasibility [122, 123].

Visceral Artery Stents

Elective surgical treatment of chronic visceral ischemia, by bypass or endarterectomy, is associated with significant morbidity and mortality [124, 125]. PTA and stenting is a potentially lower-risk alternative and has received more attention over recent years (Fig. 17.10).

Sharafuddin and colleagues stented 26 stenotic or occluded mesenteric vessels in 25 patients [126]. The majority of the stents were balloon-expandable (Palmaz-Corinthian; Cordis; Miami, FL). They achieved immediate technical and clinical success in 96 and 88%, respectively. After a mean clinical follow-up of 15 months, sustained clinical benefit was seen in 83%, with a primary-assisted clinical benefit seen in 92%. Five deaths occurred, four of which were related to cardiopulmonary causes. The authors concluded that selective use of endovascular treatment for chronic mesenteric ischemia is reasonable, though larger comparison studies are needed to better characterize the role of the endovascular approach in this disease process.

A recent study included treatment of occluded mesenteric vessels in its findings [127]. They found equivalent patency results with treatment of occluded vessels when compared to treatment of stenotic vessels. Balloon-expandable stents were used in 80 vessels and self-expandable stents were placed in seven vessels in 65 total patients. Eighteen patients (28%) had occluded vessels treated with 1-year primary patency rates similar to that of stenotic vessels treated (63 versus 70%, respectively). Overall 1-year patency rates were primary patency 65%, primary-assisted patency 97%, and secondary patency 99%. No differences in patency were noted between vessel types or size, number of stents placed, or number of vessels treated in each patient. Overall morbidity was 30.8%, with 15.4% related to access site complications. In-hospital and 30-day mortality rate was 7.7%, with three deaths related to bowel ischemia and subsequent multisystem organ failure. Immediate symptom relief occurred in 85% of patients with 75% showing maintained symptom relief after 1 year. The authors noted higher reintervention rates in patients with chronic obstructive pulmonary disease (COPD) or those in which femoral access was used for the procedure.

The current literature includes several comparisons between endovascular and open revascularization for mesenteric ischemia. Kasirajan et al. reported results of 28 patients (32 vessels) who underwent endovascular intervention for treatment of chronic mesenteric ischemia [128]. These results were compared with their own results from a previously published series of open revascularizations on 85 patients (130 vessels). They performed angioplasty and stenting in 23 of the 28 patients with endovascular interventions. Of 26 stents placed, 23 were balloon-expandable, with the remainder self-expanding stents. They found no significant difference between the two groups in terms of morbidity, death, or recurrent stenosis. Stented patients did, however, exhibit a significantly higher incidence of recurrent symptoms. The authors concluded that patients fit for open surgery would benefit from this long-term over percutaneous angioplasty and stenting. A retrospective study by Sivamurthy and others also compared open and endovascular therapy for chronic mesenteric ischemia [129]. Sixty patients were identified over a 14-year period, with 19 undergoing an endovascular procedure for treatment. Two or more vessels were revascularized in 22 patients in the open group versus 2 in the endovascular group. Immediate technical success was 95.3% in the endovascular group versus 100% in the open group. Seventeen percent of patients in the open group had graft occlusions within 30 days. Patency at 6 months was similar between the

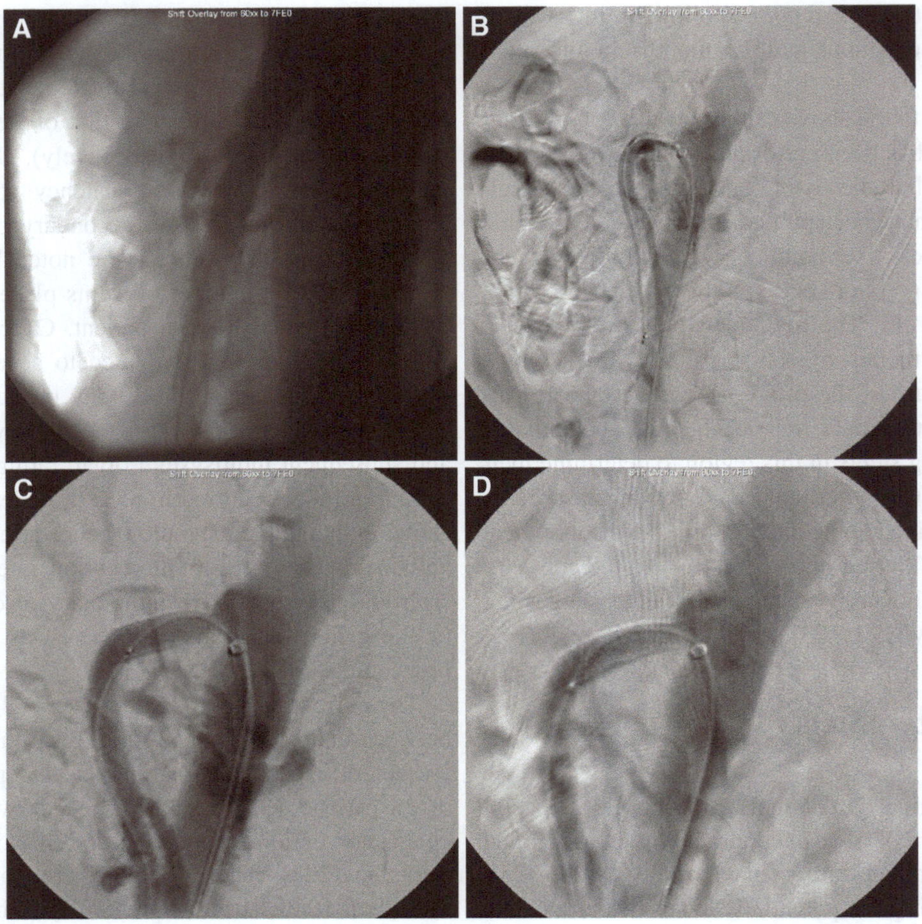

Fig. 17.10 This patient presented with postprandial pain and 20 lb weight loss over several months. **a**, Abdominal aortography revealed occlusion of the celiac artery and approximately 80% stenosis of the SMA. **b**, The SMA was cannulated with a SOS Omni catheter via right CFA access. **c**, A 6 × 17 mm balloon-expandable Express stent was placed and repeat arteriography revealed a residual stenosis proximal to the stent. **d**, A second 6 × 17 mm Express stent was placed proximal to and overlapping the previous stent, with repeat arteriography showing minimal residual stenosis. The patient remains symptom-free with widely patent stents at 1 year by duplex ultrasound and CT angiography

groups (83% for open, 68% for endovascular). Major morbidity rates were significantly higher in the open group, at 46 versus 19% in the endovascular group. No significant difference was found in 30-day mortality or cumulative survival at 3 years (15 and 62%, respectively, for open; 21 and 63%, respectively, for endovascular). Postoperative length of stay and freedom from symptom recurrence were however significantly higher in the open group. Median length of stay was 23 days for open patients as opposed to 1 day for the endovascular patients. Freedom from symptom recurrence was 68 and 59% at 1 and 2 years, respectively, for the open group. Only 27 and 20% of endovascular patients were symptom-free at 1 and 2 years, respectively. While somewhat lower symptomatic benefits were observed than those noted in previous studies [125], the authors demonstrated a clear separation between the groups in terms of a functional result. The authors concluded that while endovascular treatment offers a decreased hospital stay and morbidity with equivalent survival and patency rates as compared to open surgery, it has greater symptom recurrence and restenosis rates. They again felt that endovascular treatment should be reserved for patients not suitable for open procedures. An even more recent study yielded similar comparative results in terms of symptom recurrence between patients with operative or endovascular treatment for chronic mesenteric ischemia [130]. In-hospital major morbidity and mortality were also similar. Angioplasty and stenting of the mesenteric arteries was, however, associated with a lower primary and primary-assisted patency (58 and 65%, respectively) than operative intervention (90 and 96%, respectively) over a mean 15-month follow-up in the stent group and a mean 42-month follow-up in the open group. The authors included multiple (39%) patients with concurrent aortic revascularization procedures in their open surgical group. The authors notably had a somewhat higher complication rate in their endovascular group than the majority of the literature (29%) and a higher symptom recurrence rate in the open group than much of the literature.

Overall, the comparison data appears to reveal early benefits to endovascular treatment of CMI over open surgical treatment, but those results are ultimately diminished by the decreased long-term durability of angioplasty and stent placement. Most authors appear to agree that selective use of mesenteric stenting should be applied to patients with respect to their comorbidities and suitability for invasive surgical procedures. Large, prospective, randomized trials are unlikely to be performed due to the relative rarity of this problem. Accumulation of more data may assist in stratifying patients that will achieve benefit from mesenteric stenting.

Infectious Complications

Infectious complications are poorly reported in the literature, relegated solely to case reports due to their infrequency. A recent review of the literature summarizes the entire published experience with this entity [131]. Infection at the site of Palmaz iliac stent placement, as reported anecdotally in the current literature, can have devastating consequences including multisystem organ failure and death [132–135]. In four cases reviewed, patients manifested infectious complications within 10 days of stent placement. In two cases the infection appeared to complicate a pseudoaneurysm [132, 133]. All patients required stent removal and extra-anatomic bypass. Stent cultures grew *Staphylococcus aureus* most commonly [133–135], and a *Staphylococcus epidermidis* infection has been reported [134].

Animal studies have been performed to evaluate stent infectability in the face of a bacterial challenge. Three different studies were performed by the same group on swine models using Palmaz stents and a *S. aureus* infusion. One study involved a bacterial load immediately after stent placement and revealed 80% culture-positive stents at 3 days and 60% culture-positive stents at 3 weeks [136]. Another study featured a bacterial challenge at 4 weeks after stent placement, killing the animals 3 days later. Fifty percent of the stents placed were culture-positive [137]. Yet another study utilized prophylactic cefazolin prior to bacterial challenge at the time of stent placement and at 4 weeks after stent placement. An additional group of swine had a bacterial challenge at 3 months without prophylaxis. Stent infection rate was 17% in the prophylaxis group and 70% in the group without prophylaxis at the time of stent placement. The infection rate was 10% in the prophylaxis group versus 50% in the non-prophylaxis group in the 1-month challenge. The group challenged with bacteria at 3 months showed only 1 of 15 patent stents with evidence of infection [138]. The authors concluded that antibiotic prophylaxis is useful at the time of the procedure and at times of potential bacteremia in order to reduce the risk of stent infection. They felt stent infection rates decreased over time during times of bacteremia due to incorporation of the stent into the arterial wall. Also noted in the studies was the significant inflammatory response of the surrounding arteries of the infected stents and the high rate of thrombosis of the infected stents.

To date, there have been no randomized prospective trials to evaluate the efficacy of antibiotic prophylaxis during stent placement. Some groups do recommend use of prophylaxis before deployment and consider antibiotics while indwelling/intravascular sheaths/catheters are in place or around the time of a prolonged urokinase infusion [135].

Comments

Stents have been designed to improve the results of PTA, especially concentrating on perceived problem areas. One can, therefore, expect the complication rate of stenting to be that associated with PTA plus any problems associated with the more frequent catheter exchanges required and the deployment of the stent. In general, this translates into a procedural mortality of 0–4% and complication rate of 5–20%, depending on the indication for stent placement [35, 40, 48, 53].

The indications for stent deployment have been adequately enumerated in the text, but the contraindications have not been mentioned. Patients who are not considered candidates are usually refused stent therapy because of the possibility of doing harm. Vessel rupture after PTA may be made worse by stenting open the defect, as it is known that branches originating from major vessels often stay open after a stent has been placed across them, though covered stents can exclude the area of rupture successfully. The design stiffness of the Palmaz and possibly the Gianturco stent makes them less than ideal for use in tortuous vessels. The entrance vessel must be of sufficient diameter to allow sheath placement; otherwise, there is significant damage to the luminal surface of the vessel. Aneurysmal disease is considered a relative contraindication to stent placement for occlusive disease because of the risk of rupture, thrombus, or embolus. However, stent grafts are increasingly being used to treat the aneurysmal disease itself. The risk of embolization must be weighed against the potential benefits of recanalization when treating long occlusions. Finally, calcified lesions not amenable to dilation at the pressures used for PTA should not be expected to be treated with a stent, because the basic technique requires a similar physical force to be applied to the atherosclerotic lesion.

The following generalizations on the placement of stents for treatment of patients with peripheral vascular arterial disease must be prefaced with the following comment. Now, many years after the introduction of stents to this field, overall patient numbers remain small. Furthermore, there are still concerns that the follow-up at 5 years and especially at 10 years seldom involves sufficient patients to provide meaningful long-term results. The reported data are increasing and suggest that stenting is a viable option, especially in high-risk patients. It is difficult to determine the long-term results of stents at this time, as there are few 10+-year studies even in the iliac system. Additionally, the overall mortality rate of patients with peripheral vascular disease is so high that many patients do not live long enough to achieve follow-up at 10+ years. The data do suggest that long and more complex lesions seem to have a shorter duration of patency and a higher rate of reintervention, regardless of the vascular bed. Technological improvements in stents may also continue to increase patency rates positively. Thus, the status of peripheral stents will continue to evolve and placement will often depend on patient and lesion characteristics.

A variety of stents have been found useful for salvage of unsuccessful iliac PTA. Because complications of PTA leave unresolved pressure gradients or unacceptable degrees of stenosis on the angiogram, the resolution of these deficiencies by stent placement has improved the early technical success of PTA to more than 90% in such cases [35, 48–50, 53–55, 64]. Even with the 1 mm or more intimal hyperplasia likely to be noted on the intraluminal surface of these stents, the occurrence of significant restenosis (50% or more diameter reduction) is quite low (about 5% at 12 months) [35, 48, 50, 64, 65]. The occurrence of progressive atherosclerotic disease distant to the stent may be of more concern (about 5% per year) [35, 48] and may help to explain the approximately 85% 2-year and 70% 4-year clinical benefit rates reported [35, 48]. These data rival overall PTA results in a markedly disadvantaged group of patients. Therefore, if one is willing to accept PTA as a good treatment for isolated iliac occlusive disease, stent use for iliac PTA salvage should also be deemed appropriate. The data is somewhat conflicted in regards to primary stent placement in the iliac system, though many have adopted this in clinical practice.

Totally occluded iliac arteries are a problem for standard PTA. The use of stents has improved the success rate to about 80% at 3 years, with a late occlusion rate no different than that for treatment of stenotic lesions [40, 48]. The problem with distal emboli after this type of intervention has not been completely solved, as the embolic rate remains 5–20% [40, 48, 53]. Operative exposure for the treatment of these lesions may help solve this problem [40].

Primary stenting of iliac lesions based on theoretic advantages is reasonable and is championed by multiple investigators [46, 139]. A 5-year angiographic patency of 93.6% would rival aortic surgical constructions and therefore would be worthwhile; however, it is yet unproven in the literature. Others have suggested reasonable patency rates in the iliac system with PTA and selective stenting practices [47, 139]. Better defining those patients not optimally served by PTA alone should be more cost-effective. Multiple studies have suggested that disease of the ipsilateral SFA and overall run-off may affect patency rates of selective stenting [139–143]. Additional studies have even demonstrated reduced primary patency rates in women as compared to men [142–148]. The literature also increasingly suggests that primary stenting is more beneficial in longer lesions (TASC C and D) [139, 149, 150]. Approximately 65% of patients are served well for 5 years without a stent; the additional risk, intravascular hardware, and cost to improve the results in only one-third of patients seem excessive. A cost-effectiveness analysis has been done and concluded that PTA with selective stent placement is more cost-effective than either PTA alone or primary stenting [151]. Sullivan et al. identified patency of the SFA as the most important variable associated with both early and late success of primary iliac artery stent placement. Those patients with infrainguinal disease may be best served with immediate distal reconstruction because they are not likely to derive significant benefit from iliac stenting alone [43].

As the diameter of the artery decreases, so does the long-term success of PTA. Stent deployment in the femoral artery was undertaken to improve long-term patency (i.e., prevent restenosis). Even with stringent anticoagulation regimens, it has not accomplished this goal. Significant intimal hyperplasia, often occurring within the first 12 months after deployment, has been demonstrated in more than 20% of cases [49, 55, 65, 84] if one eliminates the 20–40% rate of early occlusive events [55, 86]. In a prospective study comparing stent use to simple PTA, comparable patency rates could be obtained only after extensive reinterventions in the stent group [86]. Proper anticoagulation to decrease early thrombosis and some method of controlling intimal hyperplasia may be required to salvage stent use at this site [49, 65, 84, 88, 89]. There are data to suggest that the larger diameter proximal SFA fares better than the smaller diameter distal SFA and popliteal artery, but even so the clinical utility is questionable [66, 87]. Some investigators [78, 87] have postulated that in patients with long-segment SFA disease (15 cm or more) poorer patency rates may be secondary to incomplete apposition of the stent(s) to the vessel wall, a small postdeployment luminal diameter, or decreasing flow velocity through the SFA. Moreover, intrinsic stent characteristics, including composition and thrombogenicity, may promote myointimal hyperplasia, restenosis, and thrombosis. Given the tendency to develop restenosis and require reintervention in the femoropopliteal segment, it seems reasonable to place stents selectively there for angioplasty failures only.

The use of stents in the mesenteric arteries is increasing, though data remains relatively scarce and limited to small series. As chronic mesenteric ischemia is often seen in elderly patients with multiple comorbidities, stenting appears to be a good treatment option if an operation would be poorly tolerated. Likewise, interest in infrapopliteal stenting is increasing. Given the small diameter of the vessels in this area, it is difficult to expect long-term patencies to approach those of distal bypass grafts with reversed saphenous vein. The opportunity exists, however, to achieve good limb salvage results in patients with critical limb ischemia while minimizing morbidity in this generally unhealthy population. Further advancement in stent designs may augment long-term patency rates in this area. Vigilant surveillance protocols will likely be critical in maintaining patency in the tibial arteries, regardless of whether PTA or stent placement is used.

The guidelines defined by the FDA phase II multicenter Wallstent trial called for 6 months of warfarin therapy to maintain the prothrombin time at 1.5 times control, but currently the need for long-term anticoagulation for femoropopliteal stent deployment is challenged. In a nonrandomized retrospective study, White et al. reported acceptable early and intermediate patency rates without the need for long-term anticoagulation [79]. One criticism of this study was the failure to provide a group of patients for comparison. Also, the segment length targeted for stent deployment was relatively short, at 2.7 cm.

Potential areas of investigation to improve stent results have been reviewed by Palmaz [17]. Better methods to manage the inherent thrombogenicity of the stent are critical, especially in small-diameter arteries [16, 17, 19]. Inhibiting unwanted tissue proliferation is an active area of research critical not only to this device but to essentially all vascular interventions [16, 17, 61, 88, 89, 152, 153]. Eliminating the offending device might be an alternate approach; the use of absorbable materials or stent removal when the job at hand is accomplished are two options [16–18]. Until more work is accomplished in these areas, the use of stents will be confined to large-diameter vessels (probably more than 6 mm in diameter) and to cases of PTA salvage where the risk/benefit ratio of the procedure favors stent use.

It remains to be seen how often endoprosthesis infection occurs. Catastrophic complications may be prevented by the use of prophylactic antibiotics, especially when stent deployment is via the femoral route [135]. Though no randomized prospective study exists to prove its benefit, many practitioners use routine antibiotic prophylaxis in endovascular procedures. A French group assessed all stent infections for elective revascularization of the lower limbs from 1985 to 1994. Based on their cost- analysis data, they concluded that a reasonable site-specific indication for using antibiotic-impregnated stents would be femorotibial disease [154].

Summary

One should not view this summary of stent results as a condemnation of the procedure. In fact, stents have had reasonable success in providing a scaffold to maintain arterial structure and patency. Rather, it is hoped that the review brings into perspective the data available, highlights areas of concern, and provides a basis for further research to determine the appropriate lesions and patients for the use of stents. Further modification of the design materials used, coverings on the stents, improved methods of deployment, and adjuvant medical therapy will likely propel newer stent designs into an even more favorable clinical light.

References

1. Becker GJ, Katzen BT, Dake MD: Noncoronary angioplasty, *Radiology* 170:921–940, 1989.
2. Glover JL, Bendick PJ, Dilley RS et al.: Efficacy of balloon catheter dilation for lower extremity atherosclerosis, *Surgery* 91:560–565, 1982.
3. Wilson SE, Wolf GL, Cross AP: Percutaneous transluminal angioplasty versus operation for peripheral arteriosclerosis, *J Vasc Surg* 9:1–9, 1989.
4. Dotter CT: Transluminally-placed coil spring endarterial tube grafts, *Invest Radiol* 4:329–332, 1969.
5. Spence RK, Frieman DB, Gatenby R et al.: Long-term results of transluminal angioplasty of the iliac and femoral arteries, *Arch Surg* 116:1377–1386, 1981.
6. Lu C, Zarins CK, Yang C et al.: Percutaneous transluminal angioplasty for limb salvage, *Radiology* 142:337–341, 1982.
7. Johnston KW, Rae M, Hogg-Johnston SA et al.: Five-year results of a prospective study of per-cutaneous transluminal angioplasty, *Ann Surg* 4:403–413, 1987.
8. Stokes KR, Strunk HM, Campbell DR et al.: Five-year results of iliac and femoropopliteal angioplasty in diabetic patients, *Radiology* 174:977–982, 1990.
9. Cambria RP, Faust G, Gusberg R et al.: Percutaneous angioplasty for peripheral arterial occlusive disease, *Arch Surg* 122:238–287, 1987.
10. Simpsom JB, Selmon MR, Robertson GC et al.: Transluminal atherectomy for occlusive peripheral vascular disease, *Am J Cardiol* 61:96G–101G, 1988.
11. Colapinto RF, Stronell RD, Johnston WK: Transluminal angioplasty of complete iliac obstructions, *AJR* 146:859–862, 1986.
12. Andros G: Interventional technology: intraoperative strategies and techniques. In Yao JST, Pearce WH, editors: *Technologies in vascular surgery*, Philadelphia, 1992, Saunders, pp. 412–423.
13. Cragg AH, Lund G, Rysavy JA et al.: Percutaneous arterial grafting, *Radiology* 150:45–49, 1984.
14. Maass D, Zollikofer CL, Largiader F et al.: Radiological follow-up of transluminally-inserted vascular endoprostheses: an experimental study using expanding spirals, *Radiology* 152:659–663, 1984.
15. Wright KC, Wallace S, Charnasangavej C et al.: Percutaneous endovascular stents: an experimental evaluation, *Radiology* 156:69–72, 1985.
16. DeJaegere PP, de Feyter PJ: Endovascular stents: preliminary clinical results and future developments, *Clin Cardiol* 16:369–378, 1993.
17. Palmaz JC: Intravascular stents: tissue-stent interactions and design considerations, *AJR* 160:613–618, 1993.
18. Irie T, Furui S, Yamauchi T et al.: Relocatable Gianturco expandable metallic stents, *Radiology* 178:575–578, 1991.
19. Dichek DA, Neville RF, Zwiebel JA et al.: Seeding of intravascular stents with genetically engineered endothelial cells, *Circulation* 80:1347–1355, 1989.
20. Palmaz JC, Windeler SA, Garcia F et al.: Atherosclerotic rabbit aortas: expandable intraluminal grafting, *Radiology* 160:723–726, 1986.
21. Rousseau H, Joffre F, Raillat C et al.: Self-expanding endovascular stent in experimental atherosclerosis, *Radiology* 170:773–778, 1989.
22. Vorwerk D, Redha F, Neuerburg J et al.: Neointima formation following arterial placement of self-expanding stents of different radial force: experimental results, *Cardiovasc Intervent Radiol* 17:27–32, 1994.
23. Duprat G Jr, Wright KC, Charnsangavej C et al.: Flexible balloon-expanded stent for small vessels, *Radiology* 162:276–278, 1987.
24. Hallisey MJ, Meranze SG, Parker BC et al.: Percutaneous transluminal angioplasty of the abdominal aorta, *J Vasc Interv Radiol* 5:679–687, 1994.
25. Sheeran SR, Hallisey MJ, Ferguson D: Percutaneous stent placement in the abdominal aorta, *J Vasc Interv Radiol* 8:55–60, 1997.
26. Schedel H, Wissgott C, Rademaker J et al.: Primary stent placement for infrarenal aortic stenosis: immediate and midterm results, *J Vasc Interv Radiol* 15:353–359, 2004.
27. Poncyljusz W, Falkowski A, Garncarek J et al.: Primary stenting in the treatment of focal atherosclerotic abdominal aortic stenoses, *Clin Radiol* 61:691–695, 2006.
28. Simons PCG, Nawijn AA, Bruijninckx CMA et al.: Long-term results of primary stent placement to treat infrarenal

aortic stenosis, *Eur J Vasc Endovasc Surg* 32:627–633, 2006.
29. Klonaris C, Katsargyris A, Tsekouras N et al.: Primary stenting for aortic lesions: from single stenoses to total aortoiliac occlusions, *J Vasc Surg* 47:310–317, 2008.
30. Kadir S, White RI, Kaufman SL et al.: Long-term results of aortoiliac angioplasty, *Surgery* 94:10–14, 1983.
31. Walden R, Siegel Y, Rubinstein ZJ et al.: Percutaneous transluminal angioplasty, *J Vasc Surg* 3:583–590, 1986.
32. Gallino A, Mahler F, Probst P et al.: Percutaneous transluminal angioplasty of the arteries of the lower limbs: a 5-year follow-up, *Circulation* 4:619–623, 1984.
33. Palmaz JC, Richter GM, Noeldge G et al.: Intraluminal stents in atherosclerotic iliac artery stenosis: preliminary report of a multicenter study, *Radiology* 168:727–731, 1988.
34. Palmaz JC, Garcia OJ, Schatz RA et al.: Placement of balloon-expandable intraluminal stents in iliac arteries: first 171 procedures, *Radiology* 174:969–975, 1990.
35. Palmaz JC, Laborde JC, Rivera FJ et al.: Stenting of the iliac arteries with the Palmaz stent: experience from a multicenter trial, *Cardiovasc Intervent Radiol* 15:291–297, 1992.
36. Dalsing MC, Ehrman KO, Cikrit DF et al.: Iliac artery angioplasty and stents: a current experience. In Yao JST, Pearce WH, editors: *Technologies in vascular surgery*, Philadelphia, 1992, Saunders, pp. 373–387.
37. Wolf YG, Schatz RA, Knowles HJ et al.: Initial experience with the Palmaz stent for aortoiliac stenoses, *Ann Vasc Surg* 7:254–261, 1993.
38. Murphy KD, Encarnacion CE, Le VA et al.: Iliac artery stent placement with the Palmaz stent: follow-up study, *J Vasc Interv Radiol* 6:321–329, 1995.
39. Henry M, Amor M, Ethevenot G et al.: Palmaz stent placement in iliac and femoropopliteal arteries: primary and secondary patency in 310 patients with 2–4-year follow-up, *Radiology* 197:167–174, 1995.
40. Rees CR, Palmaz JC, Garcia O et al.: Angioplasty and stenting of completely occluded iliac arteries, *Radiology* 172:953–959, 1989.
41. Giles H, Lesar C, Erdoes L et al.: Balloon-expandable covered stent therapy of complex endovascular pathology, *Ann Vasc Surg* 22:762–768, 2008.
42. Scheinert D, Schroder M, Ludwig J et al.: Stent-supported recanalization of chronic iliac artery occlusions, *Am J Med* 110:708–715, 2001.
43. Sullivan TM, Childs MB, Bacharach JM et al.: Percutaneous transluminal angioplasty and primary stenting of the iliac arteries in 288 patients, *J Vasc Surg* 25:829–839, 1997.
44. Bonn J, Gardiner GA, Shapiro MJ et al.: Palmaz vascular stent: initial clinical experience, *Radiology* 174:741–745, 1990.
45. Williams JB, Watts PW, Nguyen VA et al.: Balloon angioplasty with intraluminal stenting as the initial treatment modality in aortoiliac occlusive disease, *Am J Surg* 168:202–204, 1994.
46. Richter GM, Roeren T, Brado M et al.: Results of randomized trial of PTA vs. primary stenting, *Radiology* 180:105, 1991.
47. Klein WM, van der Graaf Y, Seegers J et al.: Dutch Iliac Stent Trial: long-term results in patients randomized for primary or selective stent placement, *Radiology* 238:734–744, 2006.
48. Vorwerk D, Gunther RW: Stent placement in iliac arterial lesions: three years of clinical experience with the Wallstent, *Cardiovasc Intervent Radiol* 15:285–290, 1992.
49. Gunther RW, Vorwerk D, Bohndorf K et al.: Iliac and femoral artery stenoses and occlusions: treatment with intravascular stents, *Radiology* 172:725–730, 1989.
50. Gunther RW, Vorwerk D, Antonucci F et al.: Iliac artery stenosis or obstruction after unsuccessful balloon angioplasty: treatment with a self-expandable stent, *AJR* 156:389–393, 1991.
51. Hausegger KA, Lammer J, Fluckiger F et al.: Iliac artery stenting-clinical experience with the Palmaz stent, the Wallstent, and the Strecker stent, *Acta Radiol* 33:292–296, 1992.
52. Vowerk D, Gunther RW, Wendt G et al.: Ulcerated plaques and focal aneurysms of iliac arteries: treatment with noncovered, self-expanding stents, *AJR* 162:1421–1424, 1994.
53. Long AL, Page PE, Raynaud AC et al.: Percutaneous iliac artery stent: angiographic long-term follow-up, *Radiology* 180:771–778, 1991.
54. Raillat C, Rousseau H, Joffre F et al.: Treatment of iliac artery stenoses with the Wallstent endoprosthesis, *AJR* 154:613–616, 1990.
55. Zollikofer CL, Antonucci F, Pfyffer M et al.: Arterial stent placement with use of the Wallstent: midterm results of clinical experience, *Radiology* 179:449–456, 1991.
56. Sapoval MR, Chatellier G, Long AL et al.: Self-expandable stents for the treatment of iliac artery obstructive lesions: long-term success and prognostic factors, *AJR* 166:1173–1179, 1995.
57. Murphy TP, Webb MS, Lambiase RE et al.: Per-cutaneous revascularization of complex iliac artery stenoses and occlusions with use of Wallstents: three-year experience, *J Vasc Interv Radiol* 7:21–27, 1996.
58. Martin EC, Katzen BT, Benenati JF et al.: Multicenter trial of the Wallstent in the iliac and femoral arteries, *J Vasc Interv Radiol* 6:843–848, 1995.
59. Vorwerk D, Gunther RW: Mechanical revascularization of occluded iliac arteries with use of self-expandable endoprostheses, *Radiology* 175:411–415, 1990.
60. Vowerk D, Guenther RW, Schurmann K et al.: Primary stent placement for chronic iliac artery occlusions: follow-up results in 103 patients, *Radiology* 194:745–749, 1995.
61. Reyes R, Maynar M, Lopera J et al.: Treatment of chronic iliac artery occlusions with guide wire recanalization and primary stent placement, *J Vasc Interv Radiol* 8:1049–1055, 1997.
62. Reyes R, Carreira JM, Gude F et al.: Long-term follow-up of iliac Wallstents, *Cardiovasc Intervent Radiol* 27:624–631, 2004.
63. Schurmann K, Mahnken A, Meyer J et al.: Long-term results 10 years after iliac arterial stent placement, *Radiology* 224:731–738, 2002.
64. Kichikawa K, Uchida H, Yoshioka T et al.: Iliac artery stenosis and occlusion: preliminary results of treatment

with Gianturco expandable metallic stents, *Radiology* 177:799–802, 1990.
65. Liermann D, Strecker EP, Peters J: The Strecker stent: indications and results in iliac and femoropopliteal arteries, *Cardiovasc Intervent Radiol* 15:298–305, 1992.
66. Strecker EP, Hagen B, Liermann D et al.: Iliac and femoropopliteal vascular occlusive disease treated with flexible tantalum stents, *Cardiovasc Intervent Radiol* 16:158–164, 1993.
67. Strecker EP, Boos IB, Hagen B: Flexible tantalum stents for the treatment of iliac artery lesions: long-term patency, complications, and risk factors, *Radiology* 199:641–647, 1996.
68. Cragg AH, DeJong SC, Barnhart WH et al.: Nitinol intravascular stent: results of preclinical evaluation, *Radiology* 189:775–778, 1993.
69. Hausegger KA, Cragg AH, Lammer J et al.: Iliac artery stent placement: clinical experience with a nitinol stent, *Radiology* 190:199–202, 1994.
70. Krol KL, Saxon RR, Farhat N et al.: Clinical evaluation of the Zilver vascular stent for symptomatic iliac artery disease, *J Vasc Interv Radiol* 19:15–22, 2008.
71. Ponec D, Jaff MR, Swischuk J et al.: The nitinol SMART stent vs. Wallstent for suboptimal iliac artery angioplasty: CRISP-US trial results, *J Vasc Interv Radiol* 15:911–918, 2004.
72. Greiner A, Dessl A, Klein-Weigel P et al.: Kissing stents for treatment of complex aortoiliac disease, *Eur J Vasc Endovasc Surg* 26:161–165, 2003.
73. Mohamed F, Sarkar B, Timmons G et al.: Outcome of "kissing stents" for aortoiliac atherosclerotic disease, including the effect on the non-diseased contralateral iliac limb, *Cardiovasc Intervent Radiol* 25:472–475, 2002.
74. Mouanoutoua M, Maddikunta R, Allaqaband S et al.: Endovascular intervention of aortoiliac occlusive disease in high-risk patients using the kissing stents technique: long-term results, *Catheter Cardiovasc Interv* 60:320–326, 2003.
75. Bjorses K, Ivancev K, Riva L et al.: Kissing stents in the aortic bifurcation – a valid reconstruction for aorto-iliac occlusive disease, *Eur J Vasc Endovasc Surg* 36:424–431, 2008.
76. Houston JG, Bhat R, Ross R et al.: Long-term results after placement of aortic bifurcation self-expanding stents: 10 year mortality, stent restenosis, and distal disease progression, *Cardiovasc Intervent Radiol* 30:42–47, 2007.
77. Krepel VM, van Andel GJ, van Erp WF et al.: Percutaneous transluminal angioplasty of the femoropopliteal artery: initial and long-term results, *Radiology* 156:325–328, 1985.
78. Gray BH, Sullivan TM, Childs MB et al.: High incidence of restenosis/reocclusion of stents in the percutaneous treatment of long-segment superficial femoral artery disease after suboptimal angioplasty, *J Vasc Surg* 25:74–83, 1997.
79. White GH, Liew SC, Waugh RC et al.: Early outcome and intermediate follow-up of vascular stents in the femoral and popliteal arteries without long-term anticoagulation, *J Vasc Surg* 21:270–279, 1995.
80. Chatelard P, Guibourt C: Long-term results with a Palmaz stent in the femoropopliteal arteries, *J Cardiovasc Surg* 37(suppl 1):67–72, 1996.
81. Bergeron P, Pinot JJ, Poyen V et al.: Long-term results with the Palmaz stent in the superficial femoral artery, *J Endovasc Surg* 2:161–167, 1995.
82. Cejna M, Thurnher S, Illiasch H et al.: PTA versus Palmaz stent placement in femoropopliteal artery obstructions: a multicenter prospective randomized study, *J Vasc Interv Radiol* 12:23–31, 2001.
83. Becquemin JP, Favre JP, Marzelle J et al.: Systematic versus selective stent placement after superficial femoral artery balloon angioplasty: a multicenter prospective randomized study, *J Vasc Surg* 37:487–494, 2003.
84. Rousseau HP, Raillat CR, Joffre FG et al.: Treatment of femoropopliteal stenoses by means of self-expandable endoprostheses: midterm results, *Radiology* 172:961–964, 1989.
85. Sapoval MR, Long AL, Raynaud AC et al.: Femoropopliteal stent placement: long-term results, *Radiology* 184:833–839, 1992.
86. Do DD, Triller J, Walpoth BH et al.: A comparison study of self-expandable stents vs balloon angioplasty alone in femoropopliteal artery occlusion, *Cardiovasc Intervent Radiol* 15:306–312, 1992.
87. Strecker EP, Boos IB, Gottmann MD: Femoropoliteal artery stent placement: evaluation of long-term success, *Radiology* 205:375–383, 1997.
88. Liermann D, Bottcher HD, Kollath J et al.: Prophylactic endovascular radiotherapy to prevent intimal hyperplasia after stent implantation in femoropopliteal arteries, *Cardiovasc Intervent Radiol* 17:12–16, 1994.
89. Bottcher HD, Schopohl B, Liermann D et al.: Endovascular irradiation-a new method to avoid recurrent stenosis after stent implantation in peripheral arteries: technique and preliminary results, *Int J Radiat Oncol Biol Phys* 29:183–186, 1994.
90. Schopohl B, Leirmann D, Pohlit LJ et al.: 192Ir Endovascular brachytherapy for avoidance of intimal hyperplasia after percutaneous transluminal angioplasty and stent implantation in peripheral vessels: 6 years of experience, *Int J Radiat Oncol Biol Phys* 36:835–840, 1996.
91. Henry M, Amor M, Beyar R et al.: Clinical experience with a new nitinol self-expanding stent in peripheral arteries, *J Endovasc Surg* 3:369–379, 1996.
92. Schillinger M, Sabeti S, Loewe C et al.: Balloon angioplasty versus implantation of nitinol stents in the superficial femoral artery, *N Engl J Med* 354:1879–1888, 2006.
93. Schillinger M, Sabeti S, Dick P et al.: Sustained benefit of primary femoropopliteal stenting compared with balloon angioplasty with optional stenting, *Circulation* 115:2745–2749, 2007.
94. Krankenberg H, Schluter M, Steinkamp HJ et al.: Nitinol stent implantation versus percutaneous transluminal angioplasty in superficial femoral artery lesions up to 10 cm in length: the Femoral Artery Stenting Trial (FAST), *Circulation* 116:285–292, 2007.
95. Ferreira M, Lanziotti L, Monteiro M et al.: Superficial femoral artery recanalization with self-expanding nitinol

stents: long-term follow-up results, *Eur J Vasc Endovasc Surg* 34:702–708, 2007.
96. Duda SH, Pusich B, Richter G et al.: Sirolimus-eluting stents for the treatment of obstructive superficial femoral artery disease: six-month results, *Circulation* 106:1505–1509, 2002.
97. Duda SH, Bosiers M, Lammer J et al.: Sirolimus-eluting versus bare nitinol stent for obstructive superficial femoral artery disease: the SIROCCO II trial, *J Vasc Interv Radiol* 16:331–338, 2005.
98. Duda SH, Bosiers M, Lammer J et al.: Drug-eluting and bare nitinol stents for the treatment of atherosclerotic lesions in the superficial femoral artery: long-term results from the SIROCCO trial, *J Endovasc Ther* 13:701–710, 2006.
99. Jahnke T, Andresen R, Muller-Hulsbeck S et al.: Hemobahn stent-grafts for treatment of femoropopliteal arterial obstructions: midterm results of a prospective trial, *J Vasc Interv Radiol* 14:41–51, 2003.
100. Saxon RR, Coffman JM, Gooding JM et al.: Long-term results of ePTFE stent-graft versus angioplasty in the femoropopliteal artery: single center experience from a prospective, randomized trial, *J Vasc Interv Radiol* 14:303–311, 2003.
101. Saxon RR, Dake MD, Volgelzang RL et al.: Randomized, multicenter study comparing expanded polytetrafluoroethylene-covered endoprosthesis placement with percutaneous transluminal angioplasty in the treatment of superficial femoral artery occlusive disease, *J Vasc Interv Radiol* 19:823–832, 2008.
102. Hartung O, Otero A, Dubuc M et al.: Efficacy of Hemobahn in the treatment of superficial femoral artery lesions in patients with acute or critical ischemia: a comparative study with claudicants, *Eur J Vasc Endovasc Surg* 30:300–306, 2005.
103. Alimi YS, Hakam Z, Hartung O et al.: Efficacy of Viabahn in the treatment of severe superficial femoral artery lesions: which factors influence long-term patency? *Eur J Vasc Endovasc Surg* 35:346–352, 2008.
104. Kedora J, Hohmann S, Garrett W et al.: Randomized comparison of percutaneous Viabahn stent grafts vs. prosthetic femoral-popliteal bypass in the treatment of superficial femoral arterial occlusive disease, *J Vasc Surg* 45:10–16, 2007.
105. Saxon RR, Coffman JM, Gooding JM et al.: Long-term patency and clinical outcome of the Viabahn stent-graft for femoropopliteal artery obstructions, *J Vasc Interv Radiol* 18:1341–1350, 2007.
106. Mohan IV, Bray PJ, Harris JP et al.: Endovascular popliteal aneurysm repair: are the results comparable to open surgery? *Eur J Vasc Endovasc Surg* 32:149–154, 2006.
107. Antonello M, Frigatti P, Battocchio P et al.: Open repair versus endovascular treatment for asymptomatic popliteal artery aneurysm: results of a prospective randomized study, *J Vasc Surg* 42:185–193, 2005.
108. Curi MA, Geraghty PJ, Merino OA et al.: Mid-term outcomes of endovascular popliteal artery aneurysm repair, *J Vasc Surg* 45:505–510, 2007.
109. Rajasinghe HA, Tzilinis A, Keller T et al.: Endovascular exclusion of popliteal artery aneurysms with expanded polytetrafluoroethylene stent-grafts: early results, *Vasc Endovasc Surg* 40:460–466, 2006.
110. Tielliu IF, Verhoeven EL, Zeebregts CJ et al.: Endovascular treatment of popliteal artery aneurysms: results of a prospective cohort study, *J Vasc Surg* 41:561–567, 2005.
111. Giles KA, Pomposelli FB, Hamdan AD et al.: Infrapopliteal angioplasty for critical limb ischemia: relation of TransAtlantic InterSociety Consensus class to outcome in 176 limbs, *J Vasc Surg* 48:128–136, 2008.
112. Adam DJ, Beard JD, Cleveland T et al.: Bypass versus angioplasty in severe ischaemia of the leg (BASIL): multicentre, randomized controlled trial, *Lancet* 366:1925–1934, 2005.
113. Lofberg AM, Lorelius LE, Karacagil S et al.: The use of below-knee percutaneous transluminal angioplasty in arterial occlusive disease causing chronic critical limb ischemia, *Cardiovasc Intervent Radiol* 19:317–322, 1996.
114. Kandarpa K, Becker GJ, Hunink M et al.: Transcatheter interventions for the treatment of peripheral atherosclerotic lesions: part I, *J Vasc Interv Radiol* 12:683–695, 2001.
115. Feiring AJ, Wesolowski AA, Lade S: Primary stent-supported angioplasty for treatment of below-knee critical limb ischemia and severe claudication: early and one-year outcomes, *J Am Coll Cardiol* 44:2307–2314, 2004.
116. Tepe G, Zeller T, Heller S et al.: Self-expanding nitinol stents for treatment of infragenicular arteries following unsuccessful balloon angioplasty, *Eur Radiol* 17:2088–2095, 2007.
117. Kickuth R, Keo HH, Triller J et al.: Initial clinical experience with the 4-F self-expanding XPERT stent system for infrapopliteal treatment of patients with severe claudication and critical limb ischemia, *J Vasc Interv Radiol* 18:703–708, 2007.
118. Peregrin JH, Smirova S, Koznar B et al.: Self-expandable stent placement in infrapopliteal arteries after unsuccessful angioplasty failure: one-year follow-up, *Cardiovasc Intervent Radiol* 31:860–864, 2008.
119. Kawarada O, Yokoi Y: Dorsalis pedis artery stenting for limb salvage, *Catheter Cardiovasc Interv* 71:976–982, 2008.
120. Commeau P, Barragan P, Roquebert PO: Sirolimus for below the knee lesions: mid-term results of SiroBTK study, *Catheter Cardiovasc Interv* 68:793–798, 2006.
121. Siablis D, Karnabatidis D, Katsanos K et al.: Infrapopliteal application of paclitaxel-eluting stents for critical limb ischemia: midterm angiographic and clinical results, *J Vasc Interv Radiol* 18:1351–1361, 2007.
122. Rand T, Basile A, Cejna M et al.: PTA versus carbofilm-coated stents in infrapopliteal arteries: pilot study, *Cardiovasc Intervent Radiol* 29:29–38, 2006.
123. Peeters P, Bosiers M, Verbist J et al.: Preliminary results after application of absorbable metal stents in patients with critical limb ischemia, *J Endovasc Ther* 12:1–5, 2005.
124. Christensen MG, Lorentzen JE, Schroeder TV: Revascularization of atherosclerotic mesenteric arteries: experience in 90 consecutive patients, *Eur J Vasc Surg* 8:297–302, 1994.

125. Park WM, Cherry KJ, Chua HK et al.: Current results of open revascularization for chronic mesenteric ischemia: a standard for comparison, *J Vasc Surg* 35:853–859, 2002.
126. Sharafuddin MJ, Olson CH, Sun S et al.: Endovascular treatment of celiac and mesenteric arteries stenoses: applications and results, *J Vasc Surg* 38:692–698, 2003.
127. Sarac TP, Altinel O, Kashyap V et al.: Endovascular treatment of stenotic and occluded visceral arteries for chronic mesenteric ischemia, *J Vasc Surg* 47:485–491, 2008.
128. Kasirajan K, O'Hara PJ, Gray BH et al.: Chronic mesenteric ischemia: open surgery versus percutaneous angioplasty and stenting, *J Vasc Surg* 33:63–71, 2001.
129. Sivamurthy N, Rhodes JM, Lee D et al.: Endovascular versus open mesenteric revascularization: immediate benefits do not equate with short-term functional outcomes, *J Am Coll Surg* 202:859–867, 2006.
130. Atkins MD, Kwolek CJ, LaMuraglia GM et al.: Surgical revascularization versus endovascular therapy for chronic mesenteric ischemia: a comparative experience, *J Vasc Surg* 45:1162–1171, 2007.
131. Hogg ME, Peterson BG, Pearce WH et al.: Bare metal stent infections: case report and review of the literature, *J Vasc Surg* 46:813–820, 2007.
132. Weinberg DJ, Cronin DW, Baker AG Jr: Infected iliac pseudoaneurysm after uncomplicated percutaneous balloon angioplasty and (Palmaz) stent insertion: a case report and literature review, *J Vasc Surg* 23:162–166, 1996.
133. Chalmers N, Eadington DW, Gandanhamo D et al.: Case report: infected false aneurysm at the site of an iliac stent, *Br J Radiol* 66:946–948, 1993.
134. Therasse E, Soulez G, Cartier P et al.: Infection with fatal outcome after endovascular metallic stent placement, *Radiology* 192:363–365, 1994.
135. Deiparine MK, Ballard JL, Taylor FC et al.: Endovascular stent infection, *J Vasc Surg* 23:529–533, 1996.
136. Thibodeaux LC, James KV, Lohr JM et al.: Infection of endovascular stents in a swine model, *Am J Surg* 172:151–154, 1996.
137. Hearn AT, James KV, Lohr JM et al.: Endovascular stent infection with delayed bacterial challenge, *Am J Surg* 174:157–159, 1997.
138. Paget DS, Bukhari RH, Zayyat EJ et al.: Infectibility of endovascular stents following antibiotic prophylaxis or after arterial wall incorporation, *Am J Surg* 178:219–224, 1999.
139. Kudo T, Chandra FA, Ahn SS: Long-term outcomes and predictors of iliac angioplasty with selective stenting, *J Vasc Surg* 42:466–475, 2005.
140. Kudo T, Rigberg DA, Reil TD et al.: The influence of the ipsilateral superficial femoral artery on iliac angioplasty, *Ann Vasc Surg* 20:502–511, 2006.
141. Timaran CH, Ohki T, Gargiulo NJ III et al.: Iliac artery stenting in patients with poor distal runoff: influence of concomitant infrainguinal arterial reconstruction, *J Vasc Surg* 38:479–485, 2003.
142. Timaran CH, Prault TL, Stevens SL et al.: Iliac artery stenting versus surgical reconstruction for TASC (TransAtlantic Inter-Society Consensus) type B and type C iliac lesions, *J Vasc Surg* 38:272–278, 2003.
143. Timaran CH, Stevens SL, Freeman MB et al.: External iliac and common iliac artery angioplasty and stenting in men and women, *J Vasc Surg* 34:440–446, 2001.
144. Timaran CH, Stevens SL, Freeman MB et al.: Predictors for adverse outcome after iliac angioplasty and stenting for limb-threatening ischemia, *J Vasc Surg* 36:507–513, 2002.
145. Johnston KW, Rae M, Hogg-Johnston SA et al.: 5-year results of a prospective study of percutaneous transluminal angioplasty, *Ann Surg* 4:403–412, 1987.
146. Johnston KW: Iliac arteries: reanalysis of results of balloon angioplasty, *Radiology* 186:207–212, 1993.
147. Ballard JL, Bergan JJ, Singh P et al.: Aortoiliac stent deployment versus surgical reconstruction: analysis of outcome and cost, *J Vasc Surg* 28:94–101, 1998.
148. Laborde JC, Palmaz JC, Rivera FJ et al.: Influence of anatomic distribution of atherosclerosis on the outcome of revascularization with iliac stent placement, *J Vasc Interv Radiol* 6:513–521, 1995.
149. AbuRahma AF, Hayes JD, Flaherty SK et al.: Primary iliac stenting versus transluminal angioplasty with selective stenting, *J Vasc Surg* 46:965–970, 2007.
150. Kudo T, Chandra FA, Ahn SS: The effectiveness of percutaneous transluminal angioplasty for the treatment of critical limb ischemia: a 10-year experience, *J Vasc Surg* 41:423–435, 2005.
151. Bosch JL, Haaring C, Meyerovitz MF et al.: Cost-effectiveness of percutaneous treatment of iliac artery occlusive disease in the United States, *Am J Radiol* 175:517–521, 2000.
152. Glagov S: Intimal hyperplasia, vascular modeling, and the restenosis problem, *Circulation* 89:2888–2891, 1994.
153. Clowes AW, Reidy MA: Prevention of stenosis after vascular reconstruction: pharmacologic control of intimal hyperplasia—a review, *J Vasc Surg* 13:885–891, 1991.
154. Melliere D, Zaouche S, Becquemin JP et al.: Antibiotic-impregnated prosthesis: eclectic indications, *J Mal Vasc* 21(suppl A):139–145, 1996.

Intravascular Laser Technologies

18

Craig M. Walker

Laser is an acronym for light amplification by stimulated emission of radiation [1]. There are many types of medical lasers each of which emits a different wavelength of light energy depending on their intended application [2–4]. The 308 nanometer (nm) wavelength excimer laser light energy (Spectranetics CVX-300 Excimer Laser System, Spectranetics Corp., Colorado Springs, CO) is increasingly being utilized in the interventional therapy of peripheral vascular disease and coronary artery disease [5]. It is used to debulk (atherectomy), remove thrombus, remove infected or damaged pacemaker leads, and cross lesions that are uncrossable by guidewires or unable to be crossed with a balloon once guidewire passage has been achieved [6]. The 308 nm excimer laser energy is the only currently approved catheter-based laser device utilized for the intravascular therapy of atherosclerotic disease [7–9].

History and Evolution of Laser Atherectomy

There have been many attempts to utilize laser energy to treat atherosclerotic vascular disease. Geschwind, Nakamura, and Kvasnicka experimented with bare fiber-optic Neodymium:YAG (Nd:YAG) laser angioplasty starting in 1984 [10, 11]. In the early 1990s MCM Laboratories introduced bare laser delivery using a annular bare fiber-optic tip configuration using a pulsed dye laser initially and, subsequently, a Holmium:YAG laser operating at 2.1 μm wavelength. The first laser catheter-based system to be approved by the Food and Drug Administration (FDA) was the Trimedyne Hot-tip laser in 1987. Argon laser energy was utilized in this system to heat a metal tipped nylon catheter to facilitate crossing of total occlusions [12–14]. There was no direct interaction of laser light with plaque. The GV Medical Corp. (Minneapolis, MN) laser system utilized direct argon laser energy featuring a balloon to center the laser beam and to clear blood with flush, and optically diverged laser light [15, 16]. The GV system was also used primarily to cross total occlusions. Another medical laser was developed through a collaborative effort of Massachusetts Institute of Technology (MIT), Cleveland Clinic, and the GV Medical Corp. for laser-assisted atherectomy. The GV Medical system used a frequency-tripled Neodymium:YAG operating at 355 nm and applied multiplexing to address only specific groups of fiber optics for targeted ablation [17]. Surgical Laser Technologies Inc. (Montgomeryville, PA) (SLT laser) introduced a sapphire tip delivery system around 1990 for Nd:YAG laser light delivery in contact mode [10, 18]. The operating wavelength for the SLT laser was 1,064 nm delivered by a Medilas-2 MBB laser. HGM introduced bare fiber-optic green Argon laser light delivery for plaque ablation. The Eclipse laser used Holmium:YAG (Ho:YAG) to ablate by means of infrared vaporization. Geschwind and Dubois Rande experimented with a pulsed dye laser (408 nm) guided by computerized spectral analysis of the tissue fluorescence in an attempt to achieve targeted laser ablation ("Smart Laser"). All these initial lasers resulted in deep vascular thermal and mechanical injury and are no longer utilized (Fig. 18.1) [19–23].

C.M. Walker (✉)
Interventionist, Cardiovascular Institute of the South, Lafayette, LA, USA

T.J. Fogarty, R.A. White (eds.), *Peripheral Endovascular Interventions*,
DOI 10.1007/978-1-4419-1387-6_18, © Springer Science+Business Media, LLC 1998, 2010

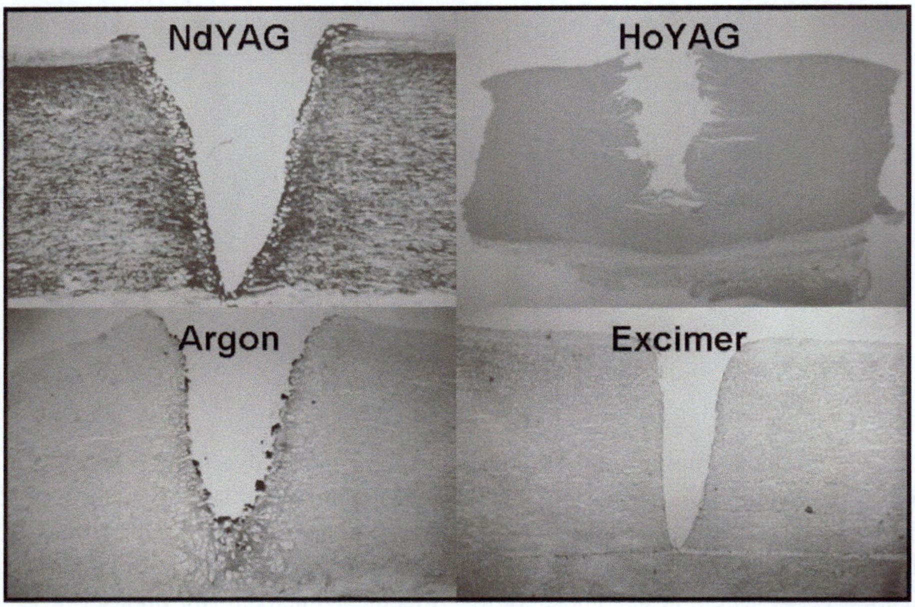

Fig. 18.1 The initial lasers resulted in deep vascular thermal and mechanical injury and are no longer utilized. (Courtesy of Spectranetics, Colorado Springs, CO.)

Advanced Interventional Systems (AIS) and Spectranetics introduced the 308 nm excimer laser (contraction of: *exc*ited d*imer*; using halogen gas as excitation medium) with fiber-optic ultraviolet laser light delivery [2, 5, 9, 24]. AIS and Spectranetics were founded independently from each other in 1984. This ultraviolet laser energy resulted in less mechanical and almost no thermal vascular injury [25]. 308 nm wavelength is absorbed by arterial plaque and thrombus. AIS was acquired by Spectranetics in 1995 and the latter is now the lone provider of endovascular laser devices.

The CVX-300 Excimer Laser System (Spectranetics Corp.), when used in combination with the fiber-optic laser catheter, laser sheath, and guiding catheter devices listed below, is currently intended for use in the following product-specific indications:

Excimer Laser Coronary Atherectomy—ELCA Catheters [26–28]

- Occluded saphenous vein bypass grafts
- Ostial lesions
- Long lesions (greater than 20 mm in length)
- Moderately calcified stenoses
- Total occlusions traversable by a guidewire
- Lesion which previously failed balloon angioplasty
- Restenosis of 316L stainless steel stent, prior to the administration of intravascular brachytherapy

Peripheral Excimer Laser Ablation—Turbo Elite Peripheral Laser Catheters [29]

- For use in the treatment of infrainguinal stenoses and occlusions

Peripheral Excimer Laser Ablation—Turbo-Booster Guiding Catheters [30]

- Designed for directing and supporting Spectranetics laser catheters for use in the treatment of infrainguinal stenoses and occlusions. Not for use in the carotid and coronary vasculature.

Pacemaker and ICD Lead Extraction—Laser Sheaths—SLS II (12, 14, and 16 F) [31]

- The laser sheath is intended for use as an adjunct to conventional lead extraction tools in patients suitable for transvenous removal of chronically implanted pacing or defibrillator leads constructed with silicone or polyurethane outer insulation.

Physics of 308 nm Excimer Laser

There are three basic requirements for any laser. These include (1) a medium, (2) a means to excite the medium with high voltage, and (3) optics consisting of a mirrored chamber with a controlled aperture through which light energy can be released [1, 2, 5, 24]. With the excimer laser, a photocoupler is utilized to deliver the energy to quartz fiber catheters.

The lasing medium is xenon gas and hydrogen chloride. As the XeCl molecule is bombarded with high voltage, electrons are displaced to outer unstable orbits [32, 33]. As the electrons return to their stable resting orbits, photons of light energy are released that measure 308 nm in wavelength. The term excimer is a contraction of "*exc*ited d*imer*" (the XeCl molecule in 308 nm lasers but any combination of an inert gas and a halogen) (Fig. 18.2).

Excimer laser energy falls in the ultraviolet light range and has a shorter wavelength than lasers of the infrared spectrum [2]. Unlike infrared lasers, excimer laser energy creates no heat in a saline system; therefore, it is referred to as the "cool laser" (Fig. 18.3).

Light energy can be absorbed, reflected, or transmitted by tissues. 308 nm light is absorbed by plaque and thrombus and to a lesser extent calcium. It has a very shallow absorption depth of 50–100 μm [5]. 308 nm light does not travel well through air but does transmit over fiber-optic catheters utilized to deliver direct excimer light energy to the catheter tip [34]. Excimer laser energy is not delivered as constant energy but is given in 125 ns bursts at frequencies up to 80/s. Energy per pulse (Fluence-milliJoules/mm^2) can also be altered.

There are three potential effects when laser energy is absorbed by tissues. These effects are (1) photochemical, (2) photothermal, and (3) photomechanical [2, 5, 7]. The photochemical effect is characterized by the fracture of billions of tissue bonds within 100 μm of the catheter tip with each 125 ns burst of energy. The photothermal effect is the result of vibration of molecules as energy is absorbed by tissue proteins. This results in the vaporization of tissue water creating steam and a vapor bubble [35–37]. This process ruptures cell membranes. As this process occurs over 100 millionths of a second, temperatures at the catheter tip seldom exceed 50°C. The photomechanical effect is a direct result of the vapor bubble. Expansion and collapse of the vapor bubble breaks down tissue and sweeps debris away from the catheter tip. Debris by-products consist of water, hydrocarbons (gasses), and small particles. Oxidative by-products are absent implying that the molecules in the tissues do not burn. Greater than 90% of particulate debris is less than 10 μm in size. The size of the vapor bubble is directly

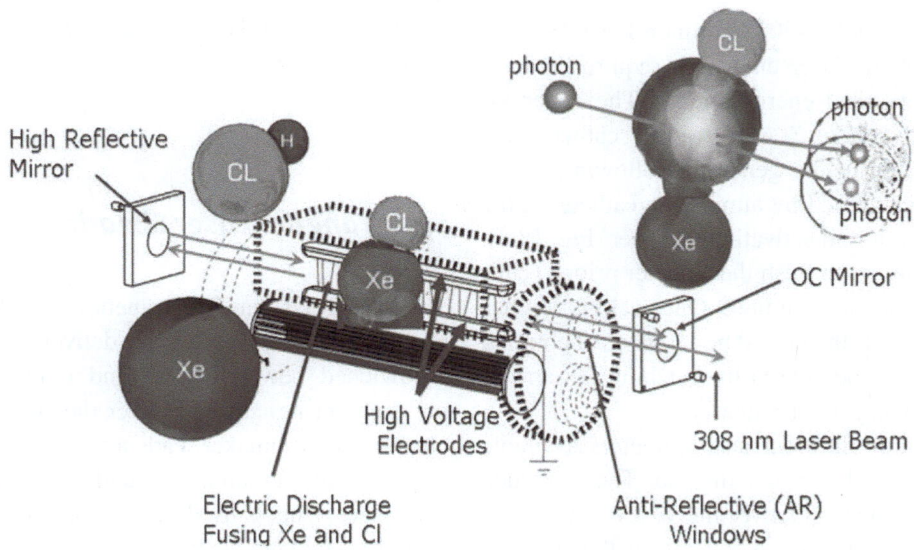

Fig. 18.2 The term excimer is a contraction of "*exc*ited d*imer*" (the XeCl molecule in 308 nm lasers but any combination of an inert gas and a halogen). (Courtesy of Spectranetics, Colorado Springs, CO.)

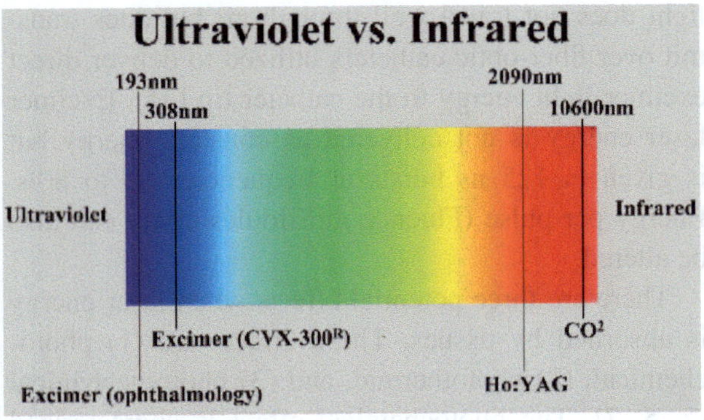

Fig. 18.3 Excimer laser energy creates no heat in a saline system; therefore, it is referred to as the "cool laser." (Courtesy of Spectranetics, Colorado Springs, CO.)

related to Fluence (energy per pulse measured in milliJoules /mm^2). The vapor bubble allows the ablation of tissue greater than the size of the catheter. The ability to cross densely calcified lesions is directly related to Frequency (pulses/s). The total energy delivered is the mathematical product of Fluence × Frequency.

Although there is no appreciable cavitation in saline or water, high-amplitude, but transient, percussion waves (which can result in dissections) can be created when laser energy is activated in an absorptive media such as contrast media.

Equipment

The Spectranetics CVX-300 Excimer Laser System is the source of the laser energy. It requires a dedicated 220 V electrical energy source. The generator has a 5 min "warm up." A fiber-optic catheter can then be connected to the generator following which the catheter is calibrated by aiming the catheter at the calibration window and activating the laser (Fig. 18.4).

It is important not to flush the catheter prior to calibration as this may cause a fault. Once calibration has been achieved, the catheter will be activated at nominal settings which can be altered by touching the arrows which adjust fluency and frequency.

There are many different laser catheters available for use in peripheral vascular disease. These include both rapid exchange and over-the-wire catheters of 0.9, 1.4, 1.7, and 2.0 mm. A 2.3 mm catheter and a 2.5 mm catheter are available in over-the-wire configurations only. Frequencies (pulse repetition rates) of up to 80 Hz can be utilized with all of the catheter sizes. A Fluence of up to 80 mJ can be used with the 0.9 mm laser catheter [38]. A Fluence of up to 45 mJ (76 mJ/mm^2) can be used with the 2.5 mm probe. All of the other catheters can utilize Fluence up to 60 mJ (Tables 18.1 and 18.2; Fig. 18.5).

Subsequent to the two largest trials utilizing excimer laser-assisted angioplasty in the treatment of peripheral vascular disease [Peripheral Excimer Laser Angioplasty (PELA) and Laser Angioplasty for Critical Ischemia (LACI)] there have been multiple modifications in catheter design and energy delivery from the generator to the patient. These include (1) more fibers being incorporated into each catheter to improve energy delivery to the catheter tip (Fig. 18.6), (2) hydrophilic catheter coatings to lessen catheter drag, (3) potential frequencies of up to 80 Hz with all catheters, and (4) a "constant on" feature rather than an automatic shut off every 5 or 10 s (allowing the interventionist to determine ablation treatment times). This results in less treatment area gaps of "dottering" that were caused by inadvertent advancement of the laser probe while energy is off (Fig. 18.7).

In addition to the laser catheters themselves, Turbo-Booster guiding catheters are now available. These catheters eccentrically displace laser catheters to allow the creation of larger channels. There is a 7F model (used with a 1.7 mm laser probe) that can create channels of up to 4.75 mm and an 8F model (used with a 2 mm laser probe) that can create channels up to 5.5 mm (Fig. 18.8).

Spectranetics Laser Sheath

The SLS II System (Spectranetics) is a sheath catheter utilizing excimer laser energy delivered by glass fibers sandwiched between inner and outer polymer tubing that can be advanced over damaged, infected, or obstructive pacemaker leads and deliver 308 nm laser energy circumferentially around leads to ablate adherent tissues. This is used in conjunction with a braided mesh lead locking device to remove the leads.

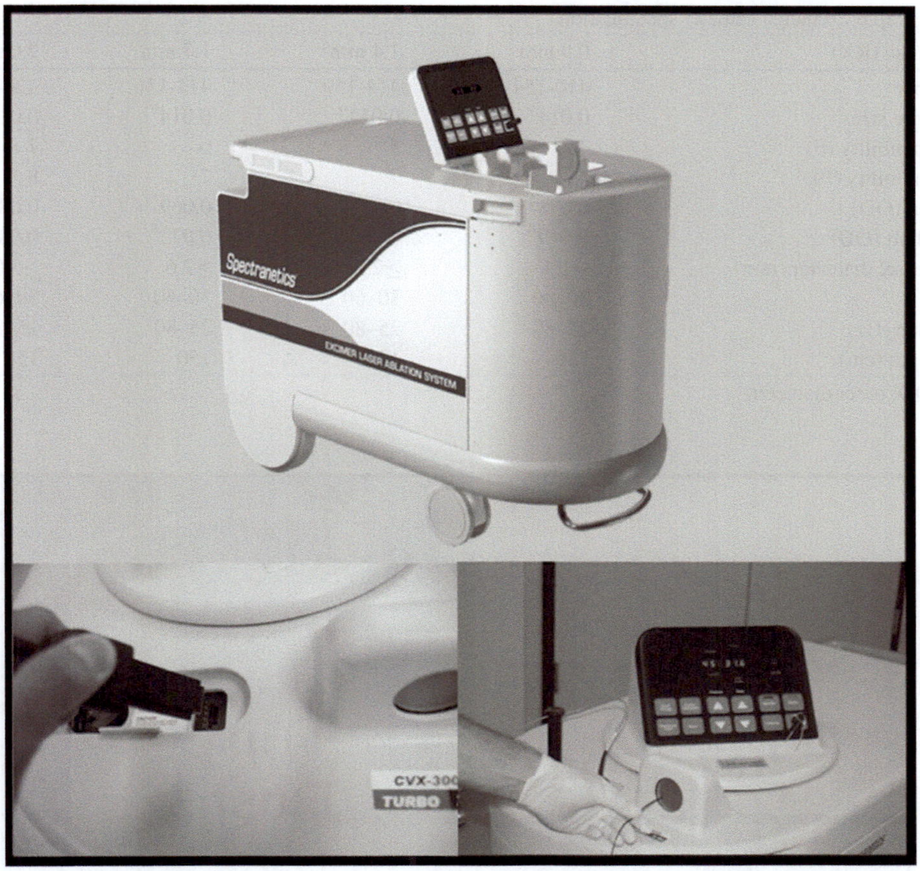

Fig. 18.4 A fiber-optic catheter can then be connected to the generator. The catheter is calibrated by aiming the catheter at the calibration window (see *lower right panel*) and activating the laser. (Courtesy of Spectranetics, Colorado Springs, CO.)

Table 18.1 Turbo elite laser catheter specifications

OTW (over the wire)	0.9 mm	1.4 mm	1.7 mm	2.0 mm	2.3 mm	2.5 mm
Model number	410-152	414-151	417-152	420-006	423-001	425-011
Maximum guidewire size	0.014″	0.014″	0.018″	0.018″	0.018″	0.018″
Sheath compatibility (F)	4	5	5	6	7	8
Guide compatibility (F)	5	7	7	8	9	10
Maximum tip (OD)	0.038″	0.055″	0.068″	0.080″	0.091″	0.101″
Maximum shaft (OD)	0.047	0.056	0.069	0.081	0.091	0.102
Min. vessel diameter (mm)	≥1.4	≥2.1	≥2.6	≥3.0	≥3.5	≥3.8
Working length (cm)	150	150	150	150	120	110
Fluence levels (mJ)	30–80	30–60	30–60	30–60	30–60	30–45
Repetition rates (Hz)	25–80	25–80	25–80	25–80	25–80	25–80
Working length (cm)	150	150	150	150	120	110
Turbo-Booster compatibility (F)	NA	7 and 8	7 and 8	8	NA	NA

F: French; OD: outer diameter.

Table 18.2 Rapid exchange catheter specifications

Rapid exchange (RX)	0.9 mm	1.4 mm	1.7 mm	2.0 mm
Model number	410-154	414-159	417-156	420-059
Max guidewire size	0.014″	0.014″	0.014″	0.014″
Sheath compatibility (F)	4	5	6	7
Guide compatibility (F)	5	7	7	8
Maximum tip (OD)	0.038″	0.057″	0.069″	0.080″
Maximum shaft (OD)	0.049″	0.062″	0.072″	0.084″
Minimum vessel diameter (mm)	≥1.4	≥2.1	≥2.6	≥3.0
Fluence	30–80	30–60	30–60	30–60
Repetition rate (Hz)	25–80	25–80	25–80	25–80
Working length (cm)	150	150	150	150

F: French; OD: outer diameter.

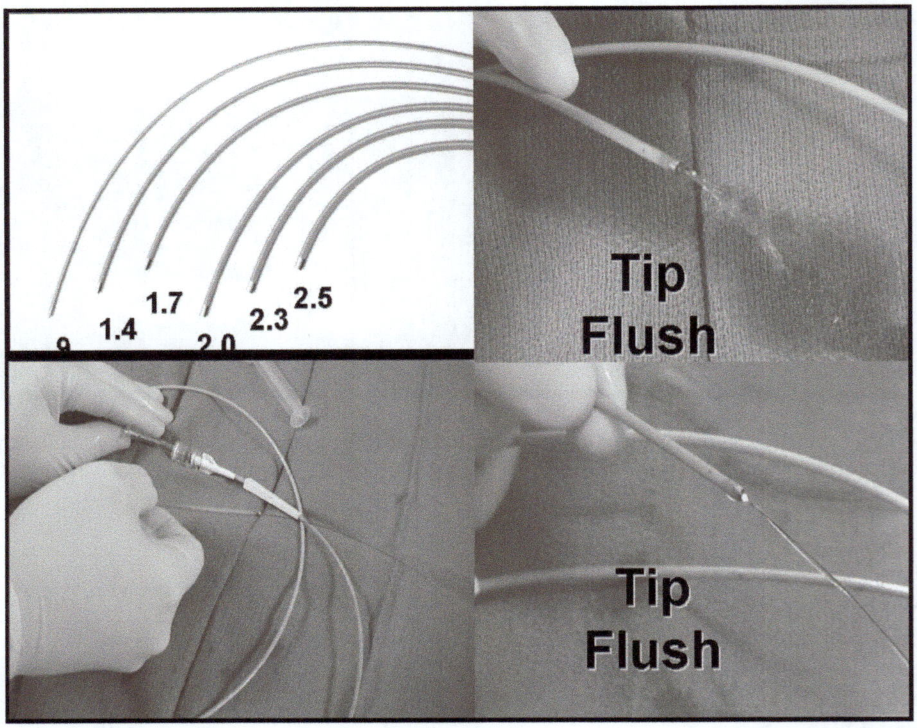

Fig. 18.5 A fluence of up to 45 mJ (76 mJ/mm^2) can be used with the 2.5 mm probe. All of the other catheters can utilize Fluence up to 60 mJ. It is required that saline be flushed through the laser catheter or guiding sheath during laser activation. (Courtesy of Spectranetics, Colorado Springs, CO.)

Using the Excimer Laser to Treat Peripheral Vascular Disease

Excimer laser is utilized in peripheral vascular disease (1) to cross lesions uncrossable with guidewires, (2) to debulk (atherectomy), and (3) to remove old and new thrombus [39–43]. The ultimate clinical outcomes are related to the final luminaldiameter achieved and the amount of intimal damage. Keys to the proper utilization of laser are simple. First and foremost is the slow advancement of the laser catheter. The maximum rate of laser ablation is 0.8 mm/s; therefore, the catheter should be advanced no faster than this to create maximal lumens [44].

As excimer laser energy creates large percussive waves in the presence of contrast media (that can result

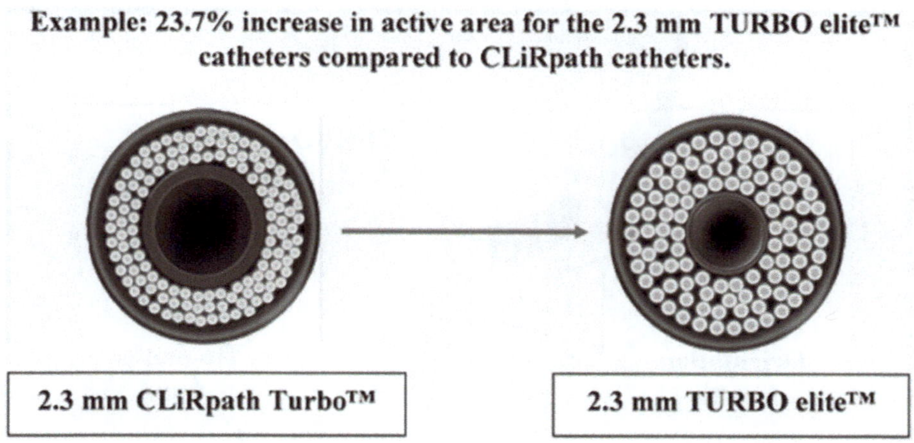

Fig. 18.6 More fibers incorporated into each catheter to improve energy delivery to the catheter tip. (Courtesy of Spectranetics, Colorado Springs, CO.)

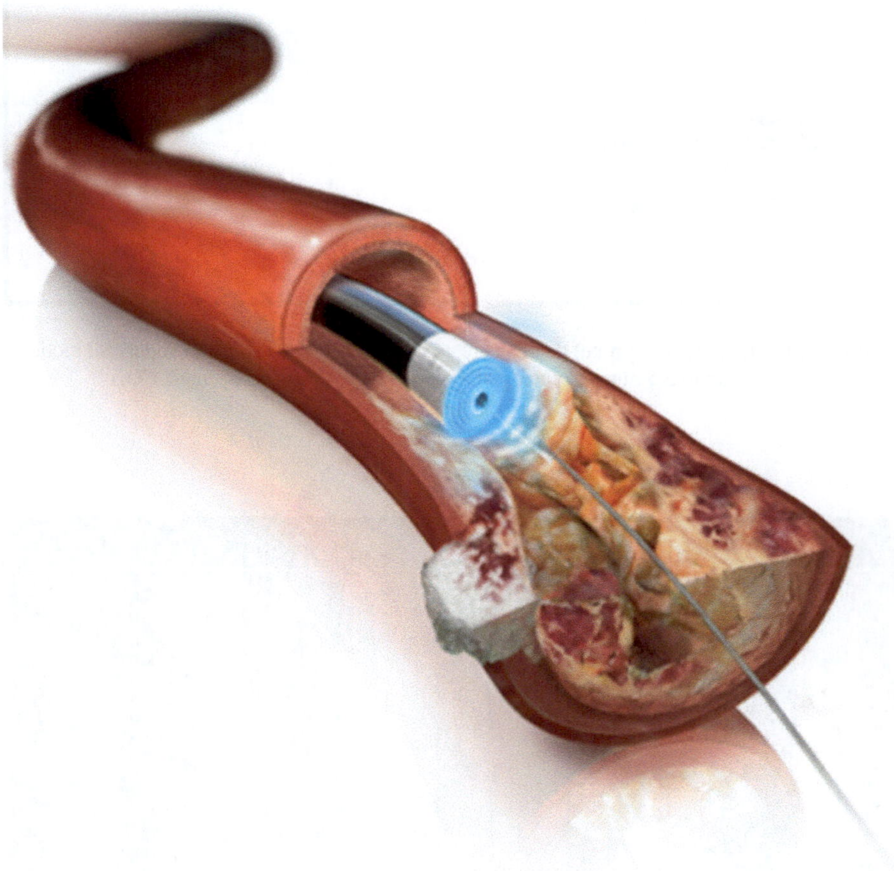

Fig. 18.7 "Dottering" caused by inadvertent advancement of the laser probe while energy is off. (Courtesy of Spectranetics, Colorado Springs, CO.)

in dissections and perforation) it is imperative to first flush all contrast from the sheath and catheters and never activate the laser in the presence of contrast media. Flushing either the catheter or the sheath with saline while lasing can clear contrast and blood from the field. This can result in less distal debris and

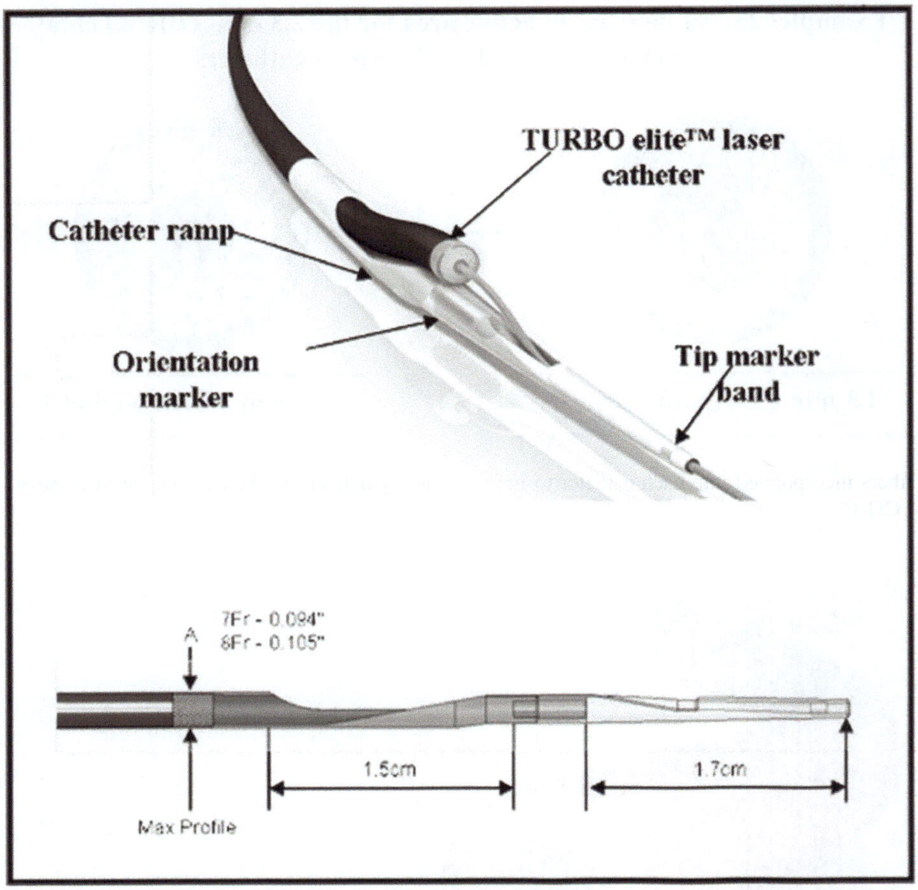

Fig. 18.8 7F model (used with a 1.7 mm laser probe) that can create channels of up to 4.75 mm and an 8F model (used with a 2 mm laser probe) that can create channels up to 5.5 mm. (Courtesy of Spectranetics, Colorado Springs, CO.)

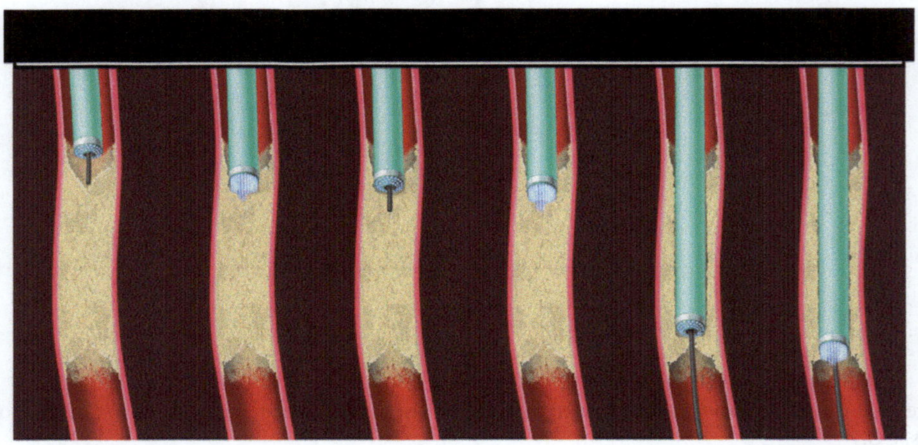

Fig. 18.9 Step-by-step technique. If the wire does not cross the laser, it is activated and advanced several more millimeters. Again wire passage is attempted. If the wire still does not cross, this sequence is repeated until crossing is achieved. If there is substantial discomfort during this sequence, one should suspect that the catheter is not making the proper intraluminal course and should be redirected. (Courtesy of Spectranetics, Colorado Springs, CO.)

vascular injury. As a general rule the laser catheter should be no larger than 2/3 the diameter of a vessel being treated (less in areas of acute bends, more in areas of instent restenosis).

In crossing total occlusions not crossable by a guidewire the "step-by-step" technique, pioneered by Professor Dr Giancarlo Biamino during the early 1990s, is utilized [45]. With this technique, a laser catheter is advanced just proximal to the total occlusion, then activated and slowly advanced at low energies while carefully monitoring for pain. After the catheter has been advanced several millimeters, the laser is inactivated and a repeat attempt at wire passage (following ablation of the proximal cap of the occlusion) is attempted. If the wire does not then cross the laser it is activated and advanced several more millimeters. Again wire passage is attempted. If the wire still does not cross this sequence is repeated until crossing is achieved. If there is substantial discomfort during this sequence one should suspect that the catheter is not making the proper intraluminal course and should be redirected (Fig. 18.9). This step-by-step technique should not be utilized in areas of acute bends.

Excimer laser energy is effective in the ablation of old and new thrombus. This author has utilized excimer laser energy alone to declot vessels and grafts of small diameter and in conjunction with a lytic flush (administered through the laser guidewire lumen while lasing) to declot large native vessels and grafts [46]. Higher Fluence settings are useful when treating thrombus as this increases the size of the vapor bubble. This author has achieved total clinical lysis in single-cath laboratory settings of less than 1 h utilizing low dose chemical lytics in conjunction with laser energy to open occluded femoral popliteal synthetic grafts (Fig. 18.10).

When utilizing the Turbo-Booster catheter the lesion is first treated with the laser catheter used with the 7F (1.7 mm) or 8F (2 mm) device over a 0.014 guidewire. Once a pilot channel has been created the laser catheter is withdrawn from the patient. The laser catheter is then loaded into the Turbo-Booster catheter. The guidewire is then placed through the tip of the Turbo-Booster catheter and into the guidewire lumen of the laser catheter. It is then advanced through the lumen of the laser catheter. The laser catheter is withdrawn several centimeters, then the entire system advanced through the sheath. The Turbo-Booster catheter is then advanced just proximal to the lesion and the laser catheter advanced over the ramp. Typically several very slow lasing passes are made directing the laser catheter toward the area of intended ablation. The 7F Turbo-Booster system can create channels up to 4.75 mm and the 8F system channels up to 5.5 mm in diameter. This author has utilized the Turbo-Booster system to treat diffuse instent restenosis and instent occlusions of the superficial femoral artery (SFA) with encouraging initial results (Fig. 18.11).

Trials

There have been many trials utilizing excimer laser energy to treat PAD that have been completed and others that are ongoing or planned. It should be noted that there were substantial improvements in equipment and technique since PELA and LACI were conducted.

Peripheral Excimer Laser Angioplasty (PELA) (1998–2002)

PELA [47, 48] was a multicenter, randomized parallel-group design study with fixed sample size comparing excimer laser atherectomy plus balloon angioplasty to balloon angioplasty in SFA occlusions. There were 13 US sites and five German sites. The trial enrolled 250 randomized patients (allocation: 129 Laser Group and 121 Balloon Group). Another 122 roll-in (non-randomized) patients were treated in training cases. CLiRpath Excimer Laser Catheters used were 2.2 and 2.5 mm over the wire models. The primary endpoint was patency at 12 months, as determined by Doppler ultrasound measurement. Clinical success was achieved if the treated artery had primary patency at 12 months without a serious adverse event (SAE) such as death, major perforation necessitating surgical repair, acute limb ischemia, unplanned amputation due to thromboembolization, myocardial infarction (Q or non-Q-wave), hematoma or false aneurysm necessitating surgical intervention, and nerve injury (Table 18.3). The authors concluded that no significant differences between the randomized groups were observed in the primary effectiveness outcome (primary patency at

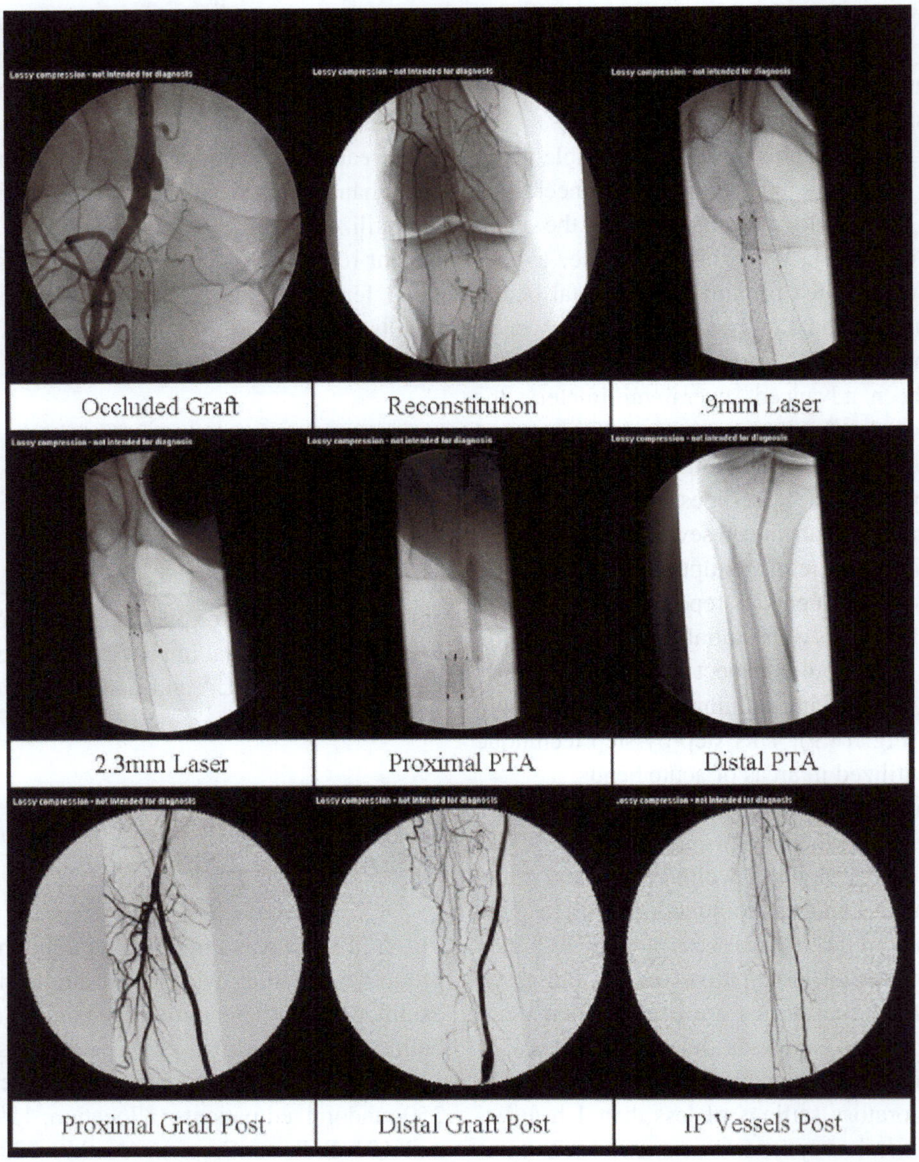

Fig. 18.10 Total clinical lysis in single-cath laboratory settings of less than 1 h utilizing low dose chemical lytics in conjunction with laser energy to open occluded femoral popliteal synthetic grafts

12 months) or in the primary safety outcome (total SAEs at 12 months). Although there was less stenting in the Laser Group, similar in-hospital and 12 month results were seen in the Laser Group and the Balloon Group. The number of patients who were reintervention-free at 12 months was not significantly different between the Laser Group and the Balloon Group. Primary patency and assisted primary patency did not differ, while secondary patency was slightly (but not significantly) higher in the Balloon Group. There was no difference in the type or number of SAEs during the procedure or during hospital stay. The SAEs adjudicated during the 12 month follow-up period did not differ in type or number.

Laser Angioplasty for Critical Ischemia (LACI Phase II) (2001–2002)

The LACI [48] trial was a multicenter prospective registry of peripheral excimer laser-assisted atherectomy

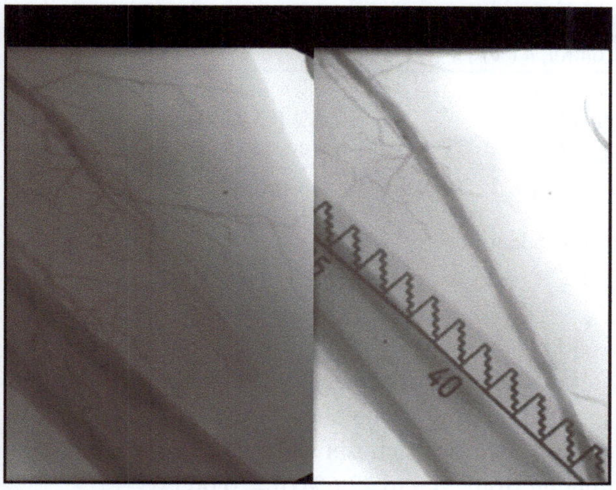

Fig. 18.11 Turbo-Booster system to treat diffuse instent restenosis and instent occlusions of the superficial femoral artery (SFA). *Left*, before (total stent occlusion); *right*, post Turbo-Booster

for the treatment of critical limb ischemia (CLI) in poor surgical candidates. Twelve US sites and three German sites enrolled patients. The historical control used is the Control Group (PTA or surgical treatment) of a randomized trial of prostaglandin in CLI patients has been described [49].

A total of 160 CLI (Rutherford Category 4–6) patients, who were non-surgical candidates, with lesions in the SFA, popliteal, and/or infrapopliteal arteries were prospectively enrolled. The Training Group contained 15 patients and the pivotal Registry Group contained 155 limbs of 145 patients, in which the mean patient age was 72 ± 10 (range 45–91) years with 53% men. There were 2.5 lesions treated per patient with an average lesion length of 16.5 cm. The Registry Group had more comorbid disease, less history of smoking, and fewer men than the Control Group. CLiRpath Excimer Laser Catheters used were both over the wire and rapid exchange models.

The primary effectiveness measure was limb salvage (freedom from major amputation) at 6 months; the primary safety measure was survival at 6 months (Table 18.4). The authors concluded that, despite containing a more morbid patient set, the Registry Group experienced higher limb salvage rate than the Control Group. Overall survival at 6 months was similar. As hypothesized in the protocol, the Registry Group demonstrated equivalence to the benchmark values provided by the Control Group while requiring 35% fewer surgical procedures during the course of the study.

In summary, LACI showed a distinctly better risk/benefit profile than the two treatment options currently available to LACI patients—medication or primary amputation. Bypass surgery, the "gold standard" for CLI, is not a good option for LACI patients, and yet LACI achieved limb salvage comparable to the "gold standard" of bypass surgery, without higher SAEs. The LACI treatment regimen showed results at least as good as large case series of PTA in CLI, despite the fact that LACI enrolled patients with far more extensive disease.

The justification for using LACI to treat CLI patients who are poor surgical candidates lies in its clinical benefit. LACI results showed greater benefit vis-à-vis any treatment strategy this patient cohort might have expected. LACI risks were lower than or not inferior to any treatment strategy this patient cohort might have expected. In fact, LACI results showed the same benefit as the best treatment strategy given to CLI patients who were (in the vast majority) good surgical candidates. LACI treatment provides an effective alternative for limb salvage in a patient population currently lacking options.

Table 18.3 Peripheral Excimer Laser Angioplasty (PELA) trial results (1998–2002)

	Laser group, *n* = 129 (%)	Balloon group, *n* = 121 (%)	Dif [95% CI]
Clinical success, 12 months	18 (14)	13 (11)	–3.3% [–11, 4.8]
Primary patency, 12 months	17 (13)	18 (15)	1.7% [–6.9, 10.3]
Secondary patency, 12 months	34 (26)	45 (37)	10.8% [–0.7, 22.3]
Any SAE	15 (12)	18 (15)	3.3% [–5.1, 11.7]
In-hospital deaths	0	0	–
In-hospital amputations	0	0	–
Death any cause, 12 months	5 (4)	4 (3)	0.6% [–4.8, 6.0]

CI: confidence interval; Mo: months; SAE: serious adverse event.

Table 18.4 Primary safety and efficacy endpoints

	Registry group, *n* (%)	Control, *n* (%)	Difference[a] [95% CI]
Patients	145 (100)	673 (100)	
Primary endpoint[b]	110 (76)	494 (73)	2.5% [−5.7, 10.6]
Death, any cause	15 (10)	96 (14)	−3.9% [−9.5, 1.7]

[a]Difference = LACI − Control = p1 − p2; SEM = p1q1/n1 + p2q2/n2; D = DEM*1.96; Corr = (1/n1 + 1/n2)2; Lo = Difference − D − Corr. Hi − Difference + D + Corr.
[b]Patients without major amputation, death, lost to follow-up, or withdrawal.

CLiRpath Excimer Laser System to Enlarge Lumen Openings (CELLO) (2006–2008)

The CELLO [50] study was a prospective, nonrandomized, registry which enrolled Rutherford category 1, 2, or 3 patients with peripheral vascular disease in the superficial femoral and popliteal arteries above the knee and who did not require intervention for infrapopliteal arteries at the time of enrollment. The objective of the study was to evaluate the safety and efficacy of the Turbo-Booster Guiding Catheter in combination with CLiRpath Excimer Laser Catheters to create larger lumens for treatment within the superficial femoral and popliteal arteries above the knee. The Turbo-Booster Guiding Catheter was cleared for marketing on June 29, 2007.

The CELLO study was designed to enroll up to 70 patients at 20 qualified investigative sites. A total of 65 patients were enrolled at 17 investigative centers. The primary efficacy endpoint is laser success, defined as achieving ≥20% average reduction in the percent diameter stenosis, post laser and prior to adjunctive therapy, based on angiographic core laboratory assessment.

The primary safety endpoint was the occurrence of major adverse events defined as clinical perforation, major dissection requiring surgery, major amputation, cerebrovascular accidents (CVA), myocardial infarction, and death at the time of the procedure, prior to release from the hospital, at 30 days, and at 6 months post procedure. The authors concluded that the primary efficacy endpoint, greater than or equal to a 20% reduction in the percent diameter stenosis post laser compared to pre-procedure was met with a sample size of 45 patients in the analysis cohort. The average percent reduction obtained for the 45 patients post all use of the bias sheath system compared to pre-procedure was 34.9% based on angiographic core laboratory analysis with 95% confidence limits ranging from 29.3 to 40.6% ($p < 0.0001$). Additionally, the training cases cohort also met the primary efficacy endpoint. On average, the training group showed a 34.3% reduction in percent diameter stenosis with 95% confidence limits ranging from 24.9 to 43.6% ($p = 0.0054$).

Sixty-three patients (97%) were available for analysis at 12 months. A peak systolic velocity (PSV) ratio of 2.0, as assessed by Duplex ultrasound core laboratory, was used to determine patency rates (<50% DS) for the analyzable cohort. The patency rate was 59% at 6 months and 54% at 12 months. Primary-assisted patency was 86% at 6 months and 76% at 12 months. Secondary-assisted patency is 100% at both 6 and 12 month intervals. The target lesion revascularization (TLR) rate was 14% at 6 months and 22% at 12 months.

Statistically significant clinical improvements were attained in the Ankle–Brachial Index (ABI), Rutherford Classification (mean value = 1.2), and Walking Impairment Questionnaire (WIQ) at both the 6 (mean value = 64.7) and 12 month (mean value = 65.1) assessments as compared to baseline (mean value = 45.6). There were no occurrences of unanticipated or major adverse events. Of the 11 reported SAEs, only one was related to the investigational procedure. The Turbo-Booster system has demonstrated efficacy and safety for the treatment of infrainguinal stenoses and occlusions.

Instent Restenosis Trial (PATENT), Ongoing

The PATENT study is a prospective multicenter registry for the evaluation of the safety and performance of the Spectranetics peripheral atherectomy laser catheters used in conjunction with Turbo-Booster catheters for the treatment of Rutherford Category 2, 3, 4 or 5 patients presenting with instent restenosis of stents implanted within femoropopliteal arteries. All enrolled subjects will be followed through to 12 months to assess the incidence of restenosis by Doppler ultrasound and major adverse events. Follow-up visits occur at 30 days and 6 and 12 month intervals. The safety endpoint is major adverse events during hospitalization and at 30 day follow-up to include death, unplanned major amputation, or target lesion revascularization. The efficacy endpoint is patency as assessed by Duplex ultrasound at 12 months post procedure. Restenosis by Doppler ultrasound is defined as a ratio of ≥2.5 using the upstream peak systolic velocity (PSV) compared with PSV in the area of greatest stenosis. Up to 100 patients will be enrolled at up to 10 sites in Germany.

AMI Trial (TAAMI), Ongoing

The TAAMI trial aims to assess whether excimer laser coronary atherectomy (ELCA) before direct infarct-related artery (IRA) stenting results in improved reperfusion success in patients presenting with acute ST wave elevation myocardial infarction (STEMI) and angiographically evident thrombus. A secondary endpoint is to validate an ELCA technique for the treatment of STEMI, at high-volume centers experienced in the treatment of acute myocardial infarction. Up to 200 patients will be enrolled and randomized to either ELCA and stenting or PTCA and stenting at investigative sites in Poland. The primary efficacy endpoint is Myocardial Blush Grade 3 (MBG3) immediately after allocated study treatment + ST wave resolution (STR) ≥70% 60 min after allocated study treatment (post guide catheter removal). The primary safety endpoint is major adverse cardiac events (MACE) defined as cardiac death, new MI, or need for reintervention (TVR, TLR, or CABG) occurring during the procedure, index hospitalization, and at the 30 day follow-up period.

EXCELLENT, Ongoing

The EXCELLENT trial is a physician-initiated prospective multicenter study on excimer laser recanalization in the treatment of long infrapopliteal lesions in patients with CLI. The study will assess the immediate and long-term angiographic patency outcomes of excimer laser recanalization (Spectranetics) + PTA in the treatment of long (≥50 mm) infrapopliteal lesions in patients with CLI. The study is a single-arm prospective multicenter study. Follow-up will be at 1, 6, and 12 months. There will be up to 60 consecutive eligible patients enrolled at up to five clinical sites in Belgium. The primary efficacy endpoint is 12 month angiographic patency for laser + PTA, as defined by <50% stenosis in the target lesion with straight line flow to the foot. The primary safety endpoint is the absence of major adverse events at the 6 month follow-up. Major adverse events are defined as death, amputation of treated limb, and target vessel revascularization.

Summary

Excimer laser utilization for the therapy of peripheral vascular disease has increased substantially. It is an effective tool for crossing lesions intraluminally and for crossing lesions uncrossable with a guidewire. It can substantially debulk de novo and instent restenosis lesions with low rates of embolic debris. It is an effective tool for removing old and new thrombus and can assist in the treatment of calcified lesions. The LACI trial demonstrated excellent success at achieving limb salvage with a very low rate of complications in a critically ill cohort of patients who would have otherwise been referred for amputation. This trial has been criticized as balloon angioplasty was frequently utilized following laser therapy and occasionally stenting was performed making it difficult to assess the exact effect of the laser. Certainly there is no argument about the subset of patients in LACI where the laser was able to cross lesions uncrossable with a guidewire or other tools. Although the PELA trial was not promising in terms of a restenosis effect there have been substantial improvements in laser therapy that are related to technique and equipment design that now allow the creation of much larger lumens in SFA disease. It will be important to determine what effects these changes will have on outcomes in SFA disease. The CELLO trial utilizing the Turbo-Booster in de novo SFA disease showed substantial debulking and sustained clinical improvement at 6 months and 1 year. The greater potential of this technology may be in the treatment of SFA instent restenosis either alone or in conjunction with some form of restenting. Excimer laser atherectomy in instent restenosis potentially has the advantage over other forms of mechanical atherectomy in instent lesions as it may not risk injuring the stent. This may allow the creation of much larger channels by removing the intimal hyperplasia and thrombus from the occluded stent. The PATENT trial may help to answer these questions. Although the potential of excimer laser energy to ablate thrombus is established, further studies are needed to determine the safety and efficacy of laser/lytic protocols to improve outcomes particularly in graft occlusions. Laser-assisted lead removal of damaged or infected pacemaker leads is well established with excellent efficacy and safety statistics.

References

1. Svelto O: *Principles of lasers*, New York, 1982, Plenium Press.
2. Splinter R, Hooper BA: *An introduction to biomedical optics*, Boca Raton, FL, 2006, Taylor & Francis.
3. Sargent M III, O'Scully M, Lamb WE: *Laser physics*, Reading, MA, 1974, Addison Wesley.
4. Goldman L, Rockwell RJ Jr: Laser systems and their applications in medicine and biology, *Adv Biomed Eng Med Phys* 1:317–382, 1968.
5. Golobic R, Bohley T, Wells LD, Sanborn TA: Clinical experience with an excimer laser angioplasty system, *Proc Diagn Ther Cardiovasc Intervent SPIE* 1425:84–91, January 20–22, 1991.
6. Verdaasdonk RM, Vos P, van Leeuwen T, Borst C et al.: Contribution of photo-thermal and photo-mechanical effects during tissue ablation by the XeCl-excimer laser, *SPIE* 2134A:333–341, 1994.
7. Tcheng JE, Wells LD, Phillips HR, Deckelbaum LI, Golobic RA: Development of a new technique for reducing pressure pulse generation during 308-nm excimer laser coronary angioplasty, *Cathet Cardiovasc Diag* 34:15–22, 1995.
8. Grundfest WS: Pulsed ultraviolet lasers and the potential for safe laser angioplasty, *Am J Surg* 150:220–226, August 1985.
9. Singleton DL, Paraskevopoulos G, Taylor RS, Higginson LAJ: Excimer laser angioplasty: tissue ablation, arterial response, and fiber optic delivery, *IEEE J Quantum Electron* QE-23(10):1772–1782, October 1987.
10 Geschwind H, Boussignac G, Teissiere B, Vielledent C, Gaston A, Becquemin JP, Mayiolini P: Percutaneous transluminal laser angioplasty in man, *Lancet* 1:844, 1984.
11. Grundfest WS, Litvack F, Forrester JS, Goldenberg T, McDermid IS, Pacala TJ et al.: Laser ablation of human atherosclerotic plaque without adjacent tissue injury, *J Am Coll Cardiol* 5:929–933, 1985.
12. Silverman SH, Khoury AL, Abela GS, Seeger JM: Effects of blood flow on laser probe temperature in human arteries, *Lasers Surg Med* 8:555–561, 1988.
13. Abela GS, Fenech A, Crea F, Conti CR: "Hot-tip": another method of laser vascular recanalization, *Lasers Surg Med* 5:327–335, 1985.
14. Verdaasdonk RM, Borst C, Boulanger LHMA et al.: Laser angioplasty with a metal laser probe ('hot tip'): probe temperature in blood, *Lasers Med Sci* 2(3):153–158, 1987.
15. Choy DSJ, Stertzer S, Loubeau JM et al.: Embolization and vessel wall perforation in Argon laser recanalization, *Lasers Surg Med* 5:297–308, 1985.
16. Nordstrom UA, Castaneda-Zuniga WR, Uindeke CC, Rasmussen TM, Burnside DK: Laser angioplasty: controlled delivery of argon laser energy, *Radiology* 167:463–465, 1988.
17. Sanborn TA, Greenfield AJ, Guben JK, Menzoian JO, LoGerfo FW, Human percutaneous laser thermal angioplasty: Initial clinical results as an adjunct to balloon angioplasty, Presented at the 40th Annual Meeting of the Society for Vascular Surgery, New Orleans, LA, June 9, 1986.
18. Ashley S, Brooks SG, Gehani AA, Kester RC, Rees MR: Experimental analysis of sapphire contact probes for ND-YAG laser angioplasty, *Angiology* 41(6):453–462, 1990.
19. Gonschior P, Hofling B, Mack B et al.: Results of directional peripheral atherectomy with reference to histology, histochemistry, and ultrastructure, *Angiology* 44:454–463, 1993.
20. Sanborn TA, Faxon DP, Haudenschild CC, Ryan TJ: Experimental angioplasty: circumferential distribution of laser thermal energy with a laser probe, *J Am Coll Cardiol* 5:934–938, 1985.
21. Geschwind H, Fabre M, Chaitman BR, Lefebvre-Villardebo M, Ladouch A, Boussignac G, Blair JD, Kennedy HL: Histopathology after Nd-YAG laser percutaneous transluminal angioplasty of peripheral arteries, *J Am Coll Cardiol* 8:1089–1095, 1986.
22. Welch AJ, Bradley AB, Torres JH, Motamedi M, Ghidoni JJ, Pearce JA, Hussein H, O'Rourke RA: Laser probe ablation of normal and atherosclerotic human aorta in vitro: a first thermographic and histologic analysis, *Circulation* 76:1353–1363, 1987.
23. Johnson DE, Hinohara T, Selmon MR et al.: Primary peripheral arterial stenoses and restenoses excised by transluminal atherectomy: a histopathologic study, *J Am Coll Cardiol* 15:419–425, 1990.
24. Waynant RW: *Lasers in medicine*, Boca Raton, FL, 2001, CRC Press.
25. Partovi F, Izatt JA, Cothren RM, Kittrell C, Thomas JE, Strikwerda S, Kramer JR, Feld MS: A model for thermal ablation of biological tissue using laser irradiation, *Laser Surg Med* 7:141–154, 1987.
26. Crea F, Abela GS, Fenech A, Smith W, Pepine CJ, Conti CR: Transluminal laser irradiation of coronary arteries in live dogs: an angiographic and morphologic study of acute effects, *Arn J Card* 57(17):1–4, 1986.
27. Crea F, French A, Smith W, Conti CR, Abela GS: Laser recanalisation of acutely thrombosed coronary arteries in live dogs: early results, *J Am Coll Card* 6: 1052–1056, 1985.

28. Mehran R, Mintz GS, Satler LF et al.: Treatment of in-stent restenosis with excimer laser coronary angioplasty: mechanisms and results compared with PTCA alone, *Circulation* 96:2183–2189, 1997.
29. http://www.spectranetics.com/index.php?option=com_content&task=view&id=136&Itemid=174
30. http://www.fda.gov/cdrh/pdf7/K071226.pdf
31. http://www.accessdata.fda.gov/scripts/cdrh/cfdocs/cfPMA/PMA.cfm?ID=13302
32. Rockwell RJ Jr: Design and functions of laser systems for biomedical applications, *Ann NY Acad Sci* 168:459–471, 1969.
33. Feynman RP, Leighton RB, Sands M: *The Feynman lectures on physics*, vol. III, Reading, MA, 1965, Addison Wesley Publishing Company, pp. 3.1–3.13, chap 3.
34. Thyagarajan K, Sharma A, Ghatak AK: Efficient coupling of incoherent light into optical fibers and bundles, *Appl Optics* 17:2416–2419, 1987.
35. Grundfest W, Litvack F, Goldenberg T, Forrester J, Laudenslager JB, Pacala TJ, McDermid IS: Excimer laser angioplasty: potential application of new technologies. Conference on Lasers and Electro-Optics, San Francisco, CA, June 1986
36. Grundfest WS, Litvack IF, Morgenstern L, Forrester JS, McDermid IS, Pacala TJ, Rider DM, Laudenslager JB: The effect of excimer laser radiation on human atherosclerotic aorta: amelioration of laser induced thermal damage. Conference on Lasers and Electro-Optics, Anaheim, CA, June 1984.
37. Laudenslager JB, McDermid IS, Pacala TJ, Goldenberg T, Litvack F, Grundfest W, Forrester J, Effect of 308 nm XeCl laser pulse duration on fiber-optic transmission and biologic tissue ablation. Conference on Lasers and Electro-Optics, San Francisco, CA, June 1986.
38. http://www.fda.gov/cdrh/pdf5/K052296.pdf
39. Dotter C, Judkins M: Transluminal treatment of atherosclerotic obstruction: description of a new technique and a preliminary report of its application, *Circulation* 30:654–670, 1964.
40. Hughes K, Domenig CM, Hamdan AD et al.: Bypass to plantar and tarsal arteries: an acceptable approach to limb salvage, *J Vasc Surg* 40:1149–1157, 2004.
41. Sanborn TA, Faxon DP, Keiiett MA, Ryan TJ: Percutaneous coronary laser thermal angioplasty, *J Am Coll Cardiol* 8:1437–1440, 1986.
42. Coulter A: AIS excimer angioplasty device approaches approval after tortuous development route, *J Clin Laser Med Surg* 9(6):405–407, December 1991.
43. Margolis JR, Mehta SM: Excimer laser coronary angioplasty, *Am J Cardiol* 69:3F–11F, 1992.
44. Topaz O: In Topol EJ, editor: *Laser angioplasty: textbook of international cardiology*, ed. 4, Philadelphia, PA, 2002, WB Saunders, pp. 675–703.
45. Walker CM: Laser assisted thrombolysis of occluded femoral-popliteal bypass grafts. Accepted. International Congress XXII on Endovascular Interventions, Scottsdale, AZ, February 10–14, 2008.
46. Walker CM: Turbo-Booster laser for treatment of diffuse SFA instent restenosis. Accepted. International Congress XXII on Endovascular Interventions, Scottsdale, AZ, February 10–14, 2008.
47. Spectranetics Corporation. FDA final report and clinical summary: the PELA trial – peripheral excimer laser angioplasty. Internal Corporate Communication, February 2004.
48. Laird JR, Zeller T, Biamino G, Scheinert D et al.: Limb salvage following laser-assisted angioplasty for critical limb ischemia: results of the LACI multicenter trial, *J Endovasc Ther* 13:1–11, 2006.
49. The ICAI Study Group: Prostanoids for chronic critical leg ischemia. A randomized, controlled, open label trial with prostaglandin EI. Ischemia Cronica degli Inferiori. *Ann Intern Med* 130(5):412, 1999.
50. Dave RM: CELLO study: 6 month results. Oral Presentation, TCT October 2007. TCTMD.COM

Endovascular Devices for Abdominal Aortic Aneurysms

19

Arash Keyhani and Rodney A. White

The field of vascular surgery entered an era of change with the introduction of stent graft for the repair of the abdominal aortic aneurysm (AAA). The first reported case by Dr. Parodi in 1991 sparked an interest in minimal invasive, catheter-driven therapeutic intervention of high-risk patients [1, 2]. The early grafts were physician-made devices employing available stents and vascular graft material. These prototypes were aortic–aortic tube grafts made to treat aneurysms with proximal and distal aortic fixation. The technology limited the number of qualified aortic anatomies suitable for these devices. Nevertheless, these first-generation devices only proved effective in short-term treatment of aneurysms as there was up to a 12% delayed aneurysm rupture within 72 months [3]. This eventually led to the formation of bifurcated devices and modular systems with iliac sealing zones, thus expanding the number of patients that could be treated. Endovascular aortic aneurysm repair (EVAR) did not reach center stage until 1999 when the Food and Drug Administration (FDA) granted approval for two industry-made devices for clinical use (AneuRx and Ancure). These second-generation endografts were designed to improve fixation and sealing leading to the improved outcome of EVAR. Further refinement in graft design and material has led to a decreased number of late complications and re-interventions. Currently there are five FDA-approved devices with several others in the early clinical trials in the United States.

The goal of the current available endograft is to exclude the aneurysm sac from the pressurized arterial flow, therefore leading to sac volume regression over time (Fig. 19.1). Each device has its own unique characteristics, but they all have several of the same basic components making up the endostent. These basic components can be categorized into the following—(1) stent configuration—modular versus unibody, (2) graft material—polyester versus polytetrafluoroethylene (ePTFE), and (3) fixation—passive fixation such as radial and columnar support versus active fixation including hooks and barbs embedding into the aortic wall (Table 19.1).

This chapter will discuss the current endovascular treatment of abdominal aortic aneurysm with the current commercially available devices and later discuss the future technology of endografts.

Patient Selection

The lessons learned from all cumulative trial data include the importance of patient selection, proper imaging with appropriate device selection, and importance of fixation in avoiding graft migration and adverse outcome [4, 5]. The most important factor for a successful endovascular repair of an aneurysm is the pre-planning stage. The pre-planning starts with an appropriate image of the abdominal aortic aneurysm.

Imaging

The optimal screening image for the assessment of the abdominal aneurysm requires a spiral CT angiography (CTA). The image quality provided is

A. Keyhani (✉)
Fellow, Department of Vascular Surgery, Harbor-UCLA Medical Center, Torrance, CA, USA

T.J. Fogarty, R.A. White (eds.), *Peripheral Endovascular Interventions*,
DOI 10.1007/978-1-4419-1387-6_19, © Springer Science+Business Media, LLC 1998, 2010

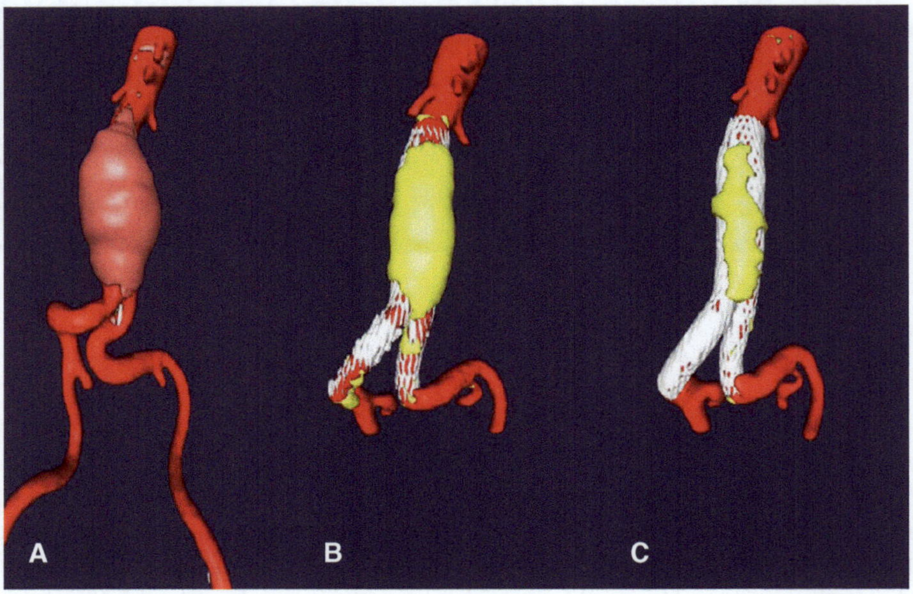

Fig. 19.1 **a**, Abdominal aortic aneurysm 5 cm in diameter with normal size iliac arteries. **b**, Six months after EVAR with AneuRx shows sac regression. **c**, Two-year follow-up reveals continued aortic remodeling with sac regression

Table 19.1 FDA-approved endovascular abdominal aortic grafts

Device	Company	Graft material	Stent material	Fixation	Suprarenal fixation
Excluder	W.L. Gore	ePTFE	Nitinol	Active/passive	No
AneuRx	Medtronic	Polyester	Nitinol	Passive	No
Talent	Medtronic	Polyester	Nitinol	Passive	Yes
Powerlink	Endologix	ePTFE	Elgiloy	Passive	Yes
Zenith	Cook	Polyester	Stainless steel	Active/passive	Yes

reflective of the available formatting ability of the CT scanner in each institution. The formatted images can vary from <1 to 5 mm thick slices depending on the image processing of the CT scanners (16–128 slicers). Three-dimensional reconstruction of the images in both sagittal and coronal views is most often obtained from the original scan when it is re-formatted. The information obtained from the initial CT scan can provide the details needed to determine the suitability of the patient's anatomy for EVAR. In the more challenging anatomies, more accurate sizing and length measurement can be obtained if the images are re-formatted to exhibit central lumen line construction. This allows the image to be re-formatted by placing the aorta as the center of reference point instead of the patient in the standard CT scans. There are different software programs and companies that can provide the accurate centerline reconstruction.

Anatomic Evaluation

Once an adequate CT scan is obtained, several key components must be evaluated to determine the likelihood for a successful EVAR. These components include (1) the anatomy of the proximal aortic neck and iliac arteries, (2) the suitability of the access arteries for device delivery, and (3) any variability in the aortoiliac branches.

Aortic Neck and Iliac Arteries

The suitability of the proximal aortic neck is the most important factor in determining the eligibility for EVAR. The current FDA-approved bifurcated devices have similar exclusion criteria for the suitability of the aortic neck. The recommendations exist to have at least

>15 mm of non-aneurismal proximal aortic neck with an angulation of <60°. In the severely angulated aortic necks, conversion to an aortouniliac with a crossover femoral–femoral artery bypass can be a viable option. Other morphologic changes associated with the aortic neck need to be recognized in determining the eligibility for EVAR. Severe calcification is not a contraindication for EVAR but additional intervention may be needed to provide secure endograft fixation. The presence of thrombus is not a contraindication with reported publications showing no increased incidence for early or late endoleaks [6]. The suprarenal fixation with open stents provide additional fixation length in the short aortic neck.

The additional fixation obtained involves placement of the bifurcated device close to the iliac bifurcation to decrease the incidence of graft migration [7]. In the aneurismal common iliac arteries several options exist to provide distal fixation points. In the ectatic common iliac arteries, several different companies have "bell-bottom" extensions available to provide adequate fixation. Other options include the exclusion of the hypogastric artery to prevent type II endoleak and extension of the limb into the external iliac artery. It is important to maintain the continuity of the hypogastric artery by having one patent antegrade flow. At the end of the chapter several devices currently under investigation will be highlighted that are aimed to address the short and angulated aortic necks.

Access Arteries

The tractability of the endograft depends on several key components involving both the delivery design of the graft along with the access vessels. The delivery access of the current devices range from 18 to 24 F and accommodates for graft diameters in the range of 14–36 mm. Three key components of the access vessel must be evaluated to determine if the device can be accessed through the femoral artery or if an iliac conduit is required. The three components include (1) access size, (2) angulation of the iliofemoral segment, and (3) degree of calcification. As a general rule, if two of the three components appear normal, then the need for iliac conduit access is minimal. In creation of the iliac conduit, a 10 mm Dacron graft is oversewn into the common iliac artery via a retroperitoneal approach and then anastomosed to the common femoral artery after device deployment. This allows for an additional bypass in severely calcified and stenotic iliac arteries. There are variabilities in the technique for the creation of the iliac conduit at different centers.

Aortoiliac Branches

In evaluation of the abdominal aneurysm, several branches must be carefully inspected prior to intervention. The flow into the superior mesenteric artery (SMA) must be evaluated on the CTA. In certain cases, the SMA may be occluded and the major arterial inflow into the small bowel is via the marginal branches off the inferior mesenteric artery (IMA). In this situation, EVAR would be contraindicated as the preservation of the IMA is essential. In other situations, accessory renal arteries may be present on the CTA throughout the aortoiliac segment. The coverage of these vessels will typically not lead to renal ischemia or renal hypertension [8]. However, the possibility for a type II endoleak does exist and must be carefully evaluated prior to EVAR.

After pre-operative evaluation is performed and the patient is deemed an endovascular candidate, the next step is choosing the right device to successfully exclude the aneurysm. The following section will focus on the characteristics of each available device and will highlight procedural outcome and midterm results.

Device Selection

Medtronic: AneuRx AAAdvantage

The current AneuRx AAAdvantage (Medtronic, Vascular, Santa Rosa, CA) device has gone through several design modifications including improvements in graft fabric material, stent design, and Xcelerant delivery system. The device has an exoskeleton made from a self-expanding nitinol stent and a high-density polyester graft with low porosity (Fig. 19.2). The device is a modular design endograft. The main body is available in sizes ranging from 20 to 28 mm

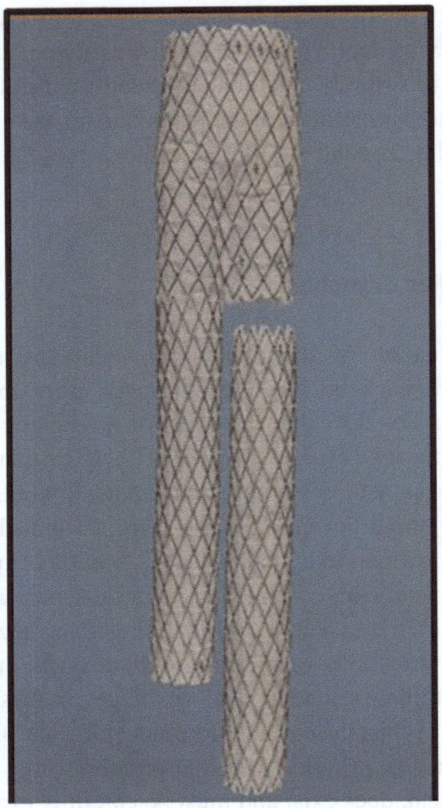

Fig. 19.2 AneuRx device: Modular bifurcated graft with nitinol exoskeleton and polyester graft fabric

(16 F–21 F delivery) with iliac limb flares ranging from 12 to 24 mm.

The AneuRx clinical trial was conducted in 19 US investigational centers from 1996 to 1999 with a total of 1,193 patients. The patient selection since the completion of the trial has been modified to include proximal aortic seal zone of 15 mm, aortic neck angulation <45°, and iliac seal zone of 25 mm.

The primary outcome measures include prevention of rupture, death from rupture, and all-cause mortality. The freedom from rupture was 97%, freedom from aneurysm-related death was 96.5%, and freedom from all-cause death was 61.5% at 5 year follow-up.

The secondary outcome measures include presence of endoleak, aneurysm sac enlargement (defined as >5 mm), along with graft migration. The reported 5 year follow-up includes 15% incidence of endoleak (mostly type II), 15% incidence of sac enlargement, and 6% graft migration. From these outcome measures, several lessons have been learned. These changes include selecting patients with >15 mm of non-aneurismal aortic neck, distal fixation of 25 mm, and neck angulation <45°. The incidence of endoleak remains high, but there is no difference in the primary endpoints that have been reported [9]. The persistence of endoleak is associated with sac enlargement, but the significance of this enlargement to the risk of aneurysm rupture is currently undefined. The incidence of graft migration has been analyzed with the AneuRx device in support of extension of the iliac limbs to the level of the hypogastric arteries for longitudinal columnar support [7, 10].

Cook—Zenith

The exoskeleton of the device is made from self-expanding stainless steel "Z" stent (Fig. 19.3). The stent is covered with a full-thickness suture-fixated polyester graft. The device is modular with a bifurcated main body and two extension limbs. The main body diameter ranges from 22 to 36 mm. The distal diameters of the extension limbs range from 8 to 24 mm. The delivery system has a tapered introducer tip and a valved sheath. The sheath sizes range from 18 to 22 F depending on the proximal diameter. The contralateral limb sheaths range from 14 to 16 F. The suprarenal fixation stent has non-covered caudally oriented barbs (10–12). Since its introduction, several steps have been taken in dealing with various technical problems such as stent disconnect and barb fractures.

In review of the current literature, the largest clinical trial comes from the United States. In the trial, 819 patients were enrolled into the open control and the endovascular arm. In all implanted devices, there was one reported late (6 months) aneurysm rupture. The conversion rate to open surgery after endovascular implantation was <1%. At 5-year follow-up, the freedom from open surgical conversion was >98% and the aneurysm-related death was 98% in standard-risk patients and 96% in high-risk subgroup [11, 12]. In addition, graft migration as defined by >5 mm movement in relation to defined landmarks was reported to be <3%. The overall late endoleak rate was 4.9%. Secondary interventions most notably to treat endoleak were performed in 153 patients. The overall incidence for re-intervention ranges from 6.8 to 14%.

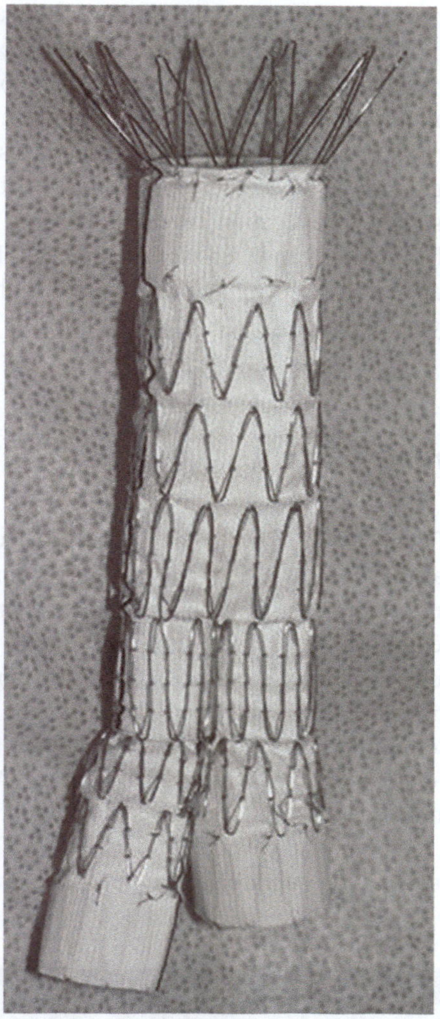

Fig. 19.3 Zenith device: Modular design with bifurcated configuration and three-component self-expanding stainless steel Z stents. There are staggered barb at the top of the graft to provide active suprarenal fixation

Endologix—Powerlink

The Powerlink device (Endologix, Inc., Irvine, CA) is a unibody, self-expanding cobalt–chromium alloy wire endoskeleton with a high-density ePTFE attached proximally and distally with polypropylene suture (Fig. 19.4). The ePTFE graft material sits on the outside of the cobalt–chromium alloy stent allowing the graft to have more movement during the cardiac cycle and reducing the stress on the endoskeleton. The device has a recently approved suprarenal proximal passive fixation using an aortic cuff extension. This allows for treatment of aortic neck diameters

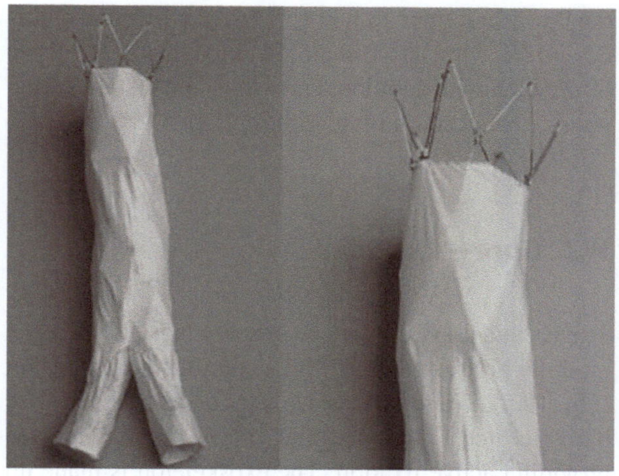

Fig. 19.4 Powerlink device: Unibody design with endoskeleton cobalt–chromium alloy wire and ePTFE graft on the outside

between 18 and 32 mm and distal iliac in the range of 10–23 mm. The device is delivered on the low-profile system (17–21 F). The SurePass pre-cannulated contralimb allows for deployment of the limb without requiring cannulation of the contralateral gate as seen in all the other modular devices.

Most of the commercially available endostents currently use the modular system allowing for variation in iliac sizes. The Powerlink has a unibody design, thus limiting the potential component separation that can occur as with other devices. The passive fixation of the device depends on the distal fixation obtained at the aortic bifurcation (anatomical fixation point) along with standard sealing zones in the iliac and aortic neck. The suprarenal bare stent configuration allows for additional proximal fixation in the larger diameter aortic necks.

In a large multicenter prospective FDA-approved clinical trial, 258 patients underwent EVAR ($N = 192$) versus open surgery ($N = 66$) between 2000 and 2003 [13]. The technical success was achieved in 97.9% of the cases. In the mean follow-up (4.1 years), there were no reported ruptures, type III/IV endoleaks, or stent fracture. There were 14.3% reported type I/II endoleaks at 72 month follow-up with the 70% of those being type II. There re-intervention rate was 14% for treating type I/II endoleak. There were 4.2% incidence of graft migration reported, all of which were in grafts initially deployed below the renal artery instead of placing the graft on the bifurcation. Other reported trials and series highlight similar results for the Powerlink stent graft [14]. The attractiveness of this device is having a true anatomical fixation at the aortic bifurcation with additional proximal and distal fixation points, therefore limiting graft migration.

W.L. Gore—Excluder

The Excluder (W.L. Gore & Assoc, Flagstaff, AZ) is a modular bifurcated graft with a contralateral extension (Fig. 19.5). There are passive fixation and angled wire barbs located at the proximal end of the main device providing active fixation. The exoskeleton is made up of nitinol stent with an inner lined ePTFE fabric. The endograft is wrapped around the delivery system with a thread that is pulled to deploy the device. The main body diameter ranges from 23 to 31.5 mm and is introduced through an 18 F (the 31.5 mm via 20 F). The contralateral limb is deployed through a 14 F sheath for iliac diameters ranging from 12 to 20 mm. The deployment of the main body may not be as accurate as other devices especially in short and angulated anatomy. The major advantage of the graft is its ability to adapt to difficult iliac anatomies as a result of thinner graft fabric.

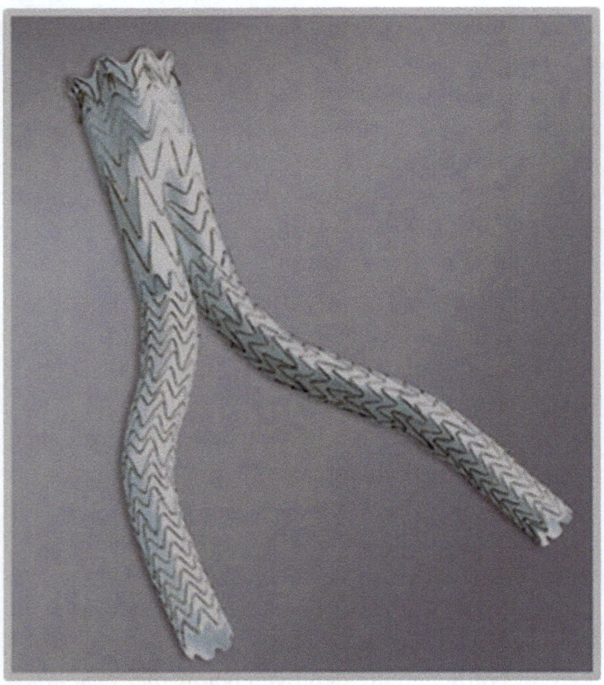

Fig. 19.5 Gore Excluder: Modular design with infrarenal active hook fixation and low porosity modified ePTFE

In the 5 year clinical data the following adverse events were reported. There are 2.6% aneurysm-related deaths, 0.4% incidence of graft migration, 10% endoleak rate, and 37% aneurysm enlargement.

There was increasing concern of a lack of sac volume regression in the results of the initial pivotal trial. The resultant investigation revealed the graft porosity as the possible cause for sac enlargement [15, 16]. The graft was therefore modified in 2004 with lower porosity ePTFE.

Medtronic—Talent

The Talent Abdominal Stent graft (Medtronic, Vascular, Santa Rosa, CA) is the only stent graft approved with an on-label indication for a proximal neck length as short as 1 cm. The Talent device is a self-expanding modular system composed of serpentine-shaped nitinol stents inlaid with a woven polyester fabric (Fig. 19.6). There is columnar support in the endograft and is more flexible than AneuRx in accommodating for aortoiliac angulation. There is also a 15 mm uncovered proximal end allowing for transrenal or suprarenal fixation. The available

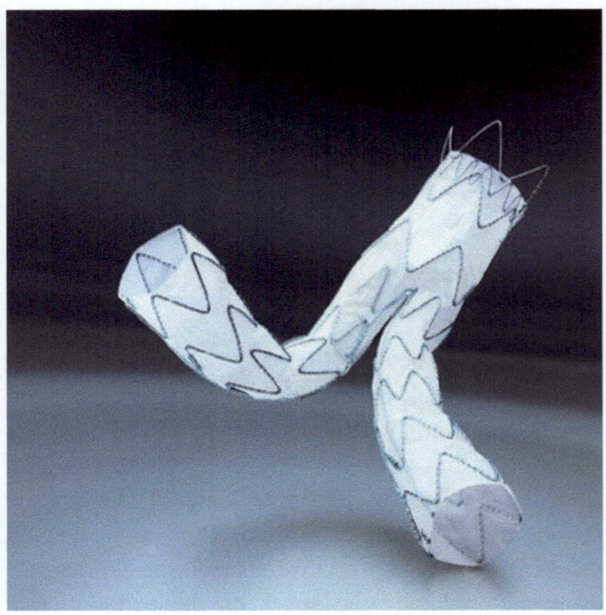

Fig. 19.6 Talent device: Modular bifurcated graft with nitinol M-shaped exoskeleton stent and polyester graft fabric. There is passive suprarenal bare stent configuration

proximal aortic neck diameters range from 22 to 36 mm (22–24 F delivery) and have tapered and flared iliac limb diameters from 8 to 24 mm.

In the longest data provided by the multicenter Talent AAA Retrospective Long-term (TARL) study, 165 patients were treated [17]. There was low aneurysm-related mortality (0.6%) and low incidence of graft migration (4.2%) at 7 years. The overall survival rate was 76% at 7 years. There were 47 secondary procedures (28%) performed including 13 (7.8%) late conversion. There were 6.1% incidence of graft thrombosis and 5.4% graft integrity (stent fracture). As a result, further refinement of the stent exoskeleton was made to reduce metal fatigue (Talent eLPS). These include the surface treatment with chemical polish of nitinol and placement of the connecting bar medially as opposed to laterally, thus improving fatigue resistance.

In the premarket approval submission with the eLPS modification (Talent Abdominal PMA), there were 166 patients treated. Analysis of the 12 month endpoint supported the overall effectiveness of the graft in treatment of patients with >10 mm length aortic neck. The incidence of graft migration was 3.6% in aortic neck between 10 and 15 mm and no migration in aortic neck >15 mm. There was 100% graft patency and <2% incidence for secondary procedural intervention.

Future of Endograft Technology

The current technology for EVAR has shown success in reducing mortality and morbidity associated with the traditional open abdominal aneurysm repair. There are significant limitations and deficiencies that still exist in the current FDA-approved devices. Therefore, there is not one superior endostent that is applicable to all patients and thus most EVAR centers use a variety of endografts. The current limitation in treatment of patients with abdominal aortic aneurysm is what the future for endovascular therapy holds. There are several stent designs that are currently under clinical investigation in dealing with these limitations. The limiting factors currently being considered are (1) short and angulated necks, (2) graft migration, (3) flexibility and conformability, (4) deliverability, and (5) late aneurysm growth associated with type II endoleak. The remaining section will highlight some of the new technologies that are currently under clinical trials in the United States and may be available in Europe.

The Aorfix stent graft (Lombard Medical, Oxfordshire, England) is designed to address the highly angulated aortic necks with tortuous iliac arteries [18]. The Aorfix is a two-part modular implant comprising of a bifurcated main body with a straight contralateral limb section (Fig. 19.7). The unique design of the graft allows for flexibility in treating aneurysm neck angulations up to 90°. The implanted device has a proximal fish mouth-shaped design with four pairs of hooks. The exoskeleton is made of nitinol circular frame with covered woven polyester allowing for a very compliant graft. The device design also allows for easy navigation in extremely tortuous iliac arteries. The flexible design allows for accurate sac exclusion in patients with severely angulated necks that were previously excluded with the current available technology.

The Aptus endovascular AAA repair system (Aptus Endosystems, Sunnyvale, CA) is designed to incorporate an independently delivered helical staple device. The graft is constructed from a robust polyester material and is fitted into a small delivery catheter (16 and 18F OD). The main body of the device is without stents allowing for conformability while the independent helical staples allow for full aortic wall penetration, thus allowing for sealing and reducing aortic neck dilatation. The iliac limbs are supported by radial stents and are conformable to the tortuous iliac arteries. The device is currently in phase II clinical trials in the United States.

The Endurant stent graft system (Medtronic Vascular, Santa Rosa, CA) has evolved to expand the applicability in previously excluded EVAR patients [19]. These include patients with highly angulated proximal necks and small and tortuous iliac arteries [20]. The device represents refinement of the current available technology in several graft designs but not in previously within the same device. The stent graft consists of polyester graft with externally supported nitinol exoskeleton (Fig. 19.7). The exoskeleton has an M-shaped design proximally to allow for improved flexibility and conformability while maintaining radial force. In addition, the suprarenal bare stent component has anchoring pins for active fixation. The delivery system is a low-profile one (smallest outerdiameter—18 F

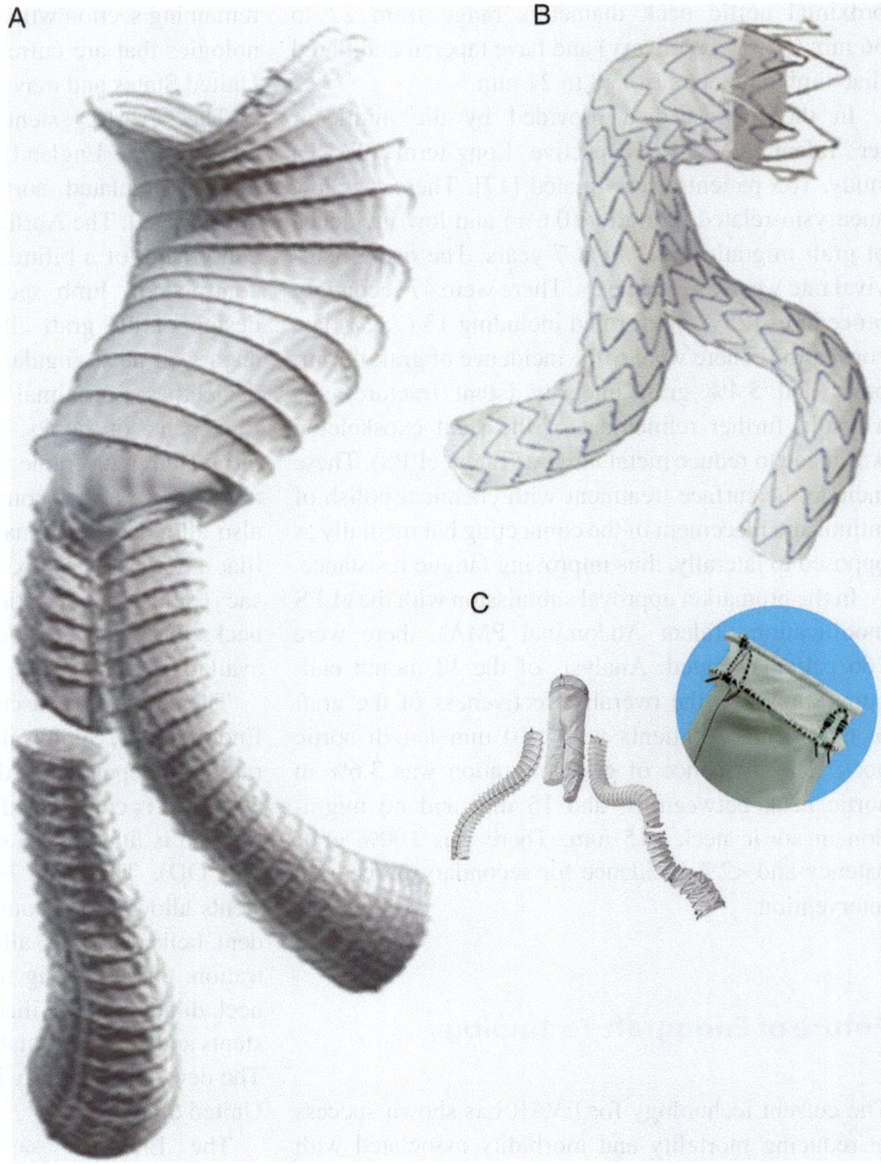

Fig. 19.7 Various stent grafts under current investigation. **a**, Aorfix, **b**, Endurant, **c**, Anaconda

OD) with hydrophilic coating. The device is currently available for use in Europe and is in phase II US trials.

The Anaconda endograft (Vascutek, Terumo) is an infrarenal stent graft consisting of woven Dacron supported by self-expanding nitinol ring [21]. The proximal part of the main body consists of two nitinol ring stents shaped like a saddle (Fig. 19.7). There is passive fixation with the radial force inserted by the nitinol stent along with active fixation comprised of four pairs of hooks. The device is also fitted with a guidewire with a magnet inside the contralateral gate allowing for easier cannulation. The proximal stent has a saddle configuration where the apex of the convexity is placed anterior–posterior and the concavity is localized laterally. This configuration allows for proximal adaptation of the stent in cases where there is eventual neck dilation allowing for the "saddle" to flatten out. The hooks placed at the cardinal points allow for active fixation and prevention of graft dislocation.

The Nellix Endovascular (Palo Alto, CA) has designed a fillable, sac-anchoring device allowing the polymer-filled endobag to fit the shape of the patient's aneurysm while providing anchoring and sealing for type II endoleak [22]. The stent is designed to treat hostile neck anatomies (lengths <1 cm and angulations >60°). The device is currently under preclinical studies.

Conclusion

Endovascular abdominal aortic aneurysm is an important technology that is able to treat patients who were previously considered to be at high risk for open aneurysm repair. The current midterm results have shown the lower perioperative morbidity and mortality associated with EVAR. In the long-term follow-ups, the incidence of non-aneurysm-related mortality is similar between the groups indicating progression of patient's non-aneurysm-related disease process. The available variety of FDA-approved endograft suggests that there is not one superior endograft available in treating all aneurysm anatomy. The complex aorta–device interaction currently being evaluated is leading to future device refinement and advancement in endovascular technology.

References

1. Parodi JC, Palmaz JC, Barone HD: Transfemoral intraluminal graft implantation for abdominal aortic aneurysms, *Ann Vas Surg* 5:491, 1991.
2. Parodi JC, Marin ML, Veith FJ: Transfemoral endovascular stented graft repair of an abdominal aortic aneurysm, *Arch Surg* 130:549, 1995.
3. Harris PL, Vallabhanensi SR, Desgranges P et al.: Incidence and risk factors of late rupture conversion and death after endovascular repair of infrarenal aortic aneurysm: EUROSTAR experience, *J Vasc Surg* 32: 739–749, 2000.
4. Sternbergh WC, Carter G, York JW et al.: Aortic neck angulation predict adverse outcome with endovascular abdominal aortic aneurysm repair, *J Vasc Surg* 35:482–486, 2002.
5. Boult M, Babidge W, Maddern G et al.: Predictors of success following endovascular aneurysm repair: mid-term results, *Eur J Vasc Endovasc Surg* 31:123–129, 2006.
6. Gitlitz DB, Ramaswami G, Kaplan D et al.: Endovascular stent-grafting in the presence of aortic neck filling defects: early clinical experience, *J Vasc Surg* 33:340–344, 2001.
7. Benharash P, Lee JT, Abilez OJ et al.: Iliac fixation inhibits both suprarenal and infrarenal aortic neck grafts, *J Vas Surg* 45:250–257, 2007.
8. Karmacharya J, Parmer SS, Antezana JN et al.: Outcomes of accessory renal artery exclusion during endovascular aneurysm repair, *J Vasc Surg* 43(1):8–13, 2006.
9. Zarins CK, White RA, Hodgson KJ et al., for the AneuRx Clinical Investigators: Endoleak as a predictor of outcome following endovascular aneurysm repair. AneuRx multicenter clinical trial, *J Vasc Surg* 32:90–107, 2002.
10. Zarins CK, Bloch DA, Crabtree T et al.: Stent graft migration after endovascular aneurysm repair: importance of proximal fixation, *J Vasc Surg* 38:1264–1271, 2003.
11. Greenberg RK, Chuter TA, Cambria R et al.: Zenith abdominal aortic aneurysm endovascular graft, *J Vasc Surg* 48:1–9, 2008.
12. Greenberg RK, Chuter TA, Sternbergh WC et al.: Zenith AAA endovascular graft: intermediate-terms results of US multicenter trial, *J Vasc Surg* 39:1209–1218, 2004.
13. Carpenter JP, the Endologix Investigators: Midterm results of the multicenter trial of the Powerlink bifurcated system for endovascular aortic aneurysm repair, *J Vasc Surg* 48:535–545, 2008.
14. Qu L, Raithel D: From clinical trials to clinical practice: 612 cases treated with the Powerlink stent-graft for endovascular repair of AAA, *J Cardiovasc Surg* 50: 131–137, 2009.
15. Fillinger M, for the Excluder Bifurcated Endoprosthesis Clinical Investigators: Three-dimensional analysis of enlarging aneurysms after endovascular abdominal aortic aneurysm repair in the Gore Excluder Pivotal clinical trial, *J Vasc Surg* 43:888–895, 2006.
16. Tanski W, Fillinger M: Outcomes of original and low-permeability Gore excluder endoprosthesis for endovascular abdominal aortic aneurysm repair, *J Vasc Surg* 45: 243–249, 2007.
17. Torsello G, Osada N, Florek HJ et al.: Long-term outcome after Talent endograft implantation from aneurysms of the abdominal aorta: A multicenter retrospective study, *J Vasc Surg* 43:277–284, 2006.
18. Balasubramaniam K, Hardman J, Horrocks M et al.: The advantage of Aorfix for endovascular repair of abdominal aortic aneurysm, *J Cardiovasc Surg* 50:139–143, 2009.
19. Verhagen HJM, Torsello G, Vries JP et al.: Endurant stent-graft system: preliminary report on an innovative treatment for challenging abdominal aortic aneurysm, *J Cardiovasc Surg* 50:153–158, 2009.
20. Patterson BO, Holt PJ, Hinchliffe R et al.: Predicting risk in elective abdominal aortic aneurysm repair: a systematic review of current evidence, *Eur J Vasc Endovasc Surg* 36:637–645, 2008.
21. Stella A, Freyrie A, Gargiulo M et al.: The advantages of Anaconda endograft for AAA, *J Cardiovasc Surg* 50: 145–152, 2009.
22. Donayre C, Kopchok GE, White RA: Fillable endovascular aneurysm repair, *EV Today* 8:64–66, 2009.

Endovascular Devices for Thoracic Aortic Aneurysms

20

Edward Diethrich

The evolution of endovascular therapy over the past two to three decades has been intimately intertwined with the introduction of new devices and technologies. While a therapeutic concept may appear applicable to treat a specific pathologic condition, without the proper tools, even a great idea may never reach clinical application. Thoracic aortic endografting for aneurysmal disease is a classic example of this situation.

Our extensive experience with thoracic endografting at the Arizona Heart Institute and Heart Hospital [1–11] has provided us an opportunity to both observe and apply new technology as it has become available, but, even more importantly, we have been able to participate in the creation and evolution of new endovascular devices. As is often the case in early-stage device development, the initial concepts and designs are developed through evaluation of a series of prototypes. No commercial products become available until extensive evaluation has been completed in both preclinical studies and, much later, clinical trials. These device studies are almost always conducted by large companies with both the financial means and the personnel to navigate the long and arduous regulatory approval process. There is, however, an opportunity outside the commercial clinical trials in the form of institutional investigations. While these are not common, they offer considerably more latitude in the early developmental stages of device design and can be useful in guiding the ultimate design and may influence the final commercial product.

E. Diethrich (✉)
Medical Director, Arizona Heart Institute and Arizona Heart Hospital, Phoenix, AZ, USA

In this chapter, we will show the progression of device development leading to the three FDA-approved commercial endografts now available for use in the thoracic aorta. Also, the concept of customization will be detailed, since it has been critical to the evolution of the technology. Finally, newer approaches to treating complex aneurysmal pathology using hybrid approaches, branched and fenestrated grafts, and unique "on-the-table" customization will be presented.

Early Endografts

Shortly after the first implantation of an abdominal aortic endograft [12], it became apparent that this new technology could be used in aneurysmal disease of the thoracic aorta as well. Of course, there were no commercially available grafts at the time, and customization was required for each case. The concept of combining a stent with a fabric tube (Dacron or PTFE) proved to work well since application in the descending thoracic aorta did not require attention to major arterial branches or the abdominal aortic bifurcation. An early case illustrates how the customized device and concept worked in a young man, who was involved in a motorcycle accident resulting in multiple injuries that included an acute transection of the descending thoracic aorta just distal to the left subclavian artery (Fig. 20.1a). A short piece of PTFE was used to line a Gianturco Z stent (without barbs), and the device was loaded into a sleeve for transfer into a long delivery sheath and was deployed across the transection (Fig. 20.1b). Both the short-term follow-up

T.J. Fogarty, R.A. White (eds.), *Peripheral Endovascular Interventions*,
DOI 10.1007/978-1-4419-1387-6_20,

at 18 months (Fig. 20.1c) and the more recent long-term follow-up examination at 9 years (Fig. 20.1d) showed excellent healing and no negative sequelae. Surprisingly, even nearly a decade later, we have no commercial device with an indication for use in this otherwise fatal condition. Since most of these injuries occur in younger people with smaller aortas, there is a problem using even the devices approved for other indications in these patients because of sizing issues. There is also a continued argument about the use of endografts in younger patients because of the lack of long-term data to support device use. Nonetheless, the application of thoracic aortic endografts in patients with acute transections is lifesaving, even though there will probably never be any level-1-based evidence to prove the worth of this technology in this segment

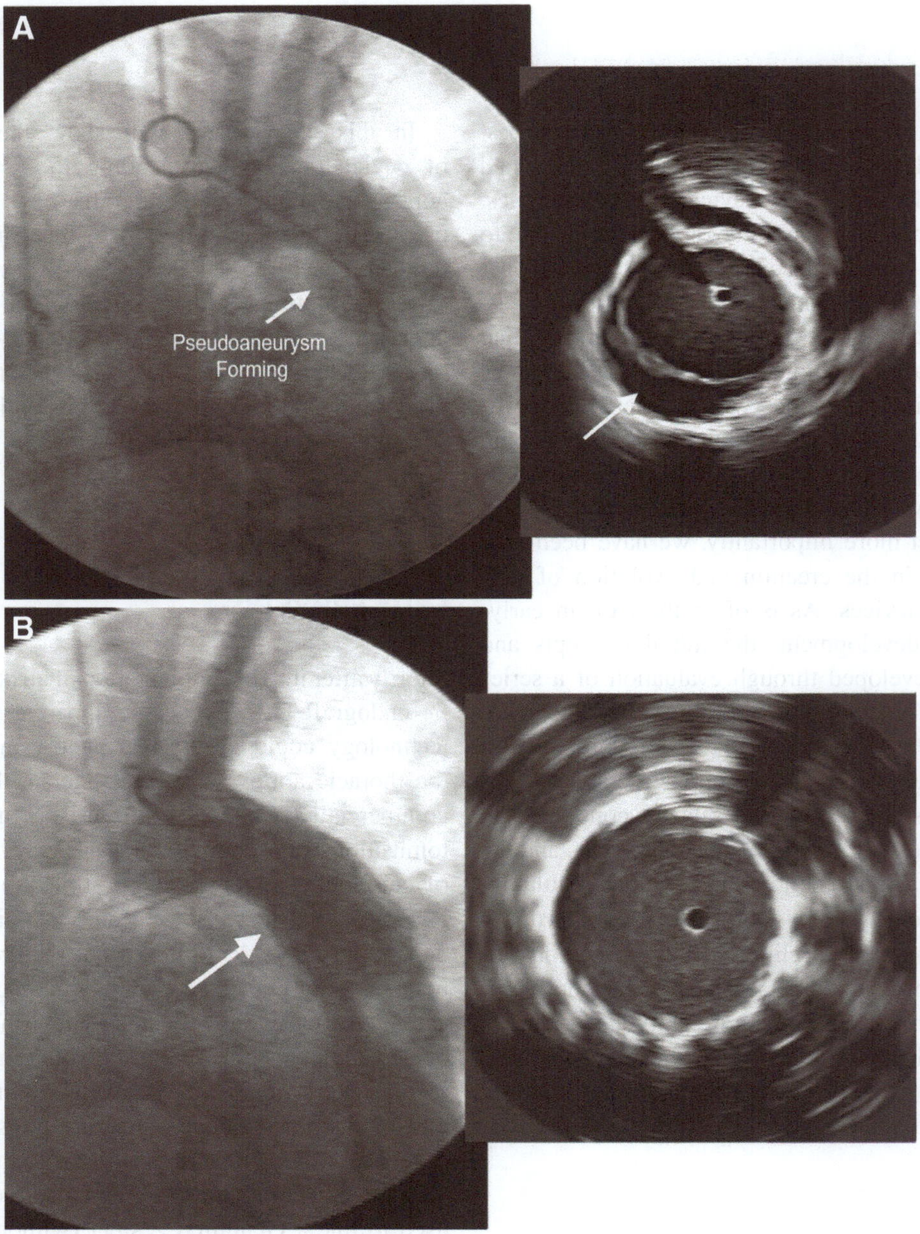

Fig. 20.1 **a**, Aortogram showing pseudoaneurysm forming after a traumatic transection of the descending thoracic aorta and an accompanying intravascular ultrasound study. **b**, Satisfactory result following deployment of an endoluminal graft. **c**, Follow-up CT showing continued resolution of the transection. **d**, Long-term (9-year) follow-up surveillance study

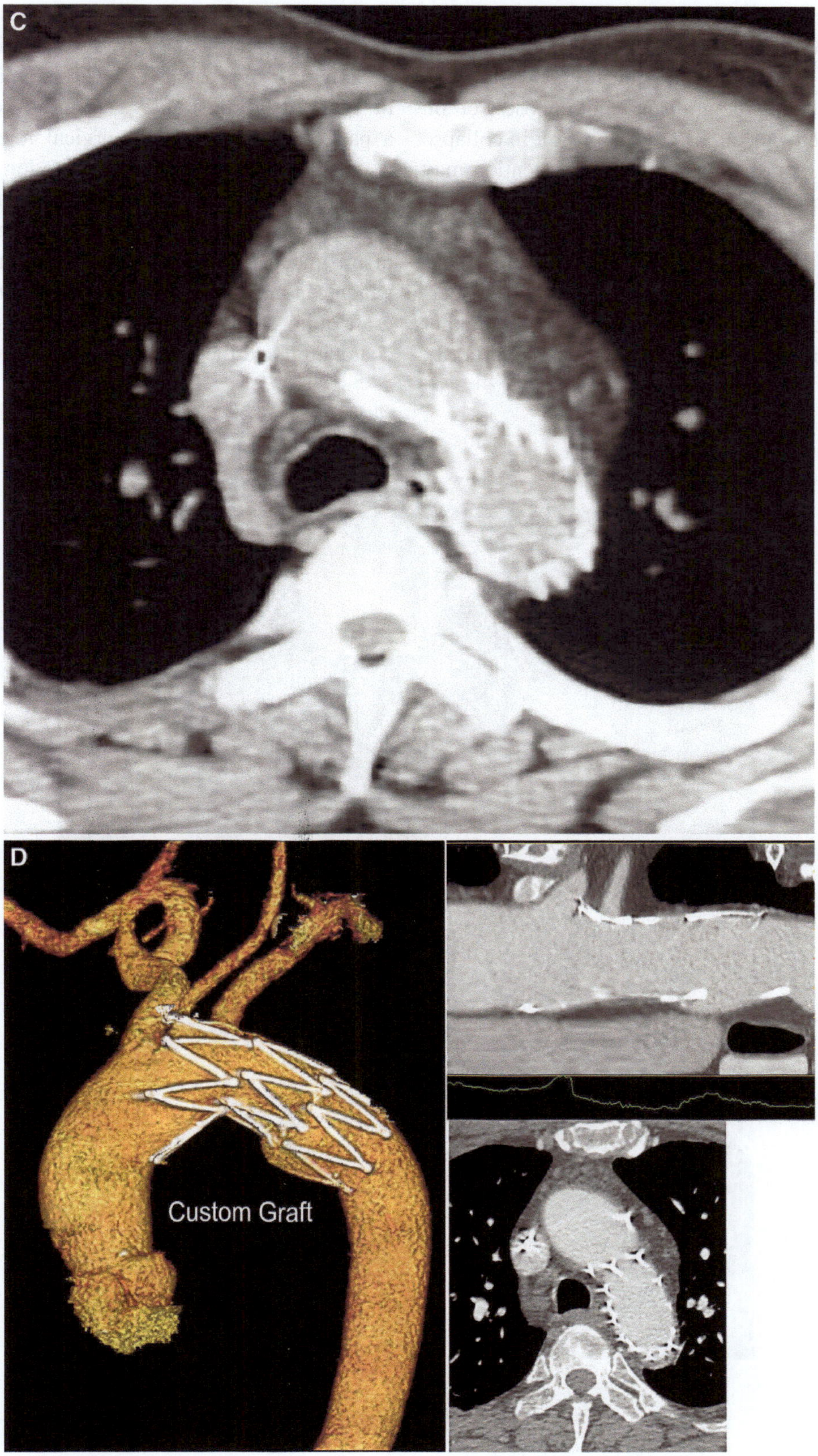

Fig. 20.1 (continued)

of the population. There is, however, one observation worth noting regarding this use of the endograft. When the endograft is applied in this location and the angle of the arch is acute, the graft may not appose well on the inner curve of the arch. This can result in collapse of the device such that a secondary intervention may be required to deploy a stent to properly appose the graft.

The use of endografts in secondary repair of congenital vascular disease in adult patients who underwent pediatric cardiac intervention has been another application for these devices in the thoracic aorta [8]. Like the transection pathologies, these cases often require some form of graft customization or the use of a hybrid approach. The CT examination shown in Fig. 20.2a illustrates a recurrent coarctation in a patient who had initial surgical repair at 6 years of age. Not only had the coarctation recurred but, more importantly, a distal aneurysm had formed and gradually expanded. This case illustrates the problem of mismatched proximal and distal aortic diameters, which can make delivery and deployment of the endograft quite challenging. In order to resolve both the coarctation and the aneurysm, three components were

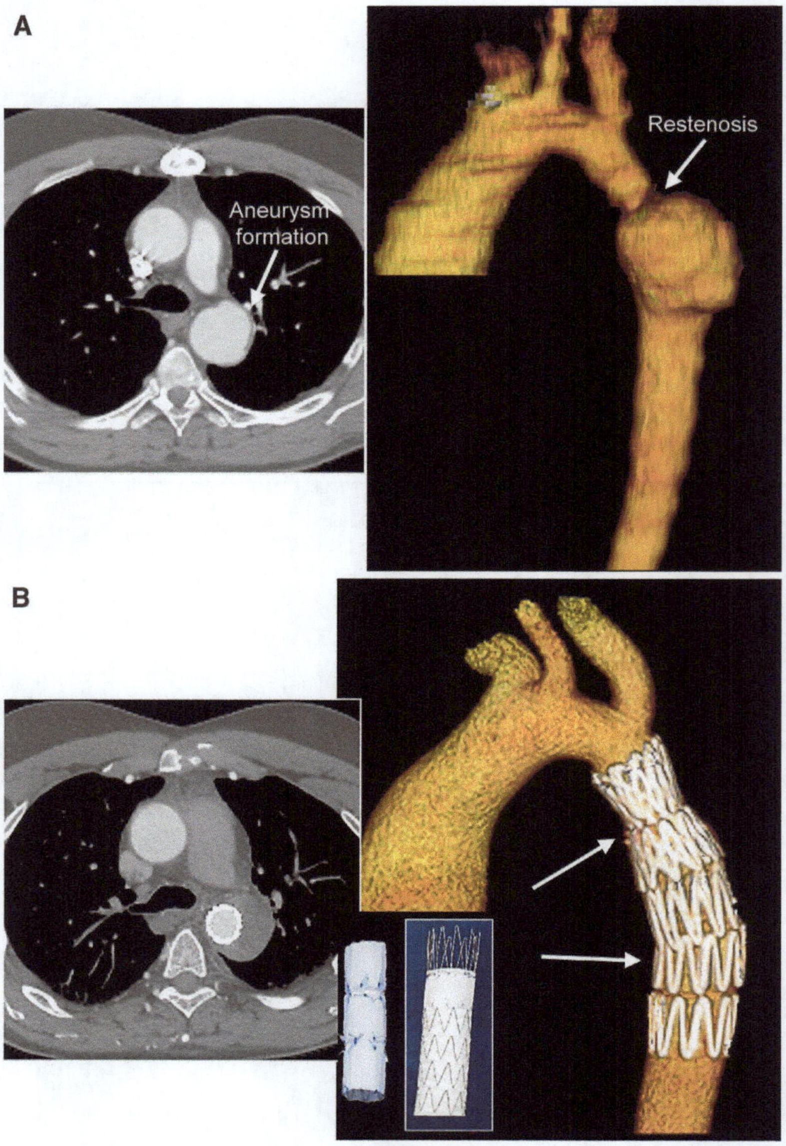

Fig. 20.2 **a**, CT showing recurrent thoracic coarctation with distal aneurysm formation. **b**, Illustration of multiple components required to treat both the coarctation and the aneurysm

required (Fig. 20.2b). A small-diameter proximal component was combined with a larger diameter distal device, and these were ultimately deployed using a Palmaz stent to correct the coarctation. New tapered commercial grafts are now becoming available for such uses, but in this example the graft still required tapering at the proximal end.

Several other complications of coarctation that may occur in adulthood have also been treated with thoracic endografts. The complication illustrated in Fig. 20.3a presented a particular problem because there was aneurysmal formation proximal and distal to the previous repair that also involved the proximal subclavian artery. The procedure entailed resection of the subclavian artery at the aortic arch through a short, supraclavicular incision. A clamp was placed at the aneurysmal origin for partial occlusion, and the stump was oversewn. A carotid–subclavian bypass restored circulation to the left arm (Fig. 20.3b). The aneurysm was excluded using overlapping endografts (Fig. 20.3c).

As technology has advanced, more complicated aneurysmal pathologies are being addressed with endografting, and combinations of classical open procedures and endovascular intervention are now often used to correct these problems [10, 13]. An unusual case is illustrated in Fig. 20.4a in a patient who, at a young age, had an open repair of an aberrant right subclavian artery, and a graft was placed between the distal aortic arch and the proximal right subclavian artery. Nearly 40 years later, the patient presented to us with an enlarging pseudoaneurysm of the distal aortic arch, as shown in Fig. 20.4b and c. Repair of the pseudoaneurysm included an open left carotid–subclavian bypass, a bypass from the right common carotid artery to the right subclavian artery (after the subclavian had been divided from the original degenerated graft and ligated), and deployment of a Gore TAG graft across the aortic arch (Fig. 20.4d). This resulted in a complete exclusion of the aneurysm (Fig. 20.4e). This case is also an example of how rerouting the supra-aortic trunks enables endografts to be deployed more proximally in the aortic arch and even into the ascending aorta as shown later in the chapter.

One of the areas of controversy involving these types of cases in which the endograft must cross the left subclavian artery concerns when left carotid–subclavian bypass or subclavian artery transposition to the left subclavian artery should be performed—whether before or at the time of endograft deployment or at all. There appears to be no consensus on the subject. We always restore left subclavian flow when a left internal mammary artery bypass is present, or when the artery will be used for coronary revascularization. Also, if the left vertebral artery is critical to perfusion for cerebral circulation, it must be preserved. This does require documentation of patency of the communicating arteries at the base of the brain. As an example, sacrificing the left subclavian artery in a patient without posterior communicating arteries (Fig. 20.5) may prove catastrophic.

Preventing neurologic complications is one of the goals in thoracic endografting, and, to date, the minimally invasive procedure is clearly showing benefit over classic open repair. There is still discussion about the advantage of documenting spinal cord blood supply in the critical areas of the descending thoracic aorta. Current imaging techniques are capable of allowing visualization of the intercostal arteries and even the artery of Adamkiewicz (Fig. 20.6a and b). There are data indicating that such identification can be useful in determining which patients should have an open repair rather than the endovascular deployment of an excluding device. We currently do not rely solely on routine preoperative imaging to make this particular decision.

Current Devices Approved for Treatment of Thoracic Aortic Aneurysms

Gore TAG

The Gore TAG endograft is comprised of an ePTFE graft with an outer self-expanding nitinol support (Fig. 20.7). This device is a flexible, self-expanding endoprosthesis that is constrained on the leading end of a delivery catheter. The system consists of two parts, the endoprosthesis and the delivery catheter. Graft sizes range in diameter from 26 to 40 mm and in length from 10 to 20 cm. The compressed profile of these devices on a delivery catheter ranges from 20 to 24 Fr. The Gore TAG® device is intended for endovascular repair of aneurysms of the descending thoracic aorta (DTA) in patients who have appropriate anatomy including adequate iliac/femoral access, aortic inner diameter in the range of 23–37 mm,

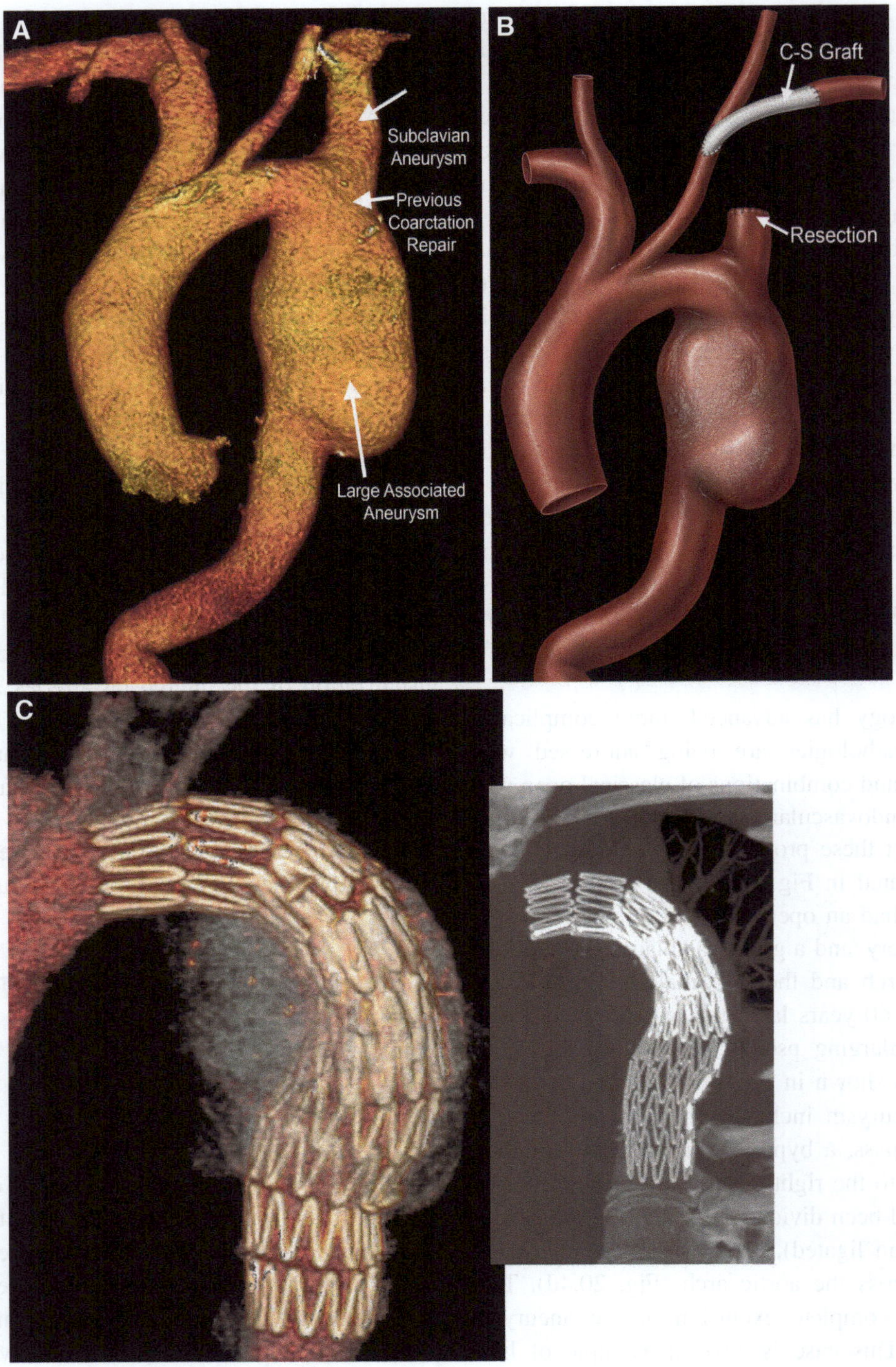

Fig. 20.3 **a**, CT showing complications following earlier coarctation repair with caudad and cephalad aneurysm formation. **b**, Drawing showing surgery component of hybrid procedure. **c**, CT showing satisfactory repair

and >2 cm non-aneurysmal aorta proximal and distal to the aneurysm.

The original Gore TAG Thoracic device received the CE mark in February 1998 and began distribution outside of the United States in December 1998. Gore discontinued distribution of the original TAG device in 2001 and began modifications to the design of the endoprosthesis. The modified TAG device received the CE mark in February 2004 and began distribution in March 2004 and was later approved by the Food and Drug Administration (FDA) in 2005.

Talent

The Talent™ Thoracic Stent Graft is composed of a series of shaped, self-expanding nitinol springs to

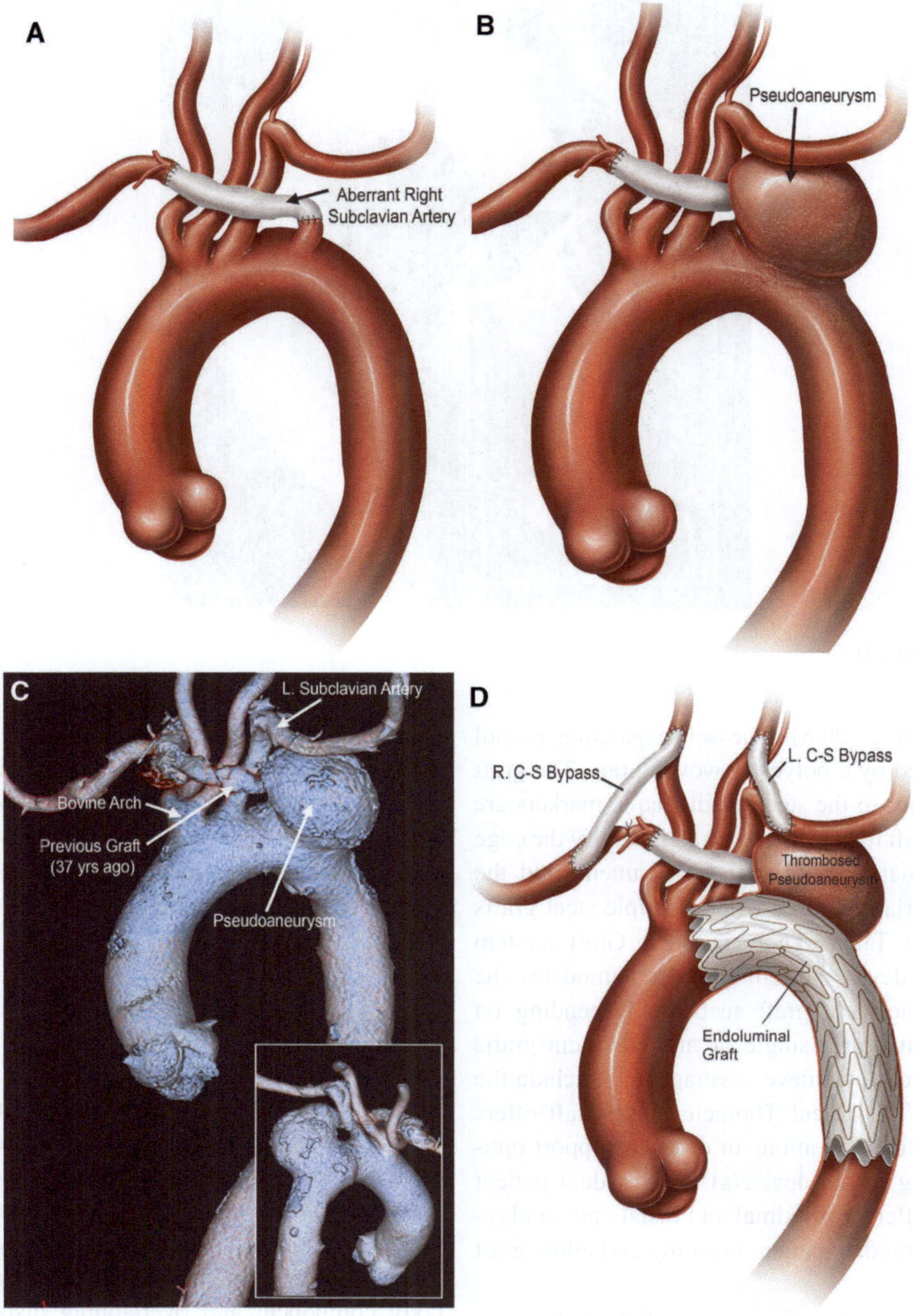

Fig. 20.4 **a**, Drawing illustrating initial repair of aberrant *right* subclavian artery. **b**, Illustration showing formation of a large pseudoaneurysm at the distal anastomotic site on the aortic arch. **c**, CT showing the pseudoaneurysm. **d**, Illustration of hybrid operative repair. **e**, Control CT showing satisfactory exclusion of the pseudoaneurysm

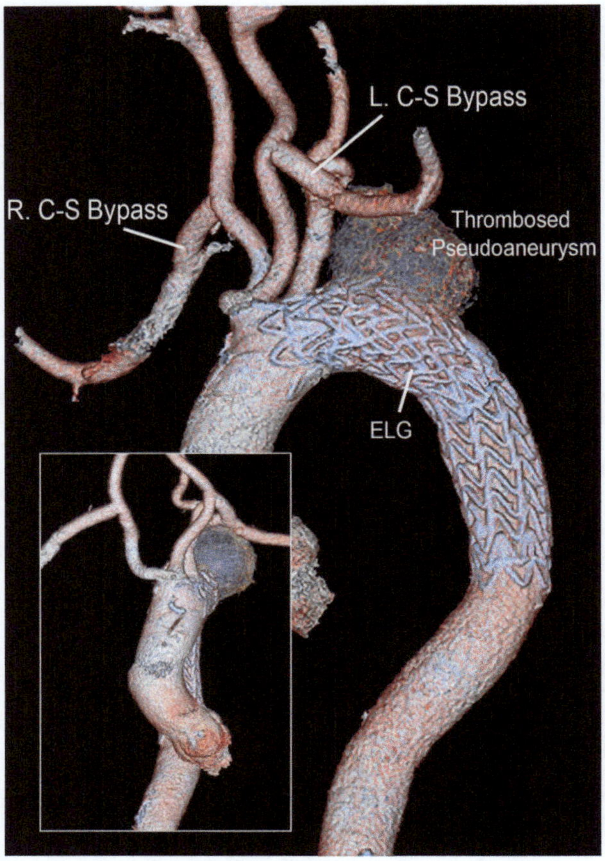

Fig. 20.4 (continued)

form a stent (Fig. 20.8). The self-expanding nitinol stent is covered by a polyester woven graft. The graft material is sewn to the stent. Radiopaque markers are sewn to the graft to help visualize and identify the edge of the graft material, stent graft alignment, and the minimum overlap required when multiple stent grafts are used. The Talent Thoracic Stent Graft System is a modular device system that accommodates the use of multiple stent graft sections. Depending on the patient's anatomy, single or multiple stent grafts may be required to achieve coverage and exclude the target lesion. The Talent Thoracic Stent Graft offers multiple graft configurations in order to support optimum matching of the device(s) to individual patient anatomies. Different proximal and distal end configurations accommodate patient anatomy and allow graft mating.

This device is indicated for the endovascular repair of fusiform aneurysms and saccular aneurysms/penetrating ulcers of the descending thoracic aorta in patients having appropriate anatomy, including iliac/femoral access vessel morphology that is compatible with vascular access techniques, devices, and/or accessories. The non-aneurysmal aortic diameter must be in the range of 18–42 mm, and non-aneurysmal aortic proximal and distal neck lengths should be >20 mm.

Zenith TX2

The Zenith TX2 TAA Endovascular Graft is a two- or one-piece cylindrical endovascular graft (Fig. 20.9). The one-piece system may consist of either a one-piece main body component or a proximal main body component (without use of a distal main body component). The two-piece system consists of a proximal main body component and overlapping distal main body component. The proximal main body components can be either tapered (by 4 mm) or non-tapered. The stent grafts are constructed of full-thickness woven

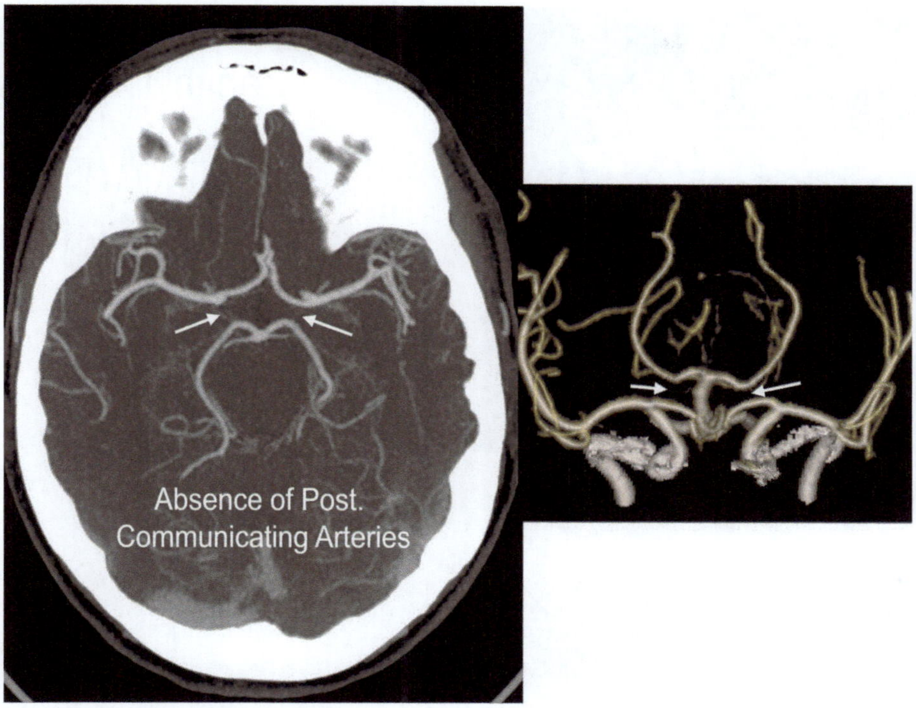

Fig. 20.5 MRA showing the importance of assessing the intracranial basilar circulation when the *left* subclavian artery is to be intentionally covered with an endograft

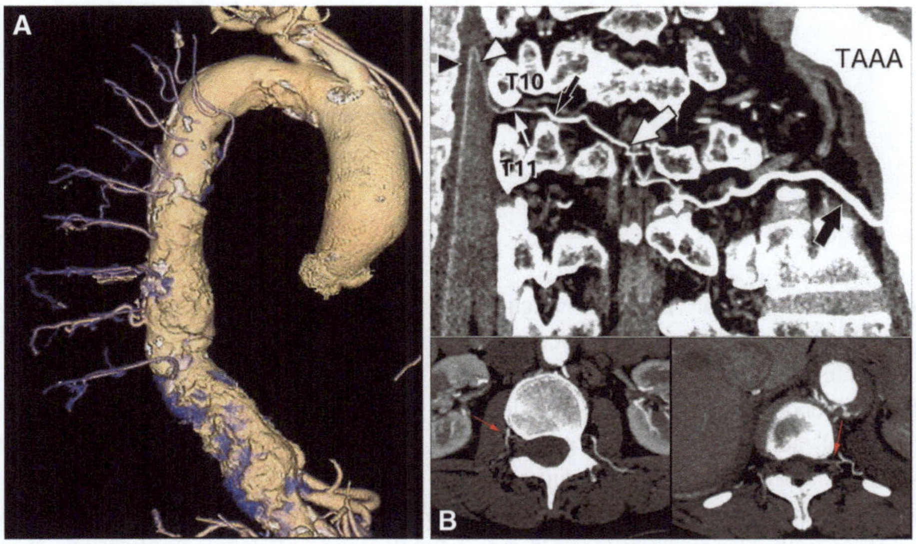

Fig. 20.6 **a**, CT illustrating intercostals arteries prior to endograft deployment. **b**, CT identification of the spinal cord blood supply

polyester fabric sewn to self-expanding stainless steel Cook-Z stents with braided polyester and monofilament polypropylene sutures. The Zenith TX2TAA Endovascular Graft is fully stented to provide stability and the force necessary to open the lumen of the graft during deployment. Additionally, the Cook-Z stents provide the necessary attachment and seal of the graft to the vessel wall. For added fixation, the covered stent is at the proximal end of the proximal main body component.

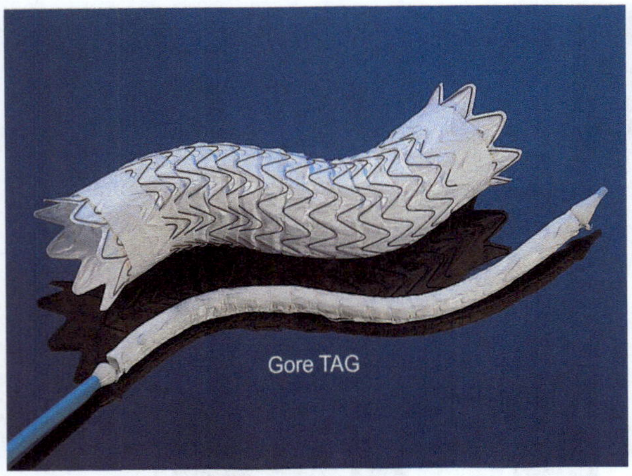

Fig. 20.7 Photograph of the Gore TAG device

Fig. 20.8 Photograph of the Talent thoracic stent graft

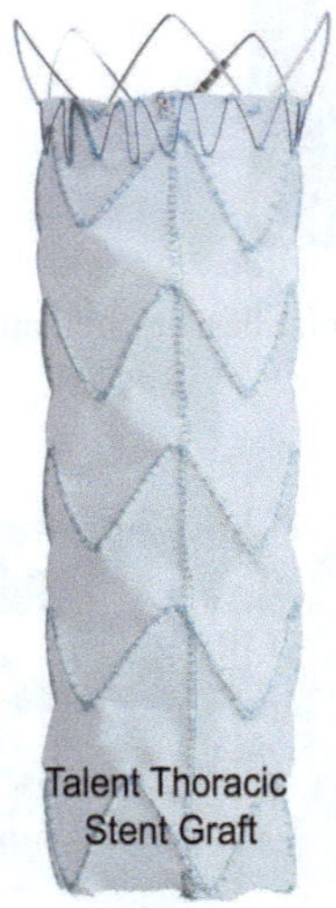

This device is indicated for the endovascular treatment of patients with aneurysms or ulcers of the descending thoracic aorta having vascular morphology suitable for endovascular repair, including adequate iliac/femoral access compatible with the required introduction systems and non-aneurysmal aortic segments (fixation sites) proximal and distal to the aneurysm or ulcer, with a length of at least 25 mm and with a diameter measured outer wall to outer wall of no greater than 38 mm and no less than 24 mm.

Off-Label Use

The approval of the above-listed devices has greatly enhanced our ability to treat thoracic aortic aneurysms.

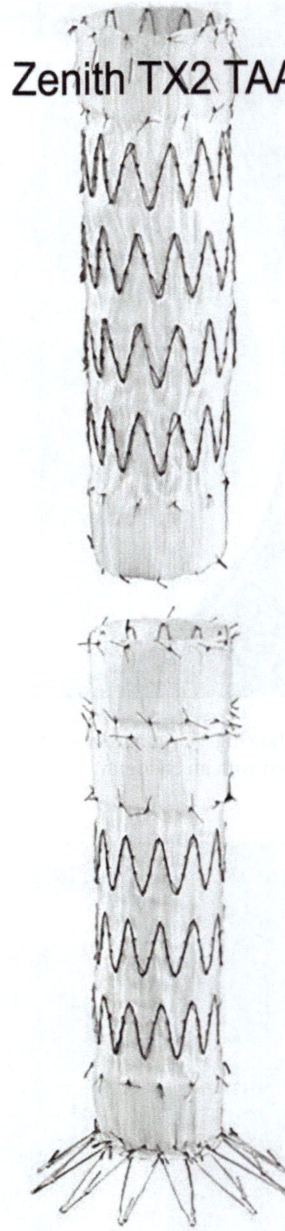

Fig. 20.9 Photograph of the Zenith TX2 device

While current labeling does not suggest broad use of the devices, "off-label" applications are very common.

Type b Dissection

One area of great interest to our team is the treatment of type b dissections. We recently reviewed the results of intervention in 324 patients who were treated

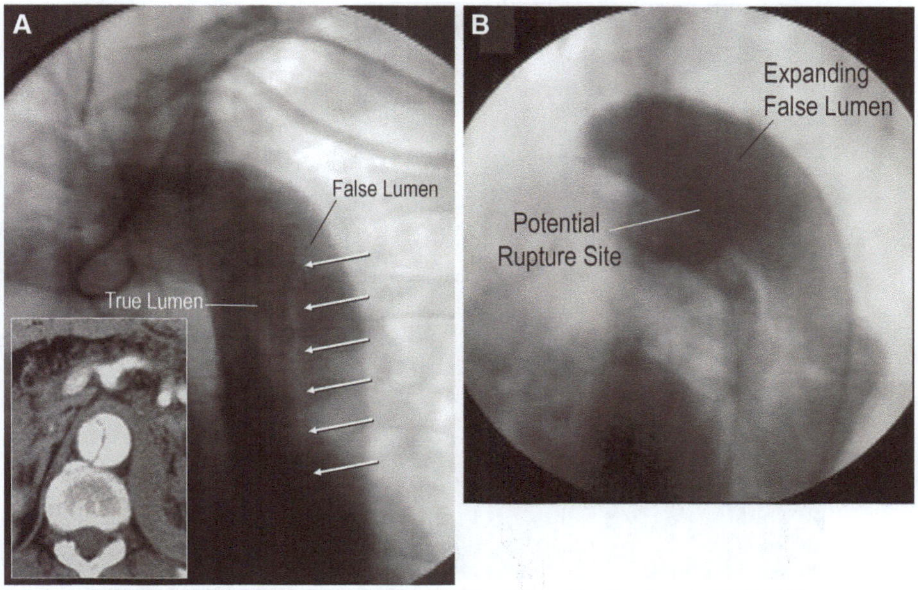

Fig. 20.10 **a**, Angiogram and CT showing true and false lumens in a type b dissection. The patient was asymptomatic but suddenly developed severe chest pain out of the hospital. **b**, Angiogram showing greatly expanded false lumen with impending rupture

with Gore Excluder graft, which is approved for treatment of abdominal aortic aneurysms [9]. Nearly half the patients in this group were treated for atherosclerotic aneurysms, but a log-rank test did not find statistical differences in actuarial survival with 30-day related mortality between aortic aneurysms and other pathologies ($P = 0.29$) or between type b dissections and other pathologies ($P = 0.97$). Late mortality was 9.6% with 31 unrelated deaths. Follow-up ranged between 1 and 70 months (average = 17 months), and the 30-day morbidity and mortality rates compared favorably with open repair.

Our position on the treatment of asymptomatic type b dissections is probably more aggressive than that of others. There is no trial published to date on regarding this subject except the INSTEAD trial, which was confounded by enrollment of a host of patients with chronic rather than acute dissections. We have encountered many patients who appear to be stable with medical treatment and then suddenly become symptomatic with expansion and rupture of the false lumen (Figs. 20.10a and b). Studies currently in progress may clarify the question of how to best treat these dissections in the future. For example, we have recently shown that both acute and chronic dissections can be effectively treated by endovascular means. When endografting includes the closure of intimal tears and resolution of false lumen antegrade flow, the true lumen of the thoracic aorta remains stable and the false lumen decreases, thus potentially reducing the risk of subsequent rupture [11].

In spite of the availability of current devices, they do not enable totally adequate treatment in complex dissections as is illustrated in Fig. 20.11a. This patient exhibited serious abdominal pain and lower limb ischemia secondary to an acute type b dissection with severe compromise of the true lumen. Deployment of a Gore TAG device from the left subclavian artery to the lower thoracic aorta did not resolve the problem due to continued true lumen compromise (Fig. 20.11b). In order to avoid placing a covered device over the visceral arterial branches, a Gianturco stent (with barbs removed, Fig. 20.11c) was used, and flow was completely restored (Fig. 20.11d). In the future, grafts will be available with uncovered components to enhance treatment of complex lesions.

Expanding into the Ascending Aorta and Arch

There is an evolving intent to use stent grafts to treat aortic pathologies in the entire arch. We have found this to be a challenging area but, as devices have

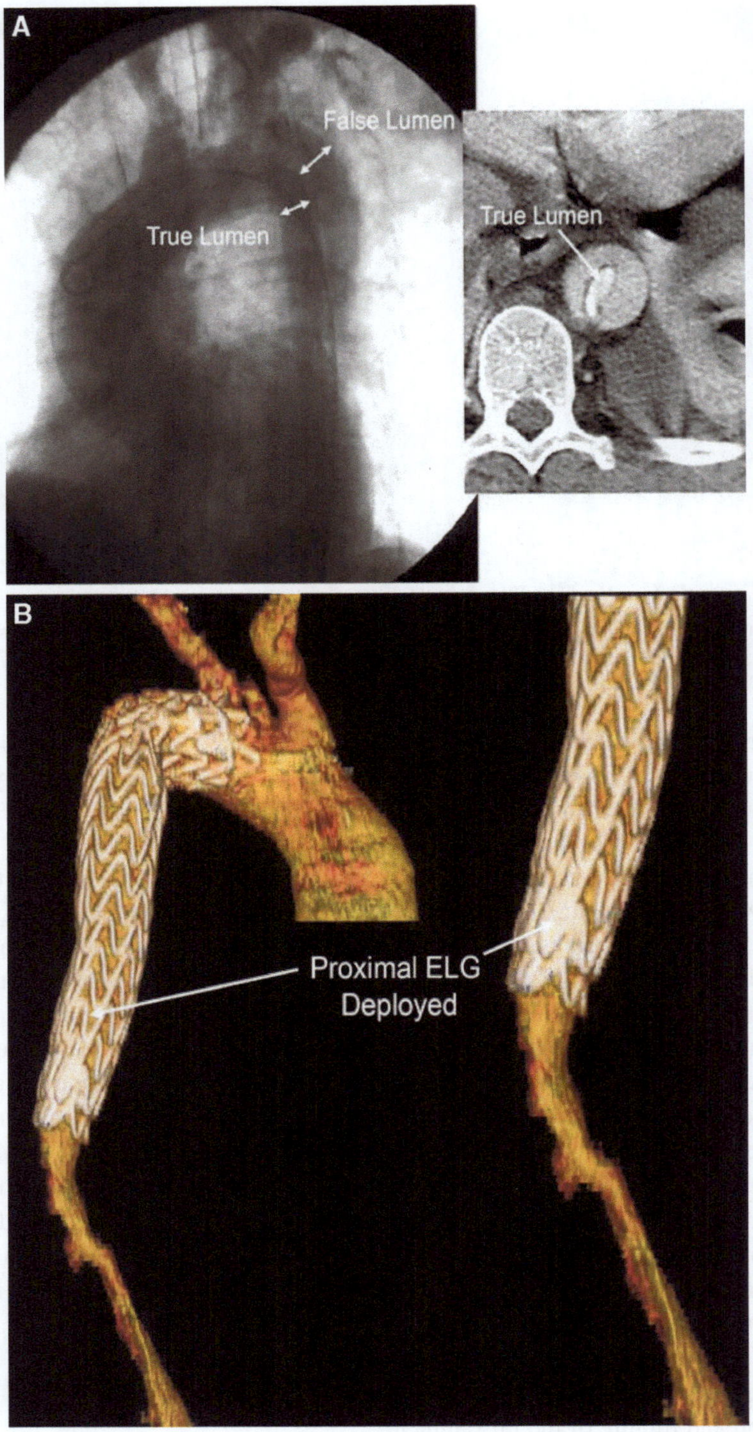

Fig. 20.11 **a**, Angiogram and CT illustrating marked compression of the true lumen, creating distal vascular compromise. **b**, CT showing incomplete resolution of the true lumen compression. **c**, Photograph showing preparation of a Gianturco Z stent with barb removal. **d**, CT and angiogram showing restoration of the true lumen and distal arterial flow

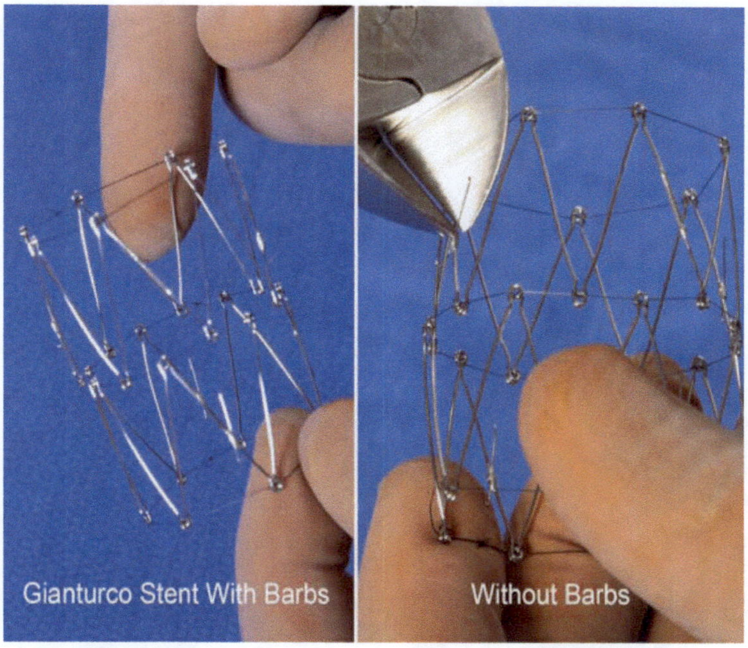

Fig. 20.11 (continued)

become available on an investigative basis (including off-label and customized device use), it is clear that in the future many of these lesions will be treated using endovascular means. Our initial experience with endografting of an ascending aneurysm occurred when we treated an aneurysm that had developed at the proximal anastomosis of a right coronary artery bypass graft (Fig. 20.12a). We treated this initially with coils but, 4 months later, the aneurysm had expanded from 6 to 10 cm. A customized endograft was deployed to exclude the aneurysm (Fig. 20.12b); a year later, CT studies confirmed the continued success (Fig. 20.12c). Several cases have now been described, and industry is developing a variety of devices for use in these locations.

Gore has designed a graft that permits side branches to be deployed into the arch vessels using a unique sleeve entry for sealing (Fig. 20.13). Customized devices by Cook have been used to deploy stent grafts into the ascending aorta with components that extend into the brachiocephalic and common carotid arteries (Fig. 20.14). Investigators in Australia are, perhaps, the most advanced with these types of techniques, no doubt due to their association with Cook Australia. Fig. 20.15 illustrates a total arch aneurysm treated with a multi-branched endograft.

When custom grafts are not available, an interesting alternative technique has been used. The main body of an endograft is deployed, and individual stent grafts are positioned alongside (thus, the name "chimney graft") to permit flow into the supra-aortic arch vessels (Fig. 20.16). This technique is also very useful with a stent graft has been inadvertently placed over a branch artery and has created end organ ischemia [14].

In an effort to extend the endografting procedure to acute type a dissections, we have used a hybrid technique with open repair of the ascending aorta and graft replacement (Fig. 20.17a) combined with arch vessel rerouting and antegrade deployment of endografts (Fig. 20.17b and c). This technique has proven useful for complete resolution of extensive dissections in one stage (Fig. 20.17d).

Conclusions

In the last decade, endografting has been used increasingly to treat a variety of problems in several different vascular territories. Although it has proven useful in the treatment of thoracic aortic pathologies, the technology is still at a relatively early developmental stage, with just three stent grafts approved by the

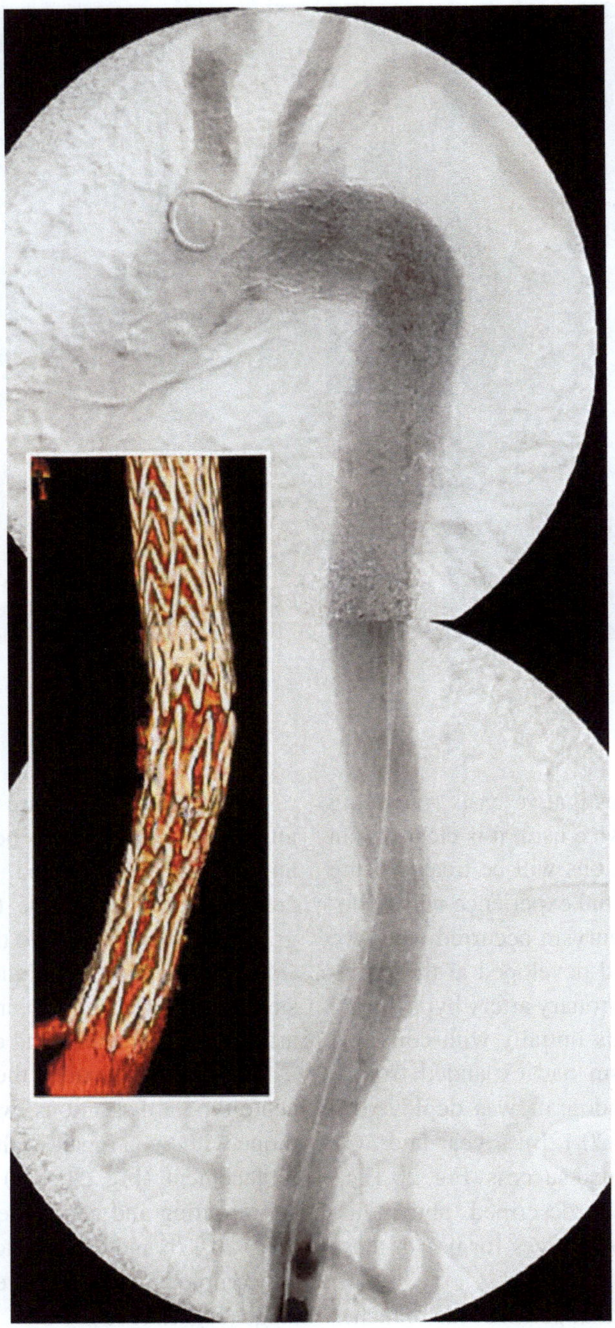

Fig. 20.11 (continued)

FDA. Thoracic endografting clearly has advantages over open surgery, including reduced rates of perioperative mortality and neurological injury, particularly in patients who are stable and do not require emergent intervention. Not all patients are suited to endovascular repair, and despite the fact that device technology has evolved considerably over the last decade, there is room for improvement in device designs.

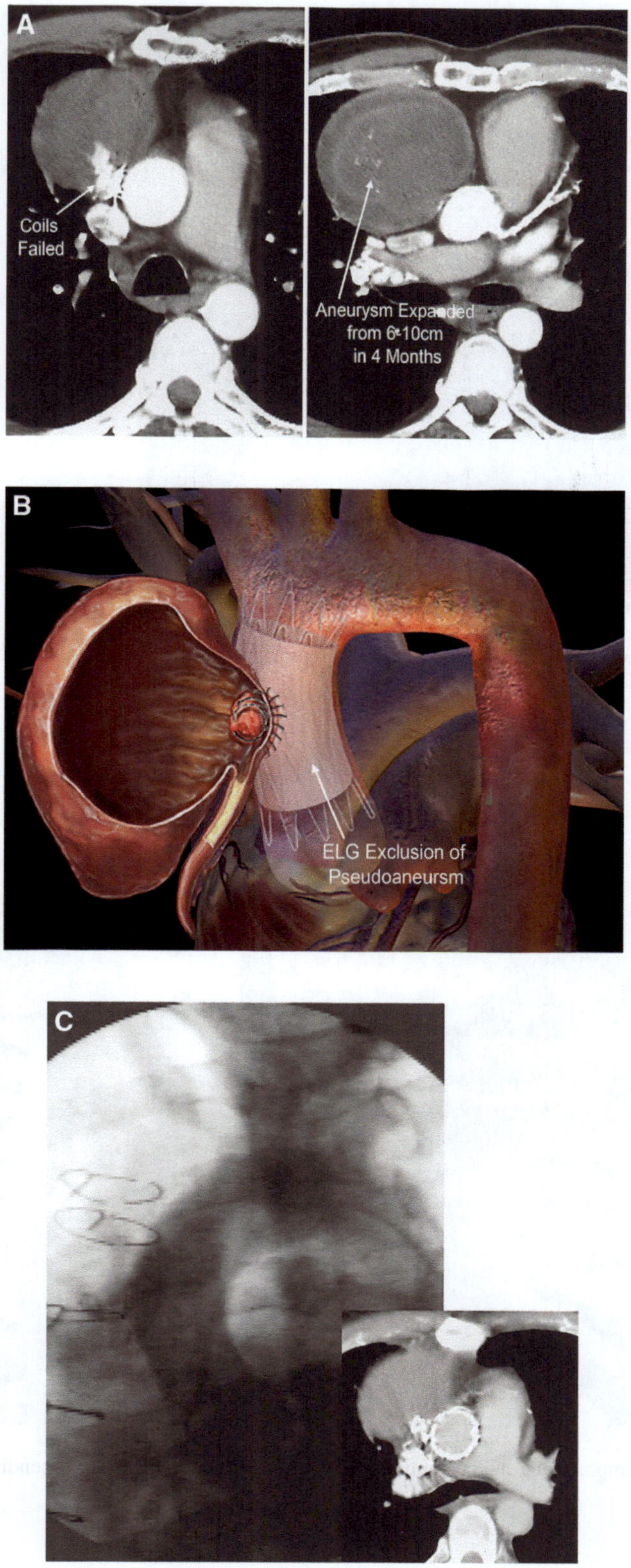

Fig. 20.12 **a**, CT showing continual expansion of an ascending arch pseudoaneurysm in spite of coil deployment to create a thrombosis. **b**, Drawing showing customized graft deployment to close the entry into the pseudoaneurysm. **c**, One-year follow-up angiogram showing exclusion of the pseudoaneurysm

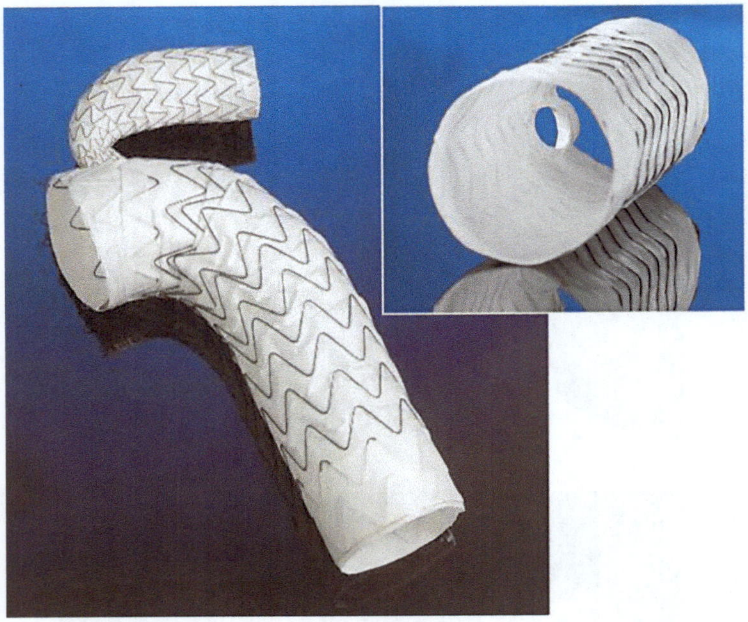

Fig. 20.13 Photograph of an experimental Gore graft to treat a thoracic arch aneurysm involving the supra-aortic trunks

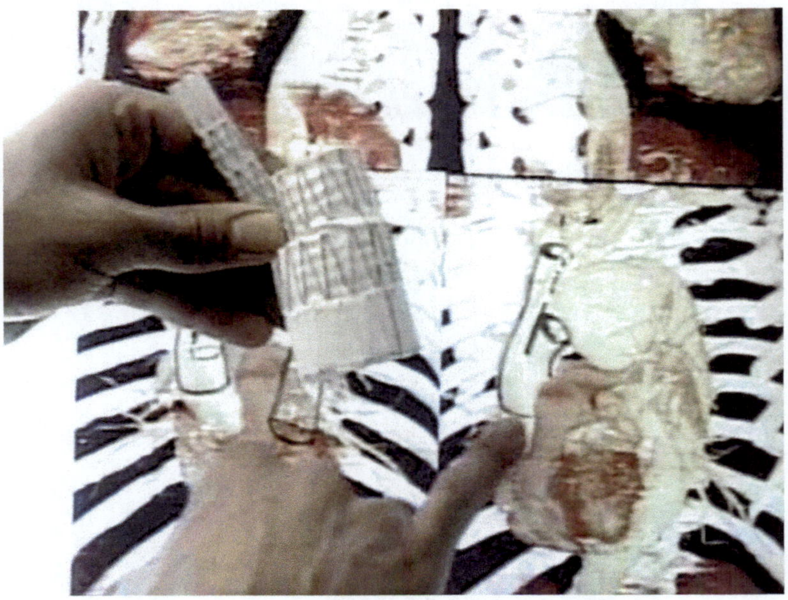

Fig. 20.14 Composite photo emphasizing the customized Cook graft for treatment of the ascending aorta with extension into the innominate artery

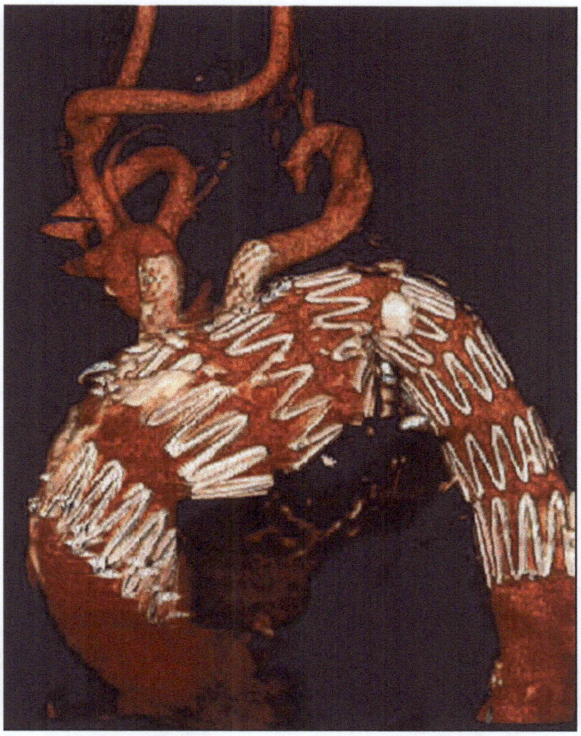

Fig. 20.15 Illustration of a total arch aneurysm treated endovascularly with a multi-branched endograft

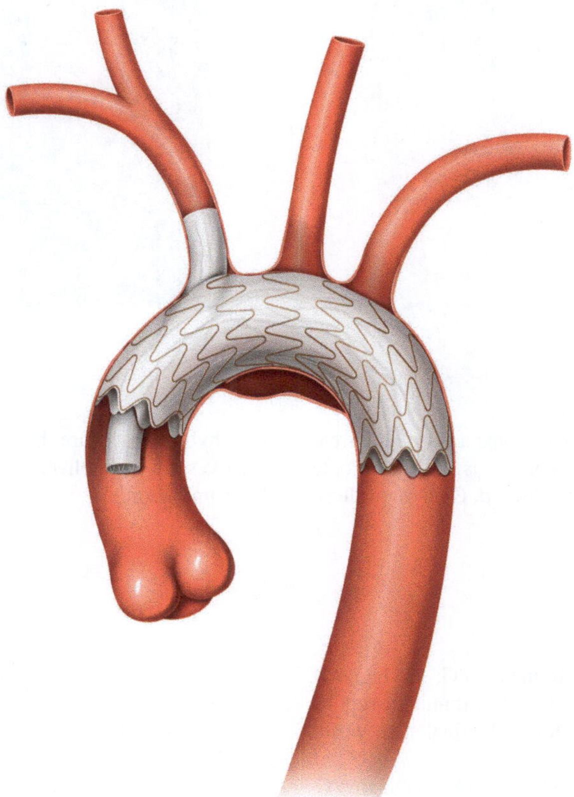

Fig. 20.16 Photograph of Chimney-Stack procedure to treat compromised flow in the arch vessels and expand the landing zones for endoluminal grafting

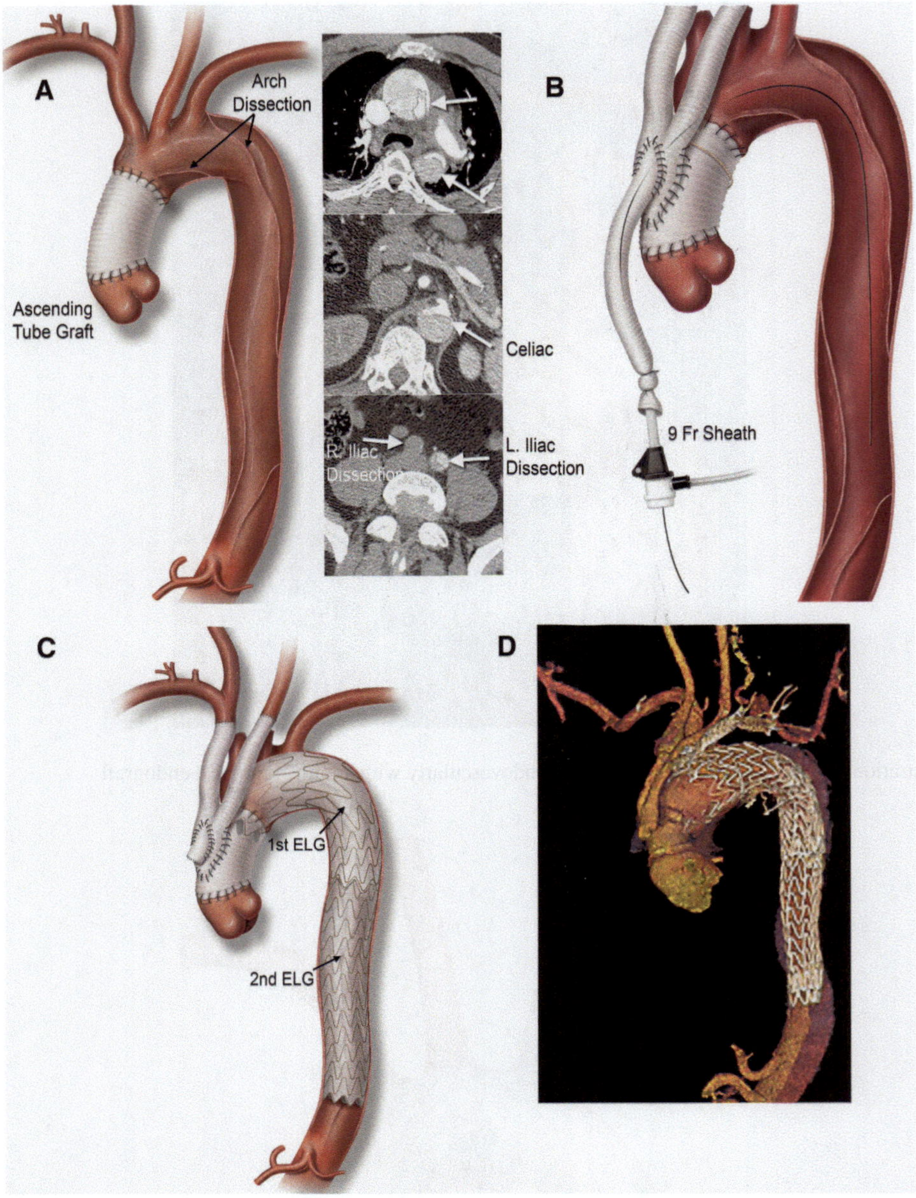

Fig. 20.17 **a**, Drawing and CT showing type a dissection treated with a hybrid procedure. **b**, After surgical repair of an ascending dissection, a bifurcated graft with a conduit is used to reroute the arch vessels and deliver an endograft in antegrade fashion. **c**, Drawing showing the completed procedure. **d**, One-year follow-up CT examination

References

1. Thompson CS, Rodriguez JA, Ramaiah VG, DiMugno L, Shafique S, Olsen D, Diethrich EB: Acute traumatic rupture of the thoracic aorta treated with endoluminal stent grafts, *J Trauma* 52:1173–1177, 2002.
2. Thompson CS, Gaxotte VD, Rodriguez JA, Ramaiah VG, Vranic M, Ravi R et al.: Endoluminal stent grafting of the thoracic aorta: initial experience with the Gore Excluder, *J Vasc Surg* 35:1163–1170, 2002.
3. Ramaiah V, Rodriguez-Lopez J, Diethrich EB: Endografting of the thoracic aorta, *J Card Surg* 18:444–454, 2003.
4. Rodriguez JA, Olsen DM, Diethrich EB: Thoracic aortic dissections: unpredictable lesions that may be treated using endovascular techniques, *J Card Surg* 18:334–350, 2003.
5. Diethrich EB: Symposium on thoracic aortic endovascular stents, part I. Editorial comment, *J Card Surg* 18:333, 2003.

6. Diethrich EB: Endovascular thoracic aortic repairs: greater experience brings rewards and new problems to challenge us, *J Endovasc Ther* 11:168–169, 2004.
7. Wheatley GH 3rd, Nunez A, Preventza O, Ramaiah VG, Rodriguez-Lopez JA, Williams J et al.: Have we gone too far? Endovascular stent-graft repair of aortobronchial fistulas, *J Thorac Cardiovasc Surg* 133(5):1277–1285, 2007.
8. Preventza O, Wheatley GH 3rd, Williams J, Hughes K, Ramaiah VG, Rodriguez-Lopez JA et al.: Endovascular approaches for complex forms of recurrent aortic coarctation, *J Endovasc Ther* 13(3):400–405, 2006.
9. Rodriguez JA, Olsen DM, Shtutman A, Lucas LA, Wheatley G, Alpern J et al.: Application of endograft to treat thoracic aortic pathologies: a single center experience, *J Vasc Surg* 46(3):413–420, 2007.
10. Diethrich EB: Technical tips for thoracic aortic endografting, *Semin Vasc Surg* 21(1):8–12, 2008.
11. Rodriguez JA, Olsen DM, Lucas L, Wheatley G, Ramaiah V, Diethrich EB: Aortic remodeling after endografting of thoracoabdominal aortic dissection, *J Vasc Surg* 47(6):1188–1194, 2008.
12. Parodi JC, Palmaz JC, Barone HD: Transfemoral intraluminal graft implantation for abdominal aortic aneurysms, *Ann Vasc Surg* 5(6):491–499, 1991.
13. Melissano G, Civilini E, Bertoglio L, Calliari F, Setacci F, Calori G et al.: Results of endografting of the aortic arch in different landing zones, *Eur J Vasc Endovasc Surg* 33(5):561–566, 2007.
14. Ohrlander T, Sonesson B, Ivancev K, Resch T, Dias N, Malina M: The chimney graft: a technique for preserving or rescuing aortic branch vessels in stent-graft sealing zones, *J Endovasc Ther* 15:427–432, 2008.

Part V

Specialized Endovascular Techniques

Critical Limb Ischemia

21

David E. Allie, Raghotham R. Patlola, Elena V. Mitran, Agostino Ingraldi, and Craig M. Walker

At the beginning of the third millennium the studies on the epidemiology of cardiovascular diseases (CVD) led to the conclusion that we are facing a very serious public health threat, that of a pandemic of cardiovascular disease. In this context, peripheral arterial disease (PAD) and its components [i.e., intermittent claudication (IC), critical limb ischemia (CLI), and acute limb ischemia (ALI)] should also be treated as a prevalent global disease [1].

A few medical domains, among them CLI, encounter at present an amazingly fast development regarding the disease management. Looking at the published papers on CLI, we are facing an explosion of publications in the last 2 years. The recent literature on CLI reveals a great awareness campaign. CLI is defined as a global epidemic and is being discussed not only as a medical problem but as a public health problem at large medical gatherings such as the Charing Cross Symposium, Paris Course on Revascularization (Euro-PCR), as well as the three annual (2005–2007) International Multidisciplinary CLI Summits of the New Cardiovascular Horizons.

The wealth of knowledge on CLI, as an integral part of the big chapter of PAD, could be divided chronologically into four periods defined by the existing documents and guidelines:

A. Second European Consensus Document on Chronic Critical Leg Ischemia based on the accumulation of literature from the beginnings until 1990 [2]. The document dedicated a large space to CLI epidemiology based on its status in the European countries as well as the US populations. All the vascular societies concerned plus the World Health Organization (WHO) elaborated the consensus document.
B. The TransAtlantic Inter Society Consensus (TASC) report published in 2000 reviewed the published literature until 1998 [3].
C. The Guidelines for the Management of Patients With Peripheral Arterial Disease (Lower Extremity, Renal, Mesenteric, and Abdominal Aortic): A Collaborative Report from the American Association for Vascular Surgery/Society for Vascular Surgery, Society for Cardiovascular Angiography and Interventions, Society for Vascular Medicine and Biology, Society of Interventional Radiology, and the ACC/AHA Task Force on Practice Guidelines covered the literature up to 2004 and was published in March 2006 [4].
D. The Intersociety Consensus for the Management of PAD (TASC II) published in January 2007 covered the literature up to May 2006 [5].

In the above-mentioned guidelines the contributing teams of experts were representing Europe, United States, Asia, Africa, Australia, in international collaborations aiming at regulating CLI. The guidelines define CLI as limb pain that occurs at rest or impending limb loss that is caused by severe compromise of blood flow to the affected extremity [6]. The patients present with lower extremity rest pain, ulceration or gangrene and a significant risk for limb loss. To date, the terms "critical limb ischemia," "chronic critical limb ischemia," and "chronic limb ischemia" are all used to describe this disease [2–5, 7, 8].

D.E. Allie (✉)
Chief, Cardiothoracic and Endovascular Surgery,
Cardiovascular Institute of the South, Lafayette, LA, USA

T.J. Fogarty, R.A. White (eds.), *Peripheral Endovascular Interventions*,
DOI 10.1007/978-1-4419-1387-6_21, © Springer Science+Business Media, LLC 1998, 2010

Epidemiology

Unfortunately, there is a lack of true (not calculated/estimated) epidemiological data regarding CLI incidence and prevalence. The answer to the real epidemiology of CLI could come from knowing the CLI geographical status. This idea was expressed in the guidelines (i.e., the need of a paper on CLI geographical status was called in the European meetings and the Transatlantic meetings) [2–5].

The search of published literature on CLI's epidemiology was conducted on Medline (1966–2008), Embase (1980–2008), Cochrane Central Register of Controlled Trials (CENTRAL), manual search of journals, meetings proceedings, clinical trials from ClinicalTrials.gov, "meta Register of Controlled Trials" (mRCT), National Center Watch and World Center Watch, and Center of Drug Evaluation and Research (CDER). An exhausting number of key words has been used, from which just a few are exemplified: atherosclerosis, epidemiology, prevalence and incidence, geographical/global/world distribution, CLI by country, CLI meetings, PAD and CLI, and peripheral vascular disease (PVD), morbidity, mortality, prognosis. Our intention was to exclude the retrieved papers dealing with CLI of other origin than atherosclerosis, but the diabetes mellitus (DM) etiology of CLI is intertwined with atherosclerotic CLI (Table 21.1) [6].

Adding to the incidence and prevalence, the data on CLI amputations due to atherosclerosis alone or the atherosclerosis plus DM project a threatening dimension of CLI. The reports on amputations due to CLI reveal a number of greater than 150,000–2,000,000 major and minor lower extremity amputations in United States and Europe yearly [9]. The amputation rate in United States has increased from 19 to 30 per 100,000 persons over the last two decades primarily, due to DM and an advancing in age population [9]. In populations over 85 years of age, the amputation rate is 140 per 100,000 persons/year with a mortality of 13–17% [9]. When referring to CLI in diabetics, statistics show that one out of every four diabetics will

Table 21.1 Retrieved CLI epidemiological data in terms of prevalence and incidence on large global geographical areas

Geographic region	CLI prevalence	CLI incidence
North America [2–5, 11]	• 1% in population >50 years (USA) • 2% in population >70 years (USA)	• Calculated incidence: 500–1,000 cases/million/year (USA) • 1.5% in population <50 years (USA) • 0.5% in men 55–65 years (USA) • 5% in population >70 years (USA)
South America [62]	• No reports	• 400 cases/million/year (Brazil)
Europe	• 500–1,000 cases/million/year (UK) [2] • 1 case in 2,500 persons (UK) [63] • 2% in the subjects with PAD (Germany) [64] • 0.1% in population aged 45–75 years (Germany) [65] • 1%/entire population/year (Sweden) [69] • 0.26% men and 0.24% women age 40–69 years (Norway) [70]	• Calculated incidence: 500–1,000 cases/million/year (Europe) [2] • 450/million/year in population >45 years (Italy) [66] • 49.8% in the contralateral limb over 6 year period (Italy) [67] • 38/100,000/year (Sweden) [68] • 0.3% in young subjects, 3.3% in age 80–84, 2.5% in age >84 years (Sweden) [69] • 0.05–0.1%/general population (Belgium) [71] • Yearly incidence 1,500–1,700 patients/year (Croatia) [72]
Asia	• Clinical studies on CLI were retrieved but no population-based studies on CLI prevalence and incidence were located	
Africa	• Clinical studies on CLI were retrieved but no population-based studies on CLI prevalence and incidence were located	
Australia	• Clinical studies on CLI were retrieved but no population-based studies on CLI prevalence and incidence were located	

CLI: critical limb ischemia.

face CLI within their lifetime, and those with CLI will have a 7–40 times greater risk of amputation [10]. An amputation is a marker for death and the 3- to 4-year mortality rate post amputation is >50–60% [3, 11]. The retrieved epidemiological data support the conclusion that CLI has no boundaries and that CLI is a pandemic of our time generated by the aging society presenting with overwhelming incidence of PAD and DM.

Clinical Presentation

CLI has a significant dimension in the medical practice, being bilateral and incurable. The clinical categories of CLI indicating the progress from asymptomatic PAD to CLI are presented by Creager and Libby as recommended by Rutherford et al. (Table 21.2). Rutherford's 1997 "standards for reports" are still used today in clinical practice [12].

The pathophysiology of CLI is determined by the abnormal microcirculation. As was hypothesized by Creager and Libby, based on the literature, few factors could be the contributors to CLI (i.e., reduced number of skin capillaries, decreased capillary perfusion, reduced blood cell deformability, increased leucocytes adhesivity, platelet aggregation and fibrinogen, microthrombosis, excessive vasoconstriction, and interstitial edema) [12]. Infrainguinal arterial blockages are the most common etiology of claudication and CLI. The superficial femoral artery (SFA) and popliteal artery (PA) pose interventional challenges. Longitudinal occlusions are common. These vessels elongate, foreshorten, bend, torque, and are externally compressible. Lesions are often calcified. Acute and chronic thrombosis is common. The infrapopliteal vessels (IP) are smaller, lesions often involve branch points, and the vessels are much less dynamic.

Table 21.2 Rutherford–Becker classification

Category	Clinical description	Objective criteria
0 1	Asymptomatic—no hemodynamically significant occlusive disease Mild claudication	Normal treadmill[a] or reactive hyperemia test
2 3	Moderate claudication Severe claudication	Completes treadmill exercise; AP after exercise >50 mmHg but ≥20 mmHg lower than resting value
4	Ischemic rest pain	Resting AP < 60 mmHg, ankle or metatarsal PVD flat or barely Pulsatile; TP < 40 mmHg
5	Minor tissue loss-nonhealing ulcer, focal gangrene with diffuse pedal ischemia	Resting AP < 60 mmHg, ankle or metatarsal PVD flat or barely Pulsatile, TP < 40 mmHg
6	Major tissue loss-extending transmetatarsal; functional foot no longer salvageable	

AP: ankle pressure; PVR: pulse volume recording; TP: toe pressure.
From Rutherford et al. [7]. with permission of Elsevier.
[a]Treadmill protocol: 2 miles/h, 12% constant grade.

The risk factors for CLI are those of general atherosclerosis: cigarette smoking, DM, dyslipidemia, hypertension, hyperhomocysteinemia, increased fibrinogen and high level of C-reactive protein, obesity, and metabolic syndrome. The classical symptoms of CLI are pain at rest, nonhealing ulcerations, and gangrene. The pain manifests as burning pain of the foot and toes, increased in intensity at night when the patients are lying down. Often patients need to dangle the legs over the side of the bed to relieve the pain, this position leading to edema of feet and ankles. One objective sign is pallor of the foot with elevation and rubor dependency. Nonhealing wounds are found in the areas of foot trauma due to improper fitting shoes or to injury. Gangrene follows necrosis and is usually present on the toes. A large portion of CLI patients suffer from severe DM and diabetic neuropathy, and both of these pathologies are major contributors to CLI and limb loss.

The battery of tests to establish the diagnosis of CLI, as recommended by the Guidelines, is presented in a protocol in Fig. 21.1 [1]. The objective diagnosis of CLI is based on the following hemodynamic parameters: ankle-brachial index of 0.4 or less, ankle systolic pressure of 50 mmHg or less, and toe systolic pressure of 30 mmHg or less.

Treatment

At present there is no single optimal treatment or "gold standard" for CLI patients [13]. Revascularization, either surgical or endovascular, aims to relieve pain,

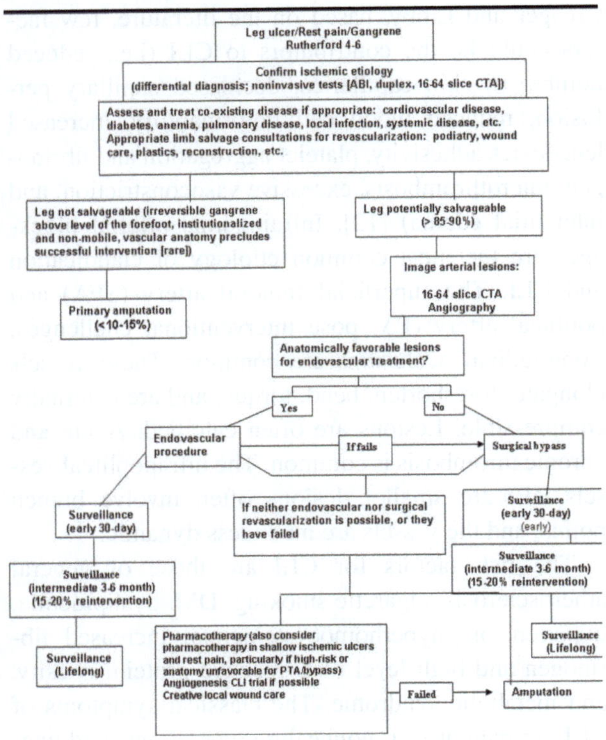

Fig. 21.1 Algorithm for establishing the diagnosis of critical limb ischemia

heal the wounds, and prevent amputation. The gold standard, open surgical revascularization, endarterectomy, or surgical infrainguinal bypass, is increasingly replaced at present by endovascular therapy. Surgical bypass techniques are used in the treatment of distal diffuse arterial occlusion. Despite limitations, infrainguinal endovascular intervention has dramatically increased as the primary therapy as well as post failed surgical intervention for claudication and CLI. New endovascular tools are being developed to cross occlusions, remove thrombus, and open vessels. Crossing long total occlusions is challenging. There have been several devices developed for crossing when available guidewires and catheters fail. A guidewire using optical reflectometry for guidance and radiofrequency ablation to cross is being evaluated [14]. Excimer laser catheters (CliRpath® Excimer Laser catheters, Spectranetics, Colorado Springs, CO) advanced via "step-by-step" technique are also used for crossing [15, 16]. Blunt dissection devices (Frontrunner XP CTO Catheter System, LuMed, Johnson & Johnson, Piscataway, NJ) mechanically spread the lumen of the vessel to allow crossing [17]. Re-entry tools with or without ultrasonic guidance allow the interventionalist to puncture back into the vessel lumen [18].

Devices to mechanically remove the clot alone or in conjunction with thrombolytics are crucial. Some devices actually aspirate thrombus, others macerate, then aspirate, and the excimer laser photoablate the thrombus [9–16, 19, 20]. Balloons, atherectomy devices, and stents are therapeutic cornerstones.

Balloons

In addition to standard balloons, cutting balloons, specialty balloons, and cryoballoons are being evaluated to lessen dissection and future intimal hyperplasia [21, 22].

Laser

The results of three clinical trials published in 2006 [Laser Angioplasty for Critical Limb Ischemia (LACI), catheter-based plaque excision with SilverHawk in critical limb ischemia], and [percutaneous transluminal (PTA) angioplasty for treatment of "below-the-knee" CLI], all using endovascular therapy in CLI patients, concluded that the excimer laser angioplasty for CLI offers high technical success and limb salvage rates in patients unfit for traditional surgical revascularization; the catheter-based plaque excision is a safe and effective revascularization method for patients with CLI, supporting further study of this intervention as a singular or adjunctive endovascular therapy for limb salvage in CLI; PTA and sirolimus-eluting stents can be considered as an effective and safe treatment of patients with CLI [23–25].

Atherectomy

Directional plaque excision allows directed excision and removal of plaque (up to 6 mm) (SilverHawk catheter, FoxHollow Technologies Inc., Redwood City, CA) [26, 27].

Stents

In the SFA and popliteal arteries, self-expanding nitinol stents are used. Stents may be bare metal, medicated, or covered. At the time of this writing several Food and Drug Administration (FDA)-approved stents for PAD in the limbs include the Zilver Vascular Stent (Cook Inc., Bloomington, IN; 2006), Viabahn Endoprosthesis (W.C. Gore & Associates, Newark, DE; 2005), Intrastent Stent (EV3 Inc., St. Paul, MN; 2004), S.M.A.R.T. and S.M.A.R.T. Control Nitinol Stent System (Cordis Corp., Warren, NJ; 2003), Intra Coil Self-Expanding Peripheral Stent (Sulzer Intratherapeutics Inc., St Paul, MN; 2002), Wallstent Iliac Endoprosthesis (Boston Scientific Inc., Natick, MA; 1996), and Palmaz Balloon Expandable Stent (Cordis Corp., Warren, NJ; 1991). Stents that are longer, more flexible, more fracture resistant, can achieve better wall apposition, and can be more accurately delivered are currently developed. There is great interest in the role that medicated stents may play, but there are no FDA-approved drug-eluting stents for limb vessels [28, 29].

Complimentary to surgery or endovascular treatment, there is the endopharmacologic treatment in CLI consisting of thrombolytics associated with glycoprotein receptor inhibitors—GP IIb/IIIa; also important interventions include lipid lowering drugs, antiplatelet therapy, analgesics, and lifestyle modification counseling [30, 31].

The management of CLI patients should also include recognition and possibility of severe coronary artery disease, cerebral vascular disease, and aortic aneurysmal disease [4]. Additionally and equally important to limb salvage as revascularization is the incorporation of an entire "multidisciplinary team" approach to limb salvage including the podiatrist, wound care specialist, diabetologist, and primary care providers. A review of the current CLI therapies will be provided.

Surgical Bypass in Critical Limb Ischemia

Distal bypass surgery (DBS) remains the "gold standard" treatment for CLI if the definition of "gold standard" requires reproducibility, good long-term results, and long-term (5–10 years) data (Fig. 21.2a–d). However, DBS has significant limitations including mortality (1.3–6.0%), wound infection (20–30%), 1–1.5% severe graft infection, myocardial infarction (3%), acute 24-month graft occlusion/stenosis (15–30%), inadequate venous conduit in 40–50% of cases, non-repeatable procedure, use of the saphenous vein which is still the most common conduit for

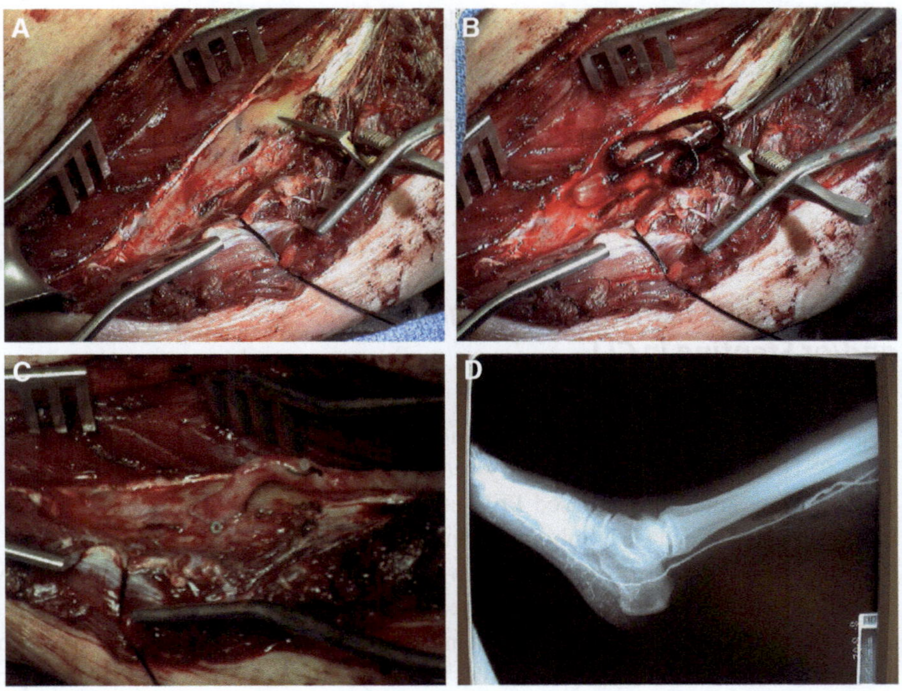

Fig. 21.2 Occluded 2.5 mm posterior tibial artery with "fresh" thrombus, **a**. Thrombus extracted using the Fogarty thrombectomy balloon catheter. Note that this simple but elegant technology was the first of all endovascular devices, **b**. Successful distal anastomosis (autologous vein). Note the metallic anastomotic graft marker which should always be placed on all anastomosis as this will facilitate future interventions by decreasing fluoroscopic time and contrast use and assist in locating grafts and "graft take offs", **c**. Angiogram demonstrating excellent patency with good posterior tibial runoff to the tarsal branches, **d**

coronary artery bypass grafting (CABG) (~50% of CLI patients will have coronary artery disease), and DBS availability as pedal bypass is a complex procedure; in addition, DBS is not available in every community [3, 32].

Excellent DBS intermediate and long-term patency and LS rates have been reported in the CLI patient with an adequate surgical target and autologous vein. Diminished but acceptable clinical results have also been reported with creative DBS strategies using arm veins, donor veins, vein cuffs, and composite grafts even in high-risk dialysis patients and in the >80 years of age group. A meta-analysis of four DBS reports published since 2001 reveals a 5-year LS rate of 65–78.1% in 1,619 CLI patients (68–100% diabetic) [33–36]. In a landmark article, Pomposelli et al. reported a decade experience with pedal bypass in 1,032 CLI patients (92% diabetic) with excellent 5- and 10-year LS rates of 78.1 and 59.8%, respectively [37]. It must be noted that these reports were from experienced institutions committed to LS.

An analysis by Hunick et al. of 4,511 patients treated with DBS revealed a 5-year patency rate of 66% in CLI with available venous conduits and 75% 5-year LS (Fig. 21.2) [38]. Samples of other studies with a mixture of conduits reveal 1-year patency rates from 33 to 92% and 5-year patency rates from 38 to 80% [39, 40]. Clearly, considering the inconsistencies in these DBS results, the known limitations of DBS, the recent improvement in percutaneous endovascular revascularization (PER) technology/results, and the fact that PER does not take away surgical options, it now may be time to debate the issue of the true contemporary "gold standard" or initial treatment for CLI.

Percutaneous Transluminal Angioplasty and/or Stenting in CLI

Improvements in wires, balloons, chronic total occlusion (CTO) crossing and re-entry catheters, and stents have resulted in increased PER utilization and improved outcomes in CLI. Subintimal angioplasty has shown high (80–90%) PS rates and LS rates >85%, but this complex technique has not gained widespread use beyond a few committed centers and the results have not been consistently reproducible. Percutaneous transluminal angioplasty (PTA)-only data in CLI is sparse and non-standardized, but several conclusions can be drawn. Dorros et al. reported tibial PTA as a primary treatment in 235 CLI patients with a 91% 5-year LS rate with low complications [41]. In a meta-analysis of five PTA reports treating 702 CLI patients, the LS rates are 79–91% with low complications and acceptable reintervention rates (9–15%) and DBS rates (2–15%) [33, 41–44]. Faglia et al. recently reported PTA as the first choice in PER in 993 diabetics with CLI. During 26 ± 15-month follow-up, 1.7% underwent major amputation with 87/993 (8.8%) experiencing clinical restenosis. A 5-year primary clinical patency rate of 88% was reported [34]. Kudo et al. very recently reported a 10-year PTA experience in 111 CLI patients with 0.9% periprocedural mortality and initial technical and clinical success of 96.4 and 92.8%, respectively [35]. The 5-year primary patency, assisted patency, and secondary patency were 31.4, 75.5, and 79.6%, respectively. The 5-year LS rate was 89.1%, concluding that PTA was safe and effective and potentially the primary treatment for CLI [35].

The role of inferior phrenic artery (IPA) stenting has expanding after poor initial experiences without dedicated tibial stents. Biamino et al. reported a 44.2% primary patency and 80% primary-assisted patency in 51 patients treated with 3–4 mm bare metal (BMS) coronary stents but with >90% LS [36]. The role of dedicated drug-eluting stents (DES) and absorbable metal stents (AMS) is now being explored. Scheinert et al. treated 30 IPAs treated with sacrolimus-coated DES (3.0–3.5 mm) versus 30 BMSs and found no difference in 6-month angiographic restenosis (60.9 versus 56.5%, $p = \mathrm{NS}$) [45]. Peeters et al. have recently investigated magnesium AMS in the IPA and reported 100% PS in 20 CLI patients with a 6-month clinical patency rate of 78.9% and LS of 94.7% [46]. A US phase I study is planned.

Laser Application in Critical Limb Ischemia

The pioneering laser work of Professor Giancarlo Biamino has lead to an understanding of the unique thrombus and atheroablative properties of pulsed excimer laser angioplasty (ELA) in contrast to earlier (now abandoned) continuous wave thermal lasers resulting in the excimer laser, now being a viable option in treating CLI. The landmark Laser Angioplasty for Critical Limb Ischemia (LACI) trial represents one of the only organized multicenter trials addressing the true CLI patient population and even today this trial has not received the true credit it deserves. The LACI trial enrolled 155 CLI limbs with 423 lesions in 15 US and German sites [47]. All patients were considered poor or non-surgical candidates with high comorbidities (Rutherford Class 4 = 29%, and 5–6 = 71%). The arteries treated included SFA = 41%, PA = 15%, and IPA = 41% with approximately 50% requiring multivessel ELA [47].

The LACI phase 2 results included procedural success (PS) = 90%; ELA delivered = 99% and this despite 8% failed wire crossing in which case the "step-by-step technique" was utilized (Fig. 21.3a); adjuvant PTA = 96% and stent = 45% overall (SFA = 61%, PA = 38%, and IPA = 16%); straight line flow to the foot = 89%; 6-month LS = 93% with very low periprocedural complications (10% overall adverse events at 6 months); and a 6-month reintervention rate of 16% with 2% requiring DBS [47].

The LACI trial demonstrated that PER in CLI can achieve high PS and 6-month LS rates (93%) in very fragile and complex CLI patients with very low complications and reinterventions, who had no other

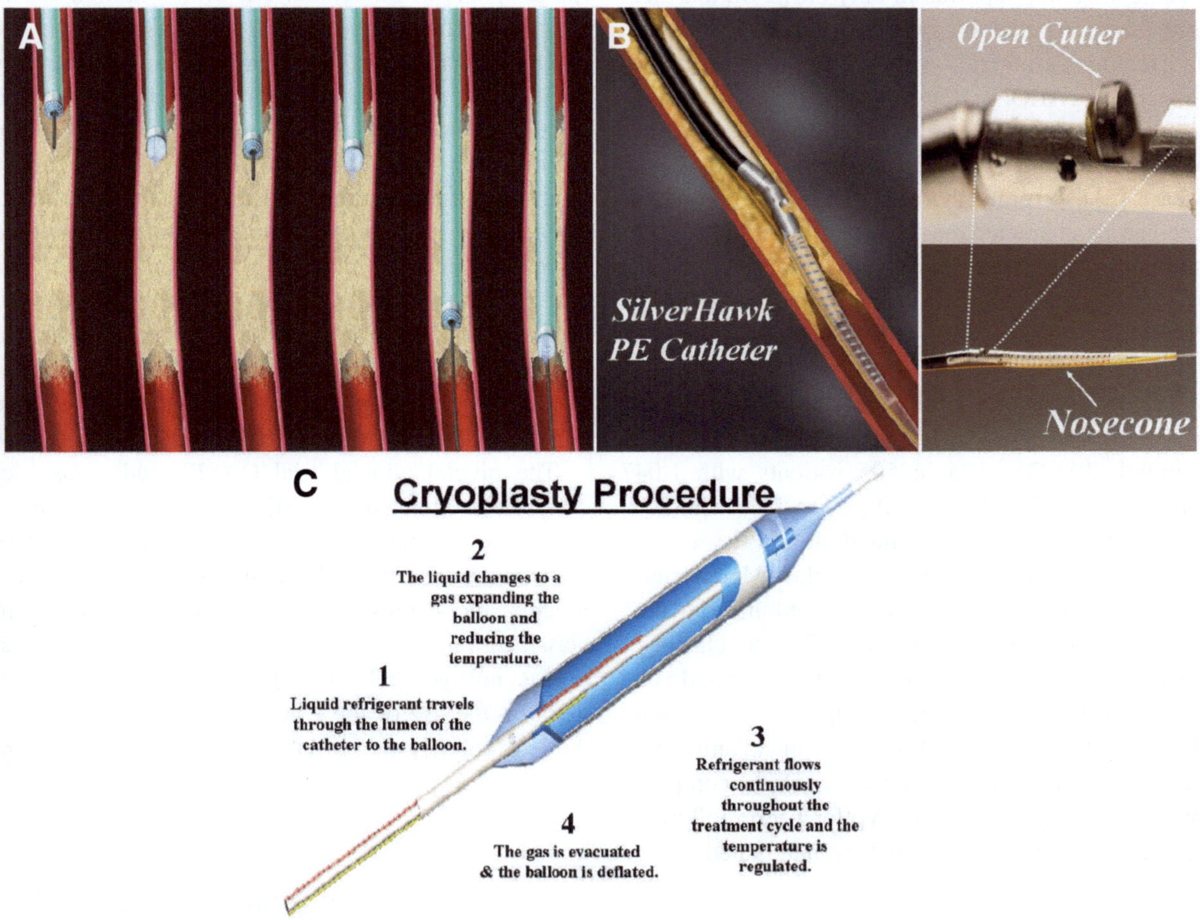

Fig. 21.3 Excimer laser catheter demonstrating the "step-by-step technique" to cross a total occlusion using laser atheroablative properties, **a**. SilverHawk PE catheter demonstrating plaque apposition and excision which is accomplished by a motorized carbide cutter blade with the plaque collected in the distal nosecone chamber, **b**. The PolarCath demonstrating the dual balloon chambers and the four steps of the cryoplasty procedure, **c**. (B courtesy of SilverHawk catheter, FoxHollow Technologies Inc., Redwood City, CA; C courtesy of PolarCath, Boston Scientific Corporation, Natick, MA.)

surgical option. Similar results have been recently reported in the "Belgium LACI" and the CIS "LACI Equivalent" studies (Fig. 21.3a) [48, 49].

Plaque Excision in Critical Limb Ischemia

The SilverHawk plaque excision (PE) catheter (FoxHollow Technologies Inc., Redwood City, CA) is a device that allows PE and retrieval without barotrauma (Fig. 21.3b). The first generation device was larger profile and better suited for the SFA and PA with a 12-month clinical primary patency of 86.8% and primary-assisted patency of 100% with 94% LS recently reported by Ramaiah et al. [50]. Adjuvant PTA/stenting was reported in only 8.6%. Similar SFA results are reported by other single centers and in the Treating Peripherals with SilverHawk: Outcomes Collection (TALON) Registry, which is a multicenter, prospective, nonrandomized observation outcomes registry collecting data on PE in treating infrainguinal disease [51]. Overall, the early TALON SFA experience can be characterized by safety with low complications (0.7% perforation, dissection A/B = 2.5% and ≥C = 0.5%, and no thrombosis or embolization), high PS (>95%), 6-month TLR rate = 11%, and low stent use (4.7%) [51].

The new lower profile catheters have further expanded PE into CLI and tibial arteries. The 12-month TALON data in 505 patients with 1,047 lesions report CLI (Rutherford ≥5) in 14% with 25% overall IPA lesions treated. Stand-alone PE was used in 74% with stenting in 5.3%. Kaplan–Meier analysis demonstrated overall 12-month freedom from TLR 80% and in 90% in IPA lesions [52]. The conclusion at a recent PE CLI Summit was that PE is safe and is an emerging effective "tool" in treating CLI. As true with all CLI treatments, a need for more clinical and objective (digital subtraction angiography [DSA]-computed tomographic angiography [CTA]) long-term follow-up was recognized and is being highly anticipated.

Orbital Atherectomy

Orbital atherectomy is the newest atherectomy procedure using the Diamondback 360°™ Orbital Atherectomy System produced by the Cardiovascular Systems Inc. (CSI) (St. Paul, MN) and approved for use in the PADs by the European Commission. For the United States, the Diamondback received FDA marketing clearance in 2005 for the treatment of stenosis in synthetic arteriovenous hemodialysis access graft. In August 2007, following successful completion of the Orbital Atherectomy System for the Treatment of Peripheral Vascular Stenosis (OASIS) Study, the FDA granted clearance to market the system as a peripheral atherectomy device for treatment of PAD [53]. The system braids plaque using an abrasive burr spinning at 80,000–200,000 rpm. The burr location is on a coil of three helically wound wires; the coil can be compressed, like a spring, with the application of pressure. The orbital path of the device is directed around the periphery of the lumen. The orbital motion allows the burr to attack the plaque as it moves. The grit size and the high rotational speed of rotational atherectomy device make tissue debris small enough to pass through circulatory system harmless, minimizing the potential for distal embolic complications. The system differs from other atherectomy devices by its unique orbiting action to remove plaque and the ability to increase lumen diameter by increasing the orbital speed. The first use of the device was on a patient in Frankfurt, Germany, on March 29, 2005. The system is indicated for use as therapy in patients with occlusive atherosclerotic disease in peripheral arteries that are acceptable candidates for percutaneous transluminal atherectomy.

The pivotal clinical trial OASIS study was successfully completed in 2007 on 124 subjects in 17 US investigational centers. The primary and secondary endpoints were achieved, and improvements in ankle–brachial blood pressure index (ABI) and Rutherford classification grade were durable at 180 days. Final results not yet published [53, 54]. Case presentations on the use of the Diamondback 360°™ Orbital Atherectomy System in PAD patients were also published [53–56].

Cryoplasty in Critical Limb Ischemia

Medical cryotherapy has been used since the late 1960s—primarily in cryosurgery where extreme cold (–10°/20°C) eliminated tissue (tumors, etc.)—but only since 1997–1998 has a vascular application been considered even though clinically arteries are known to be relatively immune to cold. The PolarCath (Boston Scientific Corporation, Natick, MA) is a novel PTA system that simultaneously dilates and rapidly cools from 37°C to –10°C the immediate tissue within contact to a known depth of only 500 μm, therefore avoiding deep wall injury with less dissection. The "freezing" occurs by the controlled inflation (20 s) of a duel balloon system with nitrous oxide instead of saline/contrast which triggers a controlled form of dilation and smooth muscle cell death (apoptosis). This results in decreased elastic recoil and negative (constrictive) remodeling and less inflammatory response, therefore less cell proliferation (less neointimal hyperplasia). Overall this results in less dissections and the need for stent use in this more controlled plaque fracture–microfracture environment (8 atm pressure, 25 s dwell time, and –10°C temperature) (Fig. 21.3c). One of the intriguing aspects of cryotherapy is that for the first time we may be delivering a true "biologic" treatment to the vessel wall that may result in positive remodeling and outcomes.

The PolarCath received FDA approval for use in the SFA and PA in September 2002 after a 15-site US and German multicenter registry reported results in 102 patients [57]. The PS was 96% with 87% receiving stand-alone therapy and 9% requiring stenting. Only 7% reported dissections ≥ type C. At 9 months, 15% required reintervention with a clinical patency of 85% [57]. Fava et al. reported 15 patients with SFA and PA lesions with a PS rate of 93% and 6 and 18 months angiographic primary patency to be 100 and 83%, respectively [58]. Moran et al. reported cryoplasty in IPA results in 20 CLI patients with 26 lesions with 6/26 lesions received adjuvant pretreatment with either PE or laser atherectomy [59]. The PS was 95% with a 95% LS and freedom from major amputation rate reported.

The recent release of smaller diameter (2.5–4.0 mm) and longer length small balloons (20–60 mm) has facilitated the PolarCath options in treating CLI. The Below-the-Knee Chill Study, a prospective multicenter trial on 108 patients with below-the-knee occlusive disease treated with cryoplasty, indicated an acute technical success in 97.3% of patients; the rate of freedom from major amputation was 93.4% at 180 days. The results led to the conclusion that cryoplasty is a safe and effective method for limb salvage [60].

Our own CIS early (3 months) data was presented recently at a PolarCath CLI Summit in which 16 patients with 29 IPAs were treated with 8/16 total occlusions requiring lesion pretreatment with laser and PE (Fig. 21.4a–d, E). The PS and 3-month LS was 100% with no complications, no ≥ C dissections, and no stents.

Treatment Strategies

Contemporary CLI treatment is in a stage of rapid evolution with several novel devices, "tools," and strategies now available that were not available just a short 3–4 years ago. The TASC CLI treatment algorithm published in 2000 is provided (Table 21.2) with several revisions considering the rapid advancements [3–5]. A low threshold for obtaining early noninvasive CTA imaging for both diagnosis and treatment planning is advised. It has been estimated that <50% of patients with primary amputations receive pre-amputation vascular imaging for revascularization and <20% DSA [61]. Additionally, it has been estimated that <50% of CLI patients undergoing an amputation are even referred for a consideration of revascularization before a primary amputation [61]. This is simply not acceptable today especially when considering the advantages of CTA versus DSA, the safety and efficacy of the emerging "tools" to accomplish PER, and the multiple recent reports of excellent (>85–90%) 3- to 5-year LS rates with both DBS and PER (Fig. 21.5a–j).

Summary

Contemporary CLI treatment is in a stage of rapid evolution with several novel devices and strategies now available to physicians. A low threshold for obtaining early, noninvasive CTA imaging for both diagnosis and treatment planning is advised. It has been estimated that <50% of patients with primary amputations receive pre-amputation vascular imaging for revascularization and <20% DSA [10]. Additionally, it has been estimated that <50% of CLI patients undergoing an amputation are even referred for consideration of revascularization before primary amputation [10]. Even less African American patients with CLI get

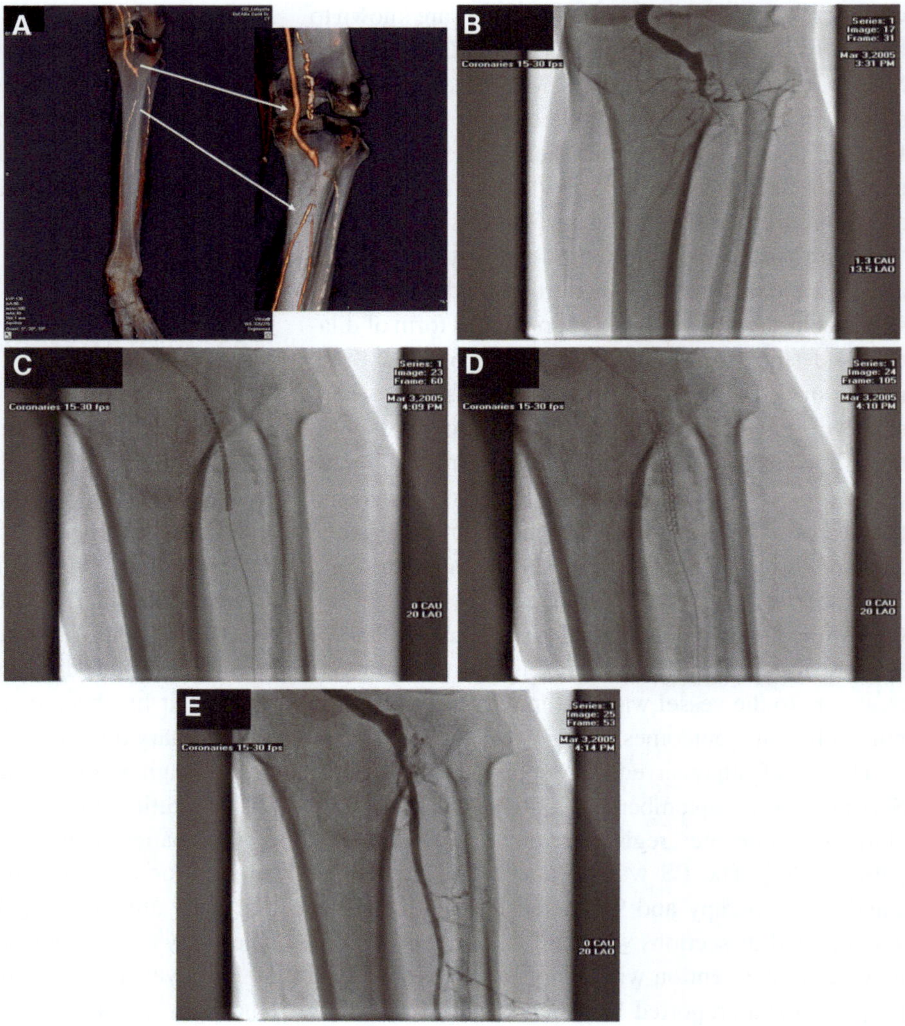

Fig. 21.4 A 64-slice CTA demonstrating total occlusion of a calcified SFA and distal PA just distal to a patent bypass graft. Note the patent runoff vessels, **a**. DSA demonstrating the flush PA occlusion, **b**. The lesion was crossed with an 0.018 guidewire and 2.0 mm laser. A PolarCath was then positioned across the remaining lesion, **c**. PolarCath balloon inflation, **d**. Excellent immediate results combining laser debulking followed by cryoplasty, **e**

referred for LS. This is simply not acceptable today, especially when considering the availability of various diagnostic modalities, the safety and efficacy of the emerging "tools" to accomplish PVI, and the multiple recent reports of excellent (>85–90%) 3- to 5-year LS rates with both DBS and PVI.

We are in the midst of a major paradigm shift in which CLI can and should be treated aggressively starting with the diagnosis and novel revascularization strategies to the multidisciplinary referral and necessary follow-up of this complex patient population. Just three to four short years ago our "tool box" for treating CLI was relatively bare as compared to today. The contemporary CLI "tool box" is armed with multiple novel PVI technologies and strategies that oftentimes can and should be used in conjunction, enabling the clinician to provide the CLI patient with a much higher likelihood of limb salvage.

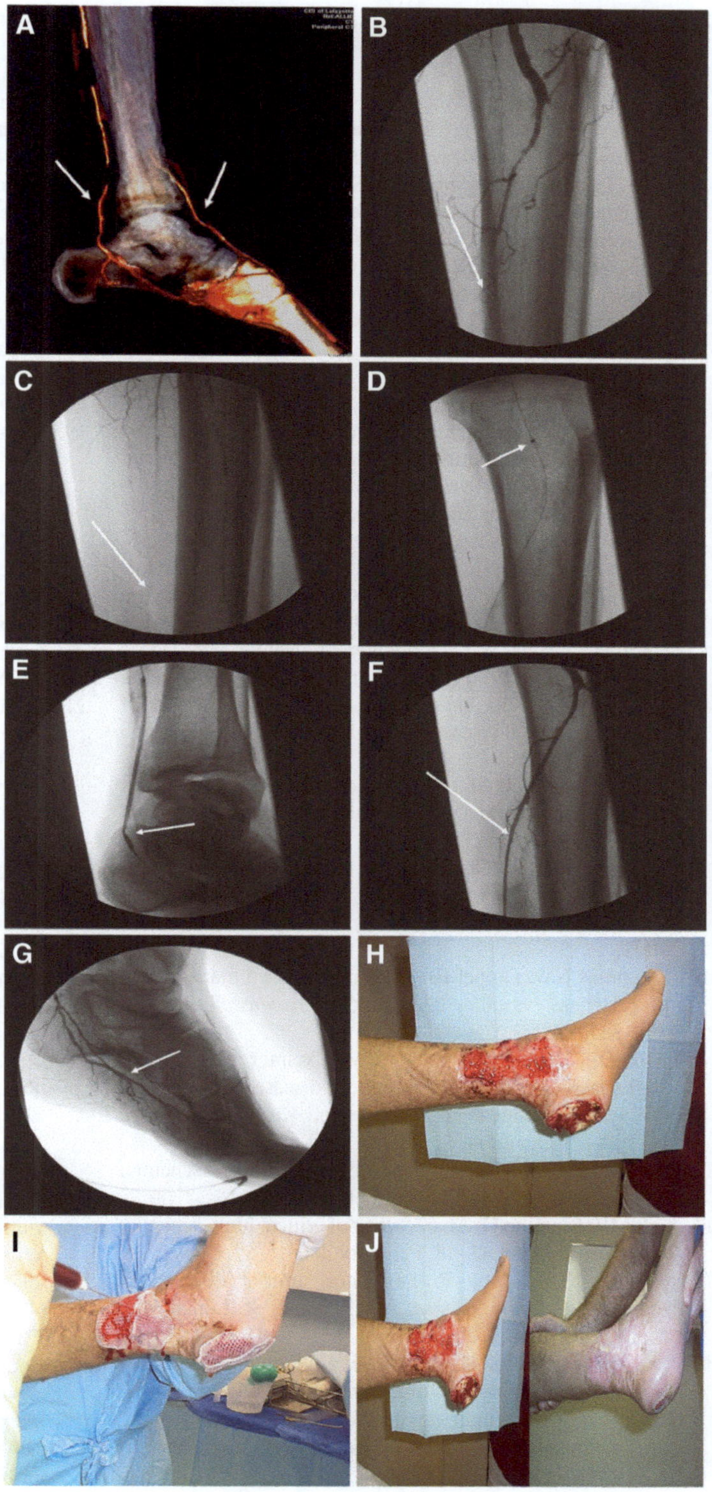

Fig. 21.5 CTA demonstrating 100% occlusion of the popliteal and all proximal infrapopliteal arteries with "pedal sparing" (*arrows*) of the foot in a patient with CLI with a diabetic foot ulcer and an ischemic ulcer of the ankle, **a**. Angiogram confirming CTA findings but without demonstrating "pedal sparing" (*arrows*), **b** and **c**. Definitive PER achieved by laser (1.4 mm)/PTA (2.5 × 120 mm), **d** and **e**. Final angiogram results revealing excellent single vessel–pedal vessel flow to the foot, **f** and **g**. The same patient 48 h after PER with ulcer and heel debridement, **h**. Bioengineered skin substitute and platelet autografting was accomplished, **i**. Limb salvage and total wound healing at 2 months, **j**

References

1. Allie DE, Hebert CJ, Mitran EV, Walker CM, Patlola RR: "Critical limb ischemia". In Heuser RR, Henry M, editors: *Textbook of peripheral vascular interventions*, ed. 2, UK, 2008, Informa Healthcare, pp. 639–647, chap 73.
2. Dormandy J, Verstraete M, Andreani D et al.: Second European consensus document on chronic critical leg ischemia, *Circulation* 84(Suppl 4):1–26, 1991.
3. Dormandy JA, Rutherford RB: TASC working group. TransAtlantic Inter-Society Consensus (TASC): management in Peripheral Arterial Disease (PAD), *J Vasc Surg* 31(1 Pt 2):S1–S296, 2000.
4. Hirsh AT, Haskal ZJ, Hertzer NR et al.: ACC/AHA guidelines for the management of patients with peripheral arterial disease (Lower extremity, renal, mesenteric, and abdominal aortic): a collaborative report from the American association for vascular surgery/society for vascular surgery, society for cardiovascular angiography and interventions, society for vascular medicine and biology, society of interventional radiology, and the ACC/AHA task force on practice, *J Am College Cardiol* 47(6):1239–1312, 2006.
5 Norgren L, Hiatt WR, Dormandy JA, Nehler MR, Harris KA, Fowkes FGR on behalf of the TASC II Working Group: the inter-society consensus for the management of peripheral arterial disease (TASC II), *J Vasc Surg* 45(Suppl. 1):S5–S67, 2007.
6. Boulton AJ, Vileikyte L, Ragnarson-Tennvall G, Apelqvist J: The global burden of diabetic foot disease, *Lancet.* 366:1719–1724, 2005.
7. Rutherford RB, Baker DJ, Ernst C et al.: Recommended standards for reports dealing with lower extremity ischemia: revised version, *J Vasc Surg* 26(3):517–538, 1997.
8. Shammas NW, Dippel EJ: Evidence – based management of peripheral vascular disease, *Curr Atheroscler Rep* 7: 358–363, 2005.
9. Allie DE, Hebert CH, Walker CM: Excimer laser-assisted angioplasty in severe infrapopliteal disease and CLI: the CIS "LACI equivalent" experience, *Vasc Dis Manage* 1(1):14–22, Oct 2004.
10. Akbari CM: Diabetes and critical limb ischemia, *Endovascular Today*, 3:66–69, February 2004.
11. Jaff MR, Biamino G: An overview of critical limb ischemia, *Endovasc Today* 3:45–48, February 2004.
12. Creager MA, Libby P: Peripheral arterial disease. In *Braunwald's heart disease*, vol. 2, ed. 7, St. Louis, MO, Mosby, 1437–1461, chap 54.
13. Bosiers M, Deloose K, Verbist J et al.: Percutaneous transluminal angioplasty for treatment of "below-the –knee" critical limb ischemia: early outcomes following the use of sirolimus-eluting stents, *J Cardiovasc Surg (Torino)* 47(2):171–176, 2006.
14. Kirvaitis RJ, Heuser RR, Das TS et al.: Usefulness of optical coherent reflectometry with guided radiofrequency energy to treat chronic total occlusions in peripheral arteries (the GRIP trial), *Am J Cardiol* 94(8):1081–1084, October 15, 2004.
15. Allie DE, Hebert CJ, Lirtzman MD et al.: Adjunctive bioengineered bi-layered cell therapy (Apligraf®) With excimer laser revascularization improves wound healing and limb salvage in critical limb ischemia, *Vasc Dis Manage* 3:185–192, January/February 2006.
16. Biamino G: The excimer laser: science fiction fantasy or practical tool? *J Endovasc Ther* 11(Suppl 2):II207–II222, 2004.
17. Orlic D, Stankovic G, Sangiorgi G et al.: Preliminary experience with the Frontrunner coronary catheter: novel device dedicated to mechanical revascularization of chronic total occlusions, *Catheter Cardiovasc Interv* 64(2):146–152, 2005.
18. Saketkhoo RR, Razavi MK, Padidar A et al.: Percutaneous bypass: subintimal recanalization of peripheral occlusive disease with IVUS guided luminal re-entry, *Tech Vasc Interv Radiol* 7(1):23–27, 2004.
19. Zehnder T, Birrer M, Do DD, Baumgartner I et al.: Percutaneous catheter thrombus aspiration for acute or subacute arterial occlusion of the legs: how much thrombolysis is needed? *Eur J Vasc Endovasc Surg* 20(1):41–46, July 2000.
20. Wildberger JE, Haage P, Bovelander J et al.: Percutaneous venous thrombectomy using the Arrow-Trerotola percutaneous thrombolytic device (PTD) with temporary caval filtration: in vitro investigations, *Cardiovasc Intervent Radiol* 28(2):221–227, 2005.
21. Albiero R, Silber S, Di Mario C et al.: RESCUT investigators. Cutting balloon versus conventional balloon angioplasty for the treatment of in-stent restenosis: results of the restenosis cutting balloon evaluation trial (RESCUT), *J Am Coll Cardiol* 43(6):943–949, March 17, 2004.
22. Joye JD: Clinical application of CryoPlasty therapy. Chapter 3: CryoPlasty therapy. In Cryoplasty therapy: new treatment strategies for infrainguinal disease and critical limb ischemia. HMP Communications, 2006, March 31, pp. 24–26. www.hmpcommunications.com .
23. Laird JR, Zeller T, Gray BH et al.: LACI investigators. Limb salvage following laser-assisted angioplasty for critical limb ischemia: results of the LACI multicenter trial, *J Endovasc Ther* 13(1):1–11, 2006.
24. Kandzari DE, Kiesz RS, Allie DE et al.: Procedural and clinical outcomes with catheter-based plaque excision in critical limb ischemia, *J Endovasc Ther* 13:12–22, 2006.
25. Bosiers M, Deloose K, Verbist J et al.: Percutaneous transluminal angioplasty for treatment of "below-the –knee" critical limb ischemia: early outcomes following the use of sirolimus-eluting stents, *J Cardiovasc Surg (Torino)* 47(2):171–176, 2006.
26. Favero L, Simpson JB, Reimers B: Treatment of an ostial and a bifurcation lesion with a new directional atherectomy device, *Heart* 90(8):e46, 2004.
27. Pershad A, Stevenson J: Directional atherectomy with the SilverHawk plaque excision device in the treatment of a proximal subclavian-vertebral artery stenosis in coronary-subclavian steal syndrome (CSSS), *J Invasive Cardiol* 16(12):723–724, 2004.
28. Duda SH, Bosiers M, Lammer J, Scheinert D et al.: Sirolimus-eluting versus bare nitinol stent for obstructive superficial femoral artery disease: the SIROCCO II trial, *J Vasc Interv Radiol* 16(3):331–338, 2005.

29. Oliva VL, Soulez G: Sirolimus-eluting stents versus the superficial femoral artery: second round, *J Vasc Interv Radiol* 16(3):313–315, 2005.
30. Allie DE, Hall PA, Shammas NW et al.: Bivalirudin in peripheral interventions. Results of the APPROVE trial and emerging role of "endopharmacology" in treating PVD, *Endovasc Today* 38:27–32, May 2005.
31. Allie DE, Hebert CJ, Lirtzman MD et al.: A safety and feasibility report of combined direct thrombin and GP IIb/IIIa inhibition with bivalirudin and tirofiban in peripheral vascular disease intervention: "treating critical limb ischemia like acute coronary syndrome", *J Invasive Cardiol* 17(8):427–432, 2005.
32. Yost ML. Peripheral arterial disease: a report by the sage group, vol. II, 2004.
33. Matsi JJ et al.: Impact of risk factors on limb salvage after angioplasty in chronic critical lower limb ischemia, *Angiology* 45:797–804, 1994.
34. Faglia E, Dalla Paola L, Clerici G et al.: Peripheral angioplasty as the first-choice revascularization procedure in diabetic patients with critical limb ischemia: prospective study of 993 consecutive patients hospitalized and followed between 1999–2003, *Euro J Vasc Endovasc Surg* 29(6):620–627, June 2005.
35. Kudo T, Chandra FA, Ahn SS: The effectiveness of percutaneous transluminal angioplasty for the treatment of critical limb ischemia: a 10-year experience, *J Vasc Surg* 41(3):423–435, March 2005.
36. Biamino G: Tibioperoneal stenting: new recanalization tools and techniques, including debulking and stenting, allow for the treatment of very complex lesions in the challenging infrageniculate region, *Endovasc Today* 3(2): 58–60, February 2004.
37. Pomposelli FB et al.: A decade of experience with dorsalis pedis artery bypass: analysis of outcome in more than 1,000 cases, *J Vasc Surg* 37:307–315, 2003.
38. Hunick MG, Wong JB et al.: Revascularization for femoropopliteal disease. A decision and cost-effectiveness analysis, *JAMA* 274:165–171, 1995.
39. Gonzalez-Fajardo JA, Vaquero C: Femorocrural bypass for limb salvage: real indications and results. In Branchereau A, Jacobs M, editors: *Critical limb ischemia*, New York, 1999, Futura Publishing Company, Inc., pp. 167–172.
40. Krajewski LP, Olin JW: Atherosclerosis of the aorta and lower extremity arteries. In Young JR, Lin JW, Bartholomew JR, editors: *Peripheral vascular disease*, ed. 2, Mosby, 1996, St. Louis, p. 227.
41. Dorros G, Jaff MR: Tibioperoneal (outflow lesion) angioplasty can be used as primary treatment in 235 patients with critical limb ischemia, *Circulation* 104:2057–2062, 2001.
42. Soder HK et al.: Prospective trial if infrapopliteal artery balloon angioplasty for critical limb ischemia: angiographic and clinical results, *JVIR* 11:1021–1031, 2000.
43. Danielsson G et al.: Percutaneous transluminal angioplasty of crural arteries: diabetes and other factors influencing outcome, *Eur J Vasc Surg* 21:432–436, 2001.
44. Lofberg AM et al.: The use of below-knee percutaneous transluminal angioplasty in arterial occlusive disease causing chronic critical limb ischemia, *Cardiovasc Intervent Radiol* 19:317–322, 1996.
45. Scheinert D, Schmidt A, Biamino G: Are drug-eluting stents better in tibial stenting? Presented at international congress XVIII annual meeting, February 2005. www.endovascularcongress.org .
46. Peeters P, Bosiers M, Verbist J: The answer for infrapopliteal lesions is absorbable metal stents. Presented at international congress XVIII annual meeting, February 2005. www.endovascularcongress.org .
47. Laird JR: Laser Angioplasty for Critical Limb Ischemia (LACI): Results of the LACI Phase 2 clinical trial. Presented at ISET annual meeting, January 2003. www.iset.com .
48. Bosiers M, Peeters P, Elset FV: Excimer laser-assisted angioplasty for critical limb ischemia: results of the LACI Belgium study, *Eur J Vasc Endovasc Surg* 29(6):613–619, June 2005.
49. Allie DE, Hebert CJ, Walker CM: Excimer laser-assisted angioplasty in severe infrapopliteal disease and CLI: the CIS "LACI Equivalent" experience, *Vasc Dis Manage* 10:14–22, October 2004.
50. Ramaiah V: One-year results of SilverHawk atherectomy of the SFA: have we tamed the SFA? Presented at international congress XVIII annual meeting, February 2005. www.endovascularcongress.org .
51. Gammon R, Fail PS, Walker CM et al.: Early results from the treating peripherals with SilverHawk: outcomes collection (TALON) registry, *Am J Cardiol* 94(suppl 6A):184E, 2004.
52. Ramaiah VG, Gammon RS, Kiesz S et al.: Mid-term results from TALON: a prospective, multi-center registry on infrainguinal plaque excision. Presented at society of vascular surgery annual meeting, June 2005. www.vascularweb.org .
53. Heuser RR: Treatment of lower extremity vascular disease: the Diamondback 360° TM orbital atherectomy system, *Expert Rev Med Devices* 5(3):279–286, May 2008.
54. Weinstock B, Dulas D:: Clinical review: a new treatment option for treating peripheral vascular stenosis: orbital atherectomy, *Vasc Dis Manage* 5(3):82–92, 2008.
55. Dave R: Orbital atherectomy for infrapopliteal occlusions. A treatment option for critical limb ischemia, *Endovasc Today* 56–60, August 2007.
56. Heuser R, Safian R, Bosier M, Turco M: Orbital Atherectomy. Initial experiences with a new system for percutaneous treatment of peripheral vascular stenosis, *Endovascular Today* September 21–26, 2006.
57. Laird JR: Interim results of the cryovascular peripheral balloon catheter system safety registry. Presented at the annual meeting of the society of radiology, April 2003.
58. Fava M, Loyola S, Polydorou A et al.: Cryoplasty for femoropopliteal arterial disease: late angiographic results in initial human experience, *J Vasc Interv Radiol* 15: 1239–1243, 2004.
59. Moran M, Joye J: Cryoplasty for critical limb ischemia: initial below-the-knee results, *Am J Cardiol* 94(suppl 6):7E, September 30, 2004.
60. Das T, McNamara T, Gray B, Sedillo GJ, Turley BR, Kollmeyer K, Rogoff M, Aruny JE: Cryoplasty therapy for limb salvage in patients with critical limb ischemia, *J Endovasc Ther* 14:753–762, 2007.

61. Allie DE, Hebert CJ, Lirtzman MD et al.: Critical limb ischemia: a global epidemic. A critical analysis of current treatment unmasks the clinical and economic costs of CLI. *Eur Interv* 1(1):75–84, May 2005.
62. Spichler D, Miranda F Jr, Spichler ES, Franco LJ: Major lower extremity amputations related to peripheral arterial disease and diabetes mellitus in the city of Rio de Janeiro. *J Vasc Brasiliero* 3:111–122, 2004.
63. The vascular surgical society of Great Britain and Ireland. Critical limb ischaemia: management and outcome. Report of a national survey. The vascular Surgical society of Great Britain and Ireland. *Eur J Vasc Endovasc Surg* 10:108–113, 1995.
64. Kröger K: Epidemiology of peripheral arterial disease in Germany, What is evident, what remains unclear? *Hamostaseologie* 26(3):193–196, 2006.
65. Kröger K, Stang A, Kondratieva J, Moebus S, Beck E, Schmermund A, Möhlenkamp S, Dragano N, Siegrist J, Jöckel KH, Erbel R: Heinz Nixdorf recall study group, prevalence of peripheral arterial disease – results of the Heinz Nixdorf recall study. *Eur J Epidemiol* 21(4): 279–285, 2006.
66. Catalano M: Epidemiology of critical limb ischaemia: North Italian data, *Eur J Med* 2(1):11–14, January 1993.
67. Faglia E, Clerici G, Mantero M, Caminiti M, Quarantiello A, Curci V, Morabito A: Incidence of critical limb ischemia and amputation outcome in contralateral limb in diabetic patients hospitalized for unilateral critical limb ischemia during 1999–2003 and followed-up until 2005, *Diabetes Res Clin Pract* 77(3):445–450, 2007.
68. Barani J, Mattiasson I, Lindblad B, Gottsäter A: Suboptimal treatment of risk factor for atherosclerosis in critical limb ischemia, *Int Angiol* 24(1):59–63, 2005.
69. Sigvant B, Wiberg-Hedman K, Bergqvist D, Rolandsson O, Andersson B, Persson E, Wahlberg E: A population-based study of peripheral arterial disease prevalence with special focus on critical limb ischemia and sex differences, *J Vasc Surg* 45(6):1185–1191, 2007.
70. Jensen SA, Vatten LJ, Myhre HO: The prevalence of chronic critical lower limb ischaemia in a population of 20,000 subjects 40–69 years of age, *Eur J Vasc Endovasc Surg* 32(1):60–65, 2006.
71. Verhaeghe R: Epidemiology and prognosis of peripheral obliterative arteriopathy, *Drugs* 56(Suppl 3):1–10, 1998.
72. Sosa T: Arterial surgery facing the 3rd millennium, *Acta Med Croatica* 55(3):103–106, 2001.

Renal Stents

22

Gregorio Sicard and Bradley Thomas

Renal artery stenosis (RAS) and ischemic kidney disease can be associated with reversible hypertension, progressive renal insufficiency, and pulmonary edema. Due to the increased clinical awareness, improvements in duplex ultrasound, computed tomography (CT), magnetic resonance imaging (MRI), and angiography, RAS has been identified with increasing frequency. RAS of greater than 50% was found in 19.2% of patients undergoing catheterization, 35–45% in patients with known peripheral vascular disease, 14–24% of patients with known cerebrovascular disease, and up to 30% of patients with coronary artery disease [1–3]. In patients with previously recognized renal insufficiency the rate of RAS has been reported as high as 24% [4] and 6.8% in patients over the age of 65 [5]. Additionally, renovascular hypertension is believed to affect 5–10% of all hypertensive patients in the United States (Table 22.1).

Table 22.1 Clinical findings that may indicate the presence of renal artery stenosis

1. Hypertension
   a. Early onset of hypertension (<30 years old)
   b. Accelerated or malignant hypertension
   c. Multidrug-resistant hypertension (three or more drugs)
2. Renal abnormalities
   a. Unexplained or worsening azotemia after administration of an ACE or ARB
   b. Reduced size of kidney (<8 cm) or a difference of >1.5 cm from one to the other
3. Other findings
   a. Sudden pulmonary edema without other etiology
   b. Abdominal bruits
   c. Multivessel coronary artery disease and refractory angina
   d. Severe PVD

The goals of therapy are usually considered to be improvement in uncontrolled hypertension, preservation or salvage of kidney function, improvement in symptoms, and improvement in quality of life. A variety of treatment options have been utilized to manage the disease. Pharmacologic therapy with multiple antihypertensive agents, usually including angiotensin-converting enzyme (ACE) inhibitors, or angiotensin receptor blockers (ARBs), calcium channel blockers, and/or beta blockers, is frequently used with the goal of normalizing blood pressure. Some clinicians also recommend statins to lower low-density lipoprotein (LDL) cholesterol and antiplatelet agents, such as aspirin or clopidogrel, to reduce rates of thrombosis. However, these medical therapies do not treat the underlying anatomic defect. Surgical revascularization, through the use of bypass or endarterectomy, represents the gold standard and has demonstrated excellent long-term durability and clinical results in terms of hypertension management and improvement of renal function [6]. However, the invasive nature of these operations have led investigators to pursue percutaneous angioplasty and stenting as a tool in the treatment of renal artery stenosis. In 1978, renal percutaneous transluminal angioplasty (PTA) was introduced by Gruntzig et al. [7], and since that time, much effort has been put forth to evaluate the efficacy of these interventions. With the introduction of self-expanding and balloon-expandable metallic stents, a new treatment that might overcome

G. Sicard (✉)
Eugene M. Bricker Professor, Surgery; Division Head of General Surgery; Section Head of Vascular Surgery; Vice Chairman, Department of Surgery, Washington University School of Medicine, St. Louis, MO, USA

T.J. Fogarty, R.A. White (eds.), *Peripheral Endovascular Interventions*,
DOI 10.1007/978-1-4419-1387-6_22,

poor angioplasty results, immediate postangioplasty complications, and restenosis became available for atherosclerotic RAS. The current standard for intervention in most patients is PTA with stent placement with open revascularization usually reserved for patients who require aortic reconstructions for aneurysmal and aortoiliac occlusive disease. The decision for any intervention must encompass an understanding of the clinical, anatomic, and physiologic considerations of the disease as well as the implications of its natural history.

Pathophysiology

The mechanism of renovascular hypertension has been well defined. Over 60 years ago, Goldblatt was able to produce sustained elevations of blood pressure in dogs after gradual reductions in renal artery blood flow by external clamps [8]. A stenosis causing an 80% reduction in the cross-sectional area of the artery induces a pressure gradient enough to cause increase in renin release from the kidney. Renin and its effects on angiotensin and aldosterone account for the elevated blood pressure of renovascular hypertension. RAS causes a reduction in renal perfusion leading to autoregulatory vasodilatation of the afferent arterioles, angiotensin II release leading to vasoconstriction of the efferent arterioles, and the systemic activation of the renin–angiotensin–aldosterone system. These are widely recognized as critical pathogenic principles involved not only in regulation of renal perfusion but also in preservation of glomerular filtration and development of renal vascular hypertension. This stenosis can be related to a variety of mechanisms, but the most common occlusive disease that affects the renal artery circulation are atherosclerosis and fibromuscular dysplasia. Other rare causes would include congenital, embolic, spontaneous dissections, and trauma but atherosclerotic lesions alone make up 80–95% of patients of renovascular hypertension. These lesions are found at the renal artery ostium, are short in length, and present most commonly in the sixth decade of life. Men are affected more often than women and, as one might expect, these patients exhibit significant pathology in the cerebrovascular, coronary, mesenteric, and peripheral vascular beds as well.

Fibromuscular Dysplasia

Fibromuscular dysplasia (FMD) is a vasculopathy that is known to affect small- and medium-sized vessels. Fibromuscular dysplasia can result in significant hypertension in women aged between 15 and 50 years but FMD accounts for <10% of cases of renovascular hypertension [9]. FMD was first described in 1938 and is frequently found to involve the distal main renal artery and its branches [9, 10]. Medial fibroplasia represents the most common dysplastic lesion and it may be indistinguishable angiographically from intimal fibroplasia. Intimal fibroplasia occurs in <10% of patients with arterial fibrodysplasia. Adventitial (periarterial) hyperplasia is the rarest type of fibrodysplastic lesion.

Although FMD has been shown to affect multiple arterial beds, the frequency of involvement in renal arteries is 60–70%, with bilateral disease occurring in 35% of patients. The natural history of renal FMD is progression in up to 37% of patients [11], but this progression only rarely results in occlusion of the renal artery [12]. Patients with FMD do demonstrate a significant decrease in mean cortical thickness and reduced renal length compared with similar patients with essential hypertension. As many as 63% of patients with FMD experience a loss of renal mass, but the incidence of renal failure remains remarkably low [11, 13]. Renal artery atherosclerosis, in contrast, is a significant cause of progressive renal dysfunction leading to ischemic nephropathy and loss of functioning renal mass [14]. The main impetus for the treatment of FMD is control of hypertension and its attendant complications. The treatment for most patients can be primarily managed medically. Revascularization is reserved for those patients who have recent onset of hypertension (<1 year), with the primary goal to cure the hypertension, those in whom blood pressure control has proved difficult, those intolerant of antihypertensive therapy, those who are not compliant with their antihypertensive medication, and those who have demonstrated a loss of renal volume leading to a diagnosis of ischemic nephropathy [15]. The primary mode of intervention is by balloon angioplasty, with surgery reserved for recalcitrant lesions. The angiographic findings in FMD are very characteristic and are depicted in Figures 22.1 and 22.2.

In general, only in the setting of a complication from angioplasty, like flow limiting dissection, should

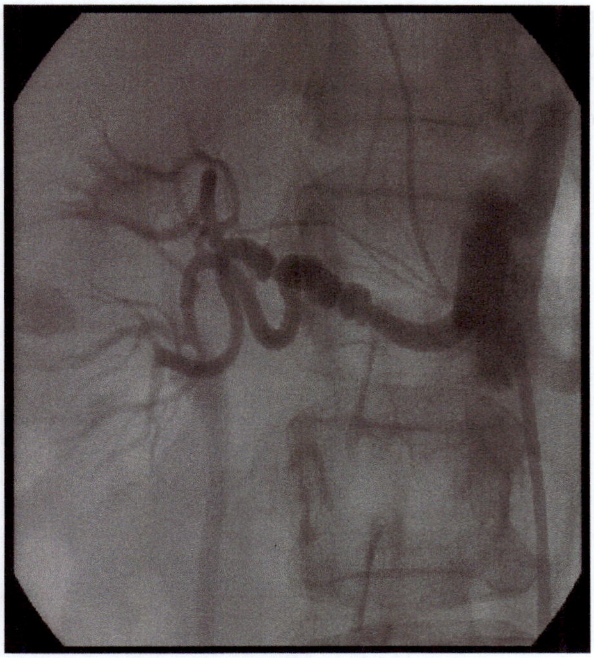

Fig. 22.1 Selective arteriogram demonstrating the string-of-beads appearance, caused by areas of relative stenoses or webs alternating with small fusiform or saccular aneurysms of the artery

stenting be employed. Few reports, however, address the factors that affect the long-term durability or clinical effectiveness of percutaneous transluminal renal angioplasty for renal artery FMD.

Takayasu's Arteritis

Nonspecific aortoarteritis, also known as Takayasu's disease, is a rare form of arteritis of unknown case that commonly involves the aorta, its major branches, and the pulmonary arteries [16]. It results in stenosis, occlusion, dilatation, or formation of aneurysms in the involved blood vessels [17]. Of these, stenosis or obstructions are the most common, frequently involving the abdominal aorta and the renal arteries, and often result in renovascular hypertension [16, 17]. The presence of obstructive renal arterial disease in patients with renovascular hypertension requires some form of revascularization to relieve systemic hypertension. Renal artery angioplasty has been described as an alternative to open reconstruction with good results [18].

Diagnosis of Renal Artery Stenosis

According to the recent American College of Cardiology [ACC]/American Heart Association [AHA] guidelines [19], diagnostic evaluations for RAS are indicated in patients with the onset of severe hypertension before the age of 30 as well as in patients

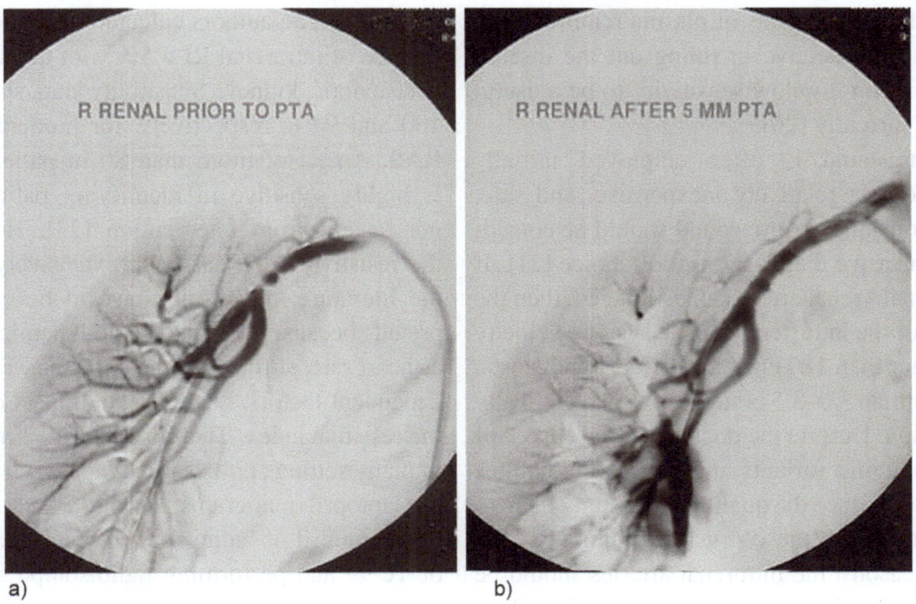

Fig. 22.2 **a**, Right renal artery in a patient with FMD prior to PTA. **b**, Same patient post PTA

with the onset of severe hypertension after the age of 55. Both of these statements are supported by Class I evidence, Level B. Furthermore, those with accelerated hypertension or drug-resistant/malignant hypertension are supported by Class I, Level C; patients with azotemia or worsening renal function associated with administration of ACE inhibitors, unexplained renal atrophy or size difference between the two kidneys >1.5 cm, and finally those with unexplained "flash" pulmonary edema are supported by all Class I, Level B. Indications for a diagnostic workup that have Class IIa evidence level B indications include patients with unexplained renal failure, and Class IIb evidence levels B and C involve patients with multivessel coronary or peripheral artery disease with unexplained congestive heart failure (CHF) or refractory angina.

Diagnostic Tools

Multiple modalities exist for the screening of RAS using non-invasive methods, including duplex ultrasonography, magnetic resonance angiography (MRA), and computed tomography angiography (CTA), and nuclear medicine studies. These various tools are used to either demonstrate the anatomic obstruction or detail the physiologic disturbance that is created by them. The original screening tests consisted of intravenous urography and measurements of plasma rennin. These measurements are effective in ruling out the disease state but suffer from too low sensitivity to be a useful screening test currently [20].

Duplex ultrasound is often employed initially because it is quick, relatively inexpensive, and safe. For these reasons duplex ultrasound should be considered the non-invasive diagnostic test of choice [21]. If the aorta and main renal artery can be imaged, then the measurement of the intrastenotic peak systolic velocity (PSV) of greater than 180 cm/s and a PSV renal/aortic ratio of greater than 3.0–3.5 is suggestive of a clinically significant lesion. Despite the documented accuracy of ultrasound, anatomic variants and large body habitus can significantly reduce the quality of the study in up to 20% of patients [22]. If these structures cannot be seen for technical reasons, the intrarenal arteries should be interrogated. The indirect method of evaluating RAS by the *tardus parvus* waveform is the easiest and most reproducible method (Fig. 22.3). "Tardus" refers to delayed or prolonged early systolic acceleration and "parvus" refers to diminished amplitude and rounding of the systolic peak.

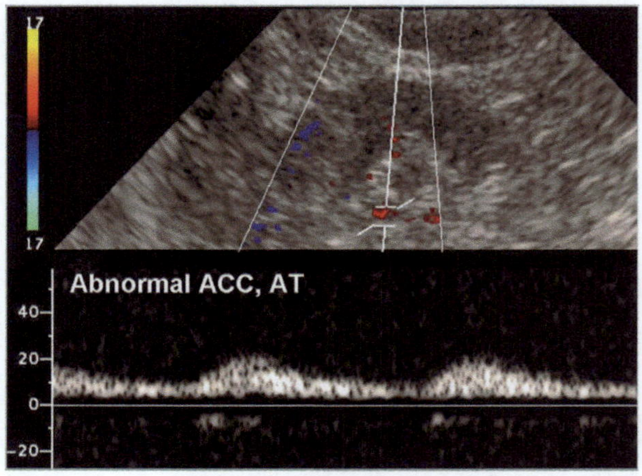

Fig. 22.3 An arterial waveform from an intrarenal interlobar artery. Note the slope of the systolic upstroke, absence of early systolic peak, and diminished amplitude of the waveform indicating a typical parvus tardus waveform

The Doppler resistive index (RI) ([peak systolic velocity–end diastolic velocity]/peak systolic velocity), introduced in 1994 by Schwerk et al., has been advanced as a useful parameter for quantifying the alterations in renal blood flow that may occur with renal disease and the functional significance of these lesions. Measurements are made in multiple parts of the kidney to ensure the most reliable assessment of perfusion. The authors calculated the side-to-side difference of intrarenal RI > 5% with the lower RI in the poststenotic kidney. Sensitivity and specificity were 100 and 94%, respectively, for moderate and severe RAS. An RI of more than 80 in patients with RAS is highly sensitive in identifying patients who will not benefit from intervention [23]. However, while the resistive index has been extensively examined in the literature, the results have to be carefully interpreted, because different hemodynamic factors, such as heart rate, stiffness of the aorta, as well as observer-dependent factors, may have an impact on the level of the resistive index. These issues have limited its utility in many settings [24, 25].

Captopril renograms, during which 25–50 mg of PO captopril is administered before administration of Tc-99 and performing radioisotope scanning, may allow for the identification of an angiotensin-II-dependent kidney. When positive, this study shows that following captopril administration there is a decrease in glomerular filtration rate (GFR) (perfusion decreased by >40%) and a slowed uptake of tracer in the ipsilateral kidney. Additionally, there is often an increased perfusion in the contralateral kidney that is thought to be a compensatory mechanism. This test is specifically less useful in cases of bilateral RAS and has a low sensitivity and specificity. Its use in widespread clinical practice has been largely abandoned.

Multidetector-row computed tomography (MDCT) can provide accurate three-dimensional reconstructions of both renal arteries and also provide additional information including the size of each kidney and shows the aortoiliac anatomy. Highly calcified lesions and previous stent placement can complicate accurate imaging but sensitivity is reported to be 95–100% [26–28]. While the risk of contrast-induced nephropathy from iodinated contrast agents for a CT is not necessarily higher than for DSA [27], the latter allows for an intervention in the setting where RAS is found.

MRA is also regarded as an excellent modality to non-invasively image the renal arteries. Gadolinium-enhanced MRA compares very favorably to DSA with 89% concordant findings when both were performed with MRA, usually overestimating the lesion when there was a discrepancy [29]. However, concerns for nephrogenic systemic fibrosis in patients with altered renal function after the administration of gadolinium [30] make the possibility of non-contrasted MRI a more attractive method (Fig. 22.4). A recent review of this non-contrasted technique found that its sensitivity was only 78% [31]. Further technical improvement such as addition of cardiac gating may increase the sensitivity of this non-contrasted technique.

When a patient presents with a high index of clinical suspicion, or with inconclusive or suggestive non-invasive testing, digital subtraction angiography (DSA) is recommended to establish the diagnosis. DSA continues to represent the gold standard to which all other methods of evaluation are compared to and allows the potential for a concomitant therapeutic intervention. A diagnostic study can be performed with an excellent safety profile in the outpatient setting, while interventions need to be admitted and monitored.

Endovascular Treatment of Renal Artery Disease

Patient Preparation

Once it has been determined that a patient's clinical picture and non-invasive imaging warrants angiography, a careful review of all available information is key to successful completion of the procedure safely, quickly, and with the use of the least amount of nephrotoxic dye. Patients who have been selected for invasive

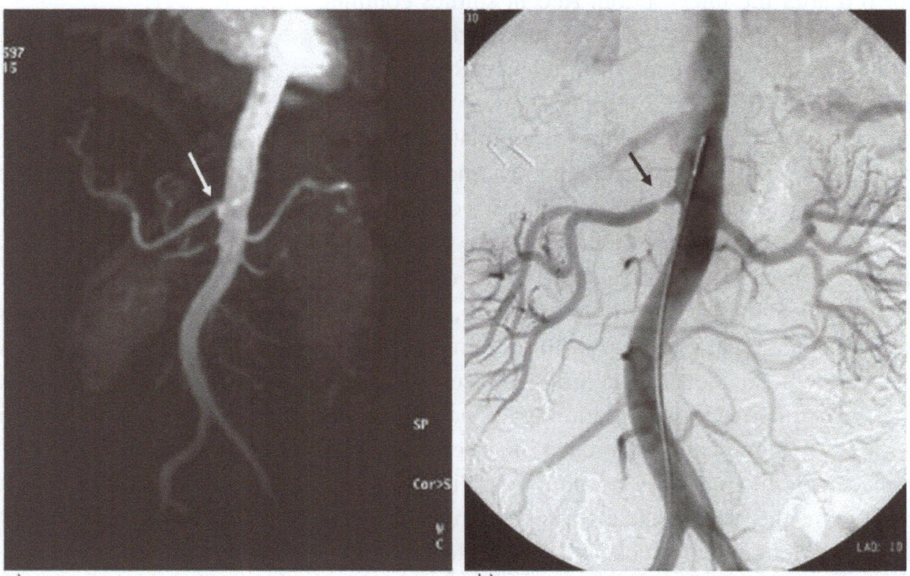

a) b)

Fig. 22.4 Side by side comparison comparing a standard gadolinium-enhanced MRA **a**, and an arteriogram, **b**. This study accurately predicted a high-grade right RAS

imaging and potential intervention are instructed to take nothing by mouth after midnight the day prior to the procedure. Coumadin should be held 4–5 days but aspirin and clopidogrel can and should be continued. Patients can take their routine medication, except for ACE inhibitors and ARBs, the morning of the intervention.

The use of iodinated contrast agents leading to nephrotoxicity has been well documented [32–36]. In fact, the derangement of excretory function as a result of contrast administration is most severe in those with preexisting dehydration, renal insufficiency, and diabetes—all of which are common in patients with RAS being considered for intervention [37–39]. The most crucial step in patient preparation is to ensure that they are adequately hydrated. Additionally, sodium bicarbonate, acetylcysteine, and the use of low-osmolarity contrast agents can be used as renal protectants.

N-Acetylcysteine (Mucomyst) is an antioxidant that acts as a scavenger of oxygen free radicals and inhibits some proteins that are implicated in contrast-mediated nephrotoxicity. Typically, patients receive 600 mg PO twice a day on the day before the study and the day after. Several randomized, controlled studies have shown its efficacy when used in combination with IV hydration, although some reports have failed to show any additional benefit [40–44].

Sodium bicarbonate infusion is also often used. A drip of 154 mEq/l is administered at 3 cc/kg for 1 h prior to the intervention and the 1 cc/kg during and for 6 h after the intervention. Recent studies continue to debate the efficacy of sodium bicarbonate infusion [45–48]. The Renal Insufficiency Radiocontrast Exposure (REINFORCE) trial reported that there is no difference between sodium bicarbonate and saline hydration when low-toxicity contrast media is used [45]. Others report no difference if *N*-acetylcysteine is used in conjunction with either saline or bicarbonate [47]. In 2008, Navaneethan et al. conducted a meta-analysis of 12 trials representing 1,854 patients and concluded that hydration with sodium bicarbonate decreases the incidence of contrast-induced nephropathy in comparison to hydration with normal saline without a significant difference in need for renal replacement therapy or in-hospital mortality [48].

Despite the current state of debates regarding the use of various agents such as renal protectants, it is good technique to minimize the volume of contrast given to patients during an intervention. In patients who have had axial imaging via CT or MRI scan, a review of the angles of takeoff of the renals from the aorta can help to reduce the number of non-selective runs. According to Kim et al., the optimal initial angle for angiographic evaluation of the origin of the renal artery and for renal artery stent placement is 30° left anterior oblique (LAO) relative to the L1 spinous process for the right renal artery and 7° LAO for the left renal artery [49]. In some patients, additional views will be necessary to optimally depict the origins of the renal arteries. Based on extensive reviews of CT scans, anteroposterior (AP) and 20° LAO for the left renal artery along with the addition of a 40° LAO view for the right renal artery are successful in the overwhelming majority of cases. Missing the optimal angle to view ostial lesions by as little as 10% can be responsible for a 5 mm foreshortening that hides the lesion from view.

In further efforts to reduce the risk of contrast-induced nephropathy (CIN), CO_2 can be used exclusively or in conjunction with iodinated contrast material to facilitate renal artery stent placement. As an imaging agent, CO_2 can facilitate the accurate placement of renal artery stents by eliminating the concern for both contrast material-associated nephropathy and allergy [50]. These attributes, along with the benefits of low CO_2 viscosity, permit unrestricted imaging, guidance, and can allow for precise stent position for those who make themselves familiar with the technique.

Access

The renal arteries are most commonly approached retrograde from the common femoral arteries. If the side of likely intervention is already known, some feel it is best to approach the lesion from the contralateral groin. Others prefer right-sided access for both sides and that is clearly a matter of operator preference. A brachial artery approach may be used for patients with very difficult or no femoral access (i.e., occluded aortoiliac system). Certain anatomy may make the arm approach more attractive as well, such as in the situation of steep downward angulation of the renal artery, as can be seen most commonly on the right side. After cannulation of the artery, we use a 0.035 in. Bentson wire. It is an excellent initial access wire as its long floppy tip is unlikely to lift plaque and cause dissection. Instead, the wire will form soft atraumatic loop that can be advanced through even a severely disease vascular bed with only a small risk. Occasionally, an MPA and an angled hydrophilic guidewire are needed. Unless the likelihood of intervention is high, a 4F flush angiographic catheter (Pigtail or Omniflush) can be advanced bare back over the wire to minimize arterial trauma or through a 4F sheath if that is preferable. However, if studies obtained prior to the procedure suggest a high likelihood of intervention, then a 6F or 7F system should generally be used.

Angiography

After review of imaging and determining the angulation needed for the image intensifier, contrast angiography can begin. As the renal arteries typically arise at the superior portion of the L1 vertebral body, the catheter should be placed at the T12–L1 interspace. Non-reflux flush catheters avoid the flow of contrast toward the celiac and superficial mesenteric artery (SMA) and helps to concentrate contrast in the aorta and renal arteries. If renal function permits a complete aortoiliac arteriogram can be obtained. This allows accessory renal arteries and other anatomic variations to be identified as well as disease along the access path. In cases where contrast load must be limited as much as possible, these initial runs can be done with CO_2 [50]. Choice of access site and the angulation of the renal artery takeoff determine the choice of guiding catheters.

Renal Artery Cannulation

Once it has been determined that a hemodynamically significant stenosis exists and an intervention is planned, the patient should be heparinized with 70 units/kg IV and the ACT should be maintained over 250 s. An intra-arterial vasodilator (100–200 μg of nitroglycerin) may also be used, although it is rarely needed. Recurve-type diagnostic catheters such as the Sos Omni Selective allow access even to renal arteries that are steeply downward oriented. Once the catheter is below the renal artery approximately 1–2 cm of the floppy tip should extend from the catheter tip. Initial renal artery entry should be done by advancing the cephalad in the same plane as the renal artery arises from the aorta. The tip of the wire can be seen to "flick" into the renal ostium. The wire can then be gently advanced through the stenosis and then supported with a diagnostic catheter. Certain lesions with a very tight stenosis may make crossing and advancing a catheter beyond a stenosis difficult or even impossible (Fig. 22.5a). In this setting it may be advantageous to convert to a coaxial technique. This technique is useful in tight ostial lesions or when acutely downward angled course makes crossing with anything other than a wire difficult. This setup involves using a 5F diagnostic catheter inside a 7F Renal Double Curve (RDC) guiding catheter. This system facilitates steering and decreases push back into the aorta. With this in mind, a diagnostic catheter can be employed in this coaxial manner to reinforce the preshaped guiding catheter. Alternatively, after gaining access with a short 6F or 7F sheath, you can perform a selective catheterization of the renal artery through an RDC guiding catheter using a steerable 0.014, 0.018, or 0.035 guidewire. Following safe crossing, the guidewire tip is placed in one of the segmental arteries and remains in that position until the completion of the procedure. Care must be taken because even a small caliber floppy nitinol wire can dissect the main renal artery or lead to arterial perforation that can promote occlusion and hemorrhage, respectively. The operator must visualize the wire tip at all times to avoid parenchymal injury. A small contrast injection at this point can confirm the intraluminal position of the catheter (Fig. 22.5b).

Angioplasty and Stenting

A variety of steel and nitinol stents have been placed in the renal arteries over the years. In 1991 Kuhn et al. described the Strecker stent in 10 patients with suboptimal angioplasty results [51]. Also in 1991, Rees et al. described the use of the hand-mounted Palmaz stent in 28 patients for the same reason [52]. Since that time, the use of premounted, flexible, lower profile stents is preferred. Boston Scientific (Express SD Renal), Cordis (GENESIS), Guidant (HERCULINK), and others offer these stents in sizes ranging from 4 to

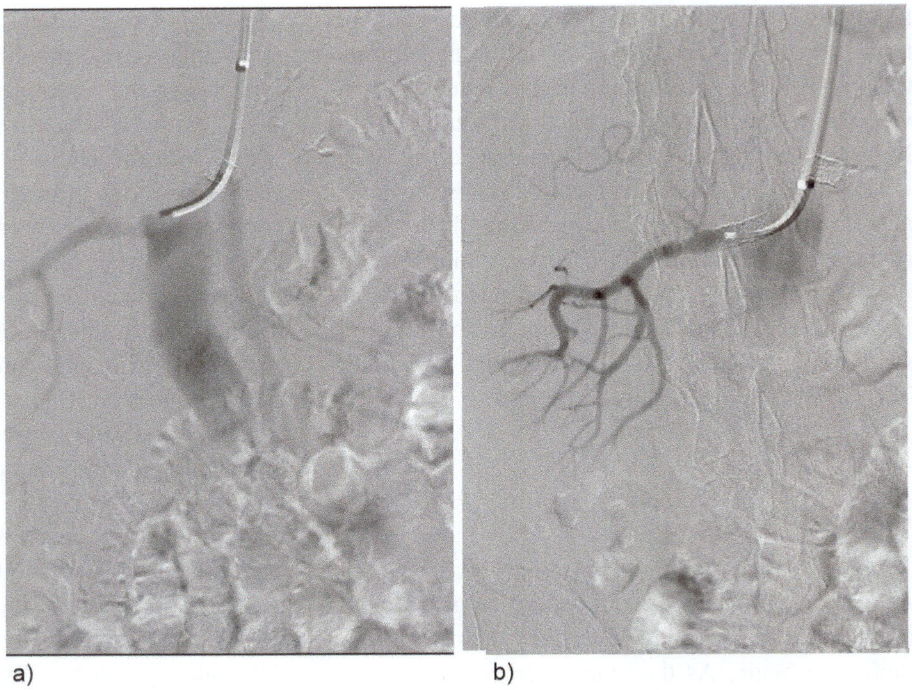

Fig. 22.5 **a**, Right renal artery stenosis demonstrated via a brachial approach with carbon dioxide. **b**, Contrast is used in small amounts post stent placement

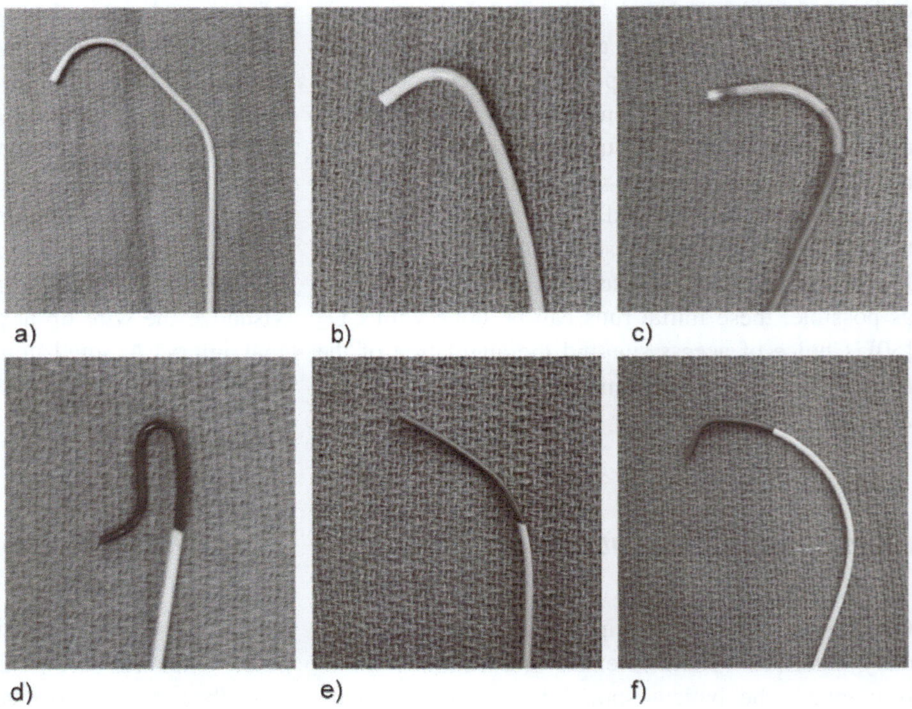

Fig. 22.6 Guide and diagnostic catheters: **a**, RDC (Cordis, Miami, FL); **b**, IM (Cordis, Miami, FL); **c**, Hockey Stick (Cordis, Miami, FL); **d**, Sos (Angiodynamics, Queensbury, NY); **e**, MPA (Cook, Bloomington, IN); and **f**, Cobra-2 (Cook, Bloomington, IN)

7 mm in a variety of lengths (Fig. 22.6). Closed cell stents may provide more radial force and many of these stents are available in a monorail system. The use of stents over angioplasty alone significantly improves the immediate success rate of the procedure in the setting of atherosclerotic disease [53–55]. This is especially true for any ostial lesion. However, avoidance of stents in renal arteries of less than 5 mm should be considered due to the higher rate of clinically significant restenosis for these smaller arteries [56–59].

Predilatation is rarely needed, but can be of use in a highly calcified lesions or those with a stenosis of >90%. If required, this can be performed with a small 3–4 mm coronary balloon. In most settings, primary stent placement is thought to help reduce distal embolization that may occur with predilation. When preparing to position the stent, having a guiding catheter in place helps facilitate balloon/catheter exchanges and allow for follow-up angiograms to be obtained while maintaining a guidewire across the lesion.

Stent Placement

Most commonly, balloon-expandable stents are chosen (typically 6–7 mm) and then loaded into the preformed 5–8F guiding catheter. The system is advanced through the vascular sheath at the groin into the renal artery over a 0.035 in. heavy duty guidewire. The stent is then exposed by withdrawing the guiding catheter from the renal artery. Another option is using a coronary type approach in which a steerable 0.014 in. wire is placed and a low-profile monorail stent balloon catheter is advanced directly into the artery. For the typical ostial lesion, the stent is positioned with the proximal end protruding into the aorta by about 1–3 mm. This helps to ensure that the overhanging plaque is completely addressed. Once the stent has been positioned, it is delivered as per instructions with an insufflation device. Care should be taken when considering placing stents on the more distal renal artery as this can complicate or preclude open surgical revascularization should it become necessary. DSA images are taken to assess the results. The images should be evaluated to determine the anatomic position of the stent, the strut structure (which provides clues about complete deployment), and distal runoff. A relatively common issue seen during this phase of the intervention would be residual narrowing of the stent. This can be treated additionally with angioplasty with a balloon that has a nominal size that is shorter than the stent that was deployed. Dilations distal to the end of the stent should be avoided to help reduce dissection and embolization. In lesions with a large amount of plaque burden, it may be impossible to achieve complete resolution of the stenosis without undue risk from repeated angioplasty attempts. If acceptable anatomic results cannot be achieved (residual stenosis <30% diameter) then open revascularization in certain settings may be preferable.

The basic techniques allow for successful stenting in the overwhelming majority of cases. However, there are certain circumstances where anatomy and pathology will require the operator to consider other options. For example, in the setting of a stenosis at the bifurcation, which usually indicates a short common renal artery, guidewires should be placed in both branches, and angioplasty only should be performed in a "kissing technique." Stents may not be feasible in some of these patients because of their anatomy; therefore, in the presence of a suboptimal result, the patient may need to be considered for open surgery.

Post Procedure Care and Follow-Up

Following completion of the intervention the patient is observed in the recovery area to monitor for any access site-related complications. Blood pressure and renal function seem to be monitored. Hypotension and bradycardia are the most common hemodynamic alteration and are most frequent during the first 2–4 h. These are usually easily managed with pharmacologic therapies and volume replacement. It is up to the operator if and when a post procedure duplex ultrasound should be obtained to establish a new baseline. During the next 2 weeks frequent blood pressure checks and readjustment of antihypertensive medications are often required.

Complications

As with any complex peripheral vascular intervention, procedural-related complications can occur. The most common complication is at the location of the access, either at the femoral or at the brachial artery. One frustrating complication is the opposite of the intent of the intervention: decline in renal function. Contrast-induced nephropathy can be temporary and resolve without any intervention, or it can be permanent resulting in the need for hemodialysis. Renal failure that is due to an excessive load of iodinated contrast can occasionally be limited with temporary dialysis.

Renal failure in this setting is not always contrast-related.

Atheroembolization during renal artery angioplasty and stenting has been postulated as a cause for the inferior renal function results observed when compared with those with surgical revascularization. Studies using distal embolic protection devices and aspiration catheters have shown that thousands of atheroembolic particles are liberated during stenting procedures [60]. The use of embolic protection devices has been advocated by some for this reason [61, 62].

Renal artery perforation and rupture is uncommon but is well described and can have fatal outcomes [63–66]. Rupture in the perioperative period is most common but has been described up to 24 h after the procedure (Fig. 22.7). It is essential that the operator recognizes this problem quickly as it can best be dealt with when sheath and wires are already in place. Simple balloon inflation may obtain a quick seal and alleviate hemodynamic instability. Placement of a covered stent is preferred but when impossible, surgical exploration may be indicated.

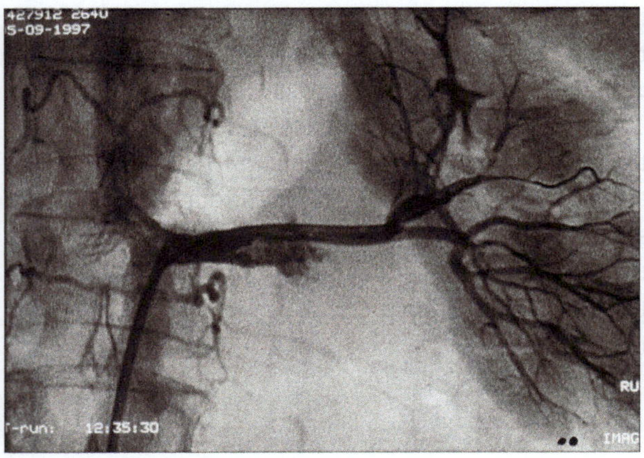

Fig. 22.7 Arteriogram demonstrating renal artery rupture and extravasation of contrast after balloon angioplasty

Perinephric hematoma (Fig. 22.8) can be caused with perforation of renal parenchyma with a guidewire. The incidence of this complication can be reduced by good technique and must be closely monitored. Assuring adequate visualization of the distal tip of the wire during the entire intervention can help to dramatically reduce the incidence of this complication. Initial management is the reversal of heparin, correction of coagulopathy, frequent exams, vitals monitoring, and often CT scans. Transfusion of packed red blood cells should be instituted in the symptomatic patient.

Current Data and Results

Immediate Technical Results

The technical success rate with renal artery intervention increases significantly with the use of stenting when compared to angioplasty alone [67, 68]. Ostial stenosis of the renal artery is continuous with atherosclerotic disease of the aorta and it is for this reason and others that balloon angioplasty alone has met with inferior results to stenting. In two of the earlier studies, successful stent placement was achieved in 83 [69] and 80% [51] of arteries, but since then multiple investigators have published reports with success rates from 94 to 100% [1, 52–54, 59, 67, 68, 70–96]. It should be considered that the definitions of "technical success" ranged from less than 10% residual stenosis to an acceptance of up to 50% residual stenosis in these publications.

Restenosis Rate

Restenosis is a well-recognized problem of percutaneous treatment of RAS. While restenosis occurs in >50% of patients treated with angioplasty alone [68, 97, 98], restenosis rates of renal artery stents are only 10–25% [52, 74, 92, 99, 100]. As expected, the risk of renal artery stent restenosis is related to stent diameter, with larger stent diameters having lower rates of restenosis. Lederman et al. demonstrated that renal stents with >4.5 mm diameter had a 12% restenosis rate while renal stents of <4.5 mm in diameter had a restenosis rate of 21%. Multiple modalities have been suggested for the treatment of instent renal artery stenosis (IRAS) [59]. Currently, reports on the treatment of instent restenosis following renal artery stent-supported angioplasty are only anecdotal and limited to either small single-center series or case reports using different treatment modalities like balloon angioplasty [101], stent-in-stent angioplasty [101], cutting balloon angioplasty [102], endovascular brachytherapy [103–106], or the placement of drug-eluting stents (Table 22.2) [107].

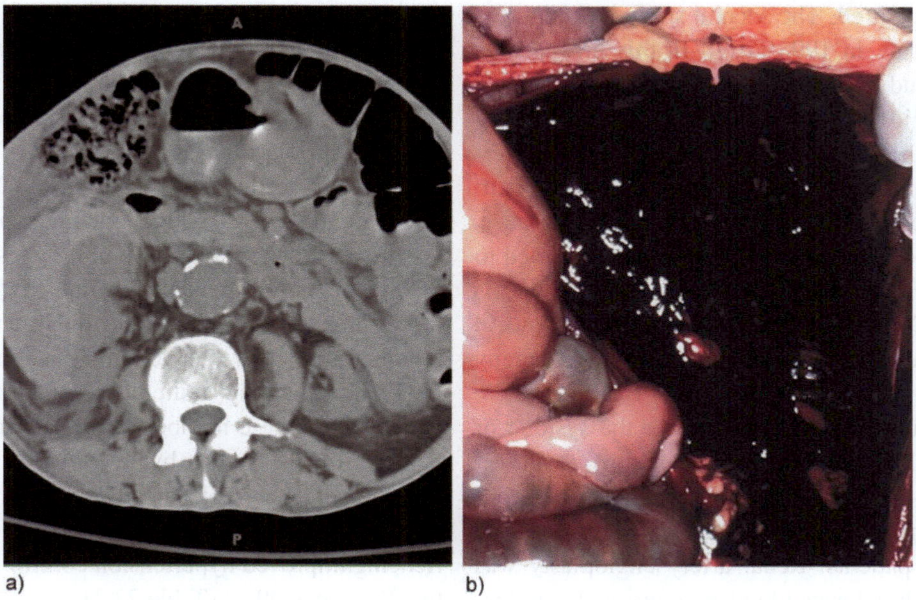

Fig. 22.8 **a**, CT scan showing a moderate perinephric hematoma managed conservatively. **b**, Large perinephric hematoma requiring open exploration

Table 22.2 Renal artery stenting: initial success and restenosis rates

Authors	Year	No. of patients	Stent type	Technical success (%)	Mean follow-up (months)	Restenosis (%)
Rees [52]	1991	28	Palmaz	27/28 (96)	7.5	7/18 (39)
Hennequin [78]	1994	21	Wallstent	25/25 (100)	29	4/20 (20)
Iannone [81]	1996	63	Varied	178/180 (99)	11.3	10/71 (14)
Blum [53]	1997	68	Palmaz	33/33 (100)	27	8/68 (11)
Harden [112]	1997	32	Palmaz	74/74 (100)	6	3/24 (12)
White [100]	1997	100	Varied	132/133 (99)	8.7	15/80 (19)
Shannon [125]	1998	21	Palmaz	21/21 (100)	9	0/16 (0)
Rundback [90]	1998	45	Palmaz	51/54 (94)	13	21/28 (25)
Dorros [54]	1998	163	Palmaz	201/202 (99)	48	NM[a]
Tuttle [67]	1998	129	Palmaz	145/148 (98)	8	7/50 (14)
Bakker [70]	1999	106	Palmaz	117/120 (98)	8	15/89 (17)
Henry [80]	1999	235	Palmaz/renal bridge	241/244 (100)	25	24/209 (11)
Isles [126]	1999	379	Varied	(96–100)[b]	6–12	49/306 (16)
Van de Ven [68]	1999	42	Palmaz	37/42 (88)	6	5/35 (14)
Lederman [59]	2001	300	Palmaz	358/358 (100)	10	23/102 (21)
Zeller [94]	2003	156	Varied	217/219 (99)	22	15/136 (11)
Sapoval [127]	2005	51	Palmaz genesis	51/51 (100)	6	6/41 (15)

[a] NM: not measured.
[b] The publication represents a review of 10 case series reports.

Randomized Controlled Studies

To date, three randomized controlled studies have been completed that compared endovascular therapy with the medical treatment of renovascular hypertension. In 1998 the Essai Multicentrique Medicaments vs. Angioplastie (EMMA) Study group published their results on 23 patients randomly assigned to undergo angioplasty and 26 to undergo medical management [108]. This study was unable to show a significant lowering of the blood pressure but the angioplasty group was able to reduce the number of hypertensive medications required. The second study was reported by Webster et al. in 1998 [109]. In this prospective, randomized study, 55 patients were randomly assigned to either angioplasty or antihypertensive management. The authors concluded that there was a modest improvement in blood pressure control, but this benefit was limited to patients who had bilateral disease. The largest prospective, randomized study reported to date was published by the Dutch Renal Artery Stenosis Intervention Cooperative Study Group [97]. Patients ($n = 106$) were assigned to either pharmacologic therapy or angioplasty, and at 12 months post treatment there was no significant difference in either the systolic or the diastolic blood pressure between the two treatment arms. A meta-analysis of these three studies was conducted by Nordmann et al. [110], reviewing the data from all 210 patients. Renal artery angioplasty was associated with a lower blood pressure and a reduction in the number of antihypertensives. Additionally, a higher renal artery patency was found in the angioplasty group at 12-month follow-up. Based on these results, the authors concluded that angioplasty has a modest but significant effect on blood pressure control.

Case Series

Blood Pressure Control

Many case series have been published evaluating the results of renal artery angioplasty and stenting in the atherosclerotic patient for the treatment of renovascular hypertension [1, 51–54, 59, 67–87, 89, 90, 92, 94, 95, 111, 112]. The basic indications for these studies were hypertension, renal insufficiency, or both. The clinical effect of successful renal artery placement on blood pressure is most often expressed in terms of cure and improvement. However, as you might expect, these terms are not uniformly described in the literature. In the majority of studies, "cure" was defined as a diastolic blood pressure of 90 mmHg or less without medication [52, 53, 69, 72, 78, 79, 81]. Other definitions of "cure" included blood pressure less than 160/95 mmHg [92], blood pressure less than 160/95 mmHg without medication [51], and systolic blood pressure less than 160 mmHg and/or diastolic blood pressure less than 90 mmHg without medication [74]. The remaining studies all had somewhat different variations of these numbers. Findings from the meta-analysis of the studies by Leertouwer [113] showed that the percentage of patients who were found to be cured ranged from 4 to 68% (mean 20%), those experiencing improved hypertension control ranged from 5 to 93% (mean 49%) (Table 22.3).

Effects on Renal Function

More uniform criteria were used to define the effect of renal arterial stenting on renal function in terms of improvement, stabilization, or decline. Most studies considered renal function to improve when the serum creatinine values decreased more than 15–20%. Renal function was considered stabilized when the serum creatinine value was less than these numbers and declined when the creatinine values increased according to these values. While the majority of earlier studies seemed to focus on the control of blood pressure as a primary endpoint, there seems to have been a shift toward discussion of preserving renal function. According to the AHA/ACC guidelines, simply slowing the decline

Table 22.3 Renal artery stenting: blood pressure control

Authors	Year	No. of patients	Mean follow-up (months)	Hypertension % Cured	Hypertension % Improved
Rees [52]	1991	28	7	11	54
Hennequin [78]	1994	21	32	14	86
Dorros [74]	1995	76	6	7	52
Iannone [81]	1996	63	10	4	35
Blum [53]	1997	68	27	16	62
Boisclair [72]	1997	33	13	6	61
Rodriguez [89]	1999	108	6	13	55
Henry [80]	1999	235	12	19	60
Zeller [94]	2004	340	34	43	46

Table 22.4 Renal artery stenting: renal function

Author	Year	Patients	% Improved	% Stable	% Declined
Rees [52]	1991	28	36	36	29
Van de Ven [92]	1995	24	33	58	8
Dorros [74]	1995	69	30	48	22
Iannone [81]	1996	63	36	46	18
Taylor [91]	1997	39	33	29	38
Blum [53]	1997	68	0	100	0
Harden [112]	1997	32	34	34	28
Boisclair [72]	1997	33	41	35	24
Paulsen [128]	1999	135	23	56	21
Isles [126]	1999	379	26	48	26
Rodriguez—Lopez [89]	1999	108	0	95	5
Henry [80]	1999	235	29	67	4
Rundback [90]	1999	45	25	43	32
Zeller [94]	2004	340	34	39	27

in renal function is enough to claim that renal artery stenting is beneficial in the setting of RAS. The majority of patients in available series showed benefit after treatment with a stabilization or improvement in renal function (Table 22.4).

A limited number of studies have focused on patients with severely compromised renal function. Zeller et al. published prospective results from treatment of 340 patients; 24 of these patients had a baseline creatine greater than 3.0 [94]. Improvement of renal function was seen in 71% and stabilization in 21%. These results are not necessarily found in other studies. When looking at all patients treated for RAS most studies have a subset of 20–30% of patients who experience a decline in renal function (Table 22.4). Dorros et al. reported a decline in renal function in 8/17 (47%) of patients with a creatine greater than 2.0. The potential reason for decline in renal function despite successful stent placement is likely multifactorial [74]. Contrast-induced nephropathy and atheroembolism [60] are among the leading culprits.

Comparison with Surgery

Renal artery bypass grafting (RABG) has long served as the mainstay for treatment of both renovascular hypertension (RVH) and ischemia-induced nephropathy. Surgery has been reported to provide a durable improvement or cure in >82% of patients with RVH [6, 114–119] and improve renal function in 43–80% of patients with ischemic nephropathy [120–123]. Mortality ranges from 0 to 4.6% for RVH and 0–7.3% for ischemic neuropathy [6, 114–123]. These numbers were reported by large referral centers with well-documented experience in the surgical management of renovascular disease. Modrall et al. were interested in identifying the operative mortality for RABG in the United States and used the Nationwide Inpatient Sample (NIS) from the Healthcare Cost and Utilization Project (HCUP) to identify all patients undergoing RABG from 2000 to 2004 [119]. This review showed that nationwide in-hospital mortality for RABG is higher than that predicted from previous reports and that in-hospital mortality was 10.0%. The in-hospital mortality for patients with chronic renal failure was 18.1%. The higher morality in this study was more reflective of RABG results outside of a few select referral centers and should be considered in open surgery. After reviewing their findings the authors concluded that factoring these data into the risk–benefit analysis for RABG may mitigate against surgical vascularization in some patients or at least referral to high-volume centers.

Future Research

The CORAL trial is currently enrolling patients to compare aggressive medical treatment with an angiotensin receptor blocker (ARB), along with a statin and aspirin, to angioplasty with stent placement followed by aggressive medical treatment with the antiplatelet agent clopidogrel [124]. Results are expected, after up to 5.5 years follow-up, in 2010. The trial is powered and designed to address many of the key questions that have been asked regarding percutaneous therapy, including effects on clinical outcomes, adverse events, and possibly through secondary analyses, the interaction of baseline features such as diagnostic test results, patient characteristics, or cointerventions with outcomes. The CORAL trial is not, however, the only study that needs to be completed to answer pertinent questions. The CORAL trial will not address the relative value of angioplasty with stent placement in patients with lower grade (<60%) athersclerotic renal artery stentosis (ARAS) nor will it address the role of angioplasty with stent placement in patients with later stage kidney disease (serum creatinine ≥ 3.0 mg/dL) as well as in certain patients with cardiovascular disease.

References

1. Gross CM, Kramer J, Waigand J et al.: Ostial renal artery stent placement for atherosclerotic renal artery stenosis in patients with coronary artery disease, *Cathet Cardiovasc Diagn* 45(1):1–8, September 1998.
2. Jean WJ, Al-Bitar I, Zwicke DL, Port SC, Schmidt DH, Bajwa TK: High incidence of renal artery stenosis in patients with coronary artery disease, *Cathet Cardiovasc Diagn* 32(1):8–10, May 1994.
3. Missouris CG, Buckenham T, Cappuccio FP, MacGregor GA: Renal artery stenosis: a common and important problem in patients with peripheral vascular disease, *Am J Med* 96(1):10–14, Jan 1994.
4. O'Neil EA, Hansen KJ, Canzanello VJ, Pennell TC, Dean RH: Prevalence of ischemic nephropathy in patients with renal insufficiency, *Am Surg* 58(8):485–490, Aug 1992.
5. Hansen KJ, Edwards MS, Craven TE et al.: Prevalence of renovascular disease in the elderly: a population-based study, *J Vasc Surg* 36(3):443–451, September 2002.
6. Cherr GS, Hansen KJ, Craven TE et al.: Surgical management of atherosclerotic renovascular disease, *J Vasc Surg* 35(2):236–245, February 2002.
7. Gruntzig A, Kuhlmann U, Vetter W, Lutolf U, Meier B, Siegenthaler W: Treatment of renovascular hypertension with percutaneous transluminal dilatation of a renal-artery stenosis, *Lancet* 1(8068):801–802, April 15, 1978.
8. Goldblatt H: Experimental renal hypertension, *Am J Med* 4(1):100–119, January 1948.
9. Safian RD, Textor SC: Renal-artery stenosis, *N Engl J Med* 344(6):431–442, February 8, 2001.
10. Leadbetter WF, Burkland CE: Hypertension in unilateral renal disease, *J Urol* 39:611, 1938.
11. Slovut DP, Olin JW: Fibromuscular dysplasia, *N Engl J Med* 350(18):1862–1871, April 29, 2004.
12. Ekelund L, Gerlock J, Molin J, Smith C: Roentgenologic appearance of fibromuscular dysplasia, *Acta Radiol Diagn (Stockh)* 19(3):433–446, 1978.
13. Goncharenko V, Gerlock AJ Jr, Shaff MI, Hollifield JW: Progression of renal artery fibromuscular dysplasia in 42 patients as seen on angiography, *Radiology* 139(1):45–51, April 1981.
14. Caps MT, Perissinotto C, Zierler RE et al.: Prospective study of atherosclerotic disease progression in the renal artery, *Circulation* 98(25):2866–2872, December 22–29, 1998.
15. Fernando D, Garasic J: Percutaneous intervention for renovascular disease: rationale and patient selection, *Curr Opin Cardiol* 19(6):582–588, November 2004.
16. Sharma S, Rajani M, Kamalakar T, Kumar A, Talwar KK: The association between aneurysm formation and systemic hypertension in Takayasu's arteritis, *Clin Radiol* 42(3):182–187, September 1990.
17. Yamato M, Lecky JW, Hiramatsu K, Kohda E: Takayasu arteritis: radiographic and angiographic findings in 59 patients, *Radiology* 161(2):329–334, November 1986.
18. Sharma S, Saxena A, Talwar KK, Kaul U, Mehta SN, Rajani M: Renal artery stenosis caused by nonspecific arteritis (Takayasu disease): results of treatment with percutaneous transluminal angioplasty, *AJR Am J Roentgenol.* 158(2):417–422, February 1992.
19. Hirsch AT, Haskal ZJ, Hertzer NR et al.: ACC/AHA 2005 Practice Guidelines for the management of patients with peripheral arterial disease (lower extremity, renal, mesenteric, and abdominal aortic): a collaborative report from the American association for vascular surgery/society for vascular surgery, society for cardiovascular angiography and interventions, society for vascular medicine and biology, society of interventional radiology, and the ACC/AHA task force on practice guidelines (writing committee to develop guidelines for the management of patients with peripheral arterial disease): endorsed by the American association of cardiovascular and pulmonary rehabilitation; national heart, lung, and blood institute; society for Vascular Nursing; TransAtlantic inter-society consensus; and vascular disease foundation, *Circulation* 113(11):e463–e654, March 21, 2006.
20. Pickering TG, Sos TA, Laragh JH, Bell GM: Percutaneous angioplasty in renovascular hypertension, *Lancet* 1(8579):234–235, January 30, 1988.
21. Olin JW, Piedmonte MR, Young JR, DeAnna S, Grubb M, Childs MB: The utility of duplex ultrasound scanning of the renal arteries for diagnosing significant renal artery stenosis, *Ann Intern Med* 122(11):833–838, June 1, 1995.
22. Radermacher J, Chavan A, Schaffer J et al.: Detection of significant renal artery stenosis with color Doppler sonography: combining extrarenal and intrarenal approaches to minimize technical failure, *Clin Nephrol* 53(5):333–343, May 2000.
23. Radermacher J, Chavan A, Bleck J et al.: Use of Doppler ultrasonography to predict the outcome of therapy for renal-artery stenosis, *N Engl J Med* 344(6):410–417, February 8, 2001.

24. Krumme B, Hollenbeck M: Doppler sonography in renal artery stenosis – does the Resistive Index predict the success of intervention? *Nephrol Dial Transplant* 22(3):692–696, March 2007.
25. Krumme B: Renal Doppler sonography – update in clinical nephrology, *Nephron Clin Pract* 103(2):c24–c28, 2006.
26. Kaatee R, Beek FJ, de Lange EE et al.: Renal artery stenosis: detection and quantification with spiral CT angiography versus optimized digital subtraction angiography, *Radiology* 205(1):121–127, October 1997.
27. Lufft V, Hoogestraat-Lufft L, Fels LM et al.: Contrast media nephropathy: intravenous CT angiography versus intraarterial digital subtraction angiography in renal artery stenosis: a prospective randomized trial, *Am J Kidney Dis* 40(2):236–242, August 2002.
28. Weise WJ, Jaffrey JB: CT angiography and magnetic resonance imaging are the best less-invasive tests for renal artery stenosis, *ACP J Club* 136(2):69, March–April 2002.
29. Law YM, Tay KH, Gan YU, Cheah FK, Tan BS: Gadolinium-enhanced magnetic resonance angiography in renal artery stenosis: comparison with digital subtraction angiography, *Hong Kong Med J* 14(2):136–141, April 2008.
30. van der Molen AJ: Nephrogenic systemic fibrosis and the role of gadolinium contrast media, *J Med Imaging Radiat Oncol* 52(4):339–350, August 2008.
31. Utsunomiya D, Miyazaki M, Nomitsu Y et al.: Clinical role of non-contrast magnetic resonance angiography for evaluation of renal artery stenosis, *Circ J* 72(10):1627–1630, October 2008.
32. Stokes JM, Bernard HR: Nephrotoxicity of iodinated contrast media: quantitative effects of high concentration upon glomerular and tubular functions, *Ann Surg* 153(2):299–309, February 1961.
33. D'Elia JA, Gleason RE, Alday M et al.: Nephrotoxicity from angiographic contrast material. A prospective study, *Am J Med* 72(5):719–725, May 1982.
34. Khoury GA, Hopper JC, Varghese Z et al.: Nephrotoxicity of ionic and non-ionic contrast material in digital vascular imaging and selective renal arteriography, *Br J Radiol* 56(669):631–635, September 1983.
35. Schwab SJ, Hlatky MA, Pieper KS et al.: Contrast nephrotoxicity: a randomized controlled trial of a nonionic and an ionic radiographic contrast agent, *N Engl J Med* 320(3):149–153, January 19, 1989.
36. Drescher P, Madsen PO: Contrast medium-induced nephrotoxicity, *AJR Am J Roentgenol* 170(2):508–509, February 1998.
37. Weisberg LS, Kurnik PB, Kurnik BR: Risk of radiocontrast nephropathy in patients with and without diabetes mellitus, *Kidney Int* 45(1):259–265, January 1994.
38. Lautin EM, Freeman NJ, Schoenfeld AH et al.: Radiocontrast-associated renal dysfunction: incidence and risk factors, *AJR Am J Roentgenol* 157(1):49–58, July 1991.
39. Manske CL, Sprafka JM, Strony JT, Wang Y: Contrast nephropathy in azotemic diabetic patients undergoing coronary angiography, *Am J Med* 89(5):615–620, November 1990.
40. Carbonell N, Blasco M, Sanjuan R et al.: Intravenous N-acetylcysteine for preventing contrast-induced nephropathy: a randomised trial, *Int J Cardiol* 115(1):57–62, January 31, 2007.
41. Heng AE, Cellarier E, Aublet-Cuvelier B et al.: Is treatment with N-acetylcysteine to prevent contrast-induced nephropathy when using bicarbonate hydration out of date? *Clin Nephrol* 70(6):475–484, December 2008.
42. Shehabi Y: Renal protection by N-acetylcysteine, *Br J Anaesth* 98(2):270, February 2007; author reply 270–271.
43. Sisillo E, Ceriani R, Bortone F et al.: N-acetylcysteine for prevention of acute renal failure in patients with chronic renal insufficiency undergoing cardiac surgery: a prospective, randomized, clinical trial, *Crit Care Med* 36(1):81–86, January 2008.
44. Wang JH, Subeq YM, Tsai WC, Lee RP, Hsu BG: Intravenous N-acetylcysteine with saline hydration improves renal function and ameliorates plasma total homocysteine in patients undergoing cardiac angiography, *Ren Fail* 30(5):527–533, 2008.
45. Adolph E, Holdt-Lehmann B, Chatterjee T et al.: Renal Insufficiency Following Radiocontrast Exposure Trial (REINFORCE): a randomized comparison of sodium bicarbonate versus sodium chloride hydration for the prevention of contrast-induced nephropathy, *Coron Artery Dis* 19(6):413–419, September 2008.
46. Brar SS, Shen AY, Jorgensen MB et al.: Sodium bicarbonate vs. sodium chloride for the prevention of contrast medium-induced nephropathy in patients undergoing coronary angiography: a randomized trial, *JAMA* 300(9):1038–1046, September 3, 2008.
47. Maioli M, Toso A, Leoncini M et al.: Sodium bicarbonate versus saline for the prevention of contrast-induced nephropathy in patients with renal dysfunction undergoing coronary angiography or intervention, *J Am Coll Cardiol* 52(8):599–604, August 19, 2008.
48. Navaneethan SD, Singh S, Appasamy S, Wing RE, Sehgal AR: Sodium bicarbonate therapy for prevention of contrast-induced nephropathy: a systematic review and meta-analysis, *Am J Kidney Dis* 53:617–27, 2009.
49. Kim PA, Khilnani NM, Trost DW, Sos TA, Lee L: Fluoroscopic landmarks for optimal visualization of the proximal renal arteries, *J Vasc Interv Radiol* 10(1):37–39, January 1999.
50. Caridi JG, Stavropoulos SW, Hawkins IF Jr: Carbon dioxide digital subtraction angiography for renal artery stent placement, *J Vasc Interv Radiol* 10(5):635–640, May 1999.
51. Kuhn FP, Kutkuhn B, Torsello G, Modder U: Renal artery stenosis: preliminary results of treatment with the Strecker stent, *Radiology* 180(2):367–372, August 1991.
52. Rees CR, Palmaz JC, Becker GJ et al.: Palmaz stent in atherosclerotic stenoses involving the ostia of the renal arteries: preliminary report of a multicenter study, *Radiology* 181(2):507–514, November 1991.
53. Blum U, Krumme B, Flugel P et al.: Treatment of ostial renal-artery stenoses with vascular endoprostheses after unsuccessful balloon angioplasty, *N Engl J Med* 336(7):459–465, February 13, 1997.

54. Dorros G, Jaff M, Mathiak L et al.: Four-year follow-up of Palmaz-Schatz stent revascularization as treatment for atherosclerotic renal artery stenosis, *Circulation* 98(7):642–647, August 18, 1998.
55. Dorros G, Prince C, Mathiak L: Stenting of a renal artery stenosis achieves better relief of the obstructive lesion than balloon angioplasty, *Cathet Cardiovasc Diagn* 29(3):191–198, July 1993.
56. Vignali C, Bargellini I, Lazzereschi M et al.: Predictive factors of in-stent restenosis in renal artery stenting: a retrospective analysis, *Cardiovasc Intervent Radiol* 28(3):296–302, May–June 2005.
57. Zeller T: Is drug-eluting stent angioplasty indicated for the treatment of atherosclerotic renal artery stenosis and restenosis? *Catheter Cardiovasc Interv* 68(1):123–124, July 2006.
58. Zeller T, Rastan A, Rothenpieler U, Muller C: Restenosis after stenting of atherosclerotic renal artery stenosis: is there a rationale for the use of drug-eluting stents? *Catheter Cardiovasc Interv* 68(1):125–130, July 2006.
59. Lederman RJ, Mendelsohn FO, Santos R, Phillips HR, Stack RS, Crowley JJ: Primary renal artery stenting: characteristics and outcomes after 363 procedures, *Am Heart J* 142(2):314–323, August 2001.
60. Edwards MS, Corriere MA, Craven TE et al.: Atheroembolism during percutaneous renal artery revascularization, *J Vasc Surg* 46(1):55–61, July 2007.
61. Edwards MS, Craven BL, Stafford J et al.: Distal embolic protection during renal artery angioplasty and stenting, *J Vasc Surg* 44(1):128–135, July 2006.
62. Holden A, Hill A: Renal angioplasty and stenting with distal protection of the main renal artery in ischemic nephropathy: early experience, *J Vasc Surg* 38(5):962–968, November 2003.
63. Axelrod DJ, Freeman H, Pukin L, Guller J, Mitty HA: Guide wire perforation leading to fatal perirenal hemorrhage from transcortical collaterals after renal artery stent placement, *J Vasc Interv Radiol* 15(9):985–987, September 2004.
64. Heye S, Vanbeckevoort D, Blockmans D, Nevelsteen A, Maleux G: Iatrogenic main renal artery injury: treatment by endovascular stent-graft placement, *Cardiovasc Intervent Radiol.* 28(1):93–94, January–February 2005.
65. Morris CS, Bonnevie GJ, Najarian KE: Nonsurgical treatment of acute iatrogenic renal artery injuries occurring after renal artery angioplasty and stenting, *AJR Am J Roentgenol* 177(6):1353–1357, December 2001.
66. Novick AC, Ziegelbaum M, Vidt DG, Gifford RW Jr, Pohl MA, Goormastic M: Trends in surgical revascularization for renal artery disease. Ten years' experience, *JAMA* 257(4):498–501, January 23–30, 1987.
67. Tuttle KR, Chouinard RF, Webber JT et al.: Treatment of atherosclerotic ostial renal artery stenosis with the intravascular stent, *Am J Kidney Dis* 32(4):611–622, October 1998.
68. van de Ven PJ, Kaatee R, Beutler JJ et al.: Arterial stenting and balloon angioplasty in ostial atherosclerotic renovascular disease: a randomised trial, *Lancet* 353(9149):282–286, January 23, 1999.
69. Wilms GE, Peene PT, Baert AL et al.: Renal artery stent placement with use of the Wallstent endoprosthesis, *Radiology* 179(2):457–462, May 1991.
70. Bakker J, Goffette PP, Henry M et al.: The Erasme study: a multicenter study on the safety and technical results of the Palmaz stent used for the treatment of atherosclerotic ostial renal artery stenosis, *Cardiovasc Intervent Radiol* 22(6):468–474, November–December 1999.
71. Baumgartner I, von Aesch K, Do DD, Triller J, Birrer M, Mahler F: Stent placement in ostial and nonostial atherosclerotic renal arterial stenoses: a prospective follow-up study, *Radiology* 216(2):498–505, August 2000.
72. Boisclair C, Therasse E, Oliva VL et al.: Treatment of renal angioplasty failure by percutaneous renal artery stenting with Palmaz stents: midterm technical and clinical results, *AJR Am J Roentgenol* 168(1):245–251, January 1997.
73. Bush RL, Najibi S, MacDonald MJ et al.: Endovascular revascularization of renal artery stenosis: technical and clinical results, *J Vasc Surg* 33(5):1041–1049, May 2001.
74. Dorros G, Jaff M, Jain A, Dufek C, Mathiak L: Follow-up of primary Palmaz-Schatz stent placement for atherosclerotic renal artery stenosis, *Am J Cardiol* 75(15):1051–1055, May 15, 1995.
75. Fiala LA, Jackson MR, Gillespie DL, O'Donnell SD, Lukens M, Gorman P: Primary stenting of atherosclerotic renal artery ostial stenosis, *Ann Vasc Surg* 12(2):128–133, March 1998.
76. Giroux MF, Soulez G, Therasse E et al.: Percutaneous revascularization of the renal arteries: predictors of outcome, *J Vasc Interv Radiol* 11(6):713–720, June 2000.
77. Halkin A, Mehran R, Casey CW et al.: Impact of moderate renal insufficiency on restenosis and adverse clinical events after paclitaxel-eluting and bare metal stent implantation: results from the TAXUS-IV Trial, *Am Heart J* 150(6):1163–1170, December 2005.
78. Hennequin LM, Joffre FG, Rousseau HP et al.: Renal artery stent placement: long-term results with the Wallstent endoprosthesis, *Radiology* 191(3):713–719, June 1994.
79. Henry M, Amor M, Henry I et al.: Stent placement in the renal artery: three-year experience with the Palmaz stent, *J Vasc Interv Radiol* 7(3):343–350, May–June 1996.
80. Henry M, Amor M, Henry I et al.: Stents in the treatment of renal artery stenosis: long-term follow-up, *J Endovasc Surg* 6(1):42–51, February 1999.
81. Iannone LA, Underwood PL, Nath A, Tannenbaum MA, Ghali MG, Clevenger LD: Effect of primary balloon expandable renal artery stents on long-term patency, renal function, and blood pressure in hypertensive and renal insufficient patients with renal artery stenosis, *Cathet Cardiovasc Diagn* 37(3):243–250, March 1996.
82. Lim ST, Rosenfield K: Renal artery stent placement: indications and results, *Curr Interv Cardiol Rep* 2(2):130–139, May 2000.
83. MacLeod M, Taylor AD, Baxter G et al.: Renal artery stenosis managed by Palmaz stent insertion: technical and clinical outcome, *J Hypertens* 13(12 Pt 2):1791–1795, December 1995.

84. Mistry S, Ives N, Harding J et al.: Angioplasty and STent for Renal Artery Lesions (ASTRAL trial): rationale, methods and results so far, *J Hum Hypertens* 21(7):511–515, July 2007.
85. Muller-Hulsbeck S, Frahm C, Behm C et al.: Low-profile stent placement with the monorail technique for treatment of renal artery stenosis: midterm results of a prospective trial, *J Vasc Interv Radiol* 16(7):963–971, July 2005.
86. Perkovic V, Thomson KR, Mitchell PJ et al.: Treatment of renovascular disease with percutaneous stent insertion: long-term outcomes, *Australas Radiol* 45(4):438–443, November 2001.
87. Raynaud AC, Beyssen BM, Turmel-Rodrigues LE et al.: Renal artery stent placement: immediate and midterm technical and clinical results, *J Vasc Interv Radiol* 5(6):849–858, November–December 1994.
88. Rocha-Singh K, Jaff MR, Lynne Kelley E: Renal artery stenting with noninvasive duplex ultrasound follow-up: 3-year results from the RENAISSANCE renal stent trial, *Catheter Cardiovasc Interv* 72(6):853–862, November 15, 2008.
89. Rodriguez-Lopez JA, Werner A, Ray LI et al.: Renal artery stenosis treated with stent deployment: indications, technique, and outcome for 108 patients, *J Vasc Surg* 29(4):617–624, April 1999.
90. Rundback JH, Gray RJ, Rozenblit G et al.: Renal artery stent placement for the management of ischemic nephropathy, *J Vasc Interv Radiol* 9(3):413–420, May–June 1998.
91. Taylor A, Sheppard D, Macleod MJ et al.: Renal artery stent placement in renal artery stenosis: technical and early clinical results, *Clin Radiol* 52(6):451–457, June 1997.
92. van de Ven PJ, Beutler JJ, Kaatee R et al.: Transluminal vascular stent for ostial atherosclerotic renal artery stenosis, *Lancet* 346(8976):672–674, September 9, 1995.
93. White CJ, Ramee SR, Collins TJ, Jenkins JS: Renal artery stent placement: indications, techniques and clinical results, *Indian Heart J* 50(Suppl 1):153–160, October 1998.
94. Zeller T, Frank U, Muller C et al.: Stent-supported angioplasty of severe atherosclerotic renal artery stenosis preserves renal function and improves blood pressure control: long-term results from a prospective registry of 456 lesions, *J Endovasc Ther* 11(2):95–106, April 2004.
95. Goncalves JA, Amorim JE, Soares Neto MM, Ribeiro AB, Lima VC: Clinical efficacy of percutaneous renal revascularization with stent placement in atherosclerotic renovascular disease, *Arq Bras Cardiol* 88(1):85–90, January 2007.
96. Mitchell JA, Subramanian R, White CJ et al.: Predicting blood pressure improvement in hypertensive patients after renal artery stent placement: renal fractional flow reserve, *Catheter Cardiovasc Interv* 69(5):685–689, April 1, 2007.
97. van Jaarsveld BC, Krijnen P, Pieterman H et al.: The effect of balloon angioplasty on hypertension in atherosclerotic renal-artery stenosis. Dutch Renal Artery Stenosis Intervention Cooperative Study Group, *N Engl J Med* 342(14):1007–1014, April 6, 2000.
98. Weibull H, Bergqvist D, Jonsson K, Hulthen L, Mannhem P, Bergentz SE: Long-term results after percutaneous transluminal angioplasty of atherosclerotic renal artery stenosis – the importance of intensive follow-up, *Eur J Vasc Surg* 5(3):291–301, June 1991.
99. Burket MW, Cooper CJ, Kennedy DJ et al.: Renal artery angioplasty and stent placement: predictors of a favorable outcome, *Am Heart J* 139(1 Pt 1):64–71, January 2000.
100. White CJ, Ramee SR, Collins TJ, Jenkins JS, Escobar A, Shaw D: Renal artery stent placement: utility in lesions difficult to treat with balloon angioplasty, *J Am Coll Cardiol* 30(6):1445–1450, November 15, 1997.
101. Bax L, Mali WP, Van De Ven PJ, Beek FJ, Vos JA, Beutler JJ: Repeated intervention for in-stent restenosis of the renal arteries, *J Vasc Interv Radiol* 13(12):1219–1224, December 2002.
102. Munneke GJ, Engelke C, Morgan RA, Belli AM: Cutting balloon angioplasty for resistant renal artery in-stent restenosis, *J Vasc Interv Radiol* 13(3):327–331, March 2002.
103. Ellis K, Murtagh B, Loghin C et al.: The use of brachytherapy to treat renal artery in-stent restenosis, *J Interv Cardiol* 18(1):49–54, February 2005.
104. Reilly JP, Ramee SR: Vascular brachytherapy in renal artery restenosis, *Curr Opin Cardiol* 19(4):332–335, July 2004.
105. Spratt JC, Leslie SJ, Verin V: A case of renal artery brachytherapy for in-stent restenosis: four-year follow-up, *J Invasive Cardiol* 16(5):287–288, May 2004.
106. Aslam MS, Balasubramanian J, Greenspahn BR: Brachytherapy for renal artery in-stent restenosis, *Catheter Cardiovasc Interv* 58(2):151–154, Februray 2003.
107. Kakkar AK, Fischi M, Narins CR: Drug-eluting stent implantation for treatment of recurrent renal artery in-stent restenosis, *Catheter Cardiovasc Interv* 68(1):118–122, July 2006; discussion 123–114.
108. Plouin PF, Chatellier G, Darne B, Raynaud A: Blood pressure outcome of angioplasty in atherosclerotic renal artery stenosis: a randomized trial. Essai Multicentrique Medicaments vs Angioplastie (EMMA) Study Group, *Hypertension* 31(3):823–829, March 1998.
109. Webster J, Marshall F, Abdalla M et al.: Randomised comparison of percutaneous angioplasty vs. continued medical therapy for hypertensive patients with atheromatous renal artery stenosis. Scottish and Newcastle Renal Artery Stenosis Collaborative Group, *J Hum Hypertens* 12(5):329–335, May 1998.
110. Nordmann AJ, Woo K, Parkes R, Logan AG: Balloon angioplasty or medical therapy for hypertensive patients with atherosclerotic renal artery stenosis? A meta-analysis of randomized controlled trials, *Am J Med* 114(1):44–50, January 2003.
111. Joffre F, Rousseau H, Bernadet P et al.: Midterm results of renal artery stenting, *Cardiovasc Intervent Radiol* 15(5):313–318, September–October 1992.
112. Harden PN, MacLeod MJ, Rodger RS et al.: Effect of renal-artery stenting on progression of renovascular renal failure, *Lancet* 349(9059):1133–1136, April 19, 1997.

113. Leertouwer TC, Gussenhoven EJ, Bosch JL et al.: Stent placement for renal arterial stenosis: where do we stand? A meta-analysis, *Radiology* 216(1):78–85, July 2000.
114. Beebe HG, MacFarlane SD: Antegrade aortorenal bypass graft: a new alternative, *Am J Surg* 155(5):647–650, May 1988.
115. Fichelle JM, Colacchio G, Farkas JC et al.: Renal revascularization in high-risk patients: the role of iliac renal bypass, *Ann Vasc Surg* 6(5):403–407, September 1992.
116. Grigoryants V, Henke PK, Watson NC, Upchurch GR Jr, Wakefield TW, Stanley JC: Iliorenal bypass: indications and outcomes following 41 reconstructions, *Ann Vasc Surg* 21(1):1–9, January 2007.
117. Hagino RT, Valentine RJ, Clagett GP: Supraceliac aortorenal bypass, *J Vasc Surg* 26(3):482–489, September 1997; discussion 490–481.
118. Lagneau P, Michel JB, Charrat JM: Use of polytetrafluoroethylene grafts for renal bypass, *J Vasc Surg* 5(5):738–742, May 1987.
119. Modrall JG, Rosero EB, Smith ST et al.: Operative mortality for renal artery bypass in the United States: results from the national inpatient sample, *J Vasc Surg* 48(2):317–322, August 2008.
120. Hansen KJ, Thomason RB, Craven TE et al.: Surgical management of dialysis-dependent ischemic nephropathy, *J Vasc Surg* 21(2):197–209, February 1995; discussion 209–111.
121. Oskin TC, Hansen KJ, Deitch JS, Craven TE, Dean RH: Chronic renal artery occlusion: nephrectomy versus revascularization, *J Vasc Surg* 29(1):140–149, January 1999.
122. Hansen KJ, Cherr GS, Craven TE et al.: Management of ischemic nephropathy: dialysis-free survival after surgical repair, *J Vasc Surg* 32(3):472–481, September 2000; discussion 481–472.
123. Marone LK, Clouse WD, Dorer DJ et al.: Preservation of renal function with surgical revascularization in patients with atherosclerotic renovascular disease, *J Vasc Surg* 39(2):322–329, February 2004.
124. Cooper CJ, Murphy TP, Matsumoto A et al.: Stent revascularization for the prevention of cardiovascular and renal events among patients with renal artery stenosis and systolic hypertension: rationale and design of the CORAL trial, *Am Heart J* 152(1):59–66, July 2006.
125. Shannon HM, Gillespie IN, Moss JG: Salvage of the solitary kidney by insertion of a renal artery stent, *AJR Am J Roentgenol* 171(1):217–222, July 1998.
126. Isles CG, Robertson S, Hill D: Management of renovascular disease: a review of renal artery stenting in ten studies, *QJM* 92(3):159–167, March 1999.
127. Sapoval M, Zahringer M, Pattynama P et al.: Low-profile stent system for treatment of atherosclerotic renal artery stenosis: the GREAT trial, *J Vasc Interv Radiol* 16(9):1195–1202, September 2005.
128. Paulsen D, Klow NE, Rogstad B et al.: Preservation of renal function by percutaneous transluminal angioplasty in ischaemic renal disease, *Nephrol Dial Transplant* 14(6):1454–1461, June 1999.

Inferior Vena Cava Filters: The Impact of Endovascular Technology

23

David Rosenthal, Eric D. Wellons, Allison B. Burkett, Paul V. Kochupura, and William Veale

Anticoagulation is the accepted therapy for patients with venous thromboembolic disease. When a contraindication to anticoagulation therapy is present, however, interruption of the inferior vena cava (IVC) can be performed to prevent pulmonary embolism (PE) as >80% of pulmonary emboli originate in the lower extremities and pelvis [1].

During the past four decades, a wide variety of permanent IVC filters (IVCFs) designed for percutaneous insertion have been developed. The commonly accepted *absolute* indications for the use of an IVCF are essentially a contraindication to or a failure of anticoagulation, while the *relative* and prophylactic indications are patients at continued high risk for PE (Table 23.1) [2]. The advent, however, of temporary or retrievable IVCFs has broadened the indications and the role of IVCFs continues to evolve, as more than half are being placed for prophylaxis against PE in patients considered high-operative risks [3]. The first removable IVCF for temporary protection from PE was proposed in 1967 [4], the same year that the Mobin-Uddin umbrella became the first endoluminal device to prevent PE [5]. It was not until 30 years later, however, that retrievable IVCFs became available in the United States when the instructions for use of three existing permanent filters were changed to allow for percutaneous retrieval [6].

The obvious advantage of a retrievable filter is that it offers protection against PE during the highest risk thromboembolic period, while avoiding the potential long-term sequelae of a permanent IVCF which includes access-site thrombosis, malposition, migration, vena cava occlusion, perforation and duodenal corrosion [7–11], but the use of such filters, especially in younger patients, is controversial [12–15].

The objective of this chapter was to report our technical and clinical results with the first US Federal and Drug Administration (FDA)-approved retrievable

Table 23.1 Indications for all vena cava filters

Absolute indications (proven VTE)
Recurrent VTE—acute or chronicdespite adequate AC
Contraindications to AC
Complication of AC
Inability to achieve/maintain therapeutic AC
Relative indications (proven VTE)
Iliocava DVT
Large, free-floating proximal DVT
Massive PE treated with thrombolysis/thrombectomy
Chronic PE treated with thromboendarterectomy
Thrombolysis for iliocaval DVT
VTE with limited cardiopulmonary reserve
Recurrent PE with filter in place
Difficulty in establishing therapeutic AC
Poor compliance with AC medications
High risk of complication of AC (such as ataxia, frequent falls)
Prophylactic indications (no VTE, primary prophylaxis not feasible[a])
Trauma patient with high risk of VTE
Surgical procedure in patient at high risk of VTE
Medical condition with high risk of VTE

AC, anticoagulation; DVT, deep venous thrombosis; PE, pulmonary embolism; VTE, venous thromboembolism, e.g., DVT and/or PE.

[a]Primary prophylaxis not feasible owing to high bleeding risk, inability to monitor the patient for VTE, etc.

D. Rosenthal (✉)
Chief, Department of Vascular Surgery, Atlanta Medical Center, Atlanta, GA, USA
e-mail: docro@mindspring.com

T.J. Fogarty, R.A. White (eds.), *Peripheral Endovascular Interventions*,
DOI 10.1007/978-1-4419-1387-6_23,

IVCFs and to evaluate the impact of endovascular technology on retrievable IVCFs.

Retrievable Inferior Vena Cava Filters

There are three retrievable IVCFs that are approved by the FDA in the United States today. These filters can be used either permanently or temporarily with subsequent retrieval for protection against PE. The first generation retrievable filters included the Günther-Tulip filter (Cook, Inc., Bloomington, IN), the Recovery filter (Bard Peripheral Vascular, Tempe, AZ), and the OptEase filter (Cordis Endovascular, Miami Lakes, FL).

Günther-Tulip Filter

The Günther-Tulip retrievable IVCF is constructed of MRI-compatible conichrome (cobalt, nickel, and chromium) with the shape of a half-basket (Fig. 23.1). The filter is 45 mm in length and has a maximum diameter of 30 mm. Four special centering wires extend outside the basket with a curvature designed to follow the IVC wall. The four wires serve to anchor the filter by small barbed anchoring hooks at the ends. Four thinner wires, shaped like tulip leaves, expand the clot-trapping area of the filter. A retrieval hook is located at the apex of the filter which allows for jugular vein percutaneous retrieval with the coaxial Günther-Tulip Retrieval Set (Cook) or a loop snare (Amplats Gooseneck; ev3, Inc., Plymouth, MN); or an En-Snare (Hatch Medical, Duluth, GA).

Recovery Filter

The Recovery nitinol filter is composed of twelve 0.13-in. nitinol wires that extend from a nitinol sleeve (Fig. 23.1). It has six arms and legs and the resting diameter of each of the arms is 30.5 mm; the resting diameter of each of the legs is 32 mm. The filter measures 4 cm in height and may be introduced via the jugular or the femoral vein and is retrieved through the jugular vein approach with the Recovery Cone Removal System (Bard Peripheral Vascular).

OptEase Filter

The nitinol, magnetic residence imaging-compatible OptEase filter (Fig. 23.1) has a unique self-centering design that provides dual-level filtration and is the only filter that is retrieved from a femoral vein approach. The filter has a symmetrical double-basket design with six straight struts connecting the proximal and the distal baskets. The filter has a maximum length of 67 mm when non-expanded and a length of 54 mm when fully deployed within a 30-mm-diameter IVC. The OptEase can be deployed from jugular and femoral approaches and hook at the inferior end of the basket allows simple retrieval with any standard loop snare.

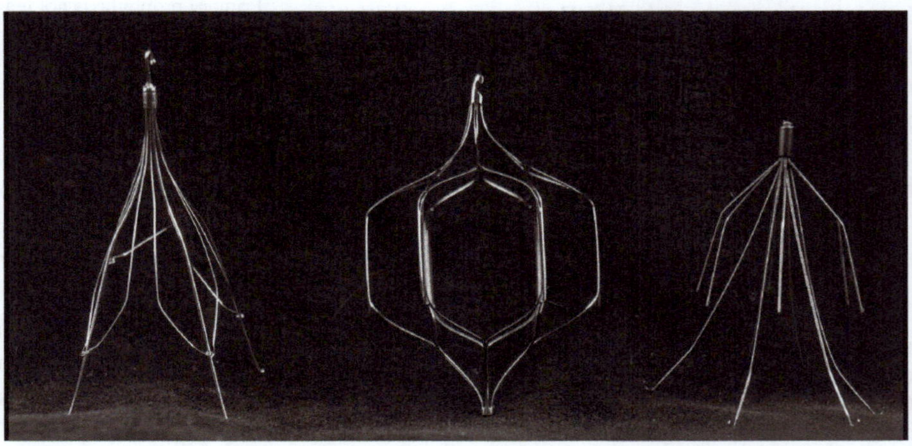

Fig. 23.1 Retrievable inferior vena cava filters

Intravascular Ultrasound-Guided IVCF Deployment

Our initial work with retrievable IVCFs was performed in multiple-trauma patients who often have injuries that preclude the standard use of anticoagulation therapy or sequential compression device prophylaxis. Intravascular ultrasound (IVUS) is a minimally invasive and accurate method of interrogating the IVC [16–19]. The ICU bedside placement of an IVCF under IVUS guidance is simple and safe, and averts the need to transport critically ill patients to the radiology department operating room.

The technique has been previously described [20], but in summary, under aseptic conditions, two femoral vena punctures were made, 1 cm apart, and two Glidewires (0.035 in.; Terumo, Somerset, NJ) were passed into the IVC. An 8-F sheath was introduced over first Glidewire (IVUS wire) and the filter's own 6-F sheath was introduced over the second Glidewire (filter wire). A 10-MHz IVUS probe (Volcano Therapeutics, Rancho Cordera, CA) was passed to the level of the right atrium. Venous anatomy was evaluated with a pull-back technique that enabled easy identification of the liver, hepatic veins, renal artery, and renal veins. The transverse IVC diameter was measured in two planes at the infrarenal location. The IVUS probe was pulled back to the level of the lowest renal vein (Fig. 23.2), and the IVC filter sheath was introduced over the second Glidewire and advanced beyond the IVUS probe. As the filter was advanced in the sheath, the IVUS identified its passage beyond the renal veins until the echogenic "scatter" from the filter disappeared. The sheath and the filter were pulled back to a point adjacent to the IVUS probe, and under continuous IVUS surveillance, the filter was deployed (Fig. 23.3).

Recently, a single-sheath technique has been reported [21]. The locations of the renal veins are identified as described above. An 8-F 55-cm Brite Tip sheath (Cordis Corp., Miami Lakes, FL) is advanced over the IVUS catheter until the radiopaque tip "covers" the ultrasound image of the catheter. The tip of the sheath is repeatedly passed across the IVUS catheter (while holding the IVUS catheter in place) to confirm the location of the 8-F sheath tip just below the renal veins.

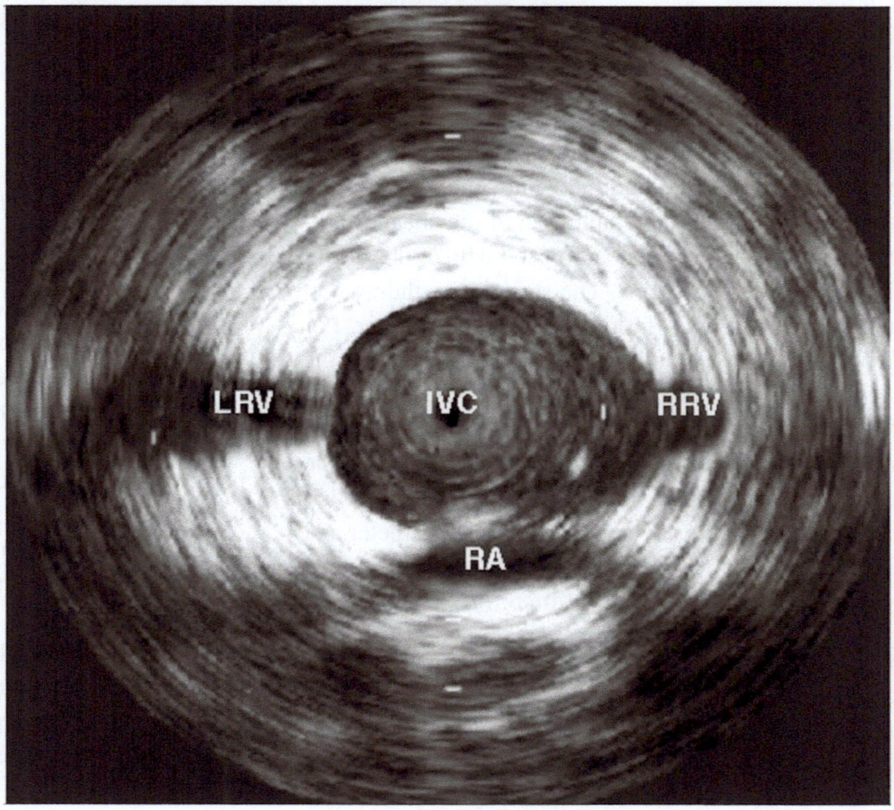

Fig. 23.2 Intravascular ultrasound image of renal artery (RA), right renal veins (RRV), left renal veins (LRV), and IVC. (From Rosenthal, et al. [22], with permission. Society for Vascular Surgery and the American Association for Vascular Surgery.)

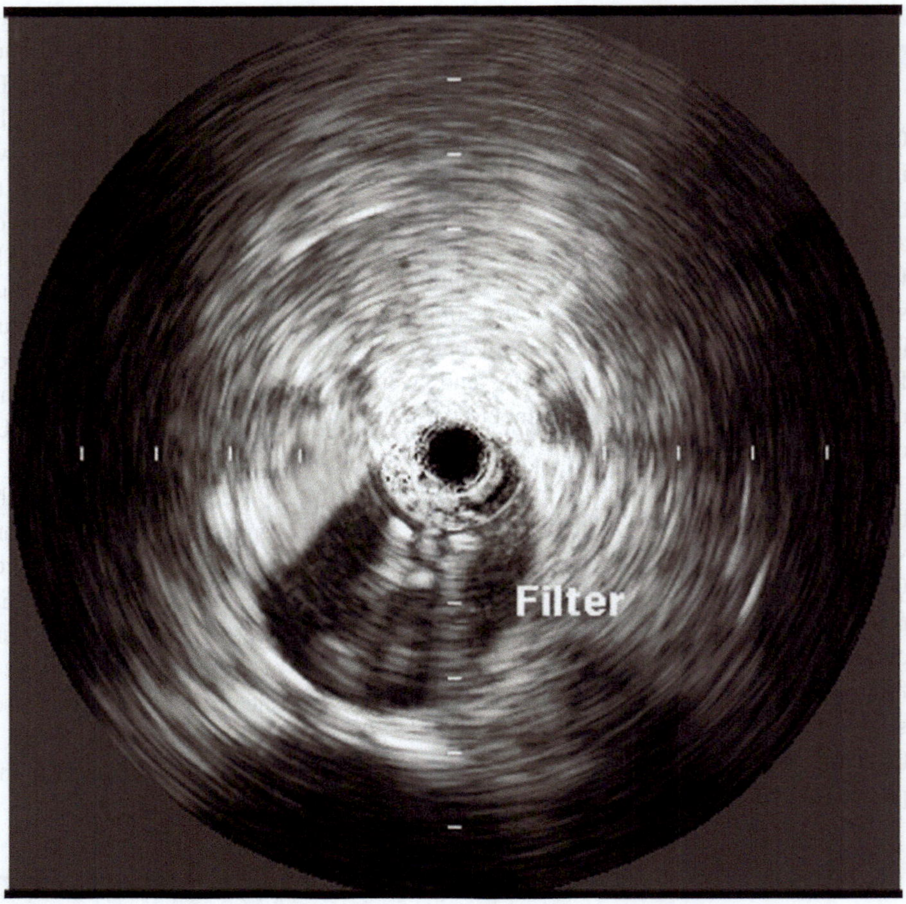

Fig. 23.3 Intravascular ultrasound image of filter deployment. Note echogenic "scatter" from filter. (From Rosenthal, et al. [22], with permission. Society for Vascular Surgery and the American Association for Vascular Surgery.)

The sheath is held in place while the IVUS catheter and the guidewire are removed. The OptEase filter can be advanced with the obturator until the mark on the obturator shaft is at the diaphragm of the sheath, indicating that the filter is in position at the tip of the sheath just below the renal veins. The sheath is withdrawn in a standard "pin-pull" fashion to deploy the filter. For deployment of the Günther-Tulip filter, the steps are the same except that there is no need to upsize the sheath for the IVUS as the femoral access delivery sheath provided with the Günther-Tulip filter is 9 F. Once the renal veins have been identified, the sheath is positioned below the renal veins and the IVUS catheter and the wire are removed. The preloaded filter is advanced into the sheath until the distal mark on the shaft is at the Tuohy-Borst valve, indicating that the tip of the filter is at the tip of the sheath. The filter delivery catheter is secured, the sheath is pulled back to the proximal mark, and the filter released in the standard manner.

Inferior Vena Cava Filter Retrieval

Filter retrieval was performed when it was deemed safe that patients could undergo anticoagulant therapy. Before filter retrieval, all patients undergo venous color-flow duplex ultrasonography of the lower extremities to rule out lower extremity DVT. All filter retrievals were performed in the catheterization laboratory via a right jugular vein approach (Recovery filter and Günther-Tulip filter) or a right femoral vein approach (OptEase filter). Before retrieval, a vena cavogram was performed to assess the IVC for trapped emboli or thrombus within the filter.

The Günther-Tulip filters were retrieved via a jugular vein approach with the Cook Retrieval Set. The hook at the apex of the filter is snared with the system's platinum wire loop snare and secured by advancing the 6-F retrieval catheter. The snare and the retrieval catheter are held in place and the filter collapsed,

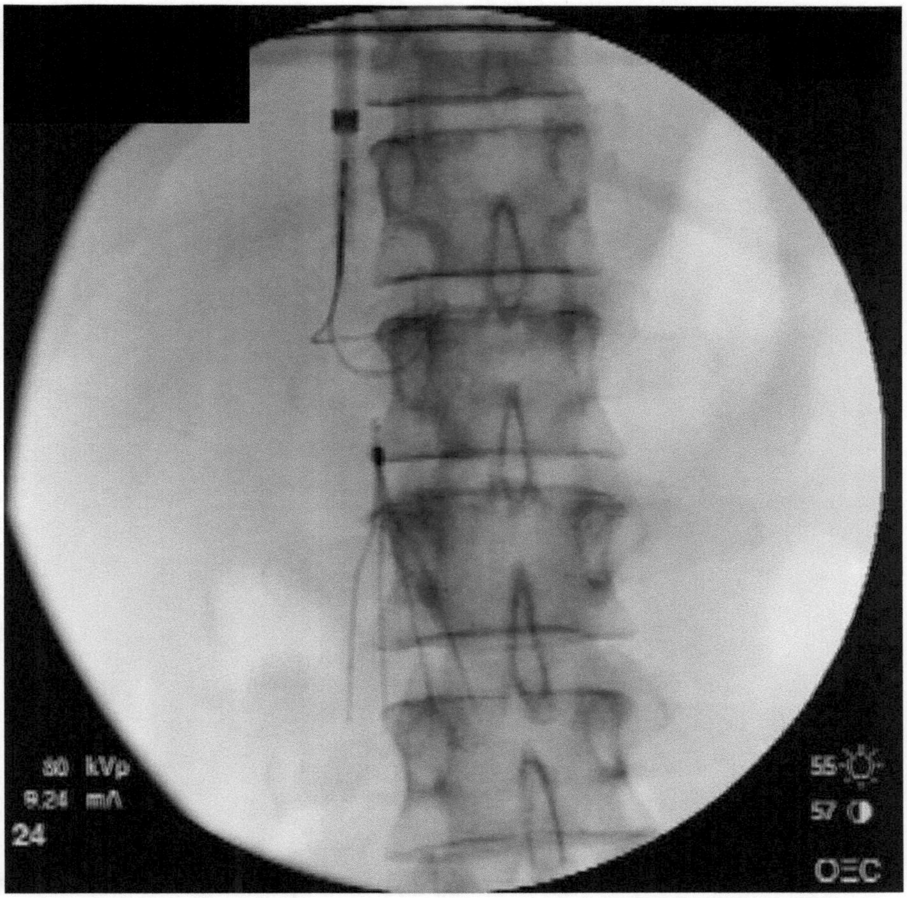

Fig. 23.4 Günther-Tulip filter retrieval

disengaging the filter from the IVC wall by advancing the outer 6-F coaxial sheath. The larger sheath (11 F) is advanced over the 6-F sheath and the collapsed filter is retrieved (Figs. 23.4, 23.5, and 23.6). The Recovery nitinol filer was retrieved via a 10-F sheath with its own Recover Cone System, which is constructed of nine metal claws covered by a urethane cover. The open diameter of the cone is 15 mm and the central lumen allows for over-the-wire placement. The OptEase filter was retrieved via a 10-F sheath using an En-Snare and is the only filter able to be retrieved via a femoral vein approach.

Phase I Study

In a Phase I study to evaluate the role and efficacy of retrievable IVCFs placed under IVUS guidance, 103 multiple-trauma patients with relative or absolute contraindications to low-dose heparin therapy or barriers to the placement of sequential compression devices underwent prophylactic placement of Günther-Tulip ($n = 38$), Recovery ($n = 30$), or OptEase ($n = 35$) retrievable IVCFs at the ICU bedside. The multiple-trauma patients had several injuries: (1) closed head injuries with prolonged immobilization ($n = 50$), (2) pelvic fractures (41), (3) spine fractures with neurologic deficit (31), (4) multiple long bone fractures (51), and (5) multiple solid organ injuries (36) [22].

All IVCFs were placed under real-time IVUS guidance at the patient's bedside. After deployment, gentle pressure was applied until hemostasis was achieved. Anterior–posterior abdominal X-rays were obtained to verify the IVCF location and position of the filter. All patients underwent femoral vein color-flow duplex ultrasound scanning within 14 days of IVCF placement to assess femoral vein patency. In patients with an initial contraindication to anticoagulation, prophylactic low molecular weight heparin was instituted as soon as it was believed to be safe by the attending surgeon. Adjunctive measures, such as pneumatic compression devices, were used whenever possible.

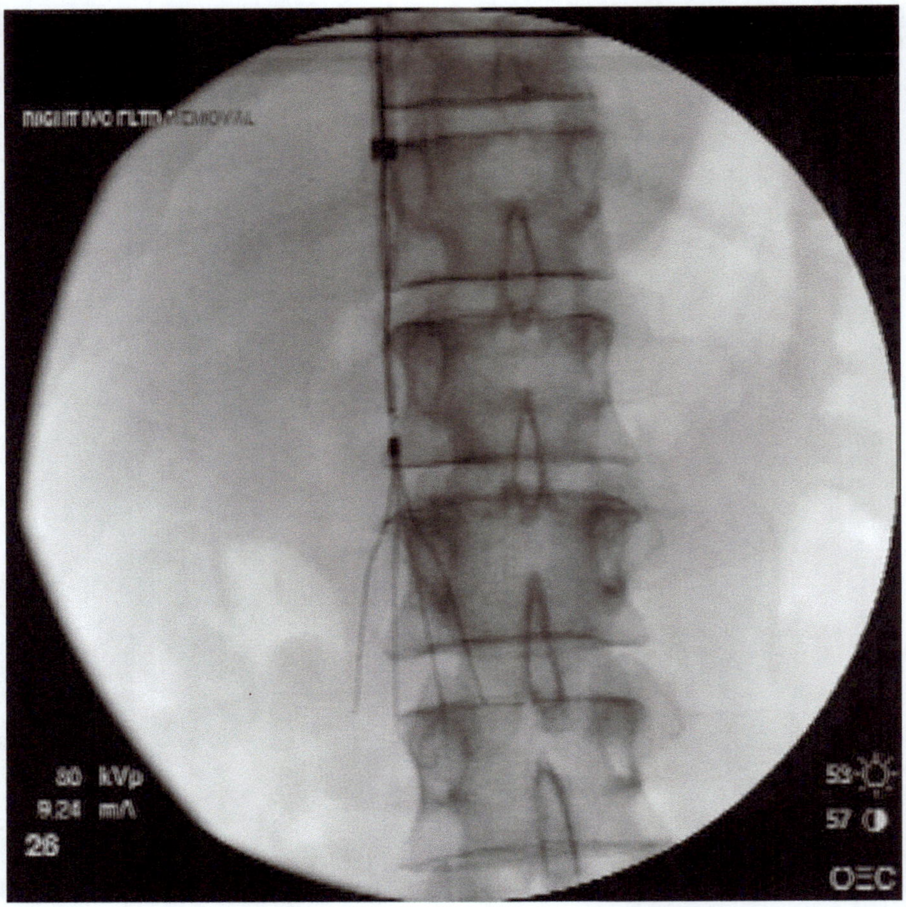

Fig. 23.5 Retrieval hook at the apex of filter is snared

Prior to filter retrieval, all patients underwent venous color-flow duplex ultrasonography of the legs to rule out lower extremity DVT and a vena cavogram to assess the IVCF for trapped emboli, filter tilt, or thrombus within the filter. A filter volume of trapped thrombus (>25%) was considered a contraindication to filter removal. After retrieval, a repeat vena cavogram was performed to evaluate the IVC for perforation, stenosis, and patency.

Patients were followed up for the development of venous thromboembolic complications until death or discharge. Complications evaluated included DVT, IVC occlusion documented by vena cavogram, or computed tomography. PE in symptomatic patients was documented by a ventilation-perfusion scan, an angiogram, or a contrast-enhanced spiral computed tomography. Complications of filter placement included migration (defined as a vertical change in location of more than 20 mm), vena cava perforation, hematoma, and insertion site venous thrombosis. Filter retrieval complications included retrieval failure, embolization of trapped thrombus, femoral vein retrieval site thrombosis, and/or hematoma.

Results

Between July 1, 2002 and July 1, 2004, 103 multiple-trauma patients underwent ICU bedside placement of retrievable IVCFs under real-time IVUS guidance. The mean age of the patients was 40 ± 2 years (range 17–68 years), and 64 (62.1%) were male. All patients sustained multiple-trauma injuries with a mean Injury Severity Score of 27.7 (± 2.2). Ninety-three (90.2%) of the patients had blunt injuries from motor vehicle crashes.

IVCFs were placed within 48 h of admission in 92 patients (89.3%). Twenty-four patients died of their injuries; 16 deaths were due to multi-system organ failure and 8 occurred after care was withdrawn because

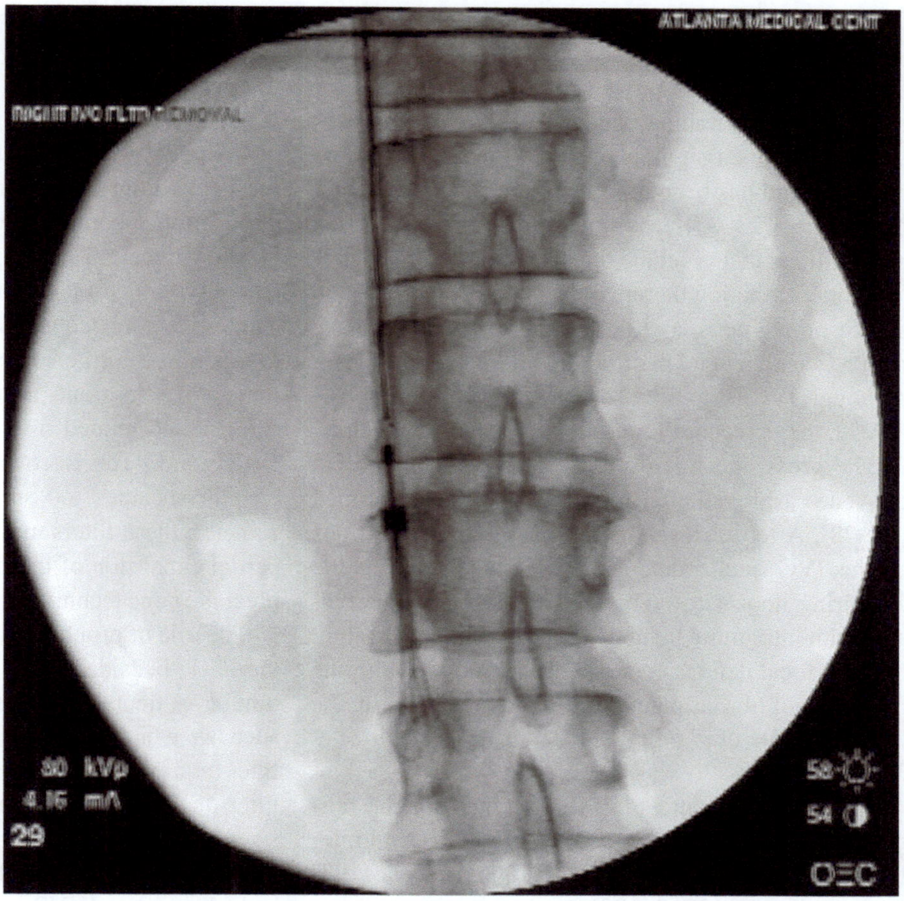

Fig. 23.6 Snare and 6-F retrieval catheter are advanced over filter, collapsing and disengaging filter from IVC wall

of irreversible brain injury. One PE, documented by contrast-enhanced spiral computed tomography, occurred after retrieval. This patient was ambulatory on the rehabilitation medicine service, but DVT prophylaxis had not been initiated. All patients underwent color-flow duplex ultrasonography within 14 days of filter placement; two femoral vein insertion site DVTs were identified. One hundred (97.1%) of IVCFs were placed without complications, as verified by post-procedure abdominal X-rays. Three IVCFs (2.9%) were misplaced in the right iliac vein early in our experience; these filters were uneventfully retrieved and replaced in the IVC within 24 h. Procedural complications included three groin hematomas (2.9%). Clinical success, defined as technical success without subsequent PE, significant filter migration or malpositioning, symptomatic caval thrombosis or other complications requiring removal or invasive intervention, occurred in 96.1% (99/103) of patients.

Filters were in place for a mean of 71 days ± 2 days (range 5–116 days) before retrieval (Günther-Tulip filters 11–116 days, Recovery filters 9–64 days, OptEase filters 5–31 days). Forty-four patients underwent uneventful retrieval of IVCFs after DVT or PE anticoagulation prophylaxis was initiated. Before filter retrieval, these patients underwent venous color-flow duplex ultrasonography of the lower extremities. Three DVTs were identified; these patients were anticoagulated. At IVCF retrieval, vena cavography identified three filters with significant (>25%) trapped thrombus within the filter. Post-retrieval vena cavography in three patients identified small defects (<1 cm) in the IVC wall without contrast extravasation. None of the vena cavograms documented contrast extravasation, penetration, or impingement on an adjacent organ or caval occlusion. Thirty-five IVCFs were not removed; 32 in patients who had continued contraindications to anticoagulation because of the severity of their injuries, while 3 filters had significant trapped thrombus within the filter. Two patients underwent catheter-mediated thrombolysis of trapped thrombus, while the third patient's injuries precluded thrombolysis.

Discussion

Despite continued improvement in the management of multi-system trauma patients, venous thromboembolism remains a significant source of morbidity and mortality and has been reported to occur in up to 58% of patients [23–25]. Multiple-trauma patients often have injuries that preclude the standard use of subclinical anticoagulation therapy or sequential compression device prophylaxis, and these treatment options have not proven beneficial in critically injured patients [26]. Although IVCFs do not prevent deep vein thrombosis (DVT), they prevent PE and its catastrophic sequelae.

The gross and microscopic changes that occur in the vena caval wall after retrieval have been described [27, 28]. After retrieval, the intima and inner portions of the IVC media demonstrate focal defects at the anchoring hook sites. These focal tears were associated with intramural hemorrhage, but complete healing of these focal defects occurs within 6 months with the formation of fibrous plaques. Intimal hyperplasia at the fixation points of various filters appears to stabilize at 3–6 weeks.

Many trauma centers have now opted for the prophylactic use of IVCFs to prevent PE in multiple-trauma patients. Although filters do not prevent DVT, they prevent PE [22, 26–28]. In these series, prophylactic IVCF placement was a safe and effective method of reducing the reported PE mortality rates by half, which emphasizes the need for protection in this generally younger population. In our series of patients, no PEs occurred while the filter was in place, which emphasizes the role of retrievable filters—they serve as an effective "bridge" to anticoagulation until venous thromboembolism prophylaxis can be initiated.

The double-puncture technique allows continuous real-time ultrasonography of the IVC and renal veins to ensure precise filter deployment. Theoretical disadvantages of this technique are the two femoral vein punctures and concern about femoral vein thrombosis. The 8-F IVUS and six IVCF catheters, however, cause defects in the femoral vein that are approximately the same size as those associated with permanent percutaneous IVCF delivery systems. Indeed, femoral vein thrombosis occurred in only 2 of our 103 patients, which is a testimony to the brief compression technique employed after filter insertion and our aggressive approach to venous thromboembolic prophylaxis, which is instituted as soon as indicated. The inadvertent deployment of three filters in the right iliac vein occurred early in our experience when the filter and sheathes were pulled distally, rather than being held in the correct position. These misplaced filters were uneventfully retrieved and were replaced in the IVC within 24 h. Venous anomalies such as IVC duplication, anomalous renal veins, and IVC transposition remain a pitfall for IVUS-guided techniques and serve as an indication for vena cavography. The single-puncture technique allows for IVUS imaging to position the filter delivery sheath and this method may prove safe and accurate for physicians already using IVUS-guided filter placement. Next generation IVCFs (i.e., The Recovery and G2, Bard) are delivered in sheathes too small (i.e., 6 F) for the IVUS catheter; these filters may "catch" in the sheath due to partial expansion of the filter in a larger sheath which precludes this technique.

The role of prophylactic retrievable IVCFs placed at the ICU "bedside" under IVUS guidance in multiple-trauma patients continues to evolve, and questions such as which patients should receive a retrievable filter and what are the long-term sequelae of the filter on IVC and femoral vein patency remain unanswered. Nevertheless, in this study of 103 patients, prophylactic temporary IVCF placement at the ICU bedside under IVUS guidance in multiple-trauma patients was simple and safe, prevented fatal PE, and served as an effective "bridge" to anticoagulation until venous thromboembolism prophylaxis could be initiated. Further investigation of this bedside technique and the role of temporary IVCFs in different patient populations is warranted.

Phase II Study

Encouraged by these results, a Phase II study was conducted to evaluate the retrieval feasibility of the Günther-Tulip filter after indwell times of more than 180 days in patients with multiple trauma. Short (<8 weeks) indwell times with early retrieval for all temporary IVCFs are preferred, as prolonged indwell times makes retrieval more difficult due to incorporation of the filter with hypertrophic scar tissue and endothelium.

Between December 1, 2003, and October 1, 2006, in an institutional review board-approved retrospective study, 117 multiple-trauma patients with relative or absolute contraindications to low-dose heparin therapy or barriers to prevent sequential compression devices underwent prophylactic placement of Günther-Tulip retrievable IVCFs [29]. Ninety-seven Günther-Tulip filters were placed at the ICU bedside under real-time intravascular ultrasound (IVUS) guidance similar to the Phase I study.

Similar to the Phase I study, prior to filter retrieval, all patients underwent venous color-flow duplex ultrasound scanning of the lower extremities to rule out DVT. All filter retrieval procedures were performed in the catheterization laboratory from a right internal jugular vein approach. Under ultrasound surveillance, the jugular vein was cannulated and a 10-F sheath placed, and the Cook retrieval system was used for retrieval. Prior to retrieval, vena cavography was performed to assess the IVCF for thrombus within the filter. As per the manufacturer's recommendation, significant thrombus (>25% of filter volume) was considered a contraindication to filter retrieval. After IVCF retrieval, repeat vena cavography was performed to evaluate the IVC for contrast extravasation, intraluminal defects, or IVC narrowing. If an IVC stenosis was identified, a contrast-enhanced CT scan was performed 6 months after retrieval.

Results

Of the 117 IVCFs implanted, 91 (77%) were successfully retrieved after a mean indwell time of 107 days (range 42–403 days). Fourteen filters were left in place permanently due to filter fixation and 12 filters were not retrieved as the patients died of their injuries; no deaths were related to IVCF placement or retrieval.

Forty-one filters had an indwell time longer than 180 days (mean 261.5 days, range 182–403 days) and make up the basis of this Phase II study. Thirty-one (76%) filters were uneventfully retrieved and 10 were left in place permanently. Pre-retrieval vena cavography identified filter tilting (compared against the long axis of IVC) in 13 filters and in all 10 filters that could not be retrieved: nine filters had a mild tilt of 10° or less and four had severe tilting of 25° or more. Of the 10 filters which could not be retrieved, four had severe tilting, four had mild tilting, and two had no tilting. All 31 prolonged indwell time filters retrieved had small strands of thrombus and hypertrophic scar/endothelium on the filter; however, these were not flow limiting and caused no defects at completion vena cavography. Sixty filters were successfully retrieved after a short (<180 days), mean indwell time of 51 days (range 42–180 days); four short indwell time filters could not be retrieved. This difference was not statistically significant ($p = 0.367$). No patients had trapped thrombus identified by vena cavography at the time of retrieval. None of the retrieved filters had structural fracture or collapse and none had migrated.

Post-retrieval vena cavagrams demonstrated no contrast extravasation, intraluminal defects, or impingement on adjacent organs.

Discussion

The ability to extend the indwell time of retrievable IVCFs affords greater protection in patients who require prolonged PE prophylaxis. Recent publications have described the placement and retrieval of optional filters, but few have reported retrievals with indwell times past 180 days. Binkert [30] reported a series of 13 patients who had Bard Recovery filters with a mean indwell time of 254 days; retrieval of all filters was performed uneventfully without complications. In this series of patients, the "rate-limiting step" for retrieval of IVCFs with indwell times extending to 403 days appears to be the amount of filter tilt. Of note in our patients was that of the 10 filters which could not be retrieved, all had some degree of tilt (six mild tilting of 10° or less, four severe tilting of 25°). A prolonged indwell time (>180 days) in the presence of severe tilting (25° or more) makes retrieval highly unlikely due to incorporation of filter components (i.e., retrieval hook, filter wires) by hypertrophic endothelial scar tissue. In this setting, the wisest course of action may be to simply leave the filter in place, especially if significant force is placed on retrieval system as indicated by straightening of the retrieval hook or "flaring" of the sheath tip. This, however, remains to be proven.

The role of retrievable IVCFs remains unproven, but the option to avoid the use of a permanent filter for what is often a temporary problem is appealing. Retrieval of IVCFs should be performed as soon as clinically indicated, but if retrieval of a Günther-Tulip filter with an indwell time longer than 180 days is considered (i.e., in "high-risk" bariatric, spinal-orthopedic and multiple-trauma patients), the patient should be ambulatory, a candidate for anticoagulation if indicated, and the filter should have less than 25° of tilt. Until then, retrieval of the Günther-Tulip filter after 180 days of indwell time appears safe.

Generation Two Retrievable Filters

The G2 filter (Bard) is an evolution of the Recovery filter. Its design was modified to include thicker leg hooks, a wider leg span, and longer arms with a more progressive angle of wires forming the arms at the filter apex with inward curves at the ends [31]. This was done in an attempt to decrease the occurrence of fatigued-related fractures, minimize IVC penetration, decrease the occurrence of tilting, and increase the resistance to migration while maintaining its extended retrievability.

In a recent trial [31], 120 patients underwent placement of the G2 filter. Patients had DVT ($n = 63$), PE ($n = 55$) or were at high risk for PE (2). Fifty-one patients met criteria for filter removal. Filter tilting (>15°) was seen in only six (12%) patients, caudal migration in two (3.9%), and no fractures or cephalic migrations were observed. Retrieval was successful in all patients with a mean implantation time of 53.4 days (range 7–242 days). The authors concluded that retrieval of the G2 filter is safe and efficacious.

The Celect IVC filter (Cook) is made of Elgiloy, an amalgam of cobalt, nickel, and chromium, is conical-shaped with a hook at the apex, and has four primary anchor wires and eight secondary wires. The secondary wires are thinner than the anchor wires and provide lateral stability and improve long-axis orientation. The tips of the secondary wires do not touch the IVC, only the curved portions of the wire. The deployment and retrieval are identical to the Günther-Tulip filter.

In the presentation at the 2008 European Congress of Radiology, workers reported on a multinational trial of patients at high risk for PE [32]. Ninety-one Celect IVCFs were placed and 48 of 50 (96%) attempted retrievals were successful. The two failures occurred in patients with indwell times of 360 and 385 days. No PEs occurred and 100% of filters were easily retrieved at 26 weeks and 89% at 52 weeks. The authors concluded that the Celect filter was easily deployed and retrieved, prevented PE, did not migrate, and is safe.

What Is on the Horizon?

As has been previously discussed, one of the major parameters in preventing retrieval of any IVCF is filter tilt. The Crux IVCF (Crux Biomedical, Menlo Park, CA) is a unique, low-profile (6F), self-centering and retrievable (via both jugular and femoral access) IVCF [33].

The Crux IVCF is constructed of two nitinol spiral elements crimped at the ends to form a symmetric double-loop helical structure. On one loop, a filter web is attached to the spiral element to capture clots. The filter is designed for either temporary or permanent use and each end has a retrieval element designed to facilitate capture by any commercial snare. The filter is delivered by a push rod through a custom 6-F introducer sheath and at deployment, the sheath is retracted, while the push rod is held stable. When deployed, the filter is designed to self-center and oppose the IVC wall along its surface and is sized to cover an IVC diameter up to 28 mm with two filter sizes available (small IVCs 17–22 mm and large IVCs 22–28 mm). Retrieval is accomplished with a double-sheath technique (6 and 10 F Cook Flexor Raabe Sheath, Bloomington, IN, 90 and 80 cm in length, respectively). The smaller sheath is advanced through the larger sheath and advanced to the level of the device. The filter retrieval tail is captured by a snare which is withdrawn into the inner sheath; the larger sheath is then advanced capturing the filter.

The Crux IVCF has several theoretical advantages over other currently available IVCFs. The conical IVCFs may have several drawbacks. First, the conical shape of the filter provides a natural tendency for the filter to tilt and the hooks to fail to engage or pull away from the IVC wall, potentially causing filter migration. Additionally, retrievability of existing conical filters may be limited by filter struts perforating the caval wall and the tilted retrieval hook apex becoming incorporated into the caval wall, making snare capture difficult or impossible. The Crux filter novel design promotes self-centering in the IVC and retrievability is rapid and easy via both jugular and femoral access. In a recent first in man trial, the results were encouraging as no complications resulting from device deployment, indwelling filters, or device retrieval occurred in a series of 10 patients. A multi-center, prospective trial will soon be initiated to evaluate the safety and efficacy of the Crux IVCF.

Conclusion

The role of retrievable IVCFs continues to evolve as they appear to be a potentially important addition in the treatment of venous thromboembolic disease. The long-term benefit of retrievable IVCFs remains to be proved, but hopefully prospective, randomized, controlled trials will delineate better the role of this exciting technology in different patient populations.

References

1. Evans AJ, Sostoman HD, Knelson MH et al.: Detection of deep venous thrombosis, *AJR Am J Roentgenol* 161:131–139, 1993.
2. Kaufman J, Kinney T, Streiff M et al.: Guidelines for the use of retrievable and convertible vena cava filters: report from the Society of Interventional Radiology multidisciplinary consensus conference, *J Vasc Interv Radiol* 17:449–459, 2006.
3. Khansarinia S, Dennis JW, Veldenz HC et al.: Prophylactic Greenfield filter placement in selected high-risk trauma patients, *J Vasc Surg* 22:231–235, 1995.
4. Williams R, Schenk W: A removable intracaval filter for prevention of pulmonary embolism: early experience with the use of the Eichelter catheter in patients, *Surgery* 68:999–1008, 1970.
5. Mobin-Uddin K, Smith PE, Martines LO, Lombardo CR: The Mobin-Uddin vena cava filter for the prevention of pulmonary embolus, *Surg Forum* 18:209–211, 1967.
6. Kaufman J: Retrievable vena cava filters, *Tech Vasc Interv Radiol* 7:96–104, 2004.
7. Rodriguez JL, Lopez JM, Proctor MC et al.: Early placement of prophylactic vena caval filters in injured patients at high risk for pulmonary embolism, *J Trauma* 35:637–641, 1993.
8. Offner PJ, Hawkes A, Madayag R et al.: The role of temporary inferior vena cava filters in critically ill surgical patients, *Arch Surg* 138:591–595, 2003.
9. Geertz WH, Code KI, Jay RM, Chen E, Szalai JP: A prospective study of venous thromboembolism after major trauma, *N Engl J Med* 331:1601–1606, 1994.
10. Blebea J, Wilson R, Waybill P, Neumyer MM, Blebea JS, Anderson KM et al.: Deep venous thrombosis after percutaneous insertion of vena caval filters, *J Vasc Surg* 30:831–838, 1999.
11. Becker DM: Inferior vena cava filters: indication, safety, effectiveness, *Arch Intern Med* 152:1985–1994, 1992.
12. Decousus H, Leizorovicz A, Parent F et al.: A clinical trial of vena caval filters in the prevention of pulmonary embolism in patients with proximal deep-vein thrombosis, *N Engl J Med* 338:409–415, 1998.
13. Mohan CR, Hoballah JJ, Sharp WJ et al.: Comparative efficacy and complications of vena caval filters, *J Vasc Surg* 21:235–246, 1995.
14. Crochet DP, Stora O, Ferry D et al.: Vena Tech-LGM filter: long-term results of a prospective study, *Radiology* 188:857–860, 1993.
15. Athanasoulis CA: Complications of vena cava filters, *Radiology* 188:614–615, 1993.
16. Bonn J, Liu JB, Eschelman DJ, Sullivan KL, Pinheiro LW, Gardiner GA Jr: Intravascular ultrasound as an alternative to positive-contrast vena cavography prior to filter placement, *J Vasc Interv Radiol* 10:834–839, 1999.
17. Ashley DW, Gamblin TC, Burch ST, Solis MMJ: Accurate deployment of vena cava filters; comparison of intravascular ultrasound and contrast venography, *J Trauma* 50:975–981, 2001.
18. Matsuura JH, White RA, Kopchak G, Nishinian G, Woody JD, Rosenthal D et al.: Vena caval filter placement by intravascular ultrasound, *Cardiovasc Surg* 9:571–574, 2001.
19. Oppar WF, Chiou AC, Matsumura JS: Intravascular ultrasound-guided vena cava filter placement, *J Endovasc Surg* 6:285–287, 1999.
20. Wellons ED, Matsuura JH, Shuler FW, Franklin JS, Rosenthal D: Bedside intravascular ultrasound-guided vena cava filter placement, *J Vasc Surg* 38:755–758, 2003.
21. Jacobs DL, Motaganahall RL, Peterson BG: Bedside vena cava filter placement with intravascular ultrasound: a simple, accurate, single venous access method, *J Vasc Surg* 46:1284–1286, 2007.
22. Rosenthal D, Wellons ED, Levitt AB, Shuler FW, O'Conner RE et al.: Role of prophylactic temporary inferior vena cava filters placed at the ICU bedside under intravascular ultrasound guidance in patients with multiple trauma, *J Vasc Surg* 40:958–964, 2004.
23. Dries DJ: Activation of the clotting system and complement after trauma, *New Horz* 4:276–289, 1996.
24. Weinmann EE, Salzman EW: Deep-vein thrombosis, *N Engl J Med* 331:1630–1641, 1994.
25. Geerts WH, Jay RM, Code KJ, Chen E, Szalai JP, Saibil E et al.: A comparison of low-dose heparin with low-molecular weight heparin as prophylaxis against venous thromboembolism after major trauma, *N Engl J Med* 335:701–707, 1996.
26. de Gregario MA, Gamboa P, Gimeno MJ, Madariaga B, Tobio R et al.: The Günther-Tulip retrievable filter: prolonged temporary filtration by repositioning within the inferior vena cava, *J Vasc Interv Rad* 14:1259–1265, 2003.
27. Neuerburg J, Gunther R, Rassmussen E et al.: New retrievable percutaneous vena cava filter: experimental in vitro and in vivo evaluation, *Cardiovasc Intervent Radiol* 16:224–229, 1993.
28. Asch MR: Initial experience in humans with a new retrievable inferior vena cava filter, *Radiology* 222:835–855, 2002.
29. Rosenthal D, Wellons ED, Hancock SM, Burkett AB: Retrievability of the Günther Tulip vena cava filter after dwell times longer than 180 days in patients with multiple trauma, *J Endovasc Ther* 14:406–410, 2007.
30. Binkert CA, Sasadeus ZK, Stavropoulos SW: Retrievability of the recovery vena cava filter after indwell times longer than 180 days, *J Vasc Interv Radiol* 17:299–302, 2006.

31. Oliva VL, Perrault P, Giroux MF, Bouchard L et al.: Recovery G2 inferior vena cava filter: technical success and safety of retrieval, *J Vasc Interv Radiol* 19:884–889, 2008.
32. Oberoi R. Celect IVC filter, European Congress of Radiology 2008, from the John Radcliff Hospital, Headington, Oxford, UK.
33. Arko F III, Murphy E, Davis CM III, Rosenthal D et al.: Early clinical experience with a novel self-centering, bi-directional vena cava filter, *Vasc Dis Manage* 5:103–105, July–August 2008.

Carotid Stenting

24

Rabih A. Chaer and Peter A. Schneider

Stroke continues to be a major public health concern with more than 750,000 strokes occurring per year in the United States, making it the third most common cause of death and the leading neurologic cause of long-term disability [1]. The resultant economic burden on health-care systems is significant and only likely to grow as life expectancy increases and the elderly population continues to expand [2]. The majority of strokes are ischemic in nature, and up to one-third of ischemic strokes are a result of carotid artery atherosclerotic occlusive disease. The treatment of carotid artery stenosis is aimed at the prevention of ischemic events caused by embolization of components of the atherosclerotic plaque and less commonly by hemodynamic compromise secondary to progression to occlusion of a previously stenotic but patent internal carotid artery.

The management of carotid occlusive disease is in evolution. Carotid endarterectomy (CEA), first introduced in the 1950s, has been the established gold standard for the treatment of carotid stenosis for many years. This was affirmed by several landmark trials in the 1990s [3–11]. More recently, carotid angioplasty and stenting (CAS) emerged as a minimally invasive alternative, and several trials ensued to determine its safety and efficacy and the indications for its use. While CAS has proven to be feasible and relatively safe, the appropriate clinical setting for its preferential use over CEA continues to be the subject of ongoing clinical trials and also of many day-to-day discussions in clinical practice, since these issues are not yet resolved. The purpose of this chapter is to describe the technique of carotid stent placement with embolic protection, provide current results of treatment, and offer an assessment of the overall role of carotid stenting in the management of carotid occlusive disease.

Evolution of Carotid Angioplasty and Stenting

Balloon angioplasty of the carotid artery was first described in the late 1970s as a proposed intervention for carotid artery stenosis [12]. Initially it was promoted as a potentially safer alternative to CEA in medically high-risk patients and those with hostile neck anatomy. Early trials involving carotid angioplasty demonstrated feasibility of the technique but were not widely accepted due to small study size, relatively high complication rates, and random use of stenting to name a few. Enthusiasm was further curtailed by the concern for embolic complications associated with the procedure. Gradually, however, CAS evolved to its current form with improvements in equipment and technique, increased operator experience, and the standard use of stenting and cerebral protection.

Cerebral Protection

The utilization of embolic protection devices (EPDs) for cerebral protection became standard practice in CAS trials after several studies suggested decreased

R.A. Chaer (✉)
Assistant Professor, Division of Vascular Surgery, Department of Surgery, The University of Pittsburgh School of Medicine, Pittsburgh, PA, USA

T.J. Fogarty, R.A. White (eds.), *Peripheral Endovascular Interventions*,
DOI 10.1007/978-1-4419-1387-6_24, © Springer Science+Business Media, LLC 1998, 2010

risk of embolic complications with their use [13]. Protection devices are based on three different approaches: (1) distal filter placement, (2) distal balloon occlusion, and (3) proximal balloon occlusion, with or without flow reversal.

Filters are the most commonly utilized EPD and are positioned in the internal carotid artery distal to the target lesion. Antegrade cerebral flow is maintained through the filter during CAS. The embolic debris dislodged during the procedure are captured within the filter and then subsequently removed with retraction of the device. They typically retain fragments larger than the pore size of the filter, approximately 100 μm, but do allow passage of smaller particles. Filters are advantageous because they allow continued cerebral perfusion, particularly in patients who have inadequate collateral circulation to permit temporary carotid occlusion. Currently, several filters are FDA approved for use in the United States and include Accunet (Abbott Laboratories, Abbott Park, IL), Emboshield (Abbot Laboratories, Abbott Park, IL), FilterWire EZ (Boston Scientific Corporation, Natick MA), SpiderFx (EV3, Plymouth, MN), and Angioguard XP (Cordis-Johnson & Johnson, Miami Lakes, FL) [14–17].

In addition to filters, distal balloon occlusion can be used for embolic protection. The PercuSurge occlusion balloon (Medtronic, Santa Rosa, CA) [18] is a component of an angiographic wire that is passed through the stenotic area and inflated in the distal internal carotid artery. After the CAS procedure, the standing column of blood containing particulate matter is aspirated. The balloon is then deflated and flow is restored to the cerebral circulation. Compared to filters, distal occlusion balloons have a lower device-crossing profile. PercuSurge requires temporary interruption of cerebral perfusion while embolic debris accumulates near the occlusion balloon.

Unlike both distal filters and distal occlusion balloons, proximal balloon occlusion devices, such as the MOMA device (Invatec, Roncadelle, Italy) [19] and the Parodi Anti-Embolic System (Gore, Flagstaff, AZ), [20] do not require crossing of the stenosis. Such devices are under active investigation and provide protection by occluding the common and external carotid artery, after which collateral flow through the circle of Willis creates a back pressure that prevents antegrade flow into the internal carotid artery (ICA).

There are currently no large randomized trials to date which compare CAS with and without EPDs, and the bulk of data relies on historical comparison of results before widespread EPD usage. EPD use has, however, become standard and is currently mandated by the Centers for Medicare and Medicaid Services (CMS).

Technique: Carotid Angioplasty and Stenting with Distal Protection

The CAS procedure is comprised of the following steps: pre-procedural evaluation, femoral access, arch aortogram, selective common carotid catheterization and angiogram, carotid sheath access, crossing the carotid stenosis, filter placement, pre-dilatation, stenting, post-dilatation, completion angiogram, access site management, and post-operative care and follow-up. More detail is available regarding the technique of CAS [21].

Pre-procedural Evaluation

Patients are seen by a neurologist and an NIH stroke scale or other objective evaluation is completed prior to CAS. A CT or MRI of the brain is obtained in symptomatic patients and in those over 80 years of age to evaluate for pre-procedural cerebral pathology. Initial duplex evaluation is performed. Approved carotid stenting systems are limited at present in the United States to use in high surgical risk patients with symptomatic ≥50% stenosis or asymptomatic ≥80% stenosis. Payment issues for the CAS procedure must be explored with individual insurance carriers or regional CMS administrator. Patients are started on antiplatelet therapy: aspirin daily and clopidogrel (Plavix) 75 mg per day for 5 days prior to the procedure. In all cases, patients should have received clopidogrel (total dose 300 mg) prior to the intervention. Patients are asked to discontinue antihypertensive medication on the day of the stent procedure and these patients are best treated as the first case of the day (to avoid prolonged dehydration). Post-op hypotension and/or bradycardia is more likely in patients with underlying cardiac disease. In patients with absent femoral pulses due to aortoiliac occlusion, a transbrachial approach may be considered.

This approach is more challenging compared to the transfemoral approach, with need for a larger selection of reversed angle catheters. The brachiocephalic anatomy should be studied prior to the procedure to assess candidacy for this approach. CAS in standard surgical risk patients and those at high risk for CEA but who are asymptomatic is not currently approved for reimbursement under Medicare guidelines.

The procedure is performed under local anesthesia with minimal or no sedation to facilitate patient cooperation and continuous neurological monitoring. An arterial line is placed for continuous blood pressure monitoring and EKG leads for cardiac monitoring. External pacer pads should be readily available. Patients with severe aortic stenosis undergo placement of a temporary venous pacemaker. Patients should have a detailed explanation of the need for continuous neurological monitoring. Techniques such as squeezing a rubber toy aid in simple and effective neurological monitoring during the procedure. Due to the minimal use of sedation, patients are often apprehensive and may develop reactive systemic hypertension. Hence, it is important to document the patient's baseline blood pressure during the prior clinic visit. We avoid acutely reducing the blood pressure during the intervention with pharmacological agents, as post-stent hypotension/bradycardia is not uncommon. If antihypertensive is required, it is best to use a short-acting agent.

Obtaining a thorough understanding of the arch, carotid, and cerebral arterial anatomy prior to the procedure is optimal. This may be obtained by arteriogram or by CTA or MRA. This permits proper patient selection and procedural planning. Several anatomical factors may be considered relative contraindications to CAS, including severe arch atherosclerosis or tortuosity, diffuse common carotid artery disease or tortuosity, severe angulation of the bifurcation or kinking of the distal internal carotid artery. If the arch anatomy is well delineated prior to the procedure, the CAS procedure time may be shortened by obviating the need for an arch aortogram.

Femoral Access

The common femoral artery is the access site in the vast majority of cases, although CAS has also been performed using brachial, radial, or direct common carotid artery access. The right common femoral approach is the most convenient for catheter manipulations by the right-handed surgeon. A micropuncture set (21-gauge needle) may be used for the initial femoral access; this has significantly reduced the number of femoral access complications. Following guidewire access an introducer sheath is placed in the common femoral artery that is the same size as that intended for the carotid stent placement, usually 6Fr or 7Fr.

Aortic Arch Angiogram

Arch manipulations with guidewires, catheters, and sheaths carry a risk of neurological events. In several studies of CAS, especially early on in the experience, up to 1% of patients sustained a stroke in the contralateral hemisphere, suggesting that carotid access may be a contributor to morbidity [22, 23]. Better patient selection that avoids some of the riskiest anatomic pitfalls has helped to improve this. It is also the authors' practice to administer systemic heparin prior to any aortic arch manipulation. A 260-cm guidewire is placed in the ascending aorta followed by a pigtail catheter. An initial arch angiogram is performed with the image intensifier (I-I) in a left anterior oblique (LAO) position. The I-I is rotated until the upside down U-shape formed by the guidewire is as wide as possible, usually 30–40°. The origins of the arch vessels are better exposed in this oblique projection. The pigtail catheter is subsequently withdrawn over a 260-cm angled Glidewire. Resist attempts to leave the Glidewire in place if inadvertent selective cannulation of the common carotid artery is achieved while withdrawing the pigtail catheter from the aortic arch. It is almost impossible to withdraw the pigtail catheter from the aortic arch while maintaining Glidewire access in the common carotid artery. As few manipulations are carried out in the aortic arch and great vessels as possible, in hopes of lowering the risk of an embolic event.

Hypertension and advanced age are associated with increased tortuosity of the aortic arch. This makes no difference in the performance of CEA but directly influences the challenges posed for CAS. Negotiating the tortuous arch requires more manipulation for catheterization, a more embedded position of the exchange guidewire, and more maneuvers to achieve sheath placement. The tortuosity of the arch may be assessed very rapidly by drawing a horizontal line across the apex of the inner curvature of the arch [24]. Vessels that originate below the horizontal line at the apex of the aortic arch often are more difficult to selectively cannulate (Fig. 24.1). The authors caution against carotid stenting in the setting of a "difficult arch" until the operator has become expert with selective cannulation of the common carotid arteries in this situation. Training and credentialing documents suggest varying numbers of carotid arteriograms as a prerequisite to initiating CAS training [25, 26].

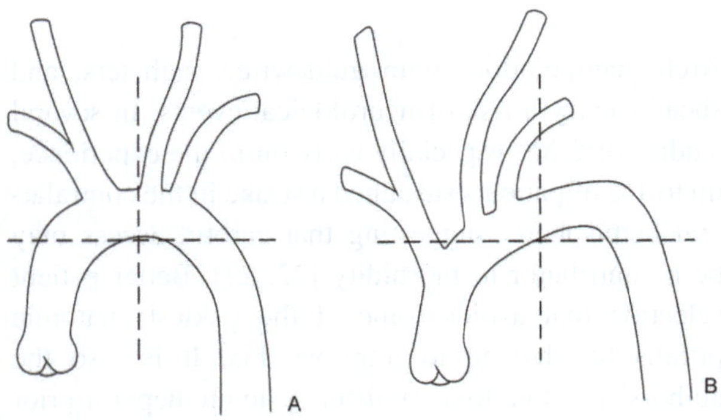

Fig. 24.1 Arch configuration. **a**, The aortic arch is evaluated with the image intensifier in the left anterior oblique projection to separate the arch branches. A *horizontal line* is drawn across the apex of the arch on the inner curvature. The uppermost point of the arch acts as a fulcrum over which the catheter must work and the sheath must be placed. **b**, The arch often becomes more tortuous with age and with hypertension. The functional result is to lengthen the arch segment from which the branches arise and put them in a position such that the artery origins are to the right and inferior to the fulcrum. By drawing the *horizontal line* across the apex of the arch on the *inner curve*, it is readily apparent that working over the fulcrum will be more challenging. The further inferior to the horizontal line the branch origin is located, the more challenging the access for catheterization and also for sheath placement (From Schneider [72], with permission.)

Selective Common Carotid Catheterization

Selective cannulation of the arch vessels can be technically challenging and is a critical portion of CAS procedures. Most intent-to-treat failures are secondary to inability to establish carotid access. Catheterization can almost always be accomplished using one of two pre-shaped catheters, a simple curve catheter such as a vertebral catheter or a complex curve catheter such as the reversed angle Vitek catheter (VTK). The image intensifier is maintained in its fixed position (LAO) and the bony landmarks may be used to guide vessel cannulation. Road mapping techniques and simple marks made with a dry-erase pen on the screen may also help guide selective common carotid artery cannulation. The catheter of first choice in most cases is a simple curve catheter such as a vertebral catheter. The angle formed by the vertebral catheter along with the tip angle on an angled Glidewire is adequate to cannulate the common carotid artery in most patients. Once the Glidewire has accessed the common carotid artery the vertebral catheter is advanced over the Glidewire for selective angiograms of the common carotid artery. Be careful to avoid inadvertently passing the guidewire into the carotid artery bifurcation. As the cerebral catheter rounds the turn from the arch into the common carotid artery, it tends to straighten out and the guidewire may "jump" forward.

Reversed angle catheters such as the VTK (Fig. 24.2) are usually required when the aortic arch is tortuous or the common carotid arteries are retroflexed toward the patient's left. Complex curve catheters, such as the VTK, are best reformed in the proximal descending aorta and then pushed proximally, especially for cannulation of the left common carotid artery. A complex curve catheter must be used for catheterizing the common carotid when it arises from the "difficult arch." The most challenging are those branches that originate from the upslope of the ascending aorta (see Fig. 24.1). Although reversed angle catheters such as VTK and Simmons are useful for catheterization, they cannot be easily advanced into the branch vessels and are often used only to access the origin of the branch vessels for a selective angiogram of the carotid arteries. Due to the reverse angle, forward motion on these catheters will only advance the catheter further proximally in the aortic arch. Catheter access to the common carotid artery following access with the reversed angle catheter usually requires a subsequent catheter exchange. This requires the Glidewire to be placed in the distal common carotid artery or the external carotid artery and the reversed angle catheter is withdrawn over the guidewire and replaced with the vertebral catheter. Reversed angle catheters have a tendency to flip the guidewire as they exit the femoral sheath, hence the Glidewire needs to be grasped immediately as the tip of the reversed angle catheter is seen exiting the femoral sheath.

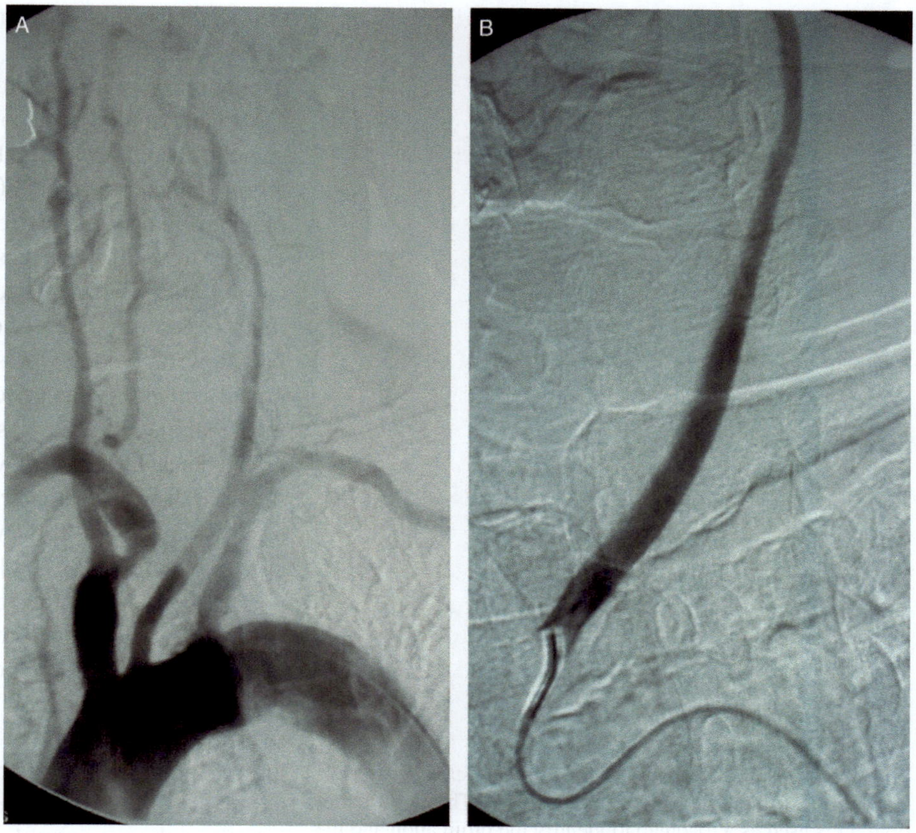

Fig. 24.2 The Vitek catheter is a complex curve catheter. It has an extra curve which allows the tip to be directed in a reverse fashion. This allows for cannulation of a difficult arch branch origin from a tortuous arch and to work over the fulcrum of the arch. **a**, In this arch configuration, the left common carotid artery is somewhat retroflexed as the artery passes toward the patient's left. **b**, The Vitek catheter is advanced into the arch and the tip of the catheter is used to cannulate the origin of the left common carotid artery (From Kasirajan and Schneider [73], with permission.)

Once selective cannulation of the common carotid artery is performed, angiograms are performed with a 10-ml syringe filled with half-strength contrast. The carotid bifurcation is best visualized in the ipsilateral oblique position (approximately 60° ipsilateral oblique) or sometimes straight lateral position. Multiple views may be needed to best open the carotid bifurcation, as the next step would involve selective cannulation of the external carotid artery. If an arteriogram or CT angiogram was performed before the CAS procedure, optimal angles for viewing the open carotid bifurcation can usually be derived from these studies. If a lateral view of the carotid bifurcation is required to open carotid bifurcation and cannulate the external carotid artery, after the exchange guidewire is anchored in place, the sheath is best advanced using an LAO view rather than a straight lateral view. This permits the operator to see the tip of the sheath advancing from the arch and into the common carotid artery and to assess real time whether there will be any difficulty with this maneuver.

Lateral and cranio-caudal AP intracranial images are obtained if they have not already been performed prior to CAS to identify any intracranial pathology and to document the intracranial circulation prior to CAS. A certain amount of experience must be gained in interpretation of intracranial images. Identifying small embolic events during or after CAS may be quite challenging.

Carotid Sheath Access

Carotid sheath access requires placement of an adequate length of exchange guidewire into the common carotid artery. This sometimes can be accomplished by placing the tip of the exchange guidewire in the distal common carotid artery but usually requires cannulation of the external carotid artery and use of this vessel to anchor the stiff guidewire (Fig. 24.3). Blind guidewire and catheter manipulation in the carotid artery must be avoided. Selective external carotid cannulation can be accomplished with a 260-cm angled Glidewire and the vertebral catheter. In case of a tight external stenosis a Tracker-18 ([BS]3Fr catheter with

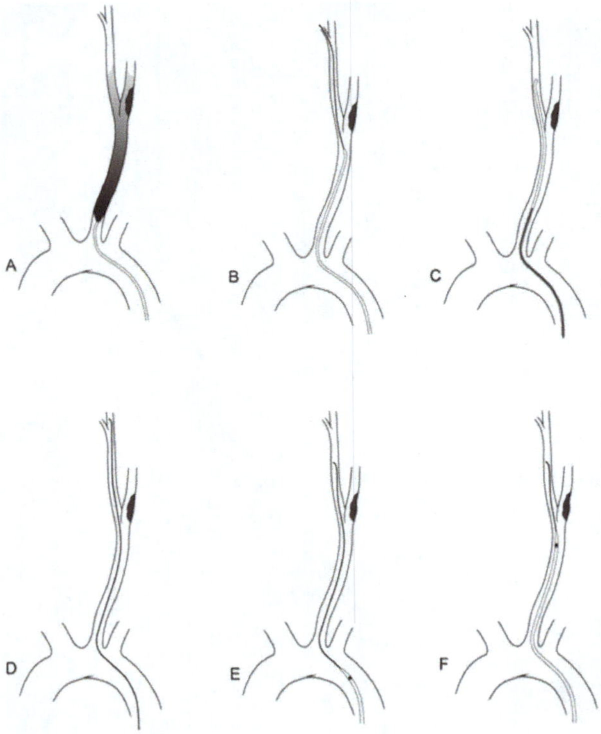

Fig. 24.3 Sheath placement. **a**, The common carotid artery is catheterized with a selective cerebral catheter. The carotid arteriogram is used as a roadmap to identify the bifurcation and the course of the external carotid artery. **b**, The steerable Glidewire is advanced through the catheter and into the external carotid artery. **c**, The cerebral catheter is advanced over the Glidewire so that the tip of the cerebral catheter is placed deep into the branches of the external carotid artery. **d**, The Glidewire is removed and a stiff exchange guidewire is placed. The cerebral catheter is then removed, leaving only the stiff exchange guidewire in place. **e**, The sheath is advanced over the stiff exchange guidewire. As the sheath rounds the turn form the arch into the common carotid artery, there may be significant force on the system and this is observed carefully. **f**, The sheath tip is advanced into the common carotid artery into a position that is stable. Care must be taken to avoid placing the tip of the dilator into the bifurcation. After the sheath is in place, the dilator and stiff guidewire are removed (From Schneider [72], with permission.)

a 0.018 wire) may be used and the 0.018 wire is then exchanged for a stiffer 0.018 guidewire (Roadrunner-Cook, Inc.) and pre-dilated with a low-profile, monorail, 2-mm balloon. The balloon is withdrawn and a vertebral catheter is passed into the external carotid artery over the Roadrunner guidewire. An attempt should be made to reach distally in the external carotid artery. This allows adequate guidewire length placed beyond the carotid bifurcation for the subsequent placement of the carotid sheath. Passage of the stiff exchange guidewire into the small external carotid artery branches must be performed with caution to avoid injury or perforation to these small branches. CAS can usually be accomplished with a 6Fr or 7Fr sheath. The Glidewire is then withdrawn from the vertebral catheter and a 260-cm Amplatz superstiff or other exchange guidewire is passed into the external carotid artery. If it is necessary to evaluate the external carotid artery with an arteriogram, contrast injections into the carotid system should not be done unless free backflow of blood is present at the hub of the diagnostic catheter. Otherwise there is a risk of pushing microbubbles into the system. In the external carotid artery, back bleeding may at times be diminished by the tight fit of the catheter in the small external carotid artery branches. In this event, the cerebral catheter is slowly withdrawn until adequate backflow is noted.

The vertebral catheter is withdrawn leaving the Amplatz guidewire in the external carotid artery. The groin sheath is removed. A 90-cm long sheath (Pinnacle Destination or Shuttle Sheath) is advanced over the Amplatz guidewire into the common carotid artery. Image the tip of the Amplatz guidewire in the external carotid artery and the last turn from the arch into the common carotid artery during sheath passage. If the tip of the advancing sheath hangs up at the turn into the common carotid artery or the tip of the guidewire moves back, it indicates that the sheath is not advancing appropriately over the guidewire. Reassess the curvature in the system and make sure that an adequate length of stiff exchange guidewire is present. Occasionally it is helpful to have the patient take a deep breath as the sheath tip is rounding the corner out of the arch and into the common carotid artery. This maneuver alters the configuration of the branch origin a bit and can offer a more favorable anatomical trajectory for sheath placement.

The dilator tip for the 90-cm carotid sheath is long and not well visualized during fluoroscopy. Identify the optimal length for the dilator to protrude from the sheath and lock the Y-adaptor on the back end of the dilator in this position. After the dilator and sheath are advanced fully into the common carotid artery, if a position closer to the bifurcation is needed, the dilator is held steady while the sheath is advanced over it. The stiff exchange guidewire and the dilator are withdrawn and the carotid angiogram is repeated through the long 6Fr or 7Fr sheath with a road map of the carotid bifurcation stenosis.

Filter Placement and Stenting

This step may be performed with any one of a variety of distal protection devices that are available. The tip of the leading guidewire is hand shaped with a curve to provide directionality for crossing the lesion. Most lesions that are isolated to the proximal internal carotid artery are posterior wall plaques. In passing the guidewire tip to cross the lesion, the best pathway is usually anterior in the proximal internal carotid artery, just behind the flow divider. Bifurcation lesions that involve the distal common carotid artery are usually more complex and less predictable. The key is to lead with the guidewire tip, do not make a loop, and be gentle in probing the lesion. After the lesion has been crossed and the filter deployed, it is pre-dilated with a 3-mm rapid exchange balloon (Fig. 24.4). Some operators routinely administer small doses of atropine (0.25–0.5 mg) before balloon dilatation, except in patients with a recurrent stenosis. The pressure used for pre-dilatation is nominal for the balloon used. Use higher pressure (14–16 atm.) in heavily calcified stenoses. The duration of the pre-dilatation depends on the appearance and behavior of the balloon. If the balloon immediately attains its full shape, the pre-dilatation time is shorter. If the balloon attains its full shape slowly, the pre-dilatation time is prolonged up to 120 s, especially in calcified lesions, which has tendency for recoiling. Observe the monitor for bradycardia if a prolonged inflation is required.

A variety of self-expanding stents, mostly constructed of nitinol, are available for use with the respective embolic protection devices. The self-expanding stent is deployed using landmarks, such as a bifurcation roadmap or the nearby vertebral bodies. The stent is placed from normal artery distal to the lesion to normal artery proximal to the lesion. The self-expanding stent is post-dilated with a 5-mm balloon or 6-mm rapid exchange balloon, depending on the size of the internal carotid artery. A 5-mm balloon PTA is almost always adequate, rarely is a 6-mm PTA required post-stent deployment. The goal is to avoid a slight overdilation, even though this is how lesions in multiple other vascular beds are treated. The difference in the carotid is that the stent is used as scaffolding, the stent provides continuous expansile energy after the procedure, and there is a desire to avoid disrupting the lesion more than necessary. The patient may again be pre-treated with a small dose of atropine to blunt the carotid sinus response to stretching. A residual stenosis of <30% may be accepted. Following stent deployment, shorter (2-cm) balloons are used to dilate the narrow portion of the stent where the residual stenosis is visible using fluoroscopy. The balloon used for

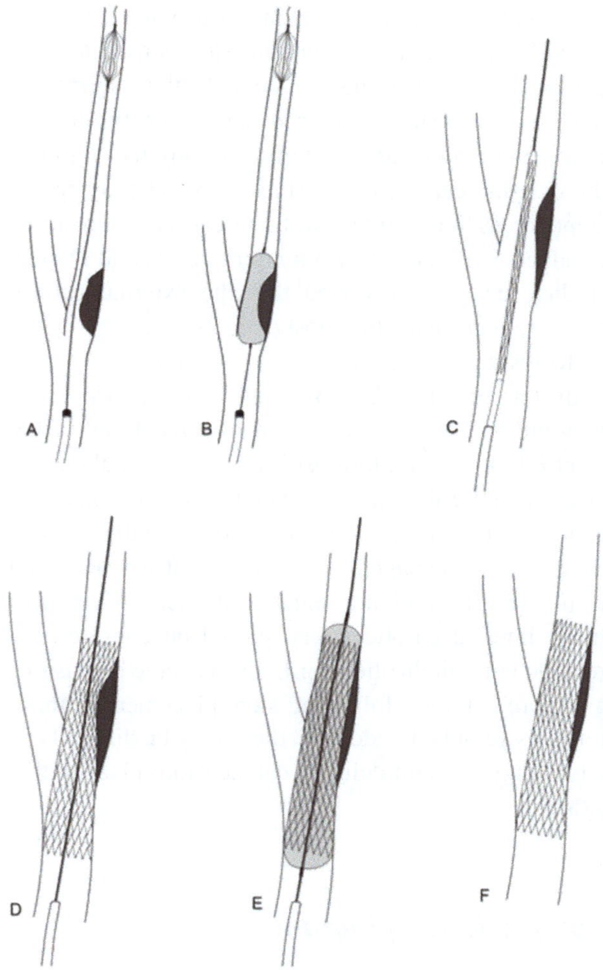

Fig. 24.4 Stent of carotid bifurcation lesion. **a**, An embolic protection filter is placed across the internal carotid artery lesion and deployed. **b**, Pre-dilation is performed after filter deployment and prior to stent placement. This is usually done with a 3- or 4-mm balloon. **c**, The stent delivery catheter is advanced across the lesion. **d**, The self-expanding stent is deployed from normal artery above the lesion to normal artery below the lesion. The stent extends from the internal to the common carotid artery in most cases and goes across the origin of the external carotid artery. **e**, Post-stent dilatation is performed, usually with a 5- or 5.5-mm balloon. Overdilation is not desirable. **f**, Completion angiography is performed showing prograde flow in the common and internal carotid arteries (From Schneider [72], with permission.)

post-stent PTA is always maintained within the stent to avoid dissection. Nominal pressure is used to fully expand the balloon and the stent. In the majority of the cases, the stent is placed across the bifurcation into the common carotid artery, crossing the origin of the external carotid artery (Fig. 24.5). Deploying the stent across the external carotid artery has not resulted in adverse events; follow-up arteriograms and Duplex studies have demonstrated that the external carotid artery remains patent in most patients.

Kinks and bends in the ICA may pose a problem with stent implants. Deploy stents across kinks only if they are isolated. Avoid placing the distal end of the stent into kinks and tortuosities of the internal carotid artery if more than a single bend is noted. Tortuosity cannot be eliminated and is displaced distally and can become more exaggerated when a stent is placed and results in stiffening of a segment of artery. A very tortuous internal carotid artery should be considered a relative contraindication for CAS, as acute occlusions are more common following stent placement in these tortuous vessels. In addition, there may be difficulty in advancing the stent delivery catheter into place in this situation.

Completion Angiogram

The filter is maintained in place until the carotid reconstruction is evaluated and continued flow through the filter is documented. Following stent placement, completion angiograms are acquired in the projection that had demonstrated the maximum stenosis. Extra attention is paid to the internal carotid artery immediately distal to the stent. Spasm in this segment may be encountered, especially where the filter is located. A small dose of intra-arterial nitroglycerine (100–200 mcg) is directly administered into the internal carotid artery, if significant spasm is encountered. Distal dissections are unusual and when present can be remedied with an additional stent of appropriate size. Reasonable prograde flow through the stented segment and the filter should be present. If there is slow flow or there is a filling defect with the filter, an aspiration catheter is used prior to filter removal. The filter retrieval catheter is passed carefully through the stent to capture the filter. Open cell stent designs have excellent contourability but also have diamond-shaped points in the lumen which can snag the retrieval catheter. If the retrieval catheter catches on the stent, do not push the catheter forward, as this will tend to withdraw the filter down toward the stent. Have the patient rotate or extend the neck to permit a straight shot of the retrieval catheter along the wire through the stented portion.

After filter retrieval, post-CAS intracranial angiograms are obtained by most operators as a routine and these may be compared with pre-operative studies. If there is any concern about the potential for kinks of the ICA distal to the stent, the carotid arteriogram is repeated without the guidewire and filter in place. The neurological status of the patient is monitored during the procedure and assessed at its conclusion.

Access Site Management

In suitable patients, access site hemostasis is achieved at the end of the procedure using one of several approved closure devices. A femoral arteriogram is performed in the oblique projection. If a calcified vessel is encountered during needle puncture, closure devices are not used. In this situation the long sheath is exchanged for a short sheath of the same caliber that is removed when the ACT is less than 180 s and manual pressure held for the appropriate time period.

Post-operative Care and Follow-Up

Patients are monitored in the hospital overnight. It is not uncommon for patients to respond to carotid sinus distension with bradycardia and hypotension. Occasionally, 24–48 h of ionotropic support is required before the carotid sinus adapts to the radial force of the self-expanding stents. Avoiding extreme oversizing of the stents helps to decrease the incidence of post-CAS bradycardia and hypotension. The presence of significant hypotension in the absence of bradycardia is unusual in the immediate post-procedure period, it is worth emphasizing that other causes (e.g., retroperitoneal bleed related to access site problems) should also be excluded as the cause.

A neurologist is routinely involved in pre-discharge evaluation and a NIH stroke scale is completed before

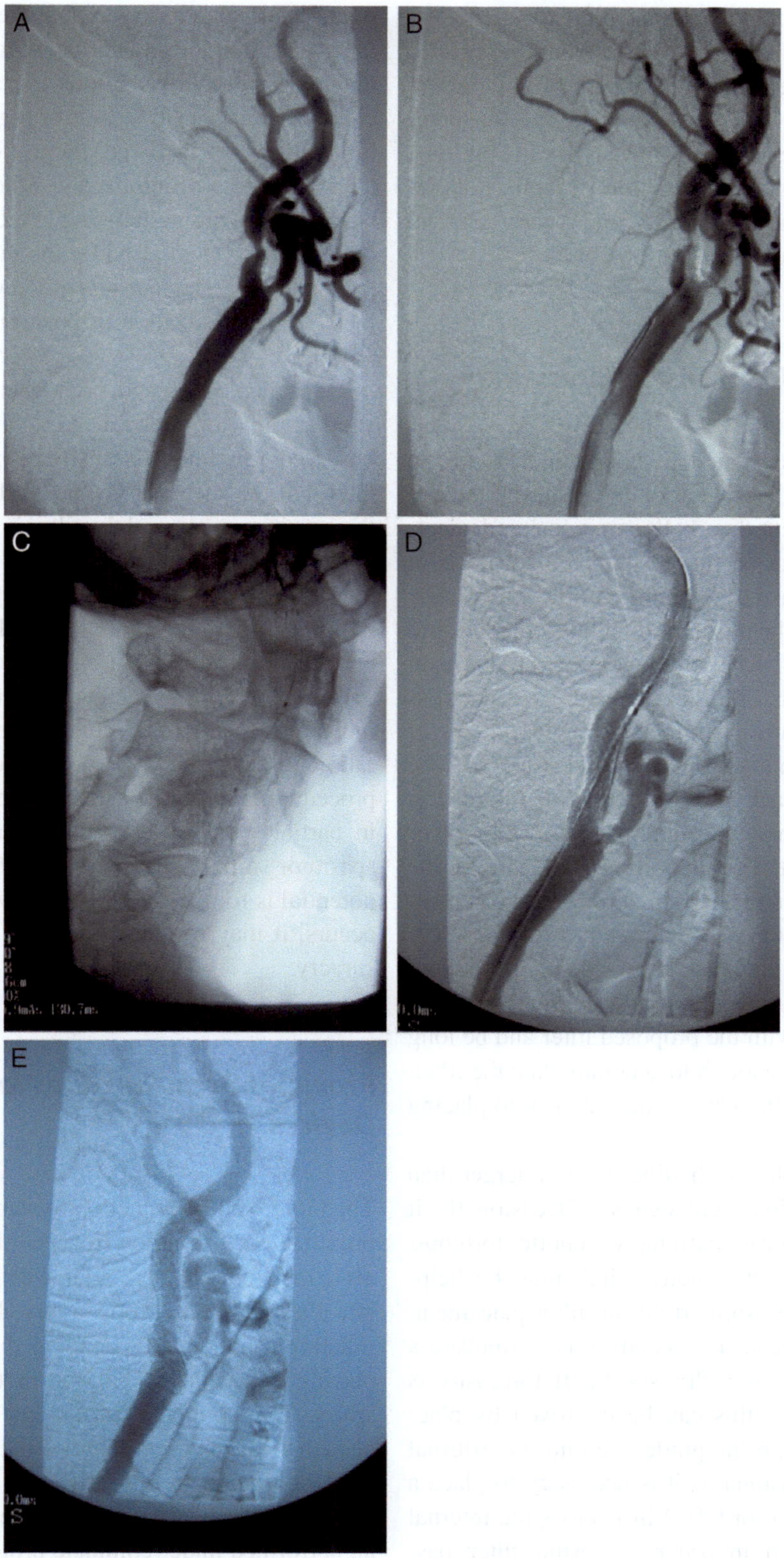

Fig. 24.5 Carotid stent placement. **a**, A symptomatic right carotid stenosis is treated in a high surgical risk patient. **b**, A guidewire tip approaches the carotid bifurcation. **c**, The distal filter has been placed, the stent is in place, and the post-stent angioplasty balloon is in place with the stent. **d**, After post-stent balloon angioplasty, a completion angiogram is performed with the filter in place. **e**, After filter removal, the stent is widely patent and supports normal prograde carotid flow

discharge. Carotid duplex is obtained if a patient sustains a neurological event or if severe internal carotid artery spasm is seen on the completion angiogram, since this may influence post-procedure management. Medications include ASA, 325 mg per day indefinitely, and clopidogrel, 75 mg per day for 1 month. Follow-up includes 1 month, 6 month, and yearly clinical evaluation and duplex examination.

Technique for Use of Distal Filters

Filter devices are designed to maintain flow in the distal ICA during the course of intervention and are substantially different than balloon occlusion devices. The filter should not be placed until the sheath is in a stable position in the common carotid artery. Any movement of the sheath after filter placement could also move the filter. After placement of the common carotid artery sheath, the filter device is placed across the target lesion into a straight, normal segment of the distal extracranial internal carotid artery. If the sheath should flip back into the arch while the filter is deployed, the filter may be withdrawn into the lesion or tangle with the stent. The supporting guidewire for the filter is not strong enough to support a readvancement of the sheath. Placing the device into a tortuous segment may be difficult and could impede filter function. The landing zone for the filter is assessed in advance; it must be reachable with the proposed filter and be long enough and straight enough to accommodate the filter. An ACT of 250 s or higher is required prior to placing filter devices.

The crossing profile of the filter is often larger than the residual lumen in a tight stenosis. Occasionally, it may be difficult to cross extremely stenotic, tortuous, or calcified lesions. A "buddy wire" may be helpful in providing extra support during filter placement. A slightly larger sheath is needed to accommodate a "buddy wire," such as a 7Fr sheath. If tortuosity is the issue, sometimes this can be improved by placing a stiff, but low-profile guidewire into the external carotid artery. Occasionally, it is necessary to place a soft guidewire (0.010 or 0.014 in.) across the internal carotid artery lesion in order to permit filter passage. Tortuosity may also be improved by having the patient change the neck position and capitalizing on the natural mobility of the carotid artery. When a very tight lesion cannot be crossed with a filter, occasionally a balloon pre-dilatation with a 2.0 or 2.5-mm diameter angioplasty balloon is required. When critically stenotic carotid lesions or highly tortuous carotid bifurcations are involved, the use of a "free-wire" filter system (e.g., Emboshield, Spider) has advantages over a fixed-wire system (e.g., Accunet, Filterwire). A "free-wire" system provides the guidewire and the filter separately. This permits guidewire crossing, placement, and optimization of position before the filter is advanced.

Once deployed, and after each step of the intervention, flow of contrast through the device must be observed. The image intensifier is positioned such that the tip of the sheath is visible on the inferior aspect of the monitor screen and the filter is visible on the superior aspect. If the device becomes filled with debris, it must be aspirated. When removing a full device, it is important not to recapture it completely, as debris may be extruded from it and embolize distally. If there is evidence of a filling defect within the filter, or some indication that it may contain debris, catheter aspiration is performed. The usual tendency during the procedure is for any tension on the guidewire to result in partial withdrawal of the filter. This may induce spasm or spill any debris that the filter holds. Another potential is for the filter to tangle with the stent. If this occurs, it may not be possible to fix it without open surgery.

Proximal Occlusion and Flow-Reversal Devices

The Gore Neuro Protection System (NPS) device is a proximal occlusion/flow-reversal device in clinical trials in the United States. A large catheter (8Fr) is placed into the common carotid artery. Flow is stopped by inflating a balloon surrounding the catheter and then placing an occlusion balloon in the external carotid artery. The common carotid artery catheter is connected to an external filter and then to the femoral vein, producing an arterio-venous fistula and reversal of flow in the internal carotid artery. Intervention can be performed under complete protection, as antegrade flow in the internal carotid artery does not occur until after the flow reversal is interrupted and the procedure is terminated.

This technique has several advantages compared to standard CAS employing distal filters. Surgeons experienced with CEA have long recognized the potential to dislodge the friable material present in carotid bifurcation plaques. Studies of carotid stenting with transcranial Doppler monitoring have demonstrated frequent embolic signals prevalent during several stages of the carotid stenting procedure including lesion crossing, pre-dilation, stent placement, and post-dilation. Diffusion-weighted MRI scans performed before and after CAS have shown evidence of lesions that may be embolic. Most filters allow particles smaller than 100 μm to pass through, resulting in multiple small, usually asymptomatic, cerebral lesions in up to 1/3 of patients using routine post-procedural diffusion-weighted MR studies of the brain. This type of distal micro-embolization, although not immediately associated with gross neurological deficits, could eventually lead to other problems, such as late cognitive impairment. Flow reversal permits CAS with the opportunity to diminish the high-intensity transits (HITs) visible on transcranial Doppler exams. Technically, the main challenges are the need for a larger carotid sheath, the need for external carotid artery occlusion, inability to control the rate of flow reversal, and identification of patients who cannot tolerate reversal of flow due to inadequate cerebral collaterals.

Registry Trials

Several registry trials have been performed and from which significant understanding has been derived about the clinical issues associated with CAS and distal filters. These registry studies are non-randomized and are intended to evaluate the safety and efficacy of specific stents and EPDs in a population of patients who are considered to be at high risk for conventional CEA. Most of the patients have been asymptomatic. Unlike very early CAS trials, modern registry trials have predefined inclusion/exclusion criteria, independent neurologic assessment, and standard use of cerebral protection. The results of these trials to date have in large part been presented at national meetings and most will be published in peer-reviewed journals in the coming months and years. Safety endpoints, such as risk of myocardial infarction, stroke, and death at 30 days, and efficacy endpoints, such as the rate of ipsilateral stroke at 30 days and 1 year, have been used routinely (Table 24.1). Technical success was achieved in greater than 97% of patients in most studies. The combined incidence at 30 days of myocardial infarction, stroke, and/or death varied between 2.1 and 8.3%, and stroke rate at 30 days ranged from 1.6 to 6.9% [23, 27–39]. A summary of the largest observational

Table 24.1 Carotid artery stenting registry trials

Registry trial	*N*	Symptomatic (%)	30-day stroke (%)	30-day death (%)	30-day MI (%)	30-day combined[a] (%)
BEACH [27]	480	25	4.4	1.5	1.0	5.8
ARCHeR[b] [23]	581	24	5.5	2.1	2.4	8.3
CABERNET[b] [28]	454	24	3.6	0.5	0.5	4.0
MAVErIC [29]	498	NR	3.6	1.0	1.8	5.2
CaRESS [30]	143	31	2.1	0.0	0.0	2.1
SECURITY[b] [31]	305	NR	6.9	0.0	0.3	7.2
PRIAMUS [32]	416	63	4.1	0.5	0.0	4.6
CREATE[b] [33]	419	17	3.3	1.9	1.0	6.2
CAPTURE [34]	3,500	14	4.8	1.8	0.9	6.3
MOMA [35]	157	NR	5.1	0.6	0.0	5.7
PASCAL [36]	113	NR	NR	NR	NR	8.0
EXACT [37]	1,500	10	3.9	1.0	0.2	4.6
CASES-PMS [38]	1,493	22	3.8	1.0	0.8	5.0
CRISTALLO [39]	124	24	1.6	2.4	0.8	4.0

MI: myocardial infarction; NR: not reported.

[a] 30-day combined = death, stroke, and/or MI. Not always additive as some individual patients experienced multiple events.

[b] Resulted in FDA device approval.

studies of CAS, including single-center case series and multi-center registries, is shown in Table 24.1.

Randomized Trials

While registry trials are invaluable in providing information pertaining to risks and adverse events associated with CAS, they are unable to offer level one comparative data between CAS and CEA. To date, randomized controlled data is limited to five completed trials [22, 40–43], and four other trials [44–47], which were terminated prior to study completion (Table 24.2).

The results of early, randomized controlled trials were mixed. The first randomized trial comparing endovascular and surgical treatments for carotid artery stenosis, Carotid and Vertebral Artery Transluminal Angioplasty Study (CAVATAS), was designed to compare balloon angioplasty alone without embolic protection to CEA in symptomatic patients. Stents were incorporated once they became available, but were utilized in only 26% of patients in the endovascular arm. For the 504 patients enrolled, there was no significant difference found in the composite stroke and/or death rate at 30 days (10.0% endovascular group vs. 9.9% CEA group) or at 3 years (14.3% endovascular group vs. 14.2% CEA group) [40]. However, this study was criticized for a number of reasons. The lack of embolic protection and 26% stent usage is in contrast to current standard practice, and the substantially higher stroke rate of 9.9% in the CEA arm makes comparison with other CEA trials difficult. The Wallstent trial followed and was the first multicenter randomized trial designed to compare CAS and CEA equivalence, but was stopped early after interim analysis revealed worse outcome in the CAS arm with combined risk of stroke and/or death at 30 days of 12.1% in the CAS group vs. 4.5% in the CEA group [44]. Notably, cerebral protection was not utilized and this was thought to contribute in part to the high risk associated with CAS in this study. More encouraging were the results of the Kentucky trials, the first of which was published in 2001 and involved symptomatic patients and the second of which was published in 2004 and involved asymptomatic patients [41, 42]. Extremely low complication rates were observed in both arms and the results of both trials suggested equivalence of CAS to CEA. However, enthusiasm was appropriately guarded since these were small, single institution studies carried out by a highly select, experienced team.

The Stenting and Angioplasty with Protection in Patients at High Risk for Endarterectomy (SAPPHIRE) trial demonstrated promise for CAS. SAPPHIRE was the first randomized trial to utilize mandatory distal embolic protection and was designed to demonstrate non-inferiority of CAS in a group of patients who were at high risk for conventional carotid endarterectomy. The majority of patients (more than 70%) were asymptomatic. The 30-day combined periprocedural adverse event rate was 4.8% for CAS patients and 9.8% for CEA patients ($p = 0.09$). At 1 year, the combined major adverse event rate was 12.2% for CAS patients and 20.1% for CEA patients ($p = 0.004$ for non-inferiority analysis, $p = 0.05$ for intention-to-treat analysis) [22]. These data strongly suggested non-inferiority of CAS for high-risk, largely asymptomatic patients. However, a few things must be noted. First, the differences in event rates between CAS and CEA were in part due to the greater association of CEA with non-Q-wave myocardial infarction. Excluding myocardial infarction, there was no significant difference found between CAS (5.5%) and CEA (8.4%) patients. Second, the high event rate noted in both groups casts serious doubt as to the appropriateness or durability of any intervention in the high-risk population, especially when the majority were asymptomatic. This concern was supported by long-term follow-up data at 3 years that revealed a substantial cumulative incidence in death from cardiac and non-neurologic causes (18.6% CAS vs. 21.0% CEA) [48]. Nevertheless, SAPPHIRE was viewed as the trial that proved the non-inferiority of CAS in high-risk patients.

As SAPPHIRE demonstrated non-inferiority in high-risk patients, two recently published multicenter, randomized European trials, Stent-Protected Angioplasty versus Carotid Endarterectomy (SPACE) and Endarterectomy Versus Stenting in Patients with Symptomatic Severe Carotid Stenosis (EVA-3S), sought to establish non-inferiority in standard-risk, symptomatic patients [46, 47]. In SPACE, the primary endpoint was ipsilateral stroke and/or death at 30 days. A variety of different stents were utilized and embolic protection was not mandated. The initial aim of the study was to enroll 950 patients per group to achieve

Table 24.2 Randomized carotid artery stenting trials

Trial	N	CAS patients	CEA patients	Year	Neurologic symptoms	30-day stroke (%)		30-day death (%)		30-day MI (%)		Primary endpoint[a] (%)		Notes
						CAS	CEA	CAS	CEA	CAS	CEA	CAS	CEA	
Naylor et al. [44].	17	7	10	1998	S	71.0	0.0	–	–	–	–	–	–	Single institution study. Trial ended prematurely after 5/7 patients in CAS arm experienced stroke at 30 days
Alberts et al. [45].	219	107	112	2001	S	12.1	3.6	–	–	–	–	12.1	3.6	Trial ended prematurely after interim analysis revealed worse outcome in CAS arm
Kentucky 1 [41]	104	53	51	2001	S	0.0	0.0	0.0	2.0	–	–	–	–	Single institution study. No EPD use
CAVATAS [40]	504	251	253	2001	S, AS	8.0	8.0	3.0	2.0	–	–	10.0	9.9	Only 26% patients in CAS arm received stents. No EPD use
SAPPHIRE [22]	334	167	167	2004	S, AS	3.6	3.1	1.2	2.5	2.4	6.1	12.2	20.1	High-risk, largely asymptomatic patients. Mandatory EPD use. Demonstrated non-inferiority of CAS to CEA
Kentucky 2 [42]	86	44	42	2004	AS	0.0	0.0	0.0	0.0	–	–	–	–	Single institution study. No EPD use
SPACE [46]	1,183	599	584	2006	S	7.5	6.2	0.7	0.9	–	–	6.8	6.3	Non-inferiority trial ended prematurely for reasons of futility. EPD use not required
EVA-3S [47]	520	261	259	2006	S	8.8	2.7	0.8	1.2	0.4	0.8	9.6	3.9	Non-inferiority trial ended prematurely for safety reasons. EPD use not initially required
CREST [43, 52]	2,500				S, AS									CAS vs. CEA. Lead-in phase results demonstrated increased adverse event risk in octogenarians. Target enrollment completed 2008
ICSS[b] [53]	1,500				S									CAS vs. CEA. Target enrollment projected 2008
ACT I[b] [54]	1,858				AS									CAS vs. CEA
ACST 2[b] [55]	5,000				AS									CAS vs. CEA
TACIT[b] [54]	3,700				AS									3-arm trial comparing CAS, CEA, and best medical management
Vienna[b] [56]	300				AS									CAS vs. best medical management

Abbreviations: ACST2: Asymptomatic Carotid Surgery Trial 2; ACT I: Asymptomatic Carotid Trial; AS: asymptomatic; CAS: carotid artery stenting; CAVATAS: Carotid and Vertebral Artery Transluminal Angioplasty Study; CEA: carotid endarterectomy; CREST: Carotid Revascularization Endarterectomy vs. Stent Trial; EPD: embolic protection device; EVA-3S: Endarterectomy Versus Stenting in Patients with Symptomatic Severe Carotid Stenosis; ICSS: International Carotid Stenting Study; MI: myocardial infarction; S: symptomatic; SAPPHIRE: Stenting and Angioplasty with Protection in Patients at High Risk for Endarterectomy; SPACE: stent-protected angioplasty vs. carotid endarterectomy; TACIT: Transatlantic Asymptomatic Carotid Intervention Trial.

[a] Primary Endpoint = 30-day stroke and/or death (Alberts, CAVATAS, SPACE, EVA-3S) *or* composite of 30-day stroke/death/MI and ipsilateral stroke and/or death at 1 year (SAPPHIRE).

[b] Trials currently enrolling.

a power of 80%. The final analysis in the SPACE trial comprised 1,183 patients and reported a primary event rate of 6.84% in the CAS group vs. 6.34% in the CEA group ($p = 0.09$ for non-inferiority analysis) [46]. SPACE CAS patients were treated variably with embolic protection; however, there were no significant differences found between those who were treated with and without. Further, in most endpoints there seemed to be a favorable trend toward the surgical arm although none were statistically significant. After this interim analysis, the steering committee decided to terminate the study on the basis of both futility and financial constraints as it was revealed that 2,500 patients would be needed to adequately power the study to achieve trial endpoints. Thus, SPACE failed to prove non-inferiority of CAS compared with CEA, and the authors concluded that CEA should remain the preferred treatment for patients with symptomatic stenosis because evidence was lacking to support equivalent or superior endovascular treatment. Subsequent subgroup analysis from SPACE revealed that this was particularly true for older patients in whom CAS was associated with a worse outcome. Investigators found that the risk of ipsilateral stroke or death increased significantly with age in the CAS group ($p = 0.001$) but not in the CEA group ($p = 0.534$) [49].

Similarly, the EVA-3S trial also failed to demonstrate non-inferiority of CAS in symptomatic patients. The primary endpoint was defined as a composite of any stroke or death occurring within 30 days after treatment. The goal was to enroll 872 patients per group to achieve a power of 80%. A variety of different stents were utilized at different centers and cerebral protection was initially not required until the safety committee instituted a protocol change as a result of a 25% 30-day rate of stroke or death in patients treated without EPDs [50]. The study randomized 527 patients and was subsequently ended prematurely for safety reasons after interim analysis revealed significantly higher 30-day event rate in the CAS group (9.6%) compared with the CEA group (3.9%) ($p = 0.01$). These results persisted at 6 months with an event rate of 11.7% in the CAS arm vs. 6.1% in the CEA group ($p = 0.02$) [47].

The EVA-3S results have been widely criticized for the significantly higher 30-day stroke rate observed in the CAS arm of the study as compared with other recently published results, namely from the SAPPHIRE trial (9.2% EVA-3S vs. 3.6% in SAPPHIRE) [22, 47]. In addition to the lack of initial EPD use in EVA-3S, the difference in reported stroke rate was also attributed to the overwhelming number of patients with asymptomatic stenosis in the SAPPHIRE trial which carries a lower risk of stroke during carotid repair than does symptomatic stenosis. Criticism for EVA-3S has also been directed at the fact that the trial did not compare groups of physicians with equal experience. Whereas the surgeons performing CEA had performed at least 25 endarterectomies within 1 year before trial entry, interventionalists were certified after performing less than half that number and were allowed to enroll study participants while completing their training and certification, a factor that could also theoretically increase stroke risk in the CAS arm. Despite these claims, however, subgroup analysis failed to show any statistically significant difference between operators based on level of experience [47]. The conclusion from the EVA-3S authors supported the notion that CEA remains an excellent option for symptomatic carotid stenosis with low complication rates that are currently not matched by CAS.

It has been challenging to collectively interpret the results of the randomized trials to date as they reached different conclusions about the safety and efficacy of CAS vs. CEA. This is not surprising in light of the fact that they differed significantly with respect to methodology including inclusion/exclusion criteria, operator experience, and technical factors. Furthermore, two of the largest trials, EVA-3S and SPACE, failed to show what they intended and were terminated prior to reaching full enrollment. Therefore, the question still remains whether CAS offers an advantage or is equivalent to CEA, and which subgroup of patients, if any, would derive the most benefit from CAS. A recent meta-analysis of all randomized trials to date found that patients who underwent CAS had a significantly higher risk of 30-day stroke and death relative to patients who underwent CEA, and that symptomatic patients treated with CAS may have fared worse than their asymptomatic counterparts [51]. The answer about the role of CAS awaits the completion of several ongoing large, multi-center randomized trials.

Ongoing Trials

Several ongoing randomized trials should help answer questions regarding the appropriate management of patients with carotid occlusive disease utilizing

CEA, CAS, or medical therapy alone. The Carotid Revascularization Endarterectomy versus Stent Trial (CREST) is a NIH-sponsored, prospective, randomized multi-center trial comparing the efficacy of CEA and CAS in both symptomatic and asymptomatic patients 43]. The primary endpoints include 30-day periprocedural composite of stroke, myocardial infarction, and death and ipsilateral stroke during the follow-up period. To address concerns from previous trials, CREST required rigorous credentialing for interventionalists performing CAS. Results from the lead-in phase have been published and demonstrate an overall 4.4% 30-day stroke and death rate for CAS 52. Of interest, results indicated increasing levels of stroke and death rates with age ($p = 0.0006$), specifically among octogenarians who experienced a 12.1% 30-day stroke and/or death rate. This was significantly above the rates observed for patients aged 70–79 (5.3%), 60–69 (1.3%), and less than 60 (1.7%). As a result, patients over 80 years of age were subsequently excluded from the trial [52]. Enrollment in CREST is complete, and results are expected in 2010.

Other ongoing trials include the International Carotid Stenting Study (ICSS), which is designed to compare efficacy of CEA and CAS in patients with symptomatic carotid stenosis and is projected to reach target enrollment of approximately 1,500 patients during late 2008 53. The Asymptomatic Carotid Trial (ACT I) 54 and the Asymptomatic Carotid Surgery Trial-2 (ACST-2) 55 are both designed to compare CEA and CAS in asymptomatic patients who are at standard risk for surgery. TACIT (Transatlantic Asymptomatic Carotid Intervention Trial) will also study exclusively asymptomatic patients and is unique in that it is a three-arm trial with two main study aims (1) to establish non-inferiority of CAS compared with CEA and (2) to establish superiority of revascularization via CEA or CAS to best medical management. TACIT seeks to enroll 3,700 patients with 1,140 patients in each revascularization arm and 1,250 patients in the medical management arm [54]. Finally, an Austrian, prospective, randomized controlled trial is currently recruiting and seeks to compare CAS with best medical management in 300 asymptomatic patients with high-grade carotid stenosis 56. The primary endpoints in all of the above-mentioned trials consist of combined myocardial infarction, stroke, and/or death within 30 days of intervention and long-term stroke-free survival.

Carotid Angioplasty and Stenting: Evolving Indications

Although CAS has proven to be a feasible and effective technique in the management of carotid artery stenosis, the appropriate clinical setting for its preferential use over CEA remains unclear and has yet to be clearly defined by the results of randomized trials. Initially CAS was proposed as an alternative to CEA in various categories of high-risk patients. CAS has also been suggested as a replacement for CEA in all patients.

High Risk for Carotid Artery Stenting

Only recently has attention focused on identification of patients who may be at high risk for complications during and after CAS. The literature includes data for octogenarians, the presence of specific vascular anatomic and lesion characteristics, and symptomatic patients. Several studies have demonstrated increased rates of stroke and death among octogenarians. The CREST trial lead-in phase reported a 30-day stroke and death rate of 12.1% for octogenarians compared with 3.2% among non-octogenarians ($p < 0.0001$), prompting the study investigators to exclude patients over 80 years of age from the study [52]. Similarly, results from Stanziale et al. indicated that CAS in octogenarians was associated with a statistically significant higher rate of adverse events at 30 days and at 1-year follow-up 57. Subgroup analysis of the SPACE trial also found that the rate of complications was significantly associated with age in the CAS group, whereas patients in the CEA group had homogenous event rates across all age groups [49]. In this study, regression analysis identified 68 years of age as the cutoff between low- and high-risk populations, reporting a combined 30-day stroke/myocardial infarction/death rate of 10.8% in older patients vs. 2.7% in younger patients. Collectively, the results indicate that CAS should be cautiously considered in the elderly population.

The etiology of increased adverse event risk for CAS procedures in the elderly remains incompletely understood. It has been suggested that adverse vascular anatomy and lesion characteristics that have the potential to increase the technical complexity of CAS may account for this finding, as recent studies have suggested that some of these complex anatomic features seem to be more prevalent among older patients [58–60]. Lin et al. found that aortic arch calcification, common carotid and innominate artery stenosis, and tortuosity of the common and internal carotid arteries were significantly more severe in patients 80 years and above [58]. Likewise, in addition to the features mentioned above, others have also found unfavorable arch elongation, severe lesion stenosis greater than 85%, and plaque ulceration to be significantly more common among patients aged 80 years and above [59, 60]. Recent work has also sought to determine the impact of these anatomic characteristics on outcome after CAS. Some variables that have been associated with increased risk of adverse events include abnormal arch anatomy, 61 vessel tortuosity, 62 long stenotic lesions (>15 mm), involvement of the internal carotid ostium, 63 and plaque echolucency [64]. It is important to note that while these anatomic and lesion characteristics are thought to be more common in the elderly population, younger patients may also have similar unfavorable risk factors. For example, Sayeed et al. reported that long stenosis and ostial involvement was associated with increased risk of stroke independent of octogenarian status [63]. Thus, the presence of certain anatomic factors that preclude safe passage and/or proper positioning of stents and EPDs must be considered high risk at any age, and this could possibly delineate a new group of patients who, in addition to the elderly, also may not be appropriate candidates for CAS.

Controversy also exists surrounding the role of CAS in managing symptomatic patients. Favorable CAS results to date from SAPPHIRE and registry trials have been achieved in populations of predominantly asymptomatic patients, and in spite of some evidence to the contrary based on retrospective data, 65 many believe that symptomatic patients comprise a high-risk category for CAS [22, 34]. As mentioned in the previous discussion, two recent randomized trials comparing CEA and CAS in exclusively symptomatic patients, SPACE and EVA-3S, were both terminated prematurely due to futility and safety concerns in the CAS arm [46, 47]. Further, the CAPTURE (Carotid Acculink/Accunet Post-approval Trial to Uncover Rare Events) post-marketing trial reported a significant increase in risk of the primary composite outcome of stroke, myocardial infarction, and/or death at 30 days among symptomatic patients (12.1%) when compared with asymptomatic patients (5.4%). Even more sobering are the numbers reported in symptomatic octogenarians who suffered a 17.1% incidence of perioperative stroke, myocardial infarction, and/or death, which is in stark contrast to the 4.6% reported risk in asymptomatic non-octogenarians [34]. The rationale behind the observed increased risk with CAS in symptomatic patients remains speculative, but many advocate the cautious application of CAS in this population at the current time.

It should be noted that most of the above-mentioned studies were relatively small in terms of patient size and absolute number of reportable adverse clinical events. Thus, interpretation of results to date is somewhat limited as only large studies are truly able to establish clear, reproducible relationships between specific patient characteristics and clinical outcomes. One novel method that has been used to overcome this limitation is the use of diffusion-weighted imaging (DWI) obtained with magnetic resonance imaging (MRI) before and after CAS [60]. The incidence of new lesions seen on DWI after CAS would likely exceed the incidence of clinical stroke, and, as such, could serve as a surrogate endpoint for clinical neurologic events. This technique has been utilized by Kastrup et al., who examined the effect of certain anatomic risk factors on the incidence of new DWI lesions after CAS. Of interest is the ability to clearly distinguish lesions that are outside the territory of the treated vessel, thus identifying sequelae of arch and proximal vessel embolization, as opposed to target lesion embolization that would be expected to produce new ipsilateral lesions. For example, the authors found that plaque ulceration was significantly associated with new ipsilateral DWI lesions, whereas aortic arch calcification and vessel tortuosity were significantly associated with new DWI lesions outside of the treated vascular territory [60]. Continuing efforts to elucidate risk factors for CAS utilizing both novel and traditional techniques are ongoing and will enable us to further refine CAS indications.

Summary of CAS Indications

The literature to date seems to support the use of CAS as a reasonable alternative to CEA in patients with anatomic factors such as history of previous neck radiation and/or surgery, recurrent stenosis, tracheostomy, spinal immobility, surgically inaccessible lesions, and contralateral laryngeal nerve palsy, in addition to patients with contralateral occlusion and severe, multiple medical comorbidities. Conversely, many would agree that CAS is best avoided in patients older than 80 years of age, those with complex vascular anatomy and specific unfavorable lesion characteristics, and possibly those with symptomatic disease. Utilizing the above-mentioned criteria a recent retrospective analysis compared high-risk patients treated with CAS to standard-risk patients treated with CEA [66]. The investigators reported comparable perioperative outcomes between the two groups, concluding that a properly selected patient population can be treated with CAS while achieving complication rates equivalent to CEA, thus reinforcing the critical importance of appropriate patient selection for CAS success.

It should be noted that to date the approved indications for reimbursement of CAS as defined by CMS have not been modified to reflect recent work and continue to support use of CAS in only "high-risk," symptomatic patients with severe stenosis. Additionally, as discussed above, a number of these high-risk categories have been challenged by several reports as being poorly predictive of adverse outcomes with CEA. It has been demonstrated that one of these "high-risk" subsets, namely advanced age, is actually predictive of poor outcomes after CAS.

Finally, it should be emphasized that for many high-risk patients, as well as asymptomatic patients, the decision to perform any form of revascularization in favor of conservative management may be more important than the choice of technique. This decision has been complicated by the fact that best medical management has improved considerably since the landmark trials of CEA vs. medical management were undertaken over a decade ago. Aspirin therapy has now been supplemented with newer antiplatelet agents, antihypertensive therapy, angiotensin-converting enzyme inhibitors, and statin therapy which collectively serve to reduce all vascular sources of morbidity and mortality. Thus, when considering any intervention, it is critical to determine whether the immediate risks attendant to the procedure are indeed significantly less than the risks associated with the natural history of the disease process and whether or not this is durable over the long term. It is possible that many high-risk and/or asymptomatic patients will ultimately be best served with medical management, a conclusion that awaits the completion of ongoing and future clinical trials.

Future Directions

The challenge for the future will continue to evolve around optimizing patient selection for CEA, CAS, or medical management alone. Ongoing prospective randomized trials will provide invaluable data on this front, but so too will examination of CEA vs. CAS in the "real-world" setting. At the most recent Society for Vascular Surgery (SVS) annual meeting, several abstracts were presented in support of this notion and addressed the frequently cited criticism that trial data is often not applicable to the general population (Vascular Annual Meeting (VAM), 2008, San Diego, CA). The SVS Vascular Registry (VR) was developed in response to the CMS National Coverage Decision on CAS, but was designed to include data for both CAS and CEA in order to allow comparison of outcomes. At the 2008 VAM, Sidawy et al. reported data on 6,403 procedures entered from 287 providers at 56 centers from July 2005 to December 2007. Risk-adjusted logistic regression analysis of the data demonstrated significantly better outcome in terms of 30-day complications following CEA as compared with CAS 67]. Similarly, other investigators utilizing the Nationwide Inpatient Sample (NIS) database examined data from 2001 through 2005 and found substantially increased stroke and death rates after CAS when compared with CEA [68–70]. Continued utilization of resources such as the SVS-VR and NIS will broaden our knowledge by serving as an outcome assessment tool for CAS and CEA in a "real-world" setting that supplements information provided by randomized trial data. The SVS recently published evidence-based clinical guidelines for the management of carotid stenosis, but the indications for CAS as a potential alternative to CEA in patients with high operative risk were weakly recommended based on low-quality evidence [71].

Conclusion

Although CEA has remained the gold standard for carotid revascularization, CAS has experienced tremendous growth over the last decade. Now a routinely performed procedure in academic and community settings, CAS annual volume is on the rise while CAS-related stroke and death rates continue to decline. As long-term data reflecting the durability of CAS begins to accumulate, greater operator experience is acquired, and new stenting technology develops, the application of CAS will continue to mature. Currently, however, the choice of CEA vs. CAS remains largely based on individual practitioner experience rather than on clear evidence-directed guidelines. This will be better defined with ongoing investigations and the emergence of new data and societal guidelines. Ultimately, the benefit of either procedure in terms of stroke prevention will depend to a significant degree on institutional outcomes with both techniques. Until additional large RCTs comparing CAS with CEA are completed, CEA should be considered the treatment of choice for standard-risk patients with carotid stenosis requiring intervention. For patients considered high risk for CEA, however, CAS is a viable alternative when performed in centers with established expertise and excellence.

References

1. Rosamond W, Flegal K, Furie K et al.: American heart association statistics committee and stroke statistics subcommittee. Heart disease and stroke statistics—2008 update: a report from the American heart association statistics committee and stroke statistics subcommittee, *Circulation* 117(4):e25–e146, January 29, 2008.
2. Carandang R, Seshadri S, Beiser A et al.: Trends in incidence, lifetime risk, severity, and 30-day mortality of stroke over the past 50 years, *JAMA* 296(24):2939–2946, 2006.
3. North American Symptomatic Carotid Endarterectomy Trial Collaborators. Beneficial effect of carotid endarterectomy in symptomatic patients with high-grade carotid stenosis, *N Engl J Med* 325:445–453, 1991
4. Barnett HJ, Taylor DW, Eliasziw M et al.: Benefit of carotid endarterectomy in patients with symptomatic moderate or severe stenosis. North American Symptomatic Carotid Endarterectomy Trial Collaborators, *N Engl J Med* 339(20):1415–1425, 1998.
5. European Carotid Surgery Trial Collaborators. Randomized trial of endarterectomy for recently symptomatic carotid stenosis: final results of the MRC European Carotid Surgery Trial (ECST), *Lancet* 351:1379–1387, 1998
6. Streifler JY, Eliasziw M, Benavente OR et al.: The risk of stroke in patients with first-ever retinal vs. hemispheric transient ischemic attacks and high-grade carotid stenosis. North American symptomatic carotid endarterectomy trial, *Arch Neurol* 52(3):246–249, 1995.
7. Eliasziw M, Streifler JY, Fox AJ et al.: Significance of plaque ulceration in symptomatic patients with high-grade carotid stenosis. North American symptomatic carotid endarterectomy trial, *Stroke* 25(2):304–308, February 1994.
8. Ferguson FF, Eliasziw M, Barr HW et al.: The North American symptomatic carotid endarterectomy trial: surgical results in 1415 patients, *Stroke* 30(9):1751–1758, September 1999.
9. Asymptomatic Carotid Surgery Trial Collaborative Group. Prevention of disabling and fatal strokes by successful carotid endarterectomy in patients without recent neurological symptoms: randomised controlled trial, *Lancet* 363:1491–1502, 2004
10. Executive Committee for the Asymptomatic Carotid Atherosclerosis Study. Endarterectomy for asymptomatic carotid stenosis, *JAMA* 273:1421–1428, 1995
11. Hobson RW, Weiss DG, Fields WS et al.: Efficacy of carotid endarterectomy for asymptomatic carotid stenosis. The veterans affairs cooperative study group, *N Engl J Med* 328:221–227, 1993.
12. Mathias K: A new catheter system for percutaneous transluminal angioplasty of carotid artery stenosis, *Fortschr Med* 95:1007–1011, 1997.
13. Kastrup A, Groschel K, Krapf H et al.: Early outcome of carotid angioplasty and stenting with and without cerebral protection devices: a systematic review of the literature, *Stroke* 34(3):813–819, 2003.
14. http://www.abbott.comAccessed August 15, 2008.
15. http://www.bostonscientific.comAccessed August 15, 2008
16. http://www.ev3.netAccessed August 15, 2008
17. http://www.cordis.comAccessed August 15, 2008
18. http://www.medtronic.comAccessed August 15, 2008.
19. http://www.invatec.comAccessed August 15, 2008.
20. http://www.goremedical.comAccessed August 15, 2008.
21. Kasirajan K: Technique of carotid bifurcation angioplasty and stent placement: how I do it. In Schneider PA, Bohannon WT, Silva MB, editors: *Carotid interventions*, New York, 2004, Marcel Dekker, pp. 149–164.
22. Yadav JS, Wholey MH, Kuntz RE et al.: Protected carotid-artery stenting versus endarterectomy in high-risk patients, *N Engl J Med* 351:1493–1501, 2004.
23. Gray WA, Hopkins LN, Yadav S et al.: Protected carotid stenting in high-surgical-risk patients: the ARCHeR results, *J Vasc Surg* 44(2):258–268, 2006.
24. Bohannon WT, Schneider PA, Silva MB: Aortic arch classification into segments facilitates carotid stenting. In Schneider PA, Bohannon WT, Silva MB, editors: *Carotid interventions*, New York, 2004, Marcel Dekker, pp. 15–22.
25. Rosenfield KM: SCAI/SVMB/SVS writing committee. Clinical competence statement on carotid stenting: training and credentialing for carotid stenting—multispecialty consensus recommendations, *J Vasc Surg* 41(1):160–168, January 2005.
26. Connors JJ 3rd, Sacks D, Furlan AJ et al.: American academy of neurology; American association of neurological surgeons; American society of interventional and

therapeutic neuroradiology; American society of neuroradiology; congress of neurological surgeons; AANS/CNS cerebrovascular section; society of interventional radiology; NeuroVascular coalition writing group. Training, competency, and credentialing standards for diagnostic cervicocerebral angiography, carotid stenting, and cerebrovascular intervention: a joint statement from the American academy of neurology, the American association of neurological surgeons, the American society of interventional and therapeutic neuroradiology, the American society of neuroradiology, the congress of neurological surgeons, the AANS/CNS cerebrovascular section, and the society of interventional radiology, *Neurology* 64(2):190–198, January 25, 2005.

27. White CJ, Iyer SS, Hopkins LN et al.: Carotid stenting with distal protection in high surgical risk patients: the BEACH trial 30 day results, *Catheter Cardiovasc Interv* 67:503–512, 2006.
28. Hopkins LN, Myla S, Grube E et al.: Carotid artery revascularization in high surgical risk patients with the NexStent and the Filterwire EX/EZ: 1 year results in the CABERNET trial, *Catheter Cardiovasc Interv* 71(7):950–960, 2008.
29. Ramee S, Higashida R: Evaluation of the Medtronic self-expanding carotid stent system with distal protection in the treatment of carotid artery stenosis: the MAVErIC trial Phase II 30-day update (abstr), *Am J Cardiol* 94:61E, 2004.
30. CaRES Steering Committee. Carotid Revascularization using Endarterectomy or Stenting Systems (CaRESS) phase I clinical trial: 1-year results, *J Vasc Surg* 42: 213–219, 2005.
31. Whitlow P: SECuRITY Investigators. SECuRITY: multicenter evaluation of carotid stenting with a distal protection filter. Carotid artery stenting with a distal-protection device safe in high-risk patients. Unpublished data, presented by Patrick L Whitlow at the 2003 Transcatheter Cardiovascular Therapeutics meeting, Washington, DC.
32. Coppi G, Moratto R, Silingardi R et al.: PRIAMUS—proximal flow blockage cerebral protection during carotid stenting: results from a multicenter Italian registry, *J Cardiovasc Surg (Torino)* 46:219–227, 2005.
33. Safian RD, Bresnahan JF, Jaff MR et al.: Protected carotid stenting in high-risk patients with severe carotid artery stenosis, *J Am Coll Cardiol* 47(12):2384–2389, 2006.
34. Gray WA, Yadav JS, Verta P et al.: The CAPTURE registry: predictors of outcomes in carotid artery stenting with embolic protection for high surgical risk patients in the early post-approval setting, *Catheter Cardiovasc Interv* 70(7):1025–1033, 2007.
35. Reimers B, Sievert H, Schuler GC et al.: Proximal endovascular flow blockage for cerebral protection during carotid artery stenting: results from a prospective multicenter registry, *Endovasc Ther* 12(2):156–165, 2005.
36. http://www.strokecenter.org/trials Accessed on 8/1/08.
37. Gray WA: EXACT/CAPTURE-2: Postmarketing carotid stent registry data. Presented at American college of cardiology 2007 scientific sessions: abstract 2409-5, March 24–27, 2007.
38. Katzen BT, Criado FJ, Ramee SR et al.: Carotid artery stenting with emboli protection surveillance study: thirty day results of the CASES-PMS study, *Catheter Cardiovasc Interv* 70(2):316–323, 2007.
39. Cremonesi A, Rubino P, Grattoni C et al.: Multicenter experience with a new "hybrid" carotid stent, *J Endovasc Ther* 15(2):186–192, 2008.
40. CAVATAS Investigators. Endovascular versus surgical treatment in patients with carotid stenosis in the Carotid and Vertebral Artery Transluminal Angioplasty Study (CAVATAS): a randomised trial, *Lancet* 357:1729–1737, 2001.
41. Brooks WH, McClure RR, Jones MR et al.: Carotid angioplasty and stenting versus carotid endarterectomy: randomized trial in a community hospital, *J Am Coll Cardiol* 38(6):1589–1595, 2001.
42. Brooks WH, McClure RR, Jones MR et al.: Carotid angioplasty and stenting versus carotid endarterectomy for treatment of asymptomatic carotid stenosis: a randomized trial in a community hospital, *Neurosurgery* 54:318–325, 2004.
43. http://www.cresttrial.orgAccessed October 1st, 2008.
44. Naylor AR, Bolia A, Abbott RJ et al.: Randomized study of carotid angioplasty and stenting versus carotid endarterectomy: a stopped trial, *J Vasc Surg* 28:326–334, 1998.
45. Alberts MJ: Results of a multicentre prospective randomized trial of carotid artery stenting vs. carotid endarterectomy, *Stroke* 32:325, 2001.
46. The SPACE Collaborative Group. Thirty-day results from the SPACE trial of stent-protected angioplasty versus carotid endarterectomy in symptomatic patients: a randomized inferiority trial, *Lancet* 368:1239–1247, 2006.
47. Mas J-L, Chatellier G, Beyssen B et al.: Endarterectomy versus stenting in patients with symptomatic severe carotid stenosis, *N Engl J Med* 355:1660–1671, 2006.
48. Gurm HS, Yadav JS, Fayad P et al.: Long-term results of carotid stenting versus endarterectomy in high-risk patients, *N Engl J Med* 358:1572–1579, 2008.
49. Stingele R, Berger J, Alfke K et al.: Clinical and angiographic risk factors for stroke and death within 30 days after carotid endarterectomy and stent-protected angioplasty: a subanalysis of the SPACE study, *Lancet Neurol* 7(3):216–222, March 2008.
50. Mas JL, Chatellier G, Beyssen B: EVA-3S Investigators. Carotid angioplasty and stenting with and without cerebral protection: clinical alert from the endarterectomy versus angioplasty in patients with symptomatic severe carotid stenosis (EVA-3S) trial, *Stroke* 35(1):e18–e20, January 2004.
51. Brahmanandam S, Ding EL, Conte MS et al.: Clinical results of carotid artery stenting compared with carotid endarterectomy, *J Vasc Surg* 47:343–349, 2008.
52. Hobson RW, Howard VJ, Roubin GS et al.: Carotid artery stenting is associated with increased complications in octogenarians: 30-day stroke and death rates in the CREST.
53. http://www.ion.ucl.ac.uk/cavatas_icss/index2.htm Accessed August 1, 2008.
54. http://www.evtoday.comAccessed August 1, 2008.
55. http://www.acst.org.ukAccessed August 1, 2008.
56. http://www.clinicaltrials.govAccessed August 1, 2008.
57. Stanziale SF, Marone LK, Boules TN et al.: Carotid artery stenting in octogenarians is associated with increased adverse outcomes, *J Vasc Surg* 43:297–304, 2006.
58. Lin SC, Trocciola SM, Rhee J et al.: Analysis of anatomic factors and age in patients undergoing carotid angioplasty and stenting, *Ann Vasc Surg* 19:798–804, 2005.

59. Lam RC, Lin SC, DeRubertis B et al.: The impact of increasing age on anatomic factors affecting carotid angioplasty and stenting, *J Vasc Surg* 45:875–880, 2007.
60. Kastrup A, Groschel K, Schnaudigel S et al.: Target lesion ulceration and arch calcification are associated with increased incidence of carotid stenting-associated ischemic lesions in octogenarians, *J Vasc Surg* 47:88–95, 2008.
61. Faggioli GL, Ferri M, Freyrie A et al.: Aortic arch anomalies are associated with increased risk of neurological events in carotid stent procedures, *Eur J Vasc Endovasc Surg* 33:436–441, 2007.
62. Faggioli GL, Ferri M, Gargiulo M et al.: Measurement and impact of proximal and distal tortuosity in carotid stenting procedures, *J Vasc Surg* 46:1119–1124, 2007.
63. Sayeed S, Stanziale SF, Wholey MH et al.: Angiographic lesion characteristics can predict adverse outcomes after carotid artery stenting, *J Vasc Surg* 47:81–87, 2008.
64. Biasi GM, Froio A, Diethrich EB et al.: Carotid plaque echolucency increases the risk of stroke in carotid stenting: the Imaging in Carotid Angioplasty and Risk of Stroke (ICAROS) study, *Circulation* 110:756–762, 2004.
65. Rhee-Moore SJ, DeRubertis BG, Lam RC et al.: Periprocedural complication rates are equivalent between symptomatic and asymptomatic patients undergoing carotid angioplasty and stenting, *Ann Vasc Surg* 22:233–237, 2008.
66. Sadek M, Hynecek RL, Sambol EB et al.: Carotid angioplasty and stenting, success relies on appropriate patient selection, *J Vasc Surg* 47:946–951, 2008.
67. Sidawy AN, Zwolak RM, White RA et al.: SVS carotid vascular registry: CAS vs. CEA outcomes comparison. www.vascularweb.org/Annual_Meeting/Abstracts/2008. Accessed June 15, 2008.
68. Wang JC, Blebea J, van Bemmelen P et al.: Increasing number of carotid stenting procedures performed with decreasing mortality—The national experience. www.vascularweb.org/Annual_Meeting/Abstracts/2008. Accessed June 15, 2008.
69. Vogel TR, Dombrovskiy VY, Haser P et al.: Carotid stenting and endarterectomy: outcomes in the US. www.vascularweb.org/Annual_Meeting/Abstracts/2008. Accessed June 15, 2008.
70. McPhee JT, Schanzer A, Messina LM et al.: Carotid artery stenting has higher post procedure stroke and mortality rates, and higher hospital charges than does carotid endarterectomy in the US 2005. www.vascularweb.org/Annual_Meeting/Abstracts/2008. Accessed June 15, 2008.
71. Hobson RW, Mackey WC, Ascher E et al.: Management of atherosclerotic carotid artery disease: clinical practice guidelines of the society for vascular surgery, *J Vasc Surg* 48:480–486, 2008.
72. Schneider PA: *Endovascular skills*, ed. 3, New York, 2008, Informa.
73. Kasirajan K, Schneider PA: Carotid bifurcation stented balloon angioplasty with cerebral protection. In Moore WS, editors: *Endovascular surgery*, Philadelphia, 2009, Saunders.

Neuroendovascular Interventions

25

Jacques E. Dion and Lucian M. Maidan

In the last two decades, the field of surgical interventional neuroradiology witnessed tremendous progress due to the introduction of new embolic materials, catheters, and, equally important, a better understanding of the anatomy and physiology of the intracranial vascular malformations. This chapter is a succinct review of the most common endovascular neurointerventions: embolization of intracranial aneurysms, treatment of intracranial vasospasm, embolization of arteriovenous malformations (AVM) and dural arteriovenous fistula (DAVF), angioplasty and stenting of intracranial and cervical stenosis, and acute stroke treatment.

Intracranial Aneurysms

Aneurysms (from the Latin *aneurysma* = dilatation) are abnormal outpouchings of a blood vessel wall, usually arterial. They have a relatively low prevalence in the general population, 6% in several postmortem studies, and 1% in angiographic studies of patients undergoing cerebral angiography for indications other than subarachnoid hemorrhage [1, 2]. Classically, there are three major types of intracranial aneurysms: saccular or berry, fusiform or atherosclerotic, and dissecting aneurysms.

The normal cerebral artery wall consists of three layers: the intima, which is the innermost endothelial layer; the media, which consists of smooth muscle; and the adventitia, the outermost layer, which consists of connective tissue.

The most common aneurysms are the saccular aneurysms, also called *true aneurysms*, because they have some of the layers of a normal blood vessel adventitia and intima, but they are missing the muscularis and internal elastic lamina, which terminate at the neck of the aneurysm. A false aneurysm or pseudoaneurysm is one where the integrity of the arterial wall has been compromised, the lumen being contained by an organized hematoma.

Although familial cerebral aneurysms were described, intracranial cerebral aneurysms are considered to be sporadically acquired [1]. A few congenital abnormalities of the intracranial arteries like persistent trigeminal artery or fenestrations are associated with an increased incidence of saccular aneurysms. There are several conditions associated with cerebral aneurysms: autosomal dominant polycystic kidney disease (5–40% of patients have intracranial aneurysms) [3], fibromuscular dysplasia, Marfan's syndrome, Ehlers–Danlos syndrome type IV, neurofibromatosis type I, and arteriovenous malformations of the brain. Uncommon causes of saccular aneurysms include infection, trauma, tumor, cocaine use, and other cerebral vascular malformations like high-flow AVMs.

Because 10–30% of patients will have multiple aneurysms [4], screening with magnetic resonance angiography is recommended for people who have two first-degree relatives with intracranial aneurysms and for all patients with autosomal dominant polycystic kidney disease [3, 5]. The multiplicity of aneurysms is strongly in favor of women, up to five times more than in males [6]. Pediatric population account for less than 2% of all intracranial aneurysms. They are more

J.E. Dion (✉)
Professor and Director, Interventional Neuroradiology, Department of Radiology, Emory University Hospital, Atlanta, GA, USA

T.J. Fogarty, R.A. White (eds.), *Peripheral Endovascular Interventions*,
DOI 10.1007/978-1-4419-1387-6_25,

frequently found in male, larger than those found in adults, and more often caused by trauma or infection.

The majority of all saccular intracranial aneurysms (up to 86%) are located in the anterior circulation: the anterior communicating artery 30%, posterior communicating artery 25%, middle cerebral artery bifurcation 20%, internal carotid artery terminus 7.5%, and the pericallosal/callosomarginal artery bifurcation 4%. In the posterior circulation (10% of all intracranial aneurysms), 7% arise from the basilar artery bifurcation, 3% arise at the origin of the posterior inferior cerebellar artery, 3.5% at the superior cerebellar artery and the anterior inferior cerebellar artery origin. Aneurysms caused by trauma or post-infections (mycotic) have a predilection for distal sites in the intracranial circulation.

The most common clinical presentation for the intracranial aneurysms is subarachnoid hemorrhage (the most common cause of subarachnoid hemorrhage is trauma). Aneurysms can cause symptoms by exerting mass effect on the surrounding structures. An acute onset of CIII palsy can be caused by enlargement of an aneurysm of the posterior communicating artery. Visual loss can be caused by an ophthalmic artery aneurysm that compresses the optic nerve. Large or partially thrombosed aneurysms can cause seizures, headaches, transient ischemic attacks, or cerebral infarction secondary to distal emboli.

Fifty to eighty percent of all aneurysms do not rupture during the course of a person's lifetime, but they are responsible for 80–90% of non-traumatic subarachnoid hemorrhages, approximately 10 cases per 100,000 people [7]. In addition, 5–15% of cases of stroke are related to ruptured intracranial aneurysms. Subarachnoid hemorrhage has 45% mortality at 30 days, 30% of survivors will have moderate-to-severe disability [8, 9]. Subarachnoid hemorrhages are twice as common in females as males, with a peak incidence in people 55–60 years old [10]. Terson's hemorrhages are unilateral or bilateral subhyaloid hemorrhages (between the retina and the vitreous membrane) present in up to 25% of patients with SAH [11].

Until the International Study of Unruptured Intracranial Aneurysms (ISUIA) was published in 1998 (2,621 patients in the retrospective component) and 2003 (1,692 patients in the prospective component), the annual risk of rupture of asymptomatic aneurysms was believed to be 1–2% per year (Table 25.1) [12]. ISUIA study found that for unruptured aneurysms smaller than 7 mm, in the anterior circulation the annual risk of rupture was 0.05% in the retrospective arm and a 5-year cumulative risk of rupture of 0% in the prospective arm. Basilar tip and posterior communicating artery aneurysms larger than 10 mm and aneurysms that are found in patients who had bled from a prior aneurysm were found to have an annual rate of rupture of up to 0.5%.

ISUIA study critics emphasized a selection bias of the aneurysms which were entered in the study because they were less likely to bleed, thus supporting a conservative management as opposed to invasive therapy.

Symptomatic unruptured aneurysms manifesting as new onset third nerve palsy, brain stem compression or visual loss caused by an ophthalmic artery aneurysm, have a 6% annual rupture rate much higher than that of incidentally discovered aneurysms. Cigarette smoking, uncontrolled hypertension, and drug use were shown to correlate with aneurysm growth and rupture [13]. Ten percent of patients with SAH die before reaching medical attention and another 50% die within 1 month, 50% of survivors have neurological deficits. There is a 2–4% risk of re-bleeding in the first 24 h after the initial event, and approximately 15–20% bleed a second time within the first 2 weeks [14]. The clinical outcome of re-bleeding is dismal, 59% (in some series up to 85%) of patients who re-bled were dead at 3 months [15]. Therefore, early treatment of the ruptured aneurysms by clipping or coiling will reduce the risk of re-bleeding. Antifibrinolytic agents before surgery were shown to decrease the risk of re-bleeding, but can increase the risk of ischemic complications [16, 17].

Defining the location, the size and the morphology of the aneurysm can be done by three major modalities: CT angiography (CTA), magnetic resonance angiography (MRA), and catheter angiography. For intracranial aneurysms CTA has reported sensitivities ranging from 0.77 to 0.97 and specificities ranging from 0.87 to 1.00, but the sensitivities for aneurysms smaller than 3 mm are 0.40–0.91. MRA is both highly sensitive and specific for the detection of intracranial aneurysms: sensitivity, 0.69–0.99; specificity, 1.00. The sensitivity of MRA drops for aneurysms less than 3 mm in diameter as low as 0.38 in one series [18, 19]. Although neurological complications can occur in 1.0–2.5% of cases, with permanent impairment in 0.1–0.5% (more common in older patients)[20, 21] the benchmark for identifying or for evaluating the

Table 25.1 Five-year risk (percentage) of rupture for intracranial aneurysms

	<7 mm, no history of SAH	<7 mm, history of SAH	7–12 mm	13–24 mm	>25 mm
Cavernous	0	0	0	3.0	6.4
ACA/MCA/ICA	0	1.5	2.6	14.5	40
P comm	2.5	3.4	14.5	18.4	50

Adapted with permission from Wiebers et al. [2].

morphological characteristics of an aneurysm is still catheter angiography. The three-dimensional catheter angiography (since 1998) improved some of the limitations of catheter angiography [22]. Non-neurological complications associated with catheter angiography include femoral artery injury 0.05–0.55%, groin hematoma 6.9–10.7%, and contrast-induced nephrotoxicity 1–2%.

The first successful cerebral angiogram on a living person was done in 1927, by the Portuguese neurologist Egas Moniz. He injected in a temporary-occluded ICA 70% solution of strontium bromide visualizing the MCA and PCA arteries; unfortunately, the patient died 8 h later. It was in 1941 that Werner reported the first successful electrothermic thrombosis of an intracranial aneurysm via a transorbital approach [23]. The first intracranial aneurysm treated with electrolytically detachable coils invented earlier by the Italian neurosurgeon Guido Guglielmi with the help of an engineer, Ivan Sepetka, was done on April 12, 1990, and dramatically changed the treatment of ruptured and unruptured aneurysms [24]. Approximately 150,000 patients have been treated with this technique worldwide since FDA approved this device in 1995. Whereas coiling was initially used for aneurysms not amenable to surgical clipping, this technique can now be used to treat most aneurysms. There are several obvious advantages of endovascular treatment of the aneurysm: no cerebral tissue manipulation (very important in the context of a ruptured aneurysm), lower cardiovascular stress especially for older patients with multiple comorbidities, leading to improved short- and long-term outcomes when compared to craniotomy.

The International Subarachnoid Aneurysm Trial (ISAT) conducted in England was a multicenter study which randomized 2,143 patients to microsurgical clipping (1,070 patients) or endovascular treatment (1,073 patients) with platinum coils, having as primary objective evaluation of the efficacy and safety of endovascular coiling to microsurgical clipping of ruptured aneurysms which are deemed treatable by both techniques. Primary end point was to determine whether endovascular treatment was reducing by 25% the proportion of patients with a Rankin scale of 3–6 at 1 year [25]. The study was stopped prematurely after a planned interim analysis found a 23.7% rate of dependency or death in the coiling cohort versus a 30.6% rate in the clipping cohort. The final conclusion was that at 1 year, there was a better chance of survival free of disability for patients with SAH treated by endovascular coiling with platinum coils. The relative risk reduction in dependency or death of patients treated by endovascular coiling versus clipping was 22.6%. The cumulative risk of re-bleeding at 1 year was 0.15% for coiling versus 0.07% for clipping [25]. An annual hemorrhage rate of 0.11% per year for coil embolization and with no late re-ruptures among those treated with surgical clipping were reported in the Cerebral Aneurysm Rerupture After Treatment (CARAT) study which was designed to directly compare re-rupture rates after subarachnoid hemorrhage in patients treated initially with coil embolization or surgical clipping [26]. For patients under 40 years of age due to the slight increased chance of recanalization after coiling that is higher than with clipping, it was found that the results of the ISAT study may favor clipping as a long-term treatment [27]. There were multiple critiques to the ISAT study: out of 9,559 patients with aneurysmal SAH only 22.4% were considered equally suitable for clipping or coiling; 97% of randomized aneurysms were in the anterior circulation (50.5% anterior communicating artery and 27% posterior communicating or anterior choroidal artery aneurysms) that were smaller than 10 mm (nearly 95%); 88% were a favorable clinical grade (1–3 according to WFNS classification); level or neurosurgeon's expertise (better outcomes with surgeons who over 30 craniotomies for aneurysms per year) [28].

There are a few anatomical aneurysmal characteristics which will decide between the endovascular treatment or craniotomy and the clipping: dome-to-neck ratio, calcification of the aneurysmal neck, intraaneurysmal thrombus, and location of the aneurysm. The dome-to-neck ratio greater than 2 makes the aneurysm favorable to classic endovascular treatment. A ratio smaller than 2 or an aneurysmal neck wider than 4 mm warrants the use of stents or balloons.

Detachable coils have several basic components: the coil (implant), the pusher, and the detachment system. The coils are made of different materials like platinum (three to four times more thrombogenic than stainless steel), platinum and polyglycolic/polylactic acid, platinum and hydrogel. The coil implant has a few basic components: the wire filament (which is the actual wire from which a coil is made and will determine the softness and conformability of the coil), the primary wind, and the secondary wind (which gives the coil the specific shape, loop size, and configuration). Another important characteristic of the coils is the ability to prevent stretching. Coils are made of a 90% platinum and 10% tungsten alloy and fall into three basic groups: framing coils, filling coils, and finishing coils.

In order to reduce the chances of aneurysmal re-treatment several manufacturers used inactive or bioactive materials to modify the surface of the platinum coil. Polyglycolic acid (PGA)/lactide is a bioabsorbable polymer which covers the platinum coil and promotes the intraneurysmal thrombus organization. A bioactive material is a hydrogel which expands five to nine times when in contact with (acidic pH in 20 min) blood, thus theoretically filling more of the aneurysm than a bare coil. Animal models of aneurysms embolized with hydrogel coils showed a healing response involving the aneurysmal wall (fibrosis and endothelialization), thus reducing the aneurysmal recurrence and stability to the natural thrombolytic process decreasing the rate of aneurysm recanalization. Several authors raised concerns that this second-generation coils were not evaluated in randomized controlled trials against bare platinum coils [29, 30]. A recent review of 27 studies concludes that there is no high-quality evidence for the safety or efficacy of bioactive or coated coils [31].

The aneurysmal sac is filled in a controlled fashion by compliant, soft materials, like platinum coils, or more recently onyx, the goal being to achieve, if possible, complete occlusion of the aneurysmal sac or partial occlusion and protection of the dome.

Endovascular coiling is performed by an interventional neuroradiologist, a neurosurgeon, or most recently by a neurologist with training in interventional radiology [32]. In our institution throughout the duration of the procedure (even for unruptured aneurysms) patients are under general anesthesia; some centers use conscious sedation to monitor the patient, in order to recognize thromboembolic complications, but also reporting lower cardiopulmonary morbidity and shorter hospital stay [33]. The coils induce thrombosis in the aneurysm via electrothrombosis (negatively charged red cells, platelets, and fibrinogen are attracted to the positively charged). After arterial access is achieved via puncture of the common femoral artery, a heparin bolus is administered intravenously for an activated coagulation time (ACT) of 250–300 s (at other institutions after the first coil is deployed) maintained by hourly heparin boluses, and aspirin 300 mg is given intrarectally to avoid thromboembolic complications. A guide catheter is placed for support as distally as possible in the internal carotid, vertebral, or even basilar artery. Under fluoroscopic guidance and using roadmap technique, a coaxial system formed by a microcatheter and a microguidewire, continuously flushed with heparinized saline (4,000 IU heparin/l of normal saline), is advanced into the aneurysm. Using a working projection that allows good visualization of the aneurysmal neck (to avoid coil protrusion in the parent vessel) coils of decreasing sizes are delivered using roadmap technique into the aneurysm cavity. First coil needs to achieve a good frame with as many loops as possible over the neck. If satisfactory position is achieved the coil is detached. Subsequently smaller diameter coils are placed in the aneurysm until there is angiographic obliteration of the aneurysm cavity by the coil mass. For the wide-neck aneurysms a semicompliant balloon is placed across the aneurysm neck and inflated during coil deployment, preventing them from herniation in the parent vessel. The balloon is deflated after each coil is placed in the aneurysm, and if their position is stable the coil is deployed [34]. Balloon-assisted remodeling can achieve up to 85% angiographic occlusion of the aneurysm in some series; however, there are some drawbacks like possible more thromboembolic complications (up to 9.8%) [35, 36] and due to increased intraaneurysmal pressure during inflation, increased theoretical risk of aneurysmal rupture (4%) [35, 37–40]. Other authors[34, 41] as well as a recent meta-analysis, however, did not find, when balloon remodeling technique was used, a higher incidence of thromboembolic events or aneurysmal rupture [42].

Self-expanding stents are used in patients with low neck-to-dome ratio aneurysms. The Neuroform stent (Boston Scientific Target) was the first available on the market [43–46]. This open-cell nitinol stent is deployed over the wire through a 3 French microcatheter across the aneurysmal neck. The Cordis Enterprise Vascular Reconstruction Device and Delivery System (Cordis Neurovascular, Miami Lakes, FL) is a closed-cell nitinol, self-expandable stent which has flared ends making it easier to navigate tortuous anatomy and stable after deployment in the parent vessel. It is intended for use with embolic coils for the treatment of wide-neck, intracranial, saccular, or fusiform aneurysms arising from a parent vessel with a diameter of more than 2.5 mm and less than 4 mm [47].

There are several concerns associated with the use of stents: neointimal hyperplasia (reaction to a foreign body) which can result in hemodynamically significant stenosis, rupture of the parent vessel (more of concerns with the balloon-mounted stents), or occlusion of small perforator branches by the struts of the stent [48, 49]. For elective stent-assisted coil embolization the patient is loaded with 300–600 mg of clopidogrel and 81–325 mg of aspirin the day before the procedure or 75 mg of clopidogrel and 81–325 mg of aspirin for 5 days prior to the procedure. Another used regimen to establish immediate platelet inhibition is a bolus of an irreversible glycoprotein receptor IIb/IIIa inhibitor, abciximab 0.25 mg/kg, followed by 0.125 mcg/kg/min for 12-h infusion [45].

For ruptured aneurysms, the use of the stents and the need of maintaining platelet inhibition are associated with higher rates of intracranial bleeds (intraventricular, intraparenchymal) especially when external ventricular draining catheters or ventriculoperitoneal shunts need to be placed [50].

In recent years, Onyx HD 500 (MicroTherapeutics) was used for embolization of large, wide-neck aneurysm. It is a liquid ethylene vinyl alcohol copolymer dissolved in an organic solvent, dimethyl sulfoxide (DMSO), and radiopaque tantalum powder [51]. The use of this liquid embolic agent involves the use of a balloon, placed in the parent vessel and left inflated for 3 min and then deflated to allow cerebral reperfusion for at least 2 min, this cycle being repeated until the aneurysm is filled and the neck is reconstructed by the spongy polymer formed by Onyx 500 HD in contact with blood [52, 53]. Stent-assisted onyx embolization was reported to achieve complete occlusion in 79% of patients with 8.2% neurological complications; recurrence, which needed re-treatment between 3 and 12 h after the initial embolization, occurred in 10% of aneurysms and was more likely in larger aneurysms [54]. However, the procedure is long (the embolic agent is injected at a rate of 0.1 ml/min) and technically more complicated (needs special DMSO-compatible catheters) and has DMSO-associated angionecrosis as risks in addition to the thromboembolic complications [55].

Complications of endovascular treatment of aneurysms include aneurysmal rupture, thromboembolic complications, or rarely infections.

Aneurysm re-rupture during the endovascular treatment can occur during different stages of the procedure from the diagnostic part of the angiogram (injector or even hand injection of the contrast material), catheterizing the aneurysm with the microguidewire and microcatheter and placing of the coils (usually the last and first coils) [56, 57]. The reported intraprocedural rupture rate is 4.1% for ruptured aneurysms compared to 0.7% for unruptured aneurysms. The intraprocedural rupture of the aneurysm is associated with a 33% risk of death and 5% risk of disability for ruptured aneurysms compared to 14% risk of death and 14% risk of disability for unruptured aneurysms; it was linked to the experience of the operator, location and size of the aneurysm (more likely to rupture are small anterior communicating artery aneurysms), and timing of the coiling in relation to presentation (more than 11 days) [58, 59]. If perforation is due to actual placement of the coil in the aneurysm, one should not withdraw the perforating coil, and thus keep open the rent, but continue to pack the aneurysm with coils. Temporary tamponade with a balloon can be attempted from the parent vessel [60]. Aneurysmal rupture is characterized by a dramatic surge in the systolic blood pressure and heart rate. Protamine, 50 mg intravenous, is given to reverse the heparin. The patient, if he does not already have an external ventricular draining catheter, should have one placed emergently, to help manage the intraventricular pressure. Mannitol 1 g/kg bolus and hyperventilation (all patients that have coil embolization of an aneurysm are mechanically ventilated at our institution) are employed routinely.

Under systemic heparinization, symptomatic thromboembolic complications during endovascular embolization occur in 2.5–24% of cases; [61, 62]

asymptomatic ischemic infarctions (restricted diffusion areas on MRI) were reported at even higher rates of 61% [63]. The platelet-rich thrombus (formed acutely on the microcatheter or on the coil mass) can be dissolved with the IIb/IIIa inhibitor, abciximab given intravenously at 0.25 mg/kg, followed by 0.125 mcg/kg/min for 12-h infusion, or locally intra-arterially [64]. For a fibrin-rich thrombus or atherosclerotic plaque fragment, several agents were used (heparin, urokinase, tissue plasminogen activator, or combination) but with variable results [65] (Figs. 25.1, 25.2, and 25.3).

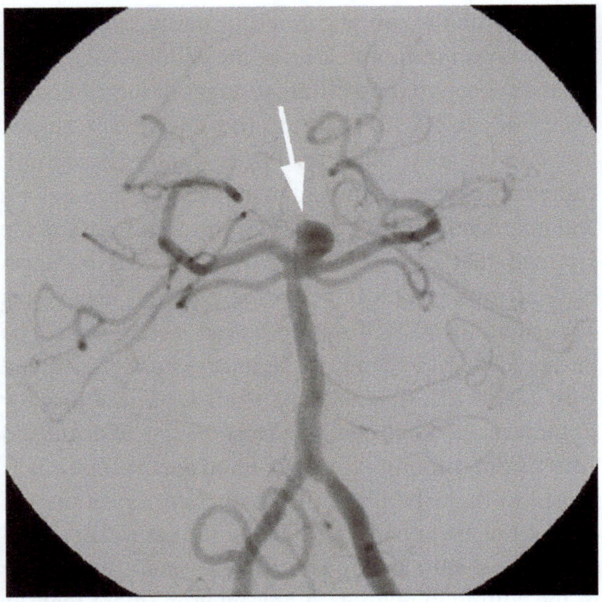

Fig. 25.1 Cerebral angiogram, left vertebral artery injection, *top* of the basilar artery aneurysm, incorporating the *left posterior* cerebral artery origin

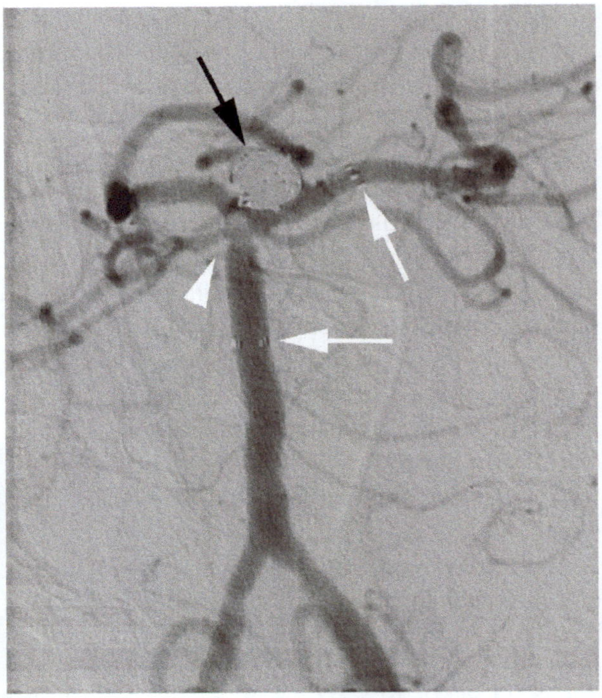

Fig. 25.2 Cerebral angiogram, AP view, left vertebral artery injection, post-stent-assisted coil embolization. The *white arrows* point at the proximal and distal ends of the Neuroform 2 stent, coil mass (*black arrow*) in the basilar artery aneurysm. The procedure was complicated by the formation of a blood clot (*white arrowhead*) that almost occluded the right superior cerebellar artery (SCA) and the distal basilar artery (BA)

Vasospasm is seen angiographically in 70% and manifests clinically in 20–30% of ruptured aneurysms, still the leading cause of morbidity and mortality with subarachnoid hemorrhage [66]. There was no statistical difference in the incidence of vasospasm between aneurysms treated by endovascular coiling or surgical clipping [67], angiographically seen after 3–5 days after the hemorrhage, peaks at 5–14 days, and resolving after 2–4 weeks [68, 69]. Despite treatment with calcium blockers like nimodipine, magnesium sulfate, and triple-H therapy, there are patients who develop refractory vasospasm; risk factors for vasospasm include the volume of subarachnoid blood, location, younger age, and history of smoking [70, 71].

It was Zubkov and colleagues in 1984 that reported first balloon angioplasty of the cerebral vessels as a treatment for vasospasm [72]. Electron microscopy studies revealed that untreated vessels in vasospasm have marked endothelial convolutions, corrugations of the internal elastic lamina, and proliferation of connective tissue in the intima when compared to the vessels treated with angioplasty [73]. When balloon angioplasty was done within 2 h of symptoms onset, there was a 70% improvement compared to 40% if the patients were treated more than 2 h after symptom onset [74]. Balloon angioplasty can be associated with major complications such as arterial dissection, thromboembolism, reperfusion hemorrhage, bleeding from unsecured aneurysms, and vessel rupture in 5% of cases [75–78].

Intra-arterial administration of calcium antagonists like verapamil and nicardipine was shown to have beneficial effects in lowering the incidence of angiographic and clinical vasospasm [79–81] (Figs. 25.4 and 25.5).

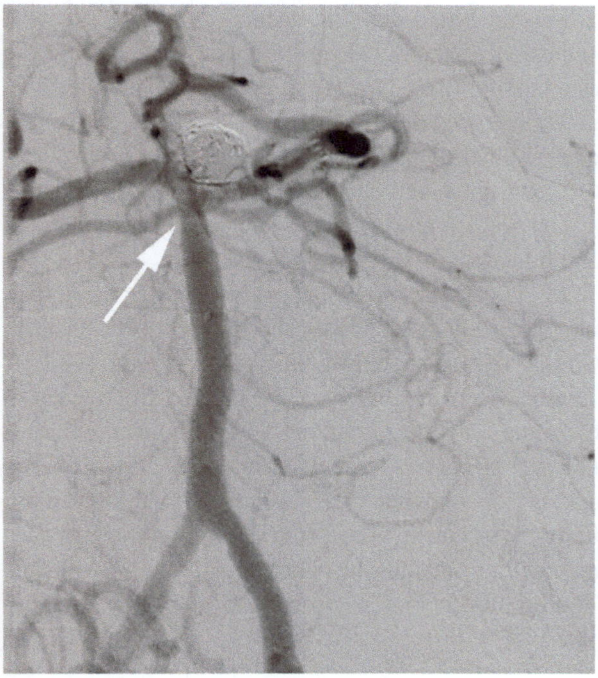

Fig. 25.3 Cerebral angiogram, AP view, left vertebral artery injection, status post-reopro IV treatment (0.25 mg/kg bolus, followed by 0.125 mcg/kg/min for 12-h infusion). Note complete resolution of the blood clot from the origin of the *right* SCA and the distal BA (*white arrow*), patient had an intact neurological exam

Arteriovenous Malformations

Arteriovenous malformations (AVM) represent 0.5% of the cerebral vascular malformations (venous angiomas 3%, capillary telangiectasias 0.9%, and cavernous angiomas 0.3%). AVMs are high-flow, shunting vascular lesions supplied by multiple arteries connected directly to the venous system without an intervening capillary bed, with dysplastic brain tissue between the vessels of the AVM nidus (Fig. 25.6) [82].

Clinically AVMs present with intracranial hemorrhage 50–60%, seizures 30% (mainly in the supratentorial locations), or progressive neurological deficit ("steal" phenomenon) [83]. The annual risk of hemorrhage for AVM is 2–4% with higher risk of re-bleeding in the first year, causing up to 30% mortality associated with a particular hemorrhage [84, 85]. The risk of hemorrhage is associated with increasing age, the size of the AVM (small AVMs bleed more frequently due to higher pressures in the feeding arteries), venous outflow stenosis, location (infratentorial and deep periventricular higher risk), and the presence of aneurysms on the arterial feeders or intranidal (2.7–14%) [86–89].

The most common grading scale designed to predict the operative risk of the AVM is the Spetzler and Martin scale [90]. In this grading scale points are assigned for the size of the AVM nidus (1 point for a nidus less than 3 cm, 2 points for a nidus size between 3 and 6 cm, and 3 points for a nidus larger than 6 cm), pattern of venous drainage (1 point for deep drainage and 0 points for superficial drainage), and the eloquence of the adjacent brain (1 point for eloquent brain and 0 points for non-eloquent brain).

Endovascular treatment of an AVM evolved since 1960 when it was done by injection of plastic microspheres, directly in a surgically exposed cervical carotid artery [91]. In 1972 a liquid embolic acrylate polymer was used to treat cerebral AVM [92].

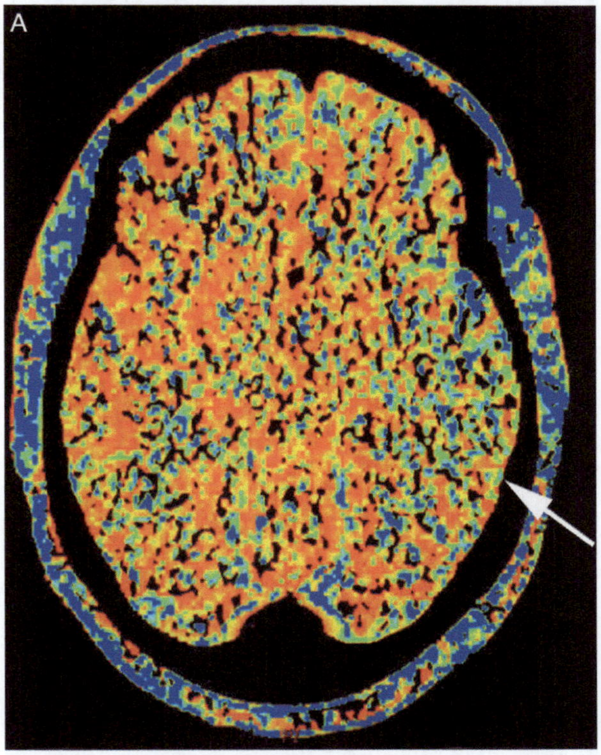

Fig. 25.4 CT perfusion of the head showing **a**, Mean Transit Time (MTT), **b**, Cerebral Blood Flow (CBF), and **c**, Cerebral Blood Volume (CBV) in a 47-year-old female with SAH, Hunt-Hess 1/Fisher 2, post-bleed day 5, post-coil embolization day 5 of a ruptured *left posterior* communicating artery aneurysm. *Arrow* points to the left temporal lobe, increased MTT, decreased CBF, and decreased CBV

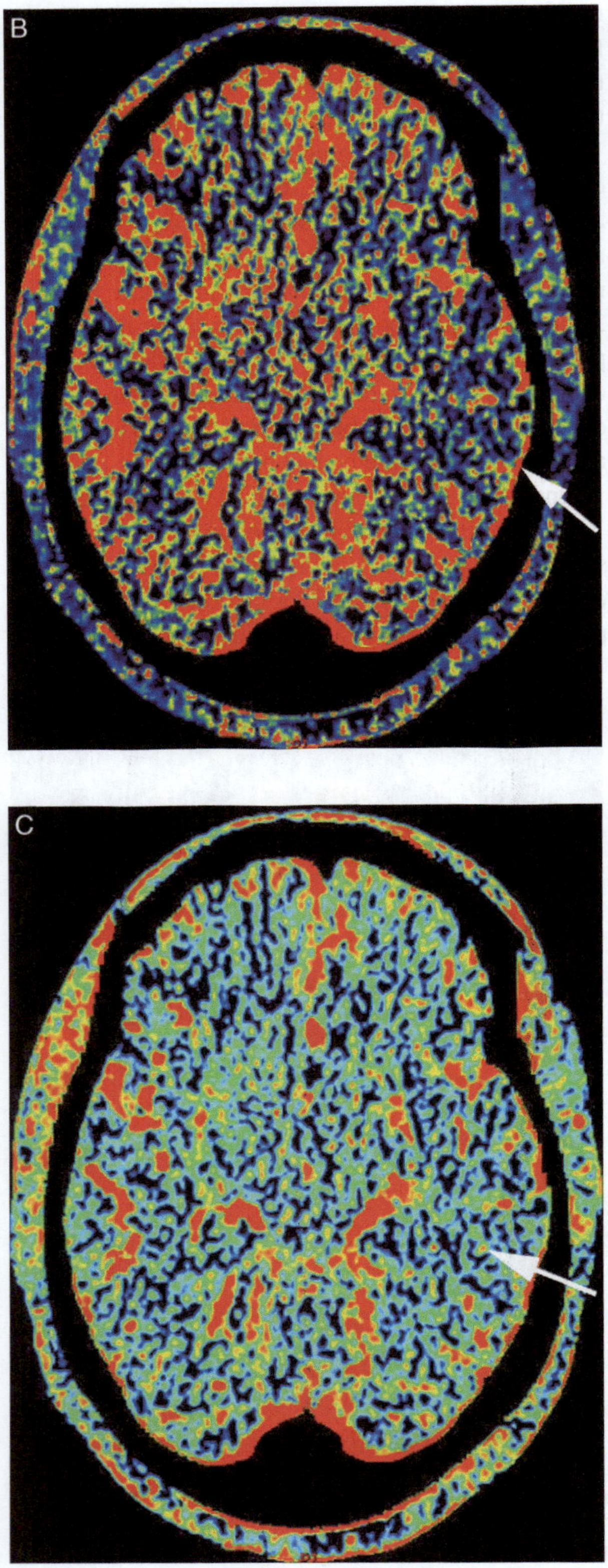

Fig. 25.4 (continued)

Several liquid embolic agents are used to achieve occlusion of the AVM, at the same time sparing the arterial supply to the normal brain parenchyma. Even in experienced hands there is a risk of permanent neurological deficit associated with these procedures; therefore some authors use pharmacologic provocative tests with different agents (amobarbital, methohexital, and lidocaine) to decrease this risk [93].

In 2000 the FDA approved a cyanoacrylate monomer, *N*-butyl cyanoacrylate (NBCA Trufill, Cordis Neurovascular, Miami Lakes, Florida) [94].

The liquid monomers of NBCA polymerize in an exogenic reaction in contact with blood (anionic initiators). NBCA is combined with several oil-based agents (iophendylate oil, more recently ethiodized oil, lipiodol) or glacial acetic acid to prolong the polymerization time and thus the penetration of the AVM nidus. The mixture comes in droplets which can end up in

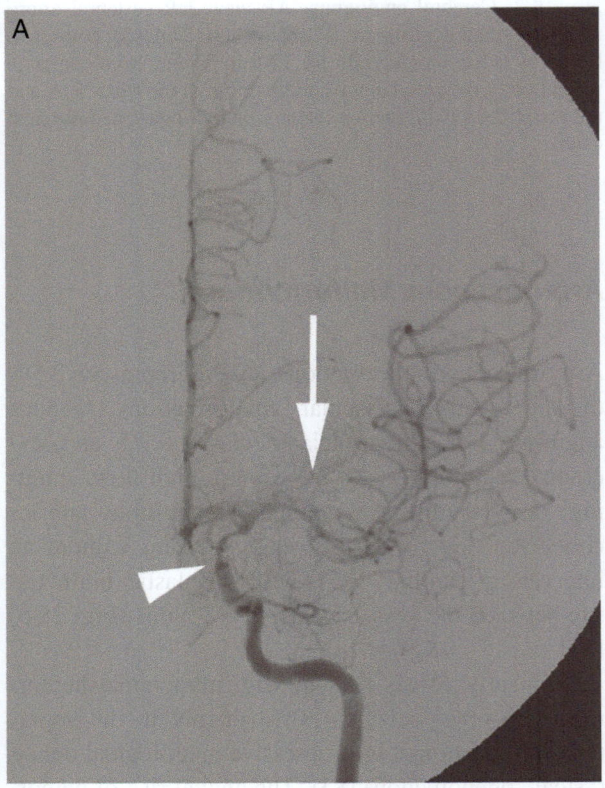

Fig. 25.5 Left internal carotid artery injection, AP view. *Arrow* points to the moderate–severe *left middle* cerebral artery vasospasm pre-balloon angioplasty **a**, then post-balloon angioplasty, **b**. The *arrowhead* points to the coil mass in the *left posterior* communicating artery superimposed on the supraclinoid left internal carotid artery

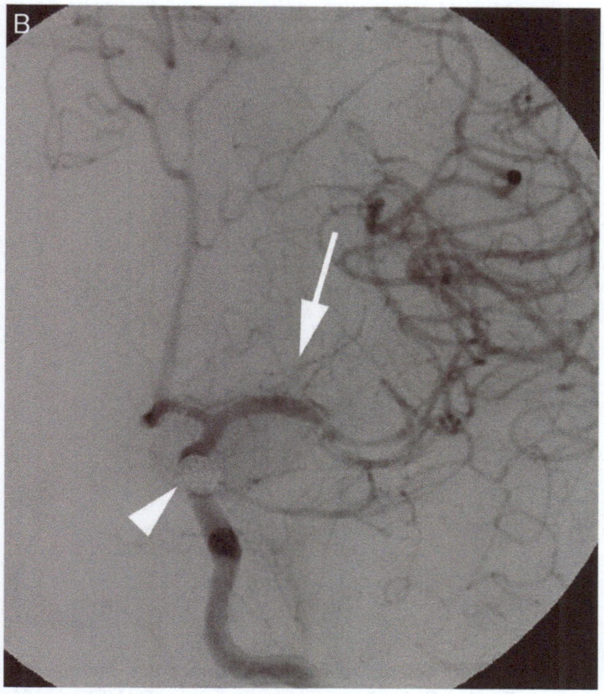

Fig. 25.5 (continued)

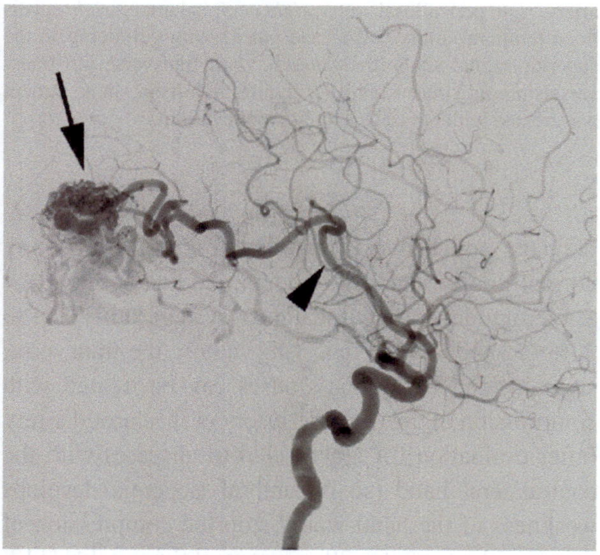

Fig. 25.6 Cerebral angiogram of the right internal carotid artery injection, lateral view. Right occipital AVM (Spetzler-Martin II) with less than 3 cm nidus (*arrow*), supplied by the *right middle* cerebral artery (*arrowhead*), and the *right posterior* cerebral artery with deep venous drainage

the systemic circulation. Tantalum powder confers the mixture radiopacity [95, 96].

The first time use of a non-adhesive ethylene vinyl alcohol copolymer (EVOH) in combination with dimethyl sulfoxide (DMSO) for cerebral AVM embolization was reported in 1990 [97]. Onyx which comes in three different concentrations of EVOH, Onyx 18 (6.0%), Onyx 20 (6.5%), and Onyx 34 (8.0%), is a premixed solution of EVOH, tantalum, and DMSO (Onyx Liquid Embolic System, Micro Therapeutics, Irvine, CA).

Due to the inability to embolize all the small arterial feeders of the AVM (thus eliminate the angiographic shunt, the abnormal early venous drainage, or any residual nidus filling), endovascular treatment alone is associated with cure rates varying between 10 and 35%. Palliative treatment is used to decrease the amount of "steal" or venous hypertension associated with a lesion causing in some cases clinical improvement. The black tantalum powder helps the surgeon to identify the abnormal vessels, and in the case of Onyx, the nidus filled with the polymer is spongy, easier to excise, thus decreasing the blood loss [98–102].

The endovascular treatment of AVMs, most of the time, is adjunctive to microsurgical resection (if able to permanently occlude the deep arterial feeders, the intranidal aneurysm, or more than 75% of the nidus) or to stereotactic radiosurgery (the smaller the AVM nidus, usually less than 10 cm^3, the higher the cure rates) [103].

Embolization of AVMs with liquid embolic material is associated with 8% neurological deficit and 1% mortality rate [104].

Dural Arteriovenous Fistulas

Dural arteriovenous fistulas (DAVFs) represent 10–15% of the intracranial vascular malformations. They are acquired lesions consisting of one or more fistulous connections within the dura mater [105].

The most common locations are the transverse/sigmoid sinus (62.6%), cavernous sinus (11.9%), superior sagittal sinus (7.4%), superior petrosal sinus (8.4%), ethmoidal sinus (5.8%), marginal sinus, and inferior petrosal sinus [106].

There are several classification systems for DAVF, most common in use are the ones by Borden and Cognard (Table 25.2).

According to the Borden classification, type I fistulas have antegrade drainage into a dural venous

Table 25.2 Cognard classification for dural AVFs

Type I	Antegrade drainage into a sinus
Type IIa	Retrograde flow into the main sinus
Type IIb	Retrograde flow into cortical veins
Type IIa+b	Retrograde flow into venous sinus and cortical veins
Type III	Direct cortical venous drainage without venous ectasia
Type IV	Direct cortical venous drainage with venous ectasia
Type V	Spinal venous drainage

Adapted with permission from Cognard et al. [160].

sinus or meningeal vein; Borden type II fistulas have both anterograde venous sinus drainage and retrograde drainage into subarachnoid veins; and finally Borden type III dural AVFs have exclusive retrograde drainage into arterialized subarachnoid veins at or on the wall of dural venous sinuses [107].

The presence of leptomeningeal drainage confers an aggressive behavior to the DAVF: type I DAVFs present with hemorrhage or progressive neurological deficits in less than 2% of cases, while type II 39% of cases and type III 79% of cases. Eighty-one percent of the patients with Borden type I DAVFs improved or were cured without treatment [108, 109] (Fig. 25.7).

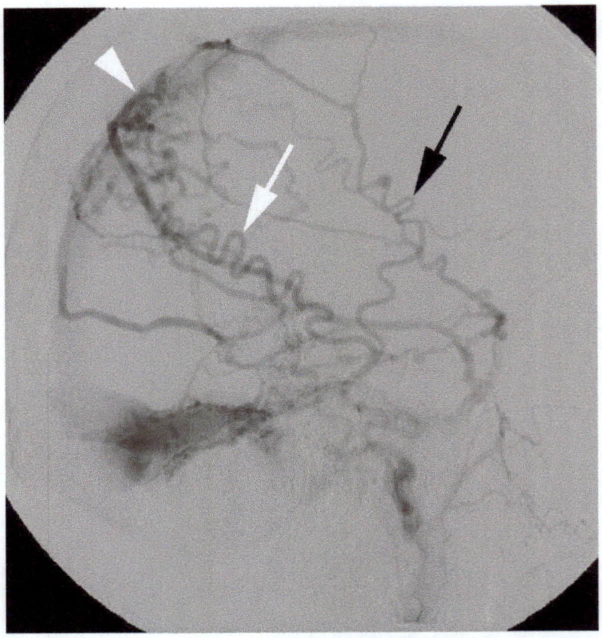

Fig. 25.7 Right internal carotid artery injection, lateral view shows a Borden II dural arteriovenous fistula (DAVF) of a 56-year-old male with 2-year history of dementia. The multiple fistulous points DAVF was supplied by the *right middle* meningeal artery, *right middle* meningeal artery, *right* meningohypophyseal artery, *right* pericallosal artery, *right* occipital artery, *right* superficial temporal artery (*white* and *black arrow*), draining in the superior sagital sinus (*arrowhead*), *right* transverse *left* transverse/sigmoid sinuses, and *left* jugular bulb/vein sinus. Patient was treated with Onyx 18 and 34 embolization

Treatment of DAVF includes observation, carotid compression, transarterial or transvenous embolization, microsurgical disconnection, and stereotactic radiosurgery. Successful treatment should obliterate the arteriovenous shunt itself as occlusion only of the venous outflow may result in increased venous hypertension in other vascular territories, potentially causing hemorrhage or worsening of the clinical symptoms [110, 111].

Transarterial embolization is effective if a microcatheter is wedged into the artery at the fistulous point, so the embolic materials like *N*-butyl cyanoacrylate (NBCA) or ethylene vinyl alcohol copolymer (Onyx) are penetrating through the fistula into the venous side, permanently occluding the shunt (Fig. 25.8). Often these lesions are able to recruit other arterial feeders so the cure can be temporary.

Transvenous embolization represents the modern endovascular therapy of intracranial DAVFs offering the best chance of cure. It should be attempted only if the dural sinus and all its pial tributaries have become arterialized, thus the risk of causing a venous infarct is low (as the sinus is defunctionalized) and if a venous drainage pouch that is separate from veins draining normal brain tissue can be identified and accessed by a microguidewire–microcatheter system [112]. Up to 30% of small DAVF involving mainly the transverse, sigmoid, and cavernous sinuses can be treated with compression of the occipital artery or the carotid artery (after evaluation for atherosclerotic disease) with the contralateral hand (so if cerebral ischemia develops weakness of the hand would stop the compression of the carotid artery), for 30 min several times a day [113, 114].

DAVF of the transverse and sigmoid sinus can be clinically asymptomatic or can cause pulse synchronous tinnitus, headache, transient ischemic attack, or intracranial hemorrhage. The arterial supply comes from the external carotid branches (transmastoid branches of the occipital artery, middle meningeal artery, neuromeningeal branches of the ascending pharyngeal artery; vertebral artery, posterior meningeal,

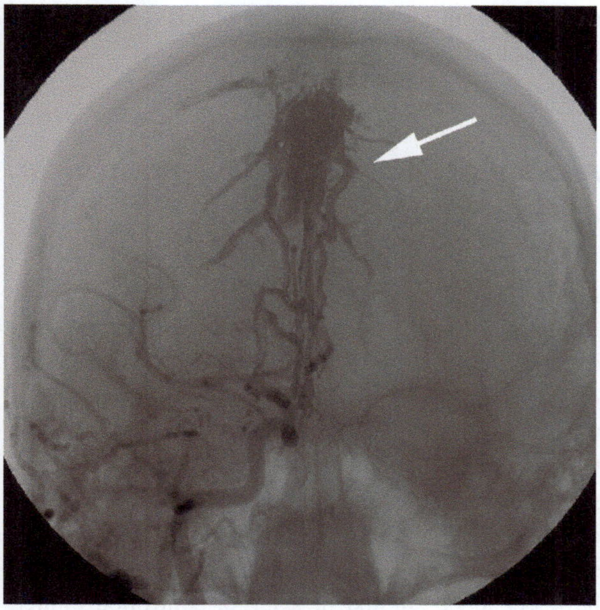

Fig. 25.8 Unsubstracted cerebral angiogram of the right internal cerebral artery injection, AP view, shows the onyx cast in the superior sagital sinus and in the superficial cerebral veins

and the artery of the falx cerebelli) and the internal carotid artery (meningohypophyseal trunk). Special attention should be paid to the direction of flow in the vein of Labbe and the point of insertion in the transverse sinus (occlusion of its takeoff in the case of antegrade drainage can increase the venous pressure).

Anterior fossa (ethmoidal) dural fistulae occur typically in males, present as frontal intraparenchymal hemorrhage, or rarely can drain in the cavernous sinus, causing chemosis and proptosis. They are supplied from the anterior and posterior ethmoidal branches of the ophthalmic artery and distal internal maxillary artery. They drain into a vein along the floor of the anterior cranial fossa, then into the superior sagittal sinus. Treatment of choice is surgical coagulation [115].

Cavernous sinus DAVF can present with proptosis, pulsatile exophthalmos, ocular bruits, chemosis, diplopia, decreased visual acuity, increased intraocular pressure, and eventually optic neuropathy. The arterial supply comes off the meningohypophyseal trunk, middle or accessory meningeal artery, the artery of foramen rotundum, and the ascending pharyngeal artery. Endovascular access into the cavernous sinus can be achieved through the inferior petrosal sinus or the enlarged superior ophthalmic vein.

Superior sagittal sinus DAVFs are rare presenting as headaches (more than 50% of patients), seizures, cerebral edema, encephalopathy, and not infrequently dementia. The arterial supply is generally bilateral derived from the middle meningeal artery, the ophthalmic artery (anterior falcine artery), or the posterior meningeal artery. These lesions are treated with a combination of endovascular techniques [116–118].

Tentorial or superior petrosal sinus dural AVF presents with intracranial hemorrhage, tinnitus, headache, and cranial nerve palsies. They have usually as arterial supply the meningohypophyseal trunk (the artery of Bernasconi–Cassinari), the middle meningeal artery (petrosal and petrosquamous branches), occipital artery, ascending pharyngeal artery, and the vertebral artery (meningeal branches) and have leptomeningeal venous drainage (pontine and perimesencephalic veins, superior petrosal sinus) [119].

Endovascular Treatment of Acute Stroke

The US Food and Drug Administration approved in 1996 the intravenous use of recombinant plasminogen activator (rt-PA) made by Genetech, South San Francisco, CA, for the treatment of acute ischemic stroke within 3 h from the symptoms onset [120]. Despite a 6.4% rate of symptomatic intracranial hemorrhage (ICH) compared to 0.6% in the placebo group, at 3 months rt-PA-treated patients were 30% more likely to have minimal or no disability compared with the placebo group.

Rapid recanalization of the occluded vessel is directly related to favorable neurological recovery [121–123]. However, in angiographic trials of IV rt-PA, the rate of recanalization of large vessels like the M1 segment of the middle cerebral artery occurred in only 25% of cases while the internal carotid artery only in 10 and 34% of the recanalized vessels will re-occlude [123–126].

The Prolyse in Acute Cerebral Thromboembolism II Trial was the only randomized trial which assessed intra-arterial fibrinolytic therapy alone (no microcatheter or microguidewire manipulation of the clot were allowed) given within 6 h of stroke symptom onset and with occlusions of the MCA. The symptomatic intracranial hemorrhage rate was 10% for the treatment group and 2% for the control group [127]. The drug used in this trial, prourokinase, did not obtain US FDA approval. Based on several large case-series cohorts which proved reasonable safety profile rt-PA is used in patients with large vessel occlusion and is supported by the American Academy of Neurology [128].

The Interventional Management of Stroke I Trial (IMS I) combined therapy of IV and IA rt-PA achieving recanalization rate of 56% with symptomatic ICH rate of 6.3% [129].

In recent years, recanalization of the occluded vessels in patients with acute ischemic stroke is attempted via mechanical rather than pharmaceutical means. The US FDA approved the first mechanical device for clot extraction in acute ischemic stroke based only on a safety study in August 2004. The X5 and X6 Merci Retriever (Concentric Medical, Mountain View, CA) were reported to achieve a recanalization rate of 48% with a 7.8% symptomatic ICH, when used within 8 h of symptoms onset. The Multi Mechanical Embolus Removal in Cerebral Ischemia Trial combined therapy of the second-generation LX Merci Retriever and rt-PA treatment (IV/IA) was assessed; the recanalization rate was increased to 69% with a symptomatic ICH of 9.0% [130, 131].

The US FDA approved in 2008 the Penumbra System (Penumbra, Alameda, CA) for thrombus removal in acute ischemic stroke within 8 h of onset. The device has three components: a reperfusion catheter, a separator, and a thrombus removal ring.

The recanalization rate is 81.6% TIMI 1 and 2 (in one study 100%) with symptomatic ICH of 11.2% [132].

IMS II trial evaluated the use of IV rt-PA followed by additional IA rt-PA and low-energy sonography via the EKOS Primo Micro-Infusion Catheter (EKOS Corp, Bothell, Wash) in patients with ischemic stroke treated within 3 h of onset. The study reported a complete recanalization rate of 68.9% in the ultrasound catheter-treated group at 2 h [133].

For a select group of patients with intracranial atherosclerosis who present with acute ischemic stroke, due to local thrombosis of the stenotic segment, primary angioplasty and stenting are promising [134]. In a retrospective case series of 9 patients, an 89% recanalization rate was achieved (TIMI 2 and 3), with no symptomatic ICH [135].

Angioplasty and Stenting for Intracranial Atherosclerosis

Intracranial atherosclerotic disease (ICAD) accounts for approximately 8–10% of ischemic strokes that occur annually in the United States and despite medical therapy it is associated with recurrent stroke rate of 20% in the first 2 years [136]. Because of their high-risk status, patients with intracranial stenosis who fail antithrombotic therapy are recommended different treatments for secondary stroke prevention, such as intracranial angioplasty or stenting, which have yet to be studied in a large, controlled clinical trial.

Balloon angioplasty for symptomatic intracranial stenosis was described by several authors since the 1980s [137, 138]. Coronary balloon-mounted stents for symptomatic intracranial lesions were associated with a 8.7% failure rate to deliver in a recent study, with periprocedural complication rate of 10.1%; 2.9% of patients developed stroke or death at 2-year follow-up [139].

Similar rates were reported previously in the Stenting of Symptomatic Atherosclerotic Lesions in the Vertebral or Intracranial Arteries (SSYLVIA) study: 6.6% periprocedural rate of stroke, 3.7% of patients had an ipsilateral stroke at 1-year follow-up [140].

The Wingspan stent system (Boston Scientific Corp) is the first stent designed for the treatment of symptomatic ICA. It is used with the Gateway PTA balloon catheter (Boston Scientific/Target) to predilate the stenotic lesion before deploying the Wingspan stent. The Wingspan stent is a self-expanding nitinol stent with a high success rate of delivery to the intracranial vasculature. Since 2005 the Wingspan stent is available under a US FDA humanitarian device exemption for patients with 50–99% stenosis who have failed medical therapy [141, 142]. Placement of the stent requires pre-medication with clopidogrel 75 mg and aspirin 81–325 mg daily for 5 days prior to the procedure (or a bolus of 300 mg of clopidogrel), followed by 6 weeks of aspirin and clopidrogel, then only aspirin indefinitely. In the multicenter Wingspan registry 6.1% of patients had a periprocedural complication, whereas an additional 10.3% developed a symptomatic restenosis in follow-up [143]. (Figs. 25.9 and 25.10).

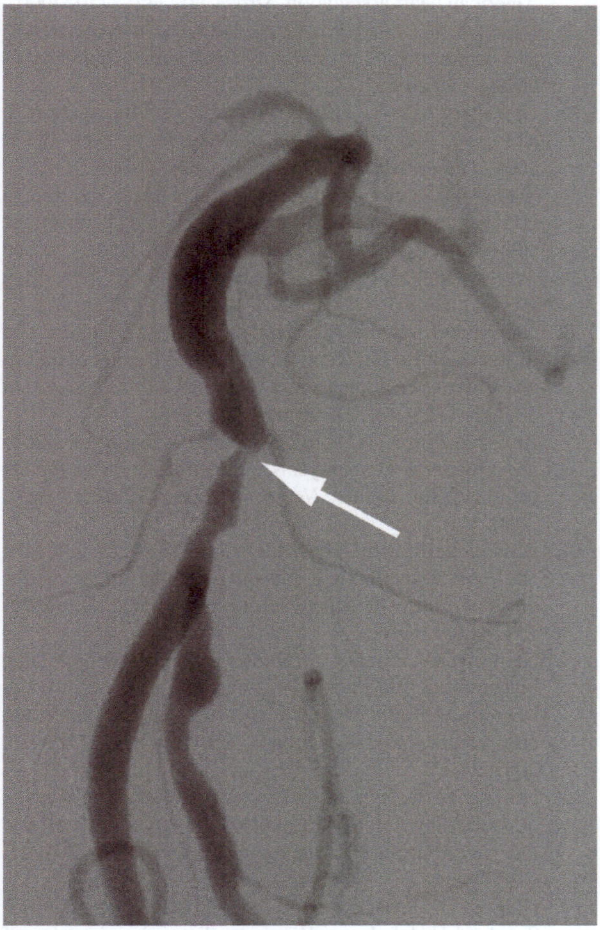

Fig. 25.9 Cerebral angiogram, left vertebral artery injection, of a symptomatic 67-year-old male on antiplatelets medication. The *white arrow* points at the mid-basilar moderate stenosis

Patient enrolling will start soon in the Stenting versus Aggressive Medical Management for Preventing Recurrent Stroke in Intracranial Stenosis (SAMMPRIS) which will compare the safety and effectiveness of either intensive medical therapy plus stenting (with the Wingspan system) or intensive medical therapy only in preventing stroke, heart attack, or death [144].

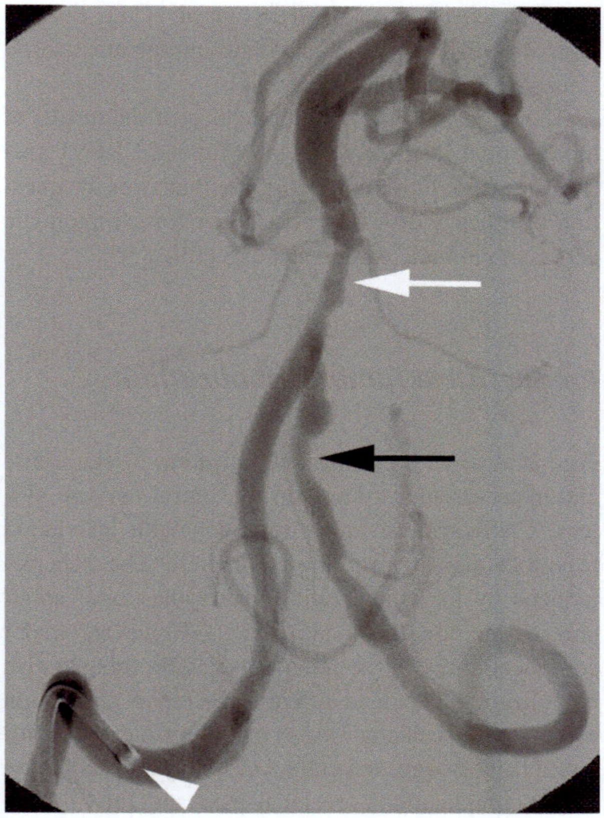

Fig. 25.10 Cerebral angiograms, left vertebral artery injection, post-Wingspan stent deployment. Note the position of the guiding catheter (*arrowhead*). The *white arrow* points at the mid-basilar post-angioplasty/stent area. The intradural segment of the left vertebral artery has multiple areas of stenosis (*black arrow*)

Carotid Angioplasty and Stenting

Stroke is the third leading cause of death in the United States, 80% of them are ischemic and 25% of all ischemic strokes are due to carotid stenosis [145].

Carotid endarterectomy (CEA) for symptomatic and asymptomatic carotid stenosis was shown in certain patients groups, to lower the risk of stroke by several large studies, if the 30-day rate of perioperative stroke or death is lower than 6% for patients with symptomatic carotid stenosis or 3% for those with asymptomatic carotid stenosis [146–148].

Several studies compared the CEA with the carotid angioplasty and stenting (CAS) [149–153]. To date, CAS may be the most advantageous in high-risk surgery patients with symptomatic carotid stenosis as indicated by the SAPPHIRE trial [151]. For the high operative risk patients with asymptomatic carotid stenosis CAS is still controversial.

The widely anticipated publication of the results of the National Institutes of Health funded CREST trial (lead-in phase closed) hopefully will answer the question of efficacy of CAS versus CEA for symptomatic and asymptomatic carotid stenosis [154, 155].

Preoperative Tumor Embolization

Preoperative endovascular embolization of skull base and hypervascular tumors of the central nervous system (CNS) achieve tumor resection with less blood loss; they are safer and more complete. The ischemia induced by the embolization makes the tumor softer and easier to resect [156–158]. However, major complications can be associated with preoperative embolization like inadvertent intracranial circulation embolization causing stroke or hemorrhage, intratumoral hemorrhage, and cranial nerve injuries; common minor complications are local pain and fever [159]. Advances in microcatheters and embolic agents make preoperative embolization an important part of the surgical treatment of a variety of CNS lesions and ultimately enhance patient care.

References

1. Schievink WI: Intracranial aneurysms, *N Engl J Med* 336:28–40, 1997.
2. Wiebers DO, Whisnant JP, Huston J III et al.: Unruptured intracranial aneurysms: natural history, clinical outcome, and risks of surgical and endovascular treatment, *Lancet* 362:103–110, 2003.
3. Yanaka K, Nagase S, Asakawa H, Matsumaru Y, Koyama A, Nose T: Management of unruptured cerebral aneurysms in patients with polycystic kidney disease, *Surg Neurol* 62:538–545, 2004.
4. Brisman JL, Song JK, Newell DW: Cerebral aneurysms, *N Engl J Med* 355(9):928–939, August 31, 2006.
5. The Magnetic Resonance Angiography in Relatives of Patients with Subarachnoid Hemorrhage Study Group. Risks and benefits of screening for intracranial aneurysms in first-degree relatives of patients with sporadic subarachnoid hemorrhage. *N Engl J Med* 341:1344–1350, 1999.
6. Ostergaard JR, Hog E: Incidence of multiple intracranial aneurysms, *J Neurosurg* 63:49–55, 1985.
7. Wijdicks EF, Kallmes DF, Manno EM, Fulgham JR, Piepgras DG: Subarachnoid hemorrhage: neurointensive care and aneurysm repair, *Mayo Clin Proc* 80:550–559, 2005.
8. Bederson JB, Awad IA, Wiebers DO et al.: Recommendations for the management of patients with unruptured intracranial aneurysms: a statement for healthcare professionals from the stroke council of the American heart association, *Stroke* 31:2742–2750, 2000.
9. Johnston SC, Selvin S, Gress DR: The burden, trends, and demographics of mortality from subarachnoid hemorrhage, *Neurology* 50:1413–1418, 1998.
10. Greenberg MS: SAH and aneurysms. In Greenberg MS, editors: *Handbook of neurosurgery*, ed. 5, New York, 2001, Thieme Medical Publishers, pp. 754–803.
11. Medele RJ, Stummer W, Mueller AJ, Steiger HJ, Reulen HJ: Terson's syndrome in subarachnoid hemorrhage and severe brain injury accompanied by acutely raised intracranial pressure, *J Neurosurg* 88(5):851–854, May 1998.
12. Unruptured intracranial aneurysms—risk of rupture and risks of surgical intervention. International study of unruptured intracranial aneurysms investigators. *N Engl J Med* 339(24):1725–1733, December 10, 1998.
13. Juvela S, Porras M, Poussa K: Natural history of unruptured intracranial aneurysms: probability and risk factors for aneurysm rupture, *Neurosurg Focus* 8(5):Preview 1, 2000.
14. Broderick JP, Brott TG, Duldner JE, Tomsick T, Leach A: Initial and recurrent bleeding are the major causes of death following subarachnoid hemorrhage, *Stroke* 25: 1342–1347, 1994.
15. Naidech AM, Janjua N, Kreiter KT, Ostapkovich ND, Fitzsimmons BF, Parra A, Commichau C, Connolly ES, Mayer SA: Predictors and impact of aneurysm rebleeding after subarachnoid hemorrhage, *Arch Neurol* 62:410–416, 2005.
16. Leipzig TJ, Redelman K, Horner TG: Reducing the risk of rebleeding before early aneurysm surgery: a possible role for antifibrinolytic therapy, *J Neurosurg* 86:220–225, 1997.
17. Hillman J, Fridriksson S, Nilsson O, Zhengquan Y, Saveland H, Jakobsson KE: Immediate administration of tranexamic acid and reduced incidence of early rebleeding after aneurysmal subarachnoid hemorrhage: a prospective randomized study, *J Neurosurg* 97:771–778, 2002.
18. Kouskouras C, Charitanti A, Giavroglou C et al.: Intracranial aneurysms: evaluation using CTA and MRA: correlation with DSA and intraoperative findings, *Neuroradiology* 46:842–850, 2004.
19. Okahara M, Kiyosue H, Yamashita M et al.: Diagnostic accuracy of magnetic resonance angiography for cerebral aneurysms in correlation with 3D-digital subtraction angiographic images: a study of 133 aneurysms, *Stroke* 33:1803–1808, 2002.
20. Heiserman JE, Dean BL, Hodak JA et al.: Neurologic complications of cerebral angiography, *AJNR Am J Neuroradiol* 15:1401–1407, 1994.
21. Dion JE, Gates PC, Fox AJ, Barnett HJ, Blom RJ: Clinical events following neuroangiography: a prospective study, *Stroke* 18:997–1004, 1987.

22. Anxionnat R, Bracard S, Ducrocq X et al.: Intracranial aneurysms: clinical value of 3D digital subtraction angiography in the therapeutic decision and endovascular treatment, *Radiology* 218:799–808, 2001.
23. Wang H, Fraser K, Wang D, Lanzino G: The evolution of endovascular therapy for neurosurgical disease, *Neurosurg Clin N Am* 16:223–229, 2005.
24. Guglielmi G, Vinuela F, Dion J, Duckwiler G: Electrothrombosis of saccular aneurysms via endovascular approach. Part 2: preliminary clinical experience, *J Neurosurg* 75:8–14, 1991.
25. Molyneux A, Kerr R, Stratton I et al.: International Subarachnoid Aneurysm Trial (ISAT) of neurosurgical clipping versus endovascular coiling in 2143 patients with ruptured intracranial aneurysms: a randomised trial, *Lancet* 360(9342):1267–1274, October 26, 2002.
26. CARAT Investigators. Rates of delayed rebleeding from intracranial aneurysms are low after surgical and endovascular treatment, *Stroke* 37:1437–1442, 2006.
27. Mitchell P, Kerr R, Mendelow AD et al.: could late rebleeding overturn the superiority of cranial aneurysm coil embolization over clip ligation seen in the international subarachnoid aneurysm trial? *J Neurosurg* 108(3):437–442, March 2008.
28. Solomon RA, Mayer SA, Tarmey JJ: Relationship between the volume of craniotomies for cerebral aneurysm performed at New York state hospitals and in-hospital mortality, *Stroke* 27:13–17, 1996.
29. Harry J: Cloft have you been smoking something that is biologically active? *AJNR Am J Neuroradiol* 27:240–242, 2006.
30. Raymond J, Guilbert F, Weill A et al.: Safety, science, and sales: a request for valid clinical trials to assess new devices for endovascular treatment of intracranial aneurysms, *AJNR Am J Neuroradiol* 25: 1128–1130, 2004.
31. White PM, Raymond J: Endovascular coiling of cerebral aneurysms using "bioactive" or coated-coil technologies: a systematic Review of the literature. AJNR Am J Neuroradiol, first published on Oct 8, 2008 as doi:10.3174/ajnr.A1324.
32. Friedman DP, Maitino AJ: Endovascular interventional neuroradiologic procedures: who is performing them, how often, and where? A survey of academic and nonacademic radiology practices, *AJNR Am J Neuroradiol* 24: 1772–1777, 2003.
33. Qureshi AI, Suri MF, Khan J et al.: Endovascular treatment of intracranial aneurysms by using Guglielmi detachable coils in awake patients: safety and feasibility, *J Neurosurg* 94:880–885, 2001.
34. Moret J, Cognard C, Weill A, Castaings L, Rey A: Reconstruction technic in the treatment of wide-neck intracranial aneurysms: long-term angiographic and clinical results: apropos of 56 cases, *J Neuroradiol* 24:30–44, 1997.
35. Sluzewski M, van Rooij WJ, Beute GN et al.: Balloon-assisted coil embolization of intracranial aneurysms: incidence, complications, and angiography results, *J Neurosurg* 105:396–399, 2006.
36. Derdeyn CP, Cross DT, Moran CJ et al.: Postprocedure ischemic events after treatment of intracranial aneurysms with Guglielmi detachable coils, *J Neurosurg* 96:837–843, 2002.
37. Lefkowitz MA, Gobin YP, Akiba Y et al.: Balloon assisted Guglielmi detachable coiling of widenecked aneurysms, Part II—clinical results, *Neurosurgery* 45(3):531–538, 1999.
38. Henkes H, Fischer S, Weber W et al.: Endovascular coil occlusion of 1811 intracranial aneurysms: early angiographic and clinical results, *Neurosurgery* 54:268–280, 2004.
39. Meyer FB: Balloon-assisted coil embolization of intracranial aneurysms, *J Neurosurg* 105:392, 2006
40. Heros RC: Complications of balloon-assisted coil embolization of intracranial aneurysms, *J Neurosurg* 105:393–395, 2006.
41. Park HK, Horowitz M, Jungreis C et al.: Periprocedural morbidity and mortality associated with endovascular treatment of intracranial aneurysms, *AJNR Am J Neuroradiol* 26:506–514, 2005.
42. Shapiro M, Babb J, Beckse T, Nelson PK: Safety and Efficacy of adjunctive balloon remodeling during endovascular treatment of intracranial aneurysms: a literature review, *AJNR Am J Neuroradiol* 29:1777–1781, 2008.
43. Howington JU, Hanel RA, Harrigan MR et al.: The Neuroform stent, the first microcatheter delivered stent for use in the intracranial circulation, *Neurosurgery* 54(1): 2–5, 2004.
44. Benitez RP, Silva MT, Klem J et al.: Endovascular occlusion of wide-necked aneurysms with a new intracranial microstent (Neuroform) and detachable coils, *Neurosurgery* 54(6):1359–1368, 2004.
45. Fiorella D, Thiabolt L, Albuquerque F, Deshmukh V, McDougall C, Rasmussen P: Antiplatelet therapy in neuroendovascular therapeutics, *Neurosurg Clin North Am* 16:517–540, 2005.
46. Fiorella D, Albuquerque FC, Han P, McDougall CG: Preliminary experience using the neuroform stent for the treatment of cerebral aneurysms, *Neurosurgery* 54:6–17, 2004.
47. Peluso JPP, van Rooij WJ, Sluzewski M, Beute GN: A new self-expandable nitinol stent for the treatment of wideneck aneurysms: initial clinical experience, *AJNR Am J Neuroradiol* 29:1405–1408, 2008.
48. Lopes DK, Ringer AJ, Boulos AS et al.: Fate of branch arteries after intracranial stenting, *Neurosurgery* 52(6):1275–1279, 2003.
49. Levy EI, Boulos AS, Hanel RA et al.: In vivo model of intracranial stent implantation: a pilot study to examine the histological response of cerebral vessels after randomized implantation of heparin-coated and uncoated endoluminal stents in a blinded fashion, *J Neurosurg* 98(3):544–553, 2003.
50. Tumialan L, Zhang J, Cawley M, Dion J, Barrow D: Intracranial hemorrhage associated with stent-assisted coil embolization of cerebral aneurysms: a cautionary report, *J Neurosurg* 108:1122–1129, 2008
51. Mandai S, Kinugasa K, Ohmoto T: Direct thrombosis of aneurysms with cellulose acetate polymer, Part I: results of thrombosis in experimental aneurysms, *J Neurosurg* 77(4):497–500, 1992.

52. Murayama Y, Vinuela F, Tateshima S et al.: Endovascular treatment of experimental aneurysms by use of a combination of liquid embolic agents and protective devices, *AJNR Am J Neuroradiol* 21(9):1726–1735, 2000.
53. Mawad ME, Cekirge S, Ciceri E et al.: Endovascular treatment of giant and large intracranial aneurysms by using a combination of stent placement and liquid polymer injection, *J Neurosurg* 96(3):474–482, 2002.
54. Molyneux AJ, Cekirge S, Saatci I et al.: Cerebral Aneurysm Multicenter European Onyx (CAMEO) trial: results of a prospective observational study in 20 European centers, *AJNR Am J Neuroradiol* 25(1):39–51, 2004.
55. Murayama Y, Vinuela F, Ulhoa A et al.: Nonadhesive liquid embolic agent for cerebral arteriovenous malformations: preliminary histopathological studies in swine rete mirabile, *Neurosurgery* 43(5):1164–1175, 1998.
56. Ricolfi F, Le Guerinel C, Blustajn J et al.: Rupture during treatment of recently ruptured aneurysms with Guglielmi electrodetachable coils, *AJNR Am J Neuroradiol* 19(9):1653–1658, 1998.
57. Vinuela F, Duckwiler G, Mawad M: Guglielmi detachable coil embolization of acute intracranial aneurysm: perioperative anatomical and clinical outcome in 403 patients, *J Neurosurg* 86(3):475–482, 1997.
58. Cloft HJ, Kallmes DF: Cerebral aneurysm perforations complicating therapy with guglielmi detachable coils: a meta-analysis, *AJNR Am J Neuroradiol* 23:1706–1709, 2002.
59. Doerfler A, Wanke I, Egelhof T, Dietrich U, Asgari S, Stolke D, Forsting M: Aneurysmal rupture during embolization with guglielmi detachable coils: causes, management, and outcome, *AJNR Am J Neuroradiol* 22:1825–1832, 2001.
60. Levy E, Koebbe CJ, Horowitz MB et al.: Rupture of intracranial aneurysms during endovascular coiling: management and outcomes, *Neurosurgery* 49(4):807–813, 2001.
61. Qureshi AI, Luft AR, Sharma M et al.: Prevention and treatment of thromboembolic and ischemic complications associated with endovascular procedures: Part II—clinical aspects and recommendations, *Neurosurgery* 46(6): 1360–1376, 2000.
62. Alexander MJ, Duckwiler GR, Gobin YP et al.: Management of intraprocedural arterial thrombus in cerebral aneurysm embolization with abciximab: technical case report, *Neurosurgery* 50(4):899–902, 2002.
63. Rordorf G, Bellon RJ, Budzik RE Jr et al.: Silent thromboembolic events associated with the treatment of unruptured cerebral aneurysms by use of Guglielmi detachable coils: prospective study applying diffusion-weighted imaging, *AJNR Am J Neuroradiol* 22(1):5–10, 2001.
64. Fiorella D, Albuquerque FC, Han P et al.: Strategies for the management of intraprocedural thromboembolic complications with abciximab (ReoPro), *Neurosurgery* 54(5):1089–1098, 2004.
65. Cronqvist M, Pierot L, Boulin A et al.: Local intraarterial fibrinolysis of thromboemboli occurring during endovascular treatment of intracerebral aneurysm: a comparison of anatomic results and clinical outcome, *AJNR Am J Neuroradiol* 19(1):157–165, 1998.
66. Qureshi AI, Dawson R, Frankel MR et al.: Recent advances in the management of vasospasm in patients with subarachnoid hemorrhage, *Neurologist* 2:53–65, 1996.
67. Rabinstein AA, Pichelmann MA, Friedman JA et al.: Symptomatic vasospasm and outcomes following aneurysmal subarachnoid hemorrhage: a comparison between surgical repair and endovascular coil occlusion, *J Neurosurg* 98:319–325, 2003.
68. Kassell NF, Sasaki T, Colohan ART et al.: Cerebral vasospasm following aneurysmal subarachnoid hemorrhage, *Stroke* 16:562–572, 1985.
69. Sundt TM Jr, Kobayashi S, Fode NC et al.: Results and complications of surgical management of 809 intracranial aneurysms in 722 cases. Related and unrelated to grade of patient, type of aneurysm, and timing of surgery, *J Neurosurg* 56(6):753–765, 1982.
70. Fisher CM, Kistler JP, Davis JM: Relation of cerebral vasospasm to subarachnoid hemorrhage visualized by computerized tomographic scanning, *Neurosurgery* 6(1):1–9, 1980.
71. Weir BK, Kongable GL, Kassell NF et al.: Cigarette smoking as a cause of aneurysmal subarachnoid hemorrhage and risk for vasospasm: a report of the cooperative aneurysm study, *J Neurosurg* 89(3): 405–411, 1998.
72. Zubkov YN, Nikiforov BM, Shustin VA: Balloon catheter technique for dilatation of constricted cerebral arteries after aneurysmal SAH, *Acta Neurochir (Wien)* 70:65–79, 1984.
73. Honma Y, Fujiwara T, Irie K et al.: Morphological changes in human cerebral arteries after percutaneous transluminal angioplasty for vasospasm caused by subarachnoid hemorrhage, *Neurosurgery* 36:1073–1080, 1995.
74. Rosenwasser RH, Armonda RA, Thomas JE et al.: Therapeutic modalities for the management of cerebral vasospasm: timing of endovascular options, *Neurosurgery* 44(5):975–980, 1999.
75. Polin RS, Coenen VA, Hansen CA et al.: Efficacy of transluminal angioplasty for the management of symptomatic cerebral vasospasm following aneurismal subarachnoid hemorrhage, *J Neurosurg* 92:284–290, 2000.
76. Rabinstein AA, Friedman JA, Nichols DA et al.: Predictors of outcome after endovascular treatment of cerebral vasospasm, *AJNR Am J Neuroradiol* 25: 1778–1782, 2004.
77. Linskey ME, Horton JA, Rao GR et al.: Fatal rupture of the intracranial carotid artery during transluminal angioplasty for vasospasm induced by subarachnoid hemorrhage. Case report, *J Neurosurg* 74:985–990, 1991.
78. Hanel RA, Lopes DK, Wehman JC, Savageau E, Levy EI, Guterman L, Hopkins LN: Endovascular treatment of intracranial aneurysms and vasospasm after aneurysmal subarachnoid hemorrhage, *Neurosurg Clin North Am* 16:317–353, 2005.
79. Badjatia N, Topcuoglu MA, Pryor JC et al.: Preliminary experience with intra-arterial nicardipine as a treatment for cerebral vasospasm, *AJNR Am J Neuroradiol* 25: 819–826, 2004.
80. Hänggi D, Turowski B, Beseoglu K, Yong M: Steiger intra-arterial nimodipine for severe cerebral vasospasm after aneurysmal subarachnoid hemorrhage: influence

on clinical course and cerebral perfusion, *AJNR Am J Neuroradiol* 29:1053–1060, June 2008.
81. Feng L, Fitzsimmons BF, Young WL, Berman MF, Lin E, Aagaard BD, Duong H, Pile-Spellman J: Intraarterially administered verapamil as adjunct therapy for cerebral vasospasm: safety and 2-year experience, *AJNR Am J Neuroradiol* 23:1284–1290, September 2002.
82. Brown RD, Wiebers DO, Forbes GS et al.: The natural history of unruptured intracranial arteriovenous malformations, *J Neurosurg* 68:352–357, 1988.
83. Mast H, Mohr JP, Osipov A et al.: "Steal" is an unestablished mechanism for the clinical presentation of cerebral arteriovenous malformation, *Stroke* 26: 1215–1220, 1995.
84. Ondra S, Troupp H, George E et al.: The natural history of symptomatic arteriovenous malformations of the brain: a 24-year follow-up assessment, *J Neurosurg* 73:387–391, 1990.
85. Hartmann A, Mast H, Mohr JP et al.: Morbidity of intracranial hemorrhage in patients with cerebral arteriovenous malformation, *Stroke* 29:931–934, 1998.
86. Nataf F, Meder JF, Roux FX et al.: Angioarchitecture associated with haemorrhage in cerebral arteriovenous malformations: a prognostic statistical model, *Neuroradiology* 39:52–58, 1997.
87. Brown RD, Wiebers DO, Forbes GS: Unruptured intracranial aneurysms and arteriovenous malformations: frequency of intracranial hemorrhage and relationship of lesions, *Neurosurgery* 73:859–863, 1990.
88. Cockroft KM, Thompson RC, Steinberg GK: Aneurysms and arteriovenous malformations, *Neurosurg Clin N Am* 9:565–576, 1998.
89. Thompson RC, Steinberg GK, Levy RP et al.: The management of patients with arteriovenous malformations and associated intracranial aneurysms, *Neurosurgery* 43: 202–211, 1998.
90. Spetzler RF, Martin NA: A proposed grading system for arteriovenous malformations, *J Neurosurg* 65:476–483, 1986.
91. Luessenhop AJ, Spence WT: Artificial embolization of cerebral arteries: report of use in a case of arteriovenous malformation, *JAMA* 172:1153–1155, 1960.
92. Zanetti PH, Sherman FE: Experimental evaluation of a tissue adhesive as an agent for the treatment of aneurysms and arteriovenous anomalies, *J Neurosurg* 36:72–79, 1972.
93. Rauch RA, Vinuela F, Dion J et al.: Preembolization functional evaluation in brain arteriovenous malformations: the superselective Amytal test, *AJNR Am J Neuroradiol* 13(1):303–308, 1992.
94. The N-BCA Trial Investigators. N-butyl cyanoacrylate embolization of cerebral arteriovenous malformations: results of a prospective, randomized, multi-center trial, *AJNR Am J Neuroradiol* 23(5):748–755, 2002.
95. Cromwell LD, Kerber CW: Modification of cyanoacrylate for therapeutic embolization: preliminary experience, *AJR Am J Roentgenol* 132(5):799–801, 1979.
96. Stoesslein F, Ditscherlein G, Romaniuk PA: Experimental studies on new liquid embolization mixtures (histoacryl-lipiodol, histoacryl-panthopaque), *Cardiovasc Intervent Radiol* 5(5):264–267, 1982.
97. Taki W, Yonekawa Y, Iwata H, Uno A, Yamashita K, Amemiya H: A new liquid material for embolization of arteriovenous malformations, *AJNR Am J Neuroradiol* 11(1):163–168, 1990.
98. Jahan R, Murayama Y, Gobin YP, Duckwiler GR, Vinters HV, Vinuela F: Embolization of arteriovenous malformations with Onyx: clinicopathological experience in 23 patients, *Neurosurgery* 48(5):984–997, 2001.
99. Niemann DB, Molyneux AJ: Embolization of brain AVMs with ethylene-vinyl alcohol copolymer dissolved in DMSO (Onyx-liquid embolic system): evidence in a prospective series of 31 patients [abstract], *J Neurosurg* 96:171A, 2002.
100. Gobin YP, Laurent A, Merienne L et al.: Treatment of brain arteriovenous malformations by embolization and radiosurgery, *J Neurosurg* 85:19–28, 1996.
101. Valavanis A, Yasargil MG: The endovascular treatment of brain arteriovenous malformations, *Adv Tech Stand Neurosurg* 24:131–214, 1998.
102. Akin ED, Perkins E, Ross IB: Surgical handling characteristics of an ethylene vinyl alcohol copolymer compared with N-butyl cyanoacrylate used for embolization of vessels in an arteriovenous malformation resection model in swine, *J Neurosurg* 98(2):366–370, 2003.
103. Gobin YP, Laurent A, Merienne L et al.: Treatment of brain arteriovenous malformations by embolization and radiosurgery, *J Neurosurg* 85:19–28, 1996.
104. Frizzel RT, Fisher WS: Cure, morbidity, and mortality associated with embolization of brain arteriovenous malformations: a review of 1246 patients in 32 series over a 35-year period, *J Neurosurg* 37:1031–1040, 1995.
105. Nishijima M, Takaku A, Endo S, Kuwayama N, Koizumi F, Sato H et al.: Etiological evaluation of dural arteriovenous malformations of the lateral and sigmoid sinuses based on histopathological examinations, *J Neurosurg* 76(4):600–606, 1992.
106. Awad IA, Little JR, Akarawi WP et al.: Intracranial dural arteriovenous malformations: factors predisposing to an aggressive neurological course, *J Neurosurg* 72:839–850, 1990.
107. Borden JA, Wu JK, Shucart WA: A proposed classification for spinal and cranial dural arteriovenous fistulous malformations and implications for treatment, *J Neurosurg* 82(2):166–179, 1995.
108. Davies MA, Ter Brugge K, Willinski R et al.: The natural history and management of intracranial dural arteriovenous fistulae. Part 2: aggressive lesions, *Intervent Neuroradiol* 3:303–311, 1997.
109. Davies MA, Saleh J, Ter Brugge K et al.: The natural history and management of intracranial dural arteriovenous fistulae. Part 1: benign lesions, *Intervent Neuroradiol* 3:295–302, 1997.
110. Soderman M, Edner G, Ericson K et al.: Gamma knife surgery for dural arteriovenous shunts: 25 years of experience, *J Neurosurg* 104:867–875, 2006.
111. Malek A, Halbach V, Higashida R, Phatouros C, Meyers P, Dowd C: Treatment of dural arteriovenous malformations and fistulas, *Neurosurg Clin N Am* 11(1): 147–166, 2000.
112. Dawson RC 3rd, Joseph GJ, Owens DS et al.: Transvenous embolization as the primary therapy for arteriovenous

fistulas of the lateral and sigmoid sinuses, *Am J Neuroradiol* 19:571–576, 1998.
113. Halbach VV, Higashida RT, Hieshima GB, Reicher M, Norman D, Newton TH: Dural fistulas involving the cavernous sinus: results of treatment in 30 patients, *Radiology* 163(2):437–442, 1987.
114. McDougall C, Halbach V, Higashida R: Treatment of dural arteriovenous fistulas, *Neurosurg Q* 7:110–134, 1997.
115. Halbach VV, Higashida RT, Hieshima GB, Wilson CB, Barnwell SL, Dowd CF: Dural arteriovenous fistulas supplied by ethmoidal arteries, *Neurosurgery* 26(5):816–823, 1990.
116. Kurl S, Saari T, Vannine R et al.: Dural arteriovenous fistulas of superior sagittal sinus: case report and review of literature, *Surg Neurol* 45:250–255, 1996.
117. Fukai J, Terada T, Kuwata T et al.: Transarterial intravenous coil embolization of dural arteriovenous fistula involving the superior sagittal sinus, *Surg Neurol* 55: 353–358, 2001.
118. Barnwell SL, Halbach VV, Dowd CF et al.: A variant of arteriovenous fistulas within the wall of dural sinuses. Results of combined surgical and endovascular therapy, *J Neurosurg* 74:199–204, 1991.
119. Cognard C, Januel AC, Silva NA Jr, Tall P: endovascular treatment of intracranial dural arteriovenous fistulas with cortical venous drainage: new management using onyx, *AJNR Am J Neuroradiol* 29:235–241, February 2008
120. The National Institute of Neurological Disorders and Stroke rt-PA Stroke Study Group. Tissue plasminogen activator for acute ischemic stroke. *N Engl J Med* 333(24):1581–1587, 1995.
121. Jansen O, Schellinger P, Fiebach J et al.: Early revascularization in acute ischemic stroke saves tissue at risk defined by MRI, *Lancet* 353:2036–2037, 1997.
122. Saqqur M, Uchino K, Demchuk A, Molina C, Garami Z, Calleja S, Akhtar N, Orouk F, Salam A, Shuaib A, Alexandrov A, and for CLOTBUST investigators: site of arterial occlusion identified by transcranial doppler predicts the response to intravenous thrombolysis for stroke, *Stroke* 38:948–954, 2007.
123. Rha J, Saver J: The impact of recanalization on ischemic stroke outcome: a meta-analysis, *Stroke* 38:967–973, 2007.
124. Molina C, Alexandrov A, Demchuk A, Saqqur M, Uchino K, Alvarez-Sabín J: Improving the predictive accuracy of recanalization on stroke outcome in patients treated with tissue plasminogen activator, *Stroke* 35: 151–156, 2004.
125. Wolpert S, Bruckmann H, Greenlee R, Wechsler L, Pessin M, del Zoppo G, and the rt-PA Acute Stroke Study Group. Neuroradiologic evaluation of patients with acute stroke treated with recombinant tissue plasminogen activator, *AJNR Am J Neuroradiol* 14:3–13, 1993.
126. Alexandrov AV, Grotta JC: Arterial reocclusion in stroke patients treated with intravenous tissue plasminogen activator, *Neurology* 59:862–867, 2002.
127. Furlan A, Higashida R, Wechsler L et al.: Intra-arterial prourokinase for acute ischemic stroke. The PROACT II Study: a randomized controlled trial, *JAMA* 282: 2003–2011, 1999.
128. Adams HP, Adams RJ, Brott T et al.: Guidelines for the early management of patients with ischemic stroke: a scientific statement from the stroke council of the American stroke association, *Stroke* 34:1056–1083, 2003.
129. IMS Trial Investigators. Combined intravenous and intra-arterial revascularization for acute ischemic stroke: the interventional management of stroke study, *Stroke* 35:904–911, 2004.
130. Smith WS, Sung G, Starkman S et al.: Safety and efficacy of mechanical embolectomy in acute ischemic stroke: results of the MERCI trial, *Stroke* 36:1432–1438, 2005.
131. Smith WS: Safety of mechanical thrombectomy and intravenous tissue plasminogen activator in acute ischemic stroke. Results of the multi Mechanical Embolus Removal in Cerebral Ischemia (MERCI) trial, part I, *AJNR Am J Neuroradiol* 27:1177–1182, 2006.
132. Bose A, Henkes H, Alfke K, Reith W, Mayer TE, Berlis A, Branca V, Sit SP, for the Penumbra Phase 1 Stroke Trial Investigators: the penumbra system: a mechanical device for the treatment of acute stroke due to thromboembolism, *AJNR Am J Neuroradiol* 29:1409–1413, 2008.
133. IMS II Trial Investigators. The interventional management of stroke (IMS) II study, *Stroke* 38:2127–2135, 2007.
134. Ringer AJ, Qureshi AI, Fessler RD et al.: Angioplasty of intracranial occlusion resistant to thrombolysis in acute ischemic stroke, *Neurosurgery* 48:1282–1288, 2001.
135. Lum C, Stys PK, Hogan MJ, Nguyen TB, Srinivasan A, Goyal M: Acute anterior circulation stroke: recanalization using clot angioplasty, *Can J Neurol Sci* 33(2):217–222, 2006.
136. Chimowitz MI, Lynn MJ, Howlett-Smith H, Stern BJ, Hertzberg VS, Frankel MR, Levine SR, Chaturvedi S, Kasner SE, Benesch CG, Sila CA, Jovin TG, Romano JG, for the Warfarin-Aspirin Symptomatic Intracranial Disease Trial Investigators: Comparison of warfarin and aspirin for symptomatic intracranial arterial stenosis, *N Engl J Med* 352:1305–1316, 2005.
137. Sundt TM Jr, Smith HC, Campbell JK, Vliestra RE, Cucchiara RF, Stanson AW: Transluminal angioplasty for basilar artery stenosis, *Mayo Clin Proc* 55:673–680, 1980.
138. O'Leary DH, Clouse ME: Percutaneous transluminal angioplasty of the cavernous carotid artery for recurrent ischemia, *AJNR Am J Neuroradiol* 5:644–645, 1984.
139. Mazighi M, Yadav J, Abou-Chebl A: Durability of endovascular therapy for symptomatic intracranial atherosclerosis, *Stroke* 39:1766–1769, 2008.
140. SSYLVIA Study Investigators. Stenting of Symptomatic Atherosclerotic Lesions in the Vertebral or Intracranial Arteries (SSYLVIA): study results, *Stroke* 35:1388–1392, 2004.
141. Bose A, Hartmann M, Henkes H, Liu HM, Teng MM, Szikora I, Berlis A, Reul J, Yu SC, Forsting M, Lui M, Lim W, Sit SP: A novel, selfexpanding, nitinol stent in medically refractory intracranial atherosclerotic stenoses: the wingspan study, *Stroke* 38:1531–1537, 2007.
142. Fiorella D, Levy EI, Turk AS, Albuquerque FC, Niemann DB, Aagaard-Kienitz B, Hanel RA, Woo H, Rasmussen PA, Hopkins LN, Masaryk TJ, McDougall CG: US multicenter experience with the wingspan stent system for the treatment of intracranial atheromatous disease: periprocedural results, *Stroke* 38:881–887, 2007.

143. Levy EI, Turk AS, Albuquerque FC, Niemann DB, Aagaard-Kienitz B, Pride L, Purdy P, Welch B, Woo H, Rasmussen PA, Hopkins LN, Masaryk TJ, McDougall CG, Fiorella DJ: Wingspan in-stent restenosis and thrombosis: incidence, clinical presentation and management, *Neurosurgery* 61:644–650, 2007.
144. Stenting versus Aggressive Medical Management for Preventing Recurrent Stroke in Intracranial Stenosis (SAMMPRIS) ClinicalTrials.gov
145. Bonita R: Epidemiology of stroke, *Lancet* 339:342–344, 1992.
146. North Am Symptomatic Carotid Endarterectomy Trial Collaborators. Beneficial effect of carotid endarterectomy in symptomatic patients with high-grade carotid stenosis, *N Engl J Med* 32(5):445–453, 1991.
147. European Carotid Surgery Trial. Randomised trial of endarterectomy for recently symptomatic carotid stenosis: final results of the MRC European Carotid Surgery Trial (ECST), *Lancet* 35(1):1379–1387, 1998.
148. Executive Committee for the Asymptomatic Carotid Atherosclerosis Study. Endarterectomy for asymptomatic carotid artery stenosis, *JAMA* 27(3):1421–1428, 1995.
149. CAVATAS Investigators. Endovascular versus surgical treatment in patients with carotid stenosis in the Carotid and Vertebral Artery Transluminal Angioplasty Study (CAVATAS): a randomized trial, *Lancet* 357:1729–1737, 2001.
150. CARESS Steering Committee. Carotid revascularization using endarterectomy or stenting systems (CARESS): phase I clinical trial, *J Endovasc Ther* 10:1021–1030, 2003.
151. Yadav JS, Wholey MD, Kuntz RE et al.: Stenting and angioplasty with protection in patients at high risk for endarterectomy investigators. Protected carotid-artery stenting versus endarterectomy in high-risk patients, *N Engl J Med* 351:1493–1501, 2004.
152. Mas JL, Chatellier G, Beyssen B et al.: EVA-3S Investigators. Endarterectomy versus stenting in patients with symptomatic severe carotid stenosis, *N Engl J Med* 355:1660–1671, 2006.
153. Ringleb PA, Allenberg J, Bruckmann H et al.: SPACE collaborative group. 30 day results from the SPACE trial of stent-protected angioplasty versus carotid endarterectomy in symptomatic patients: a randomised non-inferiority trial, *Lancet* 368:1239–1247, 2006.
154. CREST. Carotid Revascularization Endarterectomy vs Stent Trial. The Internet Stroke Center.
155. Pelz DM, Levy EI, Hopkins LN: Advances in interventional neuroradiology 2007, *Stroke* 39:268–272, 2008.
156. Gandhi D, Gemmete JJ, Ansari SA, Gujar SK: Mukherji interventional neuroradiology of the head and neck, *AJNR Am J Neuroradiol* 29:1806–1815, November 2008.
157. Choi IS, Tantivatana J: Neuroendovascular management of intracranial and spinal tumors, *Neurosurg Clin N Am* 11:167–185, 2000.
158. Abramowitz J, Dion JE, Jensen ME, Lones M, Duckwiler GR, Vinuela F, Bentson JR: Angiographic diagnosis and management of head and neck schwannomas, *AJNR Am J Neuroradiol* 12:977–984, September 1991.
159. Bendszus M, Monoranu CM, Schütz A, Nölte I, Vince GH, Solymosi L: Neurologic complications after particle embolization of intracranial meningiomas, *AJNR Am J Neuroradiol* 26:1413–1419, June 2005.
160. Cognard C, Gobin YP, Pierot L, Bailly AL, Houdart E, Casasco A et al.: Cerebral dural arteriovenous fistulas: clinical and angiographic correlation with a revised classification of venous drainage, *Radiology* 194(3):671–680, 1995.

The Current Status of Hybrid Repair of Thoracoabdominal Aortic Aneurysms

26

Christopher J. Kwolek and Rajendra Patel

The management of thoracoabdominal aortic aneurysms (TAAA) remains a significant challenge for vascular and cardiovascular specialists involved in the treatment of complex aortic disease. Until recently, open repair with visceral and intercostal reimplantation, along with adjunctive measures to decrease the incidence of spinal chord ischemia, was the only interventional option available to treat these patients (Fig. 26.1). The commercial availability of thoracic aortic stent grafts has now allowed the possibility of using endovascular techniques to treat this complex anatomy.

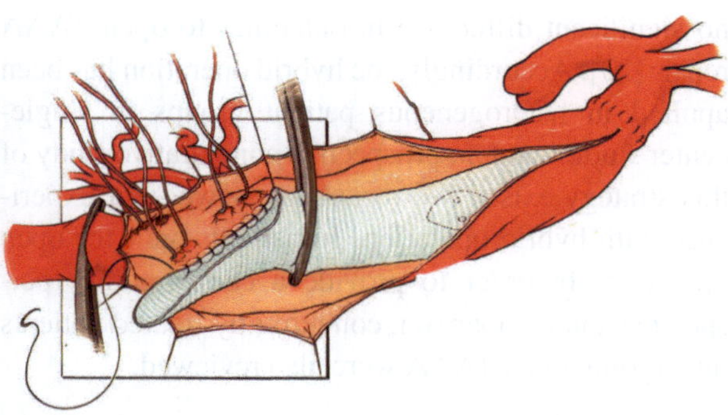

Fig. 26.1 Until recently, open repair with visceral and intercostal reimplantation, along with adjunctive measures to decrease the incidence of spinal chord ischemia, was the only interventional option available to treat these patients

C.J. Kwolek (✉)
Associate Visiting Professor, Program Director, Division of Vascular and Endovascular Surgery, Department of Surgery, Harvard Medical School, Massachusetts General Hospital, Boston, MA, USA
e-mail: ckwolek@partners.org

Current Status of Open Repair

Excellent results have been achieved in a several high-volume centers specializing in the open repair of TAAA. Invariably centers with the best results have developed specialized teams of surgeons, anesthesiologists, and critical care staff dedicated to the management of these complex patients. However, even in such institutions, the reported mortality rates of 5–10% are significantly higher than those reported for elective infrarenal abdominal aortic aneurysm (AAA) repair [1–3]. In addition, despite the use of adjunctive measures such as atriofemoral bypass, cerebrospinal fluid (CSF) drainage, and epidural cooling, spinal chord ischemia (SCI) remains a significant problem in 4–15% of patients.

In our experience, perioperative mortality has been a consistent 8% over the past 20 years [3, 4]. Additional follow-up studies have documented both favorable durability [5] and preserved functional status in long-term surviving patients [6]. However, patients unfit to withstand open operation are commonly encountered and their prognosis is poor [7]. Severe chronic obstructive pulmonary disease (COPD) often precludes open TAAA repair, yet COPD also constitutes an independent risk factor for aneurysm expansion and rupture [8, 9]. Thus, an alternative approach for treating these high-risk patients is desirable.

Furthermore, the outcomes achieved by centers of excellence have not been reproducible across a broader spectrum of institutions. Cowan recently reported a mortality rate of over 22% when evaluating the results of elective open TAAA repair in the United States [10]. This higher mortality rate was driven by the nearly two-fold increase in mortality when comparing

T.J. Fogarty, R.A. White (eds.), *Peripheral Endovascular Interventions*,
DOI 10.1007/978-1-4419-1387-6_26, © Springer Science+Business Media, LLC 1998, 2010

high-volume and low-volume institutions and high-volume vs. low-volume surgeons. Rigberg et al. recently noted an overall mortality of 19% at 1 year in the state of California, with a significant delayed mortality of 31% at 1 year for patients undergoing elective TAAA repair. With increasing age, the results were even more dramatic, with patients greater than 75 years of age having a cumulative 1-year mortality of 40% [11]. These results clearly support the concept of developing regional centers of excellence for the management of thoracic aortic disease while investigating new methods to potentially decrease the morbidity and mortality associated with treating these patients.

Endovascular Approaches to the Management of Thoracoabdominal Aortic Aneurysms

The advent of endovascular aneurysm repair (EVAR) has revolutionized the management of infrarenal AAA. Currently up to 70% of infrarenal AAAs may be treated with an endovascular approach, and it has become the preferred approach for managing high-risk patients [12, 13]. At the same time, the diffusion of this technology has allowed a broader spectrum of centers to safely treat AAA.

More recently, the availability of thoracic aortic stent grafts has allowed many centers to treat a variety of pathologies in the descending thoracic aorta including degenerative aneurysms with decreased morbidity and mortality compared with open repair [14, 15].

Thus, it would seem logical to expand the use of endovascular techniques to treat TAAA. However, the absence of a suitable proximal and distal seal zones for stent grafts in the aortic arch and the visceral abdominal segment limits its applicability in many TAAA patients. Current commercially available devices have a limited ability to deal with the visceral, renal, and arch vessels.

The successful endovascular treatment of TAAA using branched graft repair has been reported for high-risk TAAA patients [16, 17]. Recently, Chuter reported a 9.5% mortality in a high-risk cohort of patients deemed unfit for open repair. However, these custom-made devices are only available at limited sites here in the United States through the use of food and drug administration (FDA)-approved institutional device exemptions (IDEs). Thus, the availability of these grafts in the United States is currently quite limited. Furthermore, given the significant logistical, regulatory, and technical issues with custom-made branched grafts and the wide variability of visceral segment anatomy in TAAA patients, this situation is unlikely to change in the near future. Thus, the development of hybrid operations to manage complex thoracic aortic disease appears to be the most viable option at the moment for the vast majority of centers.

Hybrid operations which combine both open (typically visceral/renal debranching) and endovascular techniques were first reported in 1999 [18]. This consists of an open operation in which the visceral segment of the abdominal aorta is debranched via extra-anatomic bypass grafts originating from the distal abdominal aorta or iliac arteries to provide a distal seal zone for subsequent placement of a thoracic endograft. The endograft distal attachment site can be in the native visceral segment, in an infrarenal graft, or even in the iliac arteries [19] (Fig. 26.2).

The hybrid repair of TAAA has been suggested to have lower mortality in high-risk patients [20, 21] and is the preferred repair at certain centers [22] largely with the rationale that open operation has produced unacceptable morbidity. Other reports of hybrid TAAA repair involving visceral vessels have demonstrated no significant difference in outcomes to open TAAA repair [23]. Accordingly, the hybrid operation has been applied in heterogeneous patient groups in single-center studies and no prospective comparative study of this strategy exists. We recently reviewed our experience with hybrid operations in patients unfit for open operation. In order to provide a contemporary perspective and comparison, concurrently treated patients undergoing open TAAA were also reviewed.

Massachusetts General Hospital Results

We recently reviewed the results of 23 high-risk patients with thoracoabdominal aneurysms who underwent either mesenteric or mesenteric and renal debranching with subsequent thoracic endograft placement between June 2005 and December 2007. These patients were compared with patients who underwent an open TAA repair ($n = 77$) during the same time period [24].

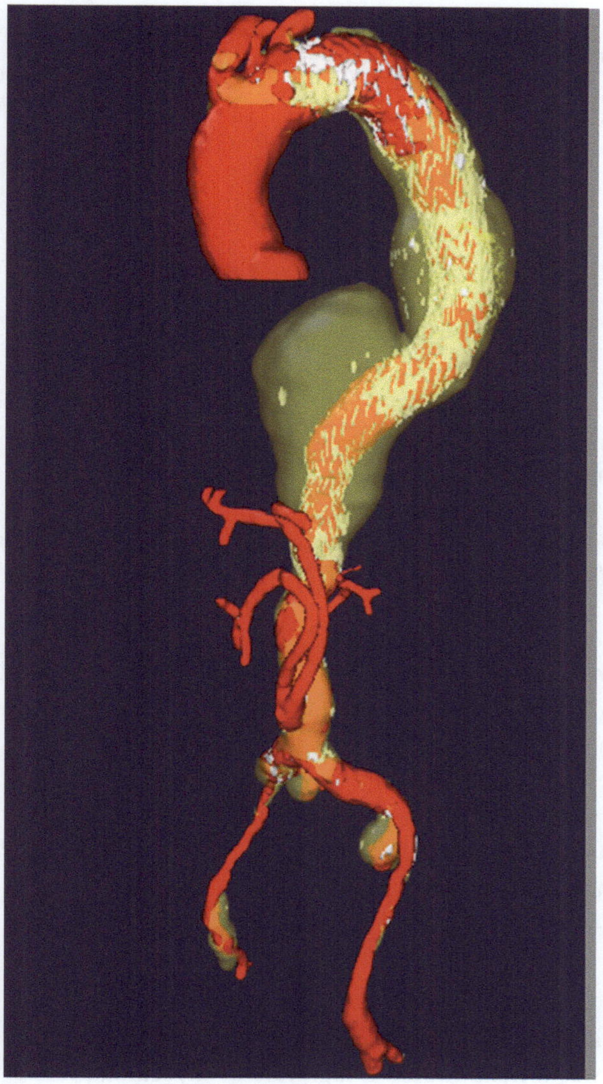

Fig. 26.2 The endograft distal attachment site can be in the native visceral segment, in an infrarenal graft, or even in the iliac arteries

Patients in the hybrid group were stratified as high risk for open repair based on advanced age/poor functional status (mean age 81 years, *n* = 14), severe oxygen-dependent COPD (*n* = 8), obesity (*n* = 2), or previous open thoracic (*n* = 4) or TAAA repair (*n* = 2) with six patients having overlapping high-risk criteria. The median age for this group was 76.6 years with a range of 59–86 years. The mean aneurysm size was 6.5 cm (range 5.2–8.5 cm); 69.6% of the hybrid patients presented on an elective basis and TAAA extent by Crawford classification was type I 9 (39%), type II 5 (22%), type III 9 (39%), and type IV 0 (0%). Hybrid TAAA repair was not considered for patients with type IV TAAA since the perceived surgical insult for debranching was felt to be equivalent to that for open repair in our institution. The majority (*n* = 13) of patients underwent staged repair with a mean interval between stages of 3 days excluding one patient who had a delayed interval of 82 days partly due to a myocardial infarction after the first surgery. Ten patients underwent a single-staged procedure.

Staged patients underwent debranching of the renal and/or mesenteric vessels first followed by placement of a thoracic endograft (W.L. Gore & Assoc., Flagstaff, Az) including coverage of the visceral vessel origins. Single-staged procedures involved the mesenteric debranching followed by the placement of the thoracic endograft. Since long-segment thoracic aortic coverage was routine, placement of a cerebrospinal fluid drainage catheter was used in all hybrid cases. Mesenteric debranching was performed via a midline laparotomy with multi-branched Dacron grafts sutured to the native infrarenal aorta (*n* = 5), infrarenal graft placed during debranching (*n* = 7), previous infrarenal graft (*n* = 8), or native iliac arteries (*n* = 3). Debranching involved all four mesenteric/renal vessels (*n* = 11), mesenteric alone (*n* = 8), or a variation in between (*n* = 4). Placement of the thoracic endograft was via the iliac arteries or conduit if the iliac artery diameter would not accommodate the device. Postoperatively all patients were placed in the intensive care unit. The cerebrospinal catheter was removed 48–72 h thereafter. Patient follow-up was at 1 month, between 3 and 6 months, and at 1 year. Preoperative SVS risk scores were calculated in a manner previously reported [25].

The open TAAA group consisted of 77 consecutive patients [Crawford extent type I 13 (17%), type II 11 (14%), type III 27 (35%), and type IV 26 (34%)] who underwent open TAAA repair during the same time period as the hybrid patients' treatment. The mean age for the patient population was 72.7 years (range 38–92 years) and the mean aneurysm size was 6.5 cm (range 4–10 cm); 74.0% underwent elective repair. Preoperative SVS scores were calculated in a similar manner as in the hybrid group. During surgery routine use of cerebrospinal catheter drainage was employed in extent I–III TAAA; details of the technical aspects of surgery have been previously reported [4]. Patients were evaluated at 1 month and at 1 year.

Demographics and clinical features of the study groups are displayed in Table 26.1. Cardiopulmonary

Table 26.1 Preoperative demographics

	Hybrid repair $n = 23$	Open repair $n = 77$	p value
Age (years)	76.6 ± 7.1	72.7 ± 10.1	0.085
Gender (male)	7 (30.4%)	36 (46.8%)	0.165
Diabetes mellitus	6 (26.1%)	8 (10.4%)	0.057
Severe COPD (oxygen dependent)	8 (34.8%)	2 (2.6%)	<0.0001
Hypertension (severe: 3 or + meds)	11 (47.8%)	18 (23.4%)	0.023
Tobacco (past or current)	16 (69.6%)	29 (37.7%)	0.007
Compensated CHF or arrhythmia	10 (43.5%)	15 (19.5%)	0.020
Creatinine, serum (>1.5 mg/dl)	5 (23.8%)	27 (35.1%)	0.434
SVS risk score	9.13 ± 3.17	6.01 ± 2.25	<0.0001

Table 26.2 Complications and disposition

	Hybrid repair $n = 23$	Open repair $n = 77$	p value
Perioperative death (30 day)	4 (17.4%)	6 (7.8%)	0.232
In-hospital death	6 (26.1%)	8 (10.4%)	0.271
Paraplegia (permanent)	1 (4.3%)	3 (3.9%)	0.983
Composite death and paraplegia (30 days)	5 (21.7%)	9 (11.7%)	0.334
Cardiac			
Myocardial infarction	5 (21.7%)	7 (9.1%)	0.14
Arrhythmia	3 (13.0%)	8 (10.4%)	0.712
Neurological			
Stroke	0 (0%)	1 (1.3%)	1
Pulmonary			
Pneumonia	4 (17.4%)	14 (18.2%)	1
Tracheostomy	1 (4.3%)	11 (14.3%)	0.286
Any reoperation	9 (39.1%)	16 (20.8%)	0.033
Length of stay (days)	14.9 (3–69)	18.3 (0–98)	0.369

comorbidities and composite SVS risk score were significantly elevated in the hybrid group. There was no significant difference in aneurysm size and non-elective operation between groups; however, the hybrid group was noted to have a higher proportion of patients with reoperative thoracic or descending TAA repairs.

The hybrid group had a greater than two-fold increase in perioperative death, but as detailed in Table 26.2, this did not achieve statistical significance. Excluding type IV TAAA from the open group did not change the trend toward higher mortality in the hybrid group (26%) vs. the open group (13%); however, this again did not achieve statistical significance ($p = 0.17$). Both groups had similar rates of paraplegia. Interestingly, the hybrid group had a significantly higher rate of any surgical re-intervention (34.8 vs. 20.8%; $p = 0.03$) such as tracheostomy, bleeding, wound disruption, endoleak, and graft thrombosis. Postoperative complication rates for renal failure, arrhythmia, and pneumonia were not different. There was a trend toward a high rate of myocardial infarction in the hybrid group (21.7 vs. 9.1%; $p = 0.14$); however, this was not statistically significant. Of note, hybrid-specific complications included a 10% graft thrombosis rate (7/70 bypass grafts) with one patient having 3/4 grafts thrombosed due to heparin-induced thrombocytopenia and 5/23 patients (22%) developing an endoleak with three patients requiring a total of four endovascular re-interventions.

Discussion

From a practical standpoint the hybrid operation has been available to most surgeons in the United States since commercial approval of the first thoracic endograft in April 2005 [15]. Given the significant morbidity and mortality of open TAAA, especially outside of high-volume centers [10], limiting the scope of the operation, especially for patients with major comorbidities, seems logical. Hybrid repair, by the avoidance of the thoracotomy, potential paralysis of the left hemidiaphragm, and cross-clamping of the aorta, has the potential to decrease overall morbidity. The potential benefit of reduced spinal cord ischemia has also been suggested [22]. Our focus was to review results in patients denied open repair similar to the original EVAR paradigm [13, 26].

A significant proportion of the hybrid patients (n = 18; 78%) were followed for a period of time, since they were not considered candidates for open operation given their comorbidities. Perhaps most notable in this regard were patients with severe COPD. In Crawford's series of 94 patients denied open operation for TAAA, 46% of patients were denied repair secondary to severe COPD [7]. In our series, 35% (n = 8) of patients undergoing hybrid TAAA repair were felt to be at high risk due to significant pulmonary comorbidity. It seems logical that avoidance of a thoracotomy and disturbance of the left hemidiaphragm function would translate into decreased pulmonary morbidity, the single most frequently occurring complication of open TAAA repair [3]. Hybrid operation may also have an advantage in the setting of redo thoracotomy by decreasing bleeding and left lung contusion [27].

Hybrid repair has also been suggested to have lower incidence of spinal cord ischemia (SCI) with paraplegia rates reported from 0 [22] to 16% [21] (Table 26.3). This argument is based on the avoidance of aortic cross-clamping and is an extension of the experience with TEVAR for repair of isolated thoracic aneurysms [28, 29]. Several comparative trials have documented a decreased risk of spinal chord ischemia with TEVAR vs. open repair of descending thoracic aortic aneurysms [28, 30]. However, our experience with TEVAR for isolated descending aneurysm did not demonstrate a difference in the incidence of SCI. Presumably this is due to our favorable results for open repair utilizing CSF drainage and epidural cooling [3, 4, 14].

In addition, the risk of SCI with TEVAR for descending aortic aneurysms would be expected to be lower than that with hybrid repair, since hybrid operations often involve long-segment thoracoabdominal coverage which has been shown to increase spinal cord ischemia rates [31]. Hybrid operations may also involve replacement of the infrarenal segment of the aorta, in addition to thoracoabdominal stent graft placement, again increasing the risk for spinal cord ischemia. While touted as a surgery of limited extent compared with open TAAA repair, hybrid repair of TAAA remains an operation of significant magnitude. Given the small numbers of patients studied in recent reports, no firm conclusions can be made regarding the benefit of hybrid operations with respect to spinal cord ischemia. In fact, the low paraplegia rates originally reported by Black et al. [22] have now increased to the 15% range [32].

Patient selection for hybrid operations has been varied in the literature. At least one center, invoking unacceptable risks of open TAAA repair, has applied hybrid operation for all TAAA [22]. Their elective 30-day mortality was 13% compared with a historic mortality of 20–30% for open repair. The majority of studies have described the hybrid operation in patients unfit for traditional open repair [20, 21, 23]. Thus, a direct comparison between the two groups is impossible, since by definition most surgeons would not agree to randomize these patients in a prospective trial. In fact, 78% of our hybrid group had been followed with TAAA prior to the study interval. They were only offered a procedure after hybrid repair became feasible from a regulatory perspective. While some centers have reported mortality rates as low as 3% [20], our own results and those of Chiesa [23] demonstrate 30-day mortality between 17 and 23% in this high-risk group (Table 26.3).

The potential for endoleaks is another significant disadvantage of hybrid repair. The relatively high incidence, 22% in our series, presumably relates to compromised fixation sites. In some instances, this could be improved by providing a longer sealing zone and routinely performing four vessel debranching. However, this approach may be limited by an unexpectedly high rate of renal/visceral graft thrombosis (10%). Even with the exclusion of one patient with heparin-induced thrombocytopenia (HIT) syndrome who thrombosed three out of four grafts, the overall thrombosis rate in our series remains at 6%. Other series have reported graft thrombosis rates between 0 and 11% [21, 23]. This is surprising given our previously reported renovisceral thrombosis rate of 1.6% in patients undergoing open TAAA repair [5] in addition to previous reports describing the reliability and durability of surgical renal artery reconstruction [33].

Table 26.3 Summary of results from previous hybrid TAAA papers

Author	Patients (n)	% Unfit for open repair	Extent I/II	Mortality (30 days)	Paraplegia	Endoleak	Debranching graft patency
Black [22]	26[a] completed	Unknown	10/62%	13% elective 23%[b] (overall)	0%	42%	98%
Chiesa [23]	13	100%	54/15%	23%	8%, $n = 1$ (delayed)	0%	100%
Zhou[c] [20]	31 (15 visceral)	100%	17/0%	3% ($n = 1$)	0%	6%	95%
Brockler [21]	28	100%	9/29%	14%	16%	18%	89% (30 days)
MGH series	23	100%	36/23%	17%	4%	22%	90%

[a]This series reported 29 patients in which hybrid was attempted with 26 patients successfully completing the hybrid and three patients having the procedure aborted.
[b]Overall mortality included the six rupture patients who died, for elective/urgent repair 30-day mortality was reported as 13%.
[c]This series included hybrid arch debranching in addition to hybrid mesenteric debranching.

The technical aspects of the reconstruction which may have contributed to the high thrombosis rates include the tunneling of grafts in a retrograde fashion while working around large undecompressed aneurysms and performing these bypasses in a redo surgical field. Technical options for the creation of debranching bypasses have been reviewed extensively elsewhere [34]. Another important consideration is whether to perform a one-stage or a two-stage procedure [19, 33].

Proponents of the single-stage approach, i.e., performing the debranching procedure and the thoracic endograft at the same operation, argue that by always placing a conduit directly on the aorta or iliac artery, access site-related complications can be minimized. In addition, once the debranching procedure has been performed, the placement of the endograft is relatively straight forward and direct surgical adjuncts can be used to facilitate identification of the distal landing zone. Disadvantages include a longer duration of operation, logistical constraints with imaging equipment, and an increased risk of renal failure given the ischemic time coupled with contrast administration.

Proponents of the two-staged approach argue that separating the two procedures allows patients to have an improved recovery period in between operations. In addition the debranching procedure can be performed in a standard open operating room (OR) while the second operation can be performed in a dedicated angiography suite. However, the increasing availability of hybrid ORs now alleviates some of these logistical issues. Finally, the two-staged approach avoids simultaneous abdominal and thoracic aortic grafting which has been correlated in some reports with an increased risk of spinal cord ischemia [35]. The disadvantages of the two-stage approach include exposure to two separate anesthetics, and the possibility of interval rupture which occurred in our very first patient and in the experience of others [21].

Limitations of the current study, similar to the majority of previously published reports of hybrid repair of TAAA, are its retrospective nature, the heterogeneity of the study groups with respect to risk factor profile and the small numbers of patients. Inclusion of the open group is more for perspective rather than comparison since a prospective randomized trial of high surgical risk patients for open repair will likely never be undertaken.

The analogy with extending EVAR and TEVAR to high-risk patients may not be as applicable to hybrid repair of TAAA. With a sobering 26% in-hospital mortality, it is clear that a conservative application of this strategy in patients unfit for conventional operation is appropriate. However, the correct comparison is not with patients fit for open repair, but rather with the natural history of medical management in patients unable to tolerate open TAAA repair. Thus, we currently reserve this procedure for large TAAA in patients with good renal function and a reasonable life expectancy.

However, debranching may also be of benefit in the treatment of lower risk operative patients who are treated in centers without extensive experience in open TAAA repair. A prospective study of hybrid TAAA repair compared to open operation in lower risk patients will be required to further define its role. This data will also serve as a comparison once more advanced endovascular techniques such as the use of branched endografts or chimney grafts placed alongside the body of the main endograft become more widely available.

References

1. Coselli JS, Bozinovski J, LeMaire SA: Open surgical repair of 2286 thoracoabdominal aortic aneurysms, *Ann Thorac Surg* 83(2):S862–S864, 2007.
2. Svensson LG, Crawford ES, Hess KR, Coselli JS, Safi HJ: Experience with 1509 patients undergoing thoracoabdominal aortic operations, *J Vasc Surg* 17(2):357–368, 1993.
3. Conrad MF, Crawford RS, Davison JK, Cambria RP: Thoracoabdominal aneurysm repair: a 20-year perspective, *Ann Thorac Surg* 83(2):S856–S861, 2007.
4. Cambria RP, Clouse WD, Davison JK, Dunn PF, Corey M, Dorer D: Thoracoabdominal aneurysm repair: results with 337 operations performed over a 15-year interval, *Ann Surg* 236(4):471–479, 2002.
5. Clouse WD, Marone LK, Davison JK, Dorer DJ, Brewster DC, LaMuraglia GM, Cambria RP: Late aortic and graft-related events after thoracoabdominal aneurysm repair, *J Vasc Surg* 37(2):254–261, 2003.
6. Crawford RS, Pedraza JD, Chung TK, Corey M, Conrad MF, Cambria RP: Functional outcome after thoracoabdominal aneurysm repair, *J Vasc Surg* 48(4):828–835, 2008.
7. Crawford ES, DeNatale RW: Thoracoabdominal aortic aneurysm: observations regarding the natural course of the disease, *J Vasc Surg* 3(4):578–582, 1986.
8. Lobato AC, Puech-Leao P: Predictive factors for rupture of thoracoabdominal aortic aneurysm, *J Vasc Surg* 27(3):446–453, 1998.
9. Juvonen T, Ergin MA, Galla JD, Lansman SL, Nguyen KH, McCullough JN, Levy D, de Asla RA, Bodian CA, Griepp RB: Prospective study of the natural history of thoracic aortic aneurysms, *Ann Thorac Surg* 63(6):1533–1545, 1997.
10. Cowan JA Jr, Dimick JB, Henke PK, Huber TS, Stanley JC, Upchurch GR Jr: Surgical treatment of intact thoracoabdominal aortic aneurysms in the US: hospital and surgeon volume-related outcomes, *J Vasc Surg* 37(6):1169–1174, 2003.
11. Rigberg DA, McGory ML, Zingmond DS, Maggard MA, Agustin M, Lawrence PF, Ko CY: Thirty-day mortality statistics underestimate the risk of repair of thoracoabdominal aortic aneurysms: a statewide experience, *J Vasc Surg* 43(2):217–222, 2006.
12. Sicard GA, Zwolak RM, Sidawy AN, White RA, Siami FS: Endovascular abdominal aortic aneurysm repair: long-term outcome measures in patients at high-risk for open surgery, *J Vasc Surg* 44(2):229–236, 2006.
13. Hua HT, Cambria RP, Chuang SK, Stoner MC, Kwolek CJ, Rowell KS, Khuri SF, Henderson WG, Brewster DC, Abbott WM: Early outcomes of endovascular versus open abdominal aortic aneurysm repair in the National Surgical Quality Improvement Program-Private Sector (NSQIP-PS), *J Vasc Surg* 41(3):382–389, 2005.
14. Stone DH, Brewster DC, Kwolek CJ, Lamuraglia GM, Conrad MF, Chung TK, Cambria RP: Stent-graft versus open-surgical repair of the thoracic aorta: mid-term results, *J Vasc Surg* 44(6):1188–1197, 2006.
15. Makaroun MS, Dillavou ED, Kee ST, Sicard G, Chaikof E, Bavaria J, Williams D, Cambria RP, Mitchell RS: Endovascular treatment of thoracic aortic aneurysms: results of the phase II multicenter trial of the GORE TAG thoracic endoprosthesis, *J Vasc Surg* 41(1):1–9, 2005.
16. Roselli EE, Greenberg RK, Pfaff K, Francis C, Svensson LG, Lytle BW: Endovascular treatment of thoracoabdominal aortic aneurysms, *J Thorac Cardiovasc Surg* 133(6):1474–1482, 2007.
17. Chuter TA, Rapp JH, Hiramoto JS, Schneider DB, Howell B, Reilly LM: Endovascular treatment of thoracoabdominal aortic aneurysms, *J Vasc Surg* 47(1):6–16, 2008.
18. Quinones-Baldrich WJ, Panetta TF, Vescera CL, Kashyap VS: Repair of type IV thoracoabdominal aneurysm with a combined endovascular and surgical approach, *J Vasc Surg* 30(3):555–560, 1999.
19. Flye MW, Choi ET, Sanchez LA, Curci JA, Thompson RW, Rubin BG, Geraghty PJ, Sicard GA: Retrograde visceral vessel revascularization followed by endovascular aneurysm exclusion as an alternative to open surgical repair of thoracoabdominal aortic aneurysm, *J Vasc Surg* 39(2):454–458, 2004.
20. Zhou W, Reardon M, Peden EK, Lin PH, Lumsden AB: Hybrid approach to complex thoracic aortic aneurysms in high-risk patients: surgical challenges and clinical outcomes, *J Vasc Surg* 44(4):688–693, 2006.
21. Bockler D, Kotelis D, Geisbusch P, Hyhlik-Durr A, Klemm K, von Tengg-Kobligk H, Kauczor HU, Allenberg JR: Hybrid procedures for thoracoabdominal aortic aneurysms and chronic aortic dissections—a single center experience in 28 patients, *J Vasc Surg* 47(4):724–732, 2008.
22. Black SA, Wolfe JH, Clark M, Hamady M, Cheshire NJ, Jenkins MP: Complex thoracoabdominal aortic aneurysms: endovascular exclusion with visceral revascularization, *J Vasc Surg* 43(6):1081–1089, 2006.
23. Chiesa R, Tshomba Y, Melissano G, Marone EM, Bertoglio L, Setacci F, Calliari FM: Hybrid approach to thoracoabdominal aortic aneurysms in patients with prior aortic surgery, *J Vasc Surg* 45(6):1128–1135, 2007.
24. Patel R, Conrad MF, Paruchuri V, Kwolek CJ, Chung T, Cambria RP: Thoracoabdominal aneurysm repair: hybrid versus open repair, *J Vasc Surg* 50(1):15–22, 2009.
25. Rutherford RB, Baker JD, Ernst C, Johnston KW, Porter JM, Ahn S, Jones DN: Recommended standards for reports dealing with lower extremity ischemia: revised version, *J Vasc Surg* 26(3):517–538, 1997.
26. Chuter TA, Gordon RL, Reilly LM, Kerlan RK, Sawhney R, Jean-Claude J, Canto CJ, LaBerge JM, Ring EJ, Wall SD, Messina LM: Abdominal aortic aneurysm in high-risk patients: short- to intermediate-term results of endovascular repair, *Radiology* 210(2):361–365, 1999.

27. Kawaharada N, Morishita K, Fukada J, Hachiro Y, Takahashi K, Abe T: Thoracoabdominal aortic aneurysm repair through redo left-sided thoracotomy, *Ann Thorac Surg* 77(4):1304–1308, 2004.
28. Greenberg R, Resch T, Nyman U, Lindh M, Brunkwall J, Brunkwall P, Malina M, Koul B, Lindblad B, Ivancev K: Endovascular repair of descending thoracic aortic aneurysms: an early experience with intermediate-term follow-up, *J Vasc Surg* 31(1 Pt 1):147–156, 2000.
29. Bavaria JE, Appoo JJ, Makaroun MS, Verter J, Yu ZF, Mitchell RS: Endovascular stent grafting versus open surgical repair of descending thoracic aortic aneurysms in low-risk patients: a multicenter comparative trial, *J Thorac Cardiovasc Surg* 133(2):369–377, 2007.
30. Matsumura JS, Cambria RP, Dake MD, Moore RD, Svensson LG, Snyder S: International controlled clinical trial of thoracic endovascular aneurysm repair with the Zenith TX2 endovascular graft: 1-year results, *J Vasc Surg* 47(2):247–257, 2008.
31. Carroccio A, Marin ML, Ellozy S, Hollier LH: Pathophysiology of paraplegia following endovascular thoracic aortic aneurysm repair, *J Card Surg* 18(4):359–366, 2003.
32. Wolfe JH: Data presented at *Houston Aortic Summit*. April 2008.
33. Cambria RP, Brewster DC, L'Italien GJ, Moncure A, Darling RC Jr, Gertler JP, La Muraglia GM, Atamian S, Abbott WM: The durability of different reconstructive techniques for atherosclerotic renal artery disease, *J Vasc Surg* 20(1):76–85, 1994.
34. Fulton JJ, Farber MA, Marston WA, Mendes R, Mauro MA, Keagy BA: Endovascular stent-graft repair of pararenal and type IV thoracoabdominal aortic aneurysms with adjunctive visceral reconstruction, *J Vasc Surg* 41(2):191–198, 2005.
35. Buth J, Harris PL, Hobo R, van Eps R, Cuypers P, Duijm L, Tielbeek X: Neurologic complications associated with endovascular repair of thoracic aortic pathology: incidence and risk factors. a study from the European Collaborators on Stent/Graft Techniques for Aortic Aneurysm Repair (EUROSTAR) registry, *J Vasc Surg.* 46(6):1103–1110, 2007.

27 Laparoscopic Aortic Surgery

Yves-Marie Dion and Thomas Joseph

Vascular surgeons have been attracted to the ideas of minimally invasive surgery and of the resulting benefits in terms of immediate survival and quality of life. This probably resulted in the initial popularity of extra-anatomical bypasses in the aorto-iliac occlusive disease [1] and the enthusiastic support for the endovascular interventions. Overall, extra-anatomic bypass for aorto-iliac occlusive disease rarely performs as well as aorto-bifemoral bypass and therefore is seldom recommended for claudication [2]. On the other hand, despite their usefulness, endovascular interventions cannot be offered to treat all vascular lesions. One cannot put aside the proven value of laparoscopy extensively studied by general surgeons who made it the procedure of choice for treatment of most intra-abdominal and intrathoracic diseases. Vascular surgeons, having to deal with lower extremity disease, who did not have much exposure to general laparoscopic surgery found the advancements of endovascular technology more appealing.

Laparoscopic vascular surgery is a recent technology which has already adapted to the stringent requirements of vascular exposure, control of blood vessels and construction of vascular anastomoses. We find it complementary to the endovascular interventions.

Y.-M. Dion (✉)
Professor, Department of Surgery, Hôpital St-François d'Assise and Lavel University, Quebec City, Canada

Evolution of Laparoscopic Vascular Surgery

The concept of laparoscopic approach to aorto-iliac disease was brought into reality for the first time in 1993 by Dion et al. [3] who reported a case of laparoscopy-assisted aorto-bifemoral bypass. This was followed by a small case series by Berens et al. [4] 2 years later. Clinical experience began after extensive work in the animal laboratory and in human cadavers on the various aspects of laparoscopic surgery [5–12]. The vascular anastomosis was first performed through strategically placed smaller incisions at the end of laparoscopic dissection. Hence the technique was called laparoscopically assisted aorto-iliac surgery [3]. The concept was conceived by many vascular surgeons and the technique evolved almost simultaneously although the following description places these in a step-wise fashion. The laparoscopically assisted procedures allowed the anastomosis to be carried out as in an open operation at the end of laparoscopic dissection [3]. Routine arterial surgery uses considerable amount of suction to keep the operating field clear. This is not feasible with laparoscopic insufflations for fear of losing the pneumoperitoneum. Berens et al. described the use of a two-bladed laparofan supported externally by a Laparo-lift robotic arm fixed to the operating table. This gasless retraction, by lifting the abdominal wall (Laparo-lift), allowed the use of suction and conventional vascular instruments introduced through stab incisions [4, 8]. The Laparo-lift could not provide adequate space to work within the abdominal cavity. On the other hand pneumoperitoneum gave a dome-shaped cavity to work with long instruments unlike the tent-like cavity provided by the Laparo-lift.

T.J. Fogarty, R.A. White (eds.), *Peripheral Endovascular Interventions*,
DOI 10.1007/978-1-4419-1387-6_27,

However, it was uncertain whether a gasless environment or a traditional insufflation approach would be the best. Carbon dioxide embolisation during laparoscopy was recognised as a potentially lethal complication [13, 14]. Dion et al. developed a model to evaluate gas embolisation under carbon dioxide pneumoperitoneum. Anaesthetised dogs with haemodynamic monitoring via an arterial line and Swan–Ganz catheter were used. The status and the amount of air embolism within the heart chambers were evaluated by trans-oesophageal echocardiography. Euvolaemic dogs were submitted to a 1 cm longitudinal incision made in the vena cava while maintaining a carbon dioxide pneumoperitoneum with pressures between 12 and 15 mmHg [7]. Eighty-two percent of the cases did not develop any embolisation while 18% had gas bubbles noted in the right heart cavities on trans-oesophageal echocardiography. Intravenous injection of 15 cc of carbon dioxide produced relatively more gas bubbles in the right heart. Massive intravenous injections of carbon dioxide (>300 cc) led to the appearance of gas bubbles in the left heart cavities and death. They also demonstrated that trans-oesophageal echocardiography was better in detecting air embolism [7]. Reported incidences of CO_2 embolism in laparoscopy in three studies were 1 in 63,845, 15 in 113,253 and 8 in 50,247 patients [15]. Pneumoperitoneum therefore was considered safe enough for vascular work and the operative steps were modified to avoid loss of pneumoperitoneum.

Following these first steps, further attempts aimed to avoid the need for minilaparotomy [8, 10]. Experimental work revolved around finding an optimum way of dissecting the vessels laparoscopically and keeping the bowel retracted while performing the arterial anastomosis. Animal experiments were carried out both in pigs and in dogs [8–10]. Both transperitoneal and retroperitoneal dissections were attempted but the retroperitoneal dissection enabled the bowel to be kept away using intact peritoneum [16]. A midline extraperitoneal approach was used by Schumaker [17]. It was modified to use a lateral retroperitoneal approach with balloon dissection in piglets placed in right lateral position [8]. The same authors successfully performed a totally laparoscopic approach in dogs while they also developed an antero-lateral retroperitoneal approach in pigs [10]. Adaptation of these techniques led to the totally laparoscopic transabdominal retrocolic approach which is used today [18, 19]. This technique, when performed with pneumoperitoneum, gave good visualisation of both the viscera in the peritoneal cavity and the vessels in the retroperitoneum while keeping the bowels retracted with the least effort. Coggia et al. also developed a totally laparoscopic technique using right lateral oblique position and left paracolic dissection [20]. This confirmed the technique developed by Dion et al. and its modifications as the preferred way of dissection in totally laparoscopic surgery [21]. The transabdominal left paracolic approach successfully avoided the problems associated with disruption of peritoneum in a totally retroperitoneal approach.

The transabdominal retroperitoneal dissection can be tedious due to difficulty in keeping the bowels retracted and is mostly used in the laparoscopy-assisted technique described by Alimi et al. To facilitate this approach, Alimi also described a bowel retractor with a metal rod inserted through a stab incision threaded into reveres of a net together with the net held using suspension threads [22].

An alternative approach called hand-assisted laparoscopic aortic surgery was developed with the introduction of hand ports that allowed insertion of the non-dominant hand while maintaining the pneumoperitoneum [23–25]. The Gelport laparoscopic system (Applied Medical) introduced into the market recently is versatile and also allows introduction of conventional instruments through it. Hand ports allowed standardisation of the minilaparotomy to the size of the hand. With this technique, tactile feedback is provided to the surgeon which helps particularly during the learning curve of laparoscopic surgery.

The totally laparoscopic operative technique used by Dion's group at Laval University, Québec City, is described later. A list of currently used approaches is given in Table 27.1.

The laparoscopic modification of routine vascular surgical instruments progressed in parallel albeit slow pace [26]. This allowed totally laparoscopic procedures to be performed. The new millennium brought robotic assistance to perform the anastomosis totally laparoscopically [27, 28].

Table 27.1 The major technical variations currently described in laparoscopic aorto-iliac reconstructions

	Assisted techniques			Totally laparoscopic techniques		
Technique	Hand assisted	Laparoscopic assisted		Laparoscopic anastomosis		Robot assisted
Incision (excluding port-sites)	≤ 7 cm, midline/ Pfannenstiel	6–9 cm or bigger, midline	5–10 cm subcostal vertical/ transverse	None	None	None
Comments	Better tactile feedback. Currently, more frequently used, especially for AAA	Variable incision		Transperitoneal retrocolic (preferred), transperitoneal retrorenal and transperitoneal available		Anastomosis with robot-assistance using any one of the previously mentioned aortic approaches

The Case for Laparoscopic Aortic Surgery

Patients with abdominal aortic aneurysm appeared to have a threefold increased risk of having postoperative incisional hernia in a systematic review of 1,132 patients who underwent abdominal aortic aneurysm repair and aorto-iliac reconstruction for occlusive disease [29]. The incidence of postoperative incisional hernia varies from 10 to 37% for aneurysm repairs and 3 to 17% for aorto-iliac reconstructions [30]. According to the UK endovascular trials, the overall 30-day mortality from open repair was 4.7% compared to 1.7% from endovascular repair [31]. At 4 years, the proportion of patients with postoperative complications were 41% in EVAR group and 9% in the open surgery group [32]. The proportion of patients who required at least one reintervention in the 4 years was 20% in EVAR group and 6% in open repair group. These differences were statistically significant on estimating the hazard ratios. One year following completion of the trial 35% of all patients who received EVAR had reported one or more postoperative complications of whom 44% needed a secondary intervention and two of whom died within 30 days of their secondary intervention [32]. The mean hospital costs per patient up to 4 years were UK Stirling 13,257 in the EVAR group compared to 9,946 in the open group (mean difference of 3,311 pounds, standard error 690) [32]. Patients will naturally benefit from endovascular repair when feasible but laparoscopic repair has demonstrated comparable results at less cost to the health system. In a review of 402 patients, Kolvenbach et al. reported a mortality of 1.8% in the aneurysm group and 1.6% in the occlusive disease group for laparoscopic-assisted repair [33]. Coggia et al. carried out a case–control study that showed better mortality (3.3% for total laparoscopy vs. 6.6% in open surgery) but relatively longer operative time, clamp time and blood loss that did not translate into poor outcome [34]. In a meta-analysis of 23 studies on aorto-iliac bypass for occlusive disease, De Vries et al. concluded that the mortality and morbidity rates of aortic bifurcation graft procedures dropped to 3.3 and 8.3% since 1975 [35]. They estimated patency rates of 91 and 86.8% for intermittent claudication and 87.5 and 81.8% for patients with critical ischaemia at 5 and 10 years, respectively [35]. An alternative to open aorto-bifemoral bypass is crossover femoro-femoral or iliofemoral and axillo-bifemoral bypass in selected cases that are not suitable for intra-abdominal procedures. In a multicentre randomised study of 143 patients, Ricco et al. concluded that the long-term patency of crossover grafts was poor compared to direct grafts [2, 36, 37]. Similarly axillofemoral bypass is associated with lower patency rates. Overall, extra-anatomic bypass rarely performs as well as aorto-bifemoral bypass in diffuse disease and therefore is seldom recommended for claudication [2]. Another open surgical alternative, though not commonly used, is aorto-iliac endarterectomy with a reported patency varying from 60 to 94% [2]. Table 27.2 compares the various open surgical approaches and their patency rates. So far, aorto-iliac reconstruction by aorto-bifemoral bypass seems to be the most durable option in aorto-iliac occlusive disease.

Table 27.2 Comparison between the open surgical techniques for aorto-iliac disease [1, 1]

Procedure	5-year patency in percentage (range) comments
Open aorto-bifemoral for claudication	91 (90–94) (limb based) 85 (85–89) (patient based)
Open aorto-bifemoral for CLI	87 (80–88) (limb based) 80 (72–82) (patient based)
Femoro-femoral crossover	75 (55–92)
Axillo unifemoral	51 (44–79)
Axillo-bifemoral	71 (50–76)
Endarterectomy	60–94 (only range available)

Limb based: patency in symptomatic limbs; Patient based: patency among the patients operated; CLI: Critical Limb Ischaemia.

The operative trauma from access route to the aorto-iliac segment could be reduced considerably by using the laparoscopic technique. Minimally invasive techniques are attractive not only for causing less postoperative pain but also for quicker recovery and the resultant monetary savings to healthcare systems [34, 38–44]. Laparoscopic aorto-iliac reconstruction in occlusive disease retains the advantages of open procedures in terms of long-term patency rates [28, 45, 46]. The Trans-Atlantic Inter-Society Consensus noted increasing interest in the laparoscopic approach [2].

The advantage of laparoscopic techniques over open surgery has been demonstrated in donor nephrectomy with better pain control, shorter hospital stay and early return to work in the donors [47, 48]. Similarly laparoscopically assisted hysterectomy was found to be associated with better pain control and less complications in gynaecology [49]. In a multicentre study Song et al. found that totally laparoscopic gastrectomy resulted in quicker recovery of bowel function [50]. In vascular surgery, Fourneau et al. compared hand-assisted surgery with open operation. They found hand-assisted laparoscopic surgery achieving significantly shorter hospital stay (7.5 vs. 8.9 days, $p = 0.005$) and better social functional recovery at 6 weeks using SF-36 survey ($p = 0.023$) [51]. In small case series hand-assisted surgery was found to favour early return of bowel function and discharge [24, 52].

The estimated learning curve in laparoscopic surgery was between 25 and 30 cases [33, 53]. This is comparable to the number of cases required for endovascular accreditation [54, 55]. In a review of laparoscopically assisted techniques, Kolvenbach et al. noted that the mortality of laparoscopic-assisted surgery was low as already stated. On comparing the hand-assisted procedures with open surgery no statistically significant difference was noted between the two groups for morbidity or mortality, but the ICU stay and length of stay were significantly longer in the open surgery group. These observations were for both aneurysmal and occlusive disease together. The median clamp time of laparoscopic-assisted reconstruction in occlusive disease was 25 (15–40) min [33].

Major case series on laparoscopic aorto-iliac reconstruction has recently been reviewed by Nio et al. [56]. Table 27.3 shows the major series published in laparoscopic repair of aorto-iliac occlusive disease and Table 27.4 describes the major series in aneurysm repair as compiled by Nio et al. The minimum operative time and clamp time reported in totally laparoscopic aorto-iliac reconstruction for occlusive disease were a mean of 193 (±58) min [45] and 57 (±21) [57] min, respectively. The maximum operative time was reported in a series of seven patients and this was a median of 390 (180–600) min [12]. The longest clamp time reported is a median of 128 (75–170) min in a series of 27 patients [22]. However, the learning curve of 25–30 cases [53], as noted above, has to be borne in mind while studying these durations. They found hand-assisted procedures taking the shortest operative times (2.5–4 h) and clamp times (less than 1 h). Clamp times were also found to be shorter for occlusive disease reflecting that only one anastomosis is performed laparoscopically. The overall mortality for laparoscopic aortic procedures (calculated for aneurysmal and occlusive disease together) was 2% (26/1044) while for occlusive disease alone, the overall mortality was 15/630 (2.4%) [56].

In the systematic review of laparoscopic vascular surgery, Nio et al. noted that the number of endovascular options for treatment of aorto-iliac disease is still growing and the role of laparoscopic vascular surgery should be considered against these ongoing developments. They concluded that wider implementation of this technique needs simplification of the procedure [56]. However, more than half of these studies fell short of the learning curve of 25–30 cases.

The laparoscopic approach offers a cheap and durable option of repair of both occlusive and aneurysmal disease of the aorto-iliac segment. It has comparable perioperative mortality and morbidity rates to both open surgery and endovascular techniques.

Table 27.3 Occlusive disease. Operative data of included studies

	Year	*N*	Operative time (min)	Clamping time (min)	Anastomosis time (min)	Hospital stay (days)	Mortality x/n	Conversion x/n
Total laparoscopic surgery								
Cau [22]	2006	72 (66abf, 4auf)	216±50[a]	57±21[a]		8 (5–42)[b]	0/72	2/72
Dooner [36]	2006	13 (abf)	390 (320–480)[nr]			7 (3–14)[nr]	0/13	3/13
Rouers [61]	2005	30 (30abf)	244±11[ac]	66±5[ac]	50±3[ac]	5± 0.3[ac]	0/30	6/30
Lin [54]	2005	68 (68af)	199±31[a]	85±32[a]		6.3±2[a]	1/68	3/68
Olinde [59]	2005	22 (20abf)	267 (199–365)[d]	90 (64–141)[d]	37 (30–56)[d]	4 (2–7)[d]	1/22	2/22
Coggia [28]	2004	93 (68abf, 25auf)	240 (150–450)[d]	68 (30–135)[d]	30 (12–90)[d]	7 (2–57)[d]	4/93	2/93
Remy [60]	2005	21 (21abf)	240 (150–420)[b]	60 (30–120)[b]	60 (30–120)[b]	7 (5–30)[b]	0/21	1/21
Dion [32]	2004	(46abf, 3if)	290±62[a]	99±28[a]	47±13[a]	5 (4–24)[a]	1/51	5/51
			193±58[a]	100±40[a]	55±13[a]	3.3±0.6[a]	0/3	0/3
Alimi [12][e]	2001	7 (5abf, 2auf)	351 (295–420)[b]	128 (75–170)[b]		11 (5–30)[b]	0/7	0/7
Said [63]	1999	7 (7abf)	390 (180–600)[b]	59 (45–110)[b]		6 (3–14)[b]	1/7	0/7
Barbera [19]	1998	24 (11abf, 5auf, 7if, 1tea)	250 (150–450)[d]	70 (55–120)[d]		(3–25)	0/24	4/24
Robot-assisted laparoscopic surgery								
Nio [6]	2005	8 (8abf)	405 (260–589)[d]	111 (85–205)[d]	74 (40–110)[d]	8 (3–57)[d]	1/8	2/8
Laparoscopic-assisted surgery								
Alimi [10]	2004	58 (52abf, 4auf, 1t, 1tea)	238 (140–420)[b]	54 (15–170)[b]		8 (3–32)[b]	2/58	1/58
Lacroix [53]	1999	10 (9abf)	350 (230–390)[d]			7 (5–13)[d]		1/10
Fabiani [39]	1997	9 (3abf, 4auf)	160 (90–240)[b]			(4–7)		2/9

Table 27.3 (continued)

	Year	*N*	Operative time (min)	Clamping time (min)	Anastomosis time (min)	Hospital stay (days)	Mortality x/n	Conversion x/n
Hand-assisted laparoscopic surgery								
Fourneaux [41]	2005	46 (45abf)	208 (155–300)[b]	28 (15–55)[bf]		6 (3–26)[b]	2/45	1/46
Debing [30][g]	2003	13 (7abf, 4abi, 1auf, 1tea)	230 (150–270)[d]	29 (23–72)[d]		6 (4–42)[d]	0/13	1/13
Wijtenburg [68][h]	2003	25 (2t, 1ai, 19abf, 3auf)	180 (120–290)[b]	37 (15–60)[b]		7 (4–15)[b]	1/25	2/25
daSilva [65]	2002	18 (18af)	191 (160–221)[b]	44 (38–50)[b]		7 (5–9)[b]	0/18	1/18
Kelly [46]	2002	8 (8abf)	234 (170–319)[b]			4 (3–5)[b]	1/8	0/8
Kolvenbach [51][e]	2000	29 (nr)	149±35.2[a]	36.4±7.9[a]		4.3±2.2[a]		

nr: not reported; t: tube repair; abi: aortobi-iliac bifurcation graft; abf: aorto-bifemoral bypass; auf: aortounifemoral graft; if: iliofemoral graft; tea: endarterectomy; ai: aorto-iliac graft; af: aortofemoral; bif: bifurcated graft.

From Nio et al. [56].

[a] Mean and standard deviation.

[b] Mean and range.

[c] Converted patients operative time 232±24*, clamping time 57±13*, anastomosis time 37± 8*, hospital stay 12.1± 2.1*.

[d] Median and range.

[e] Part of study.

[f] e-s anastomosis 28 (15–55); e-e anastomosis 69 (55–86).

[g] AAA (3) and AIOD (10).

[h] AAA (10) and AIOD (15).

Table 27.4 Aneurysm repair. Operative data of included studies

	Year	*N*	Operative time (min)	Clamping time (min)	Anastomosis time (min)	Hospital stay (days)	Mortality x/n	Conversion x/n
Total laparoscopic surgery								
Cau [22]	2006	23 (23t)	251±57[a]	101±15[a]		6 (4–12)[b]	1/23	7/23
Coggia [26]	2005	30 (13t, 17bif)	255 (170–410)[b]	80 (35–110)[b]		9 (5–37)[b]	1/30	1/30
Coggia [29]	2004	30 (11t, 15abi, 4abf)	290 (160–420)[b]	78 (35–230)[b]		9 (8–37)[b]	2/30	2/30
Kolvenbach [2]	2004	37 (nr)	227±34[a]	81±31[a]	53±9.0[a]	6.3±21.1[a]		6/37
Dion [32]	2004	7 (6abf, 1t)	299±75[a]	109±52[a]	48±23[a]	6 (3–32)[a]	0/7	1/7
Edoga [37]	1998	22 (16abf, 4abi)	391 (180–600)[c]	146 (6–286)[c]		6 (2–25)[c]	2/22	2/22
Robot-assisted laparoscopic surgery								
Kolvenbach [2]	2004	10 (8t, 2abi)	243±41[a]	96±22[a]	41±4[a]	7.3±2.4[a]		2/10
Laparoscopic-assisted surgery								
Alimi [11]	2003	24 (12t, 3abi, 8abf, 1af)	238 (155–360)[c]	76 (42–160)[c]		7 (3–21)[c]	1/24	4/24
Castronuovo [21]	2000	60 (60bif)	462 (90–690)[c]	112 (43–286)[c]		6 (1–25)[c]	3/60	3/60
Kline [47]	1998	20 (t)	246±55.2[a]			5.8±1.6[a]	0/20	2/20
Hand-assisted laparoscopic surgery								
Ferrari [40]	2006	122	257±70[a]	76±26[a]		4.4±1.7[a]	0/122	9/122
Kolvenbach [50]	2001	29 (nr)	181 (130–345)[c]	57 (44–90)[c]		6 (4–21)[c]	1/29	

t: tube repair; abi: aortobi-iliac bifurcation graft; abf: aorto-bifemoral bypass; auf: aortounifemoral graft; if: iliofemoral graft; tea: endarterectomy; ai: aorto-iliac graft; af: aortofemoral; bif: bifurcated graft; nr: not reported.

From Nio et al. [56].

[a] Mean and standard deviation.

[b] Median and range.

[c] Mean and range.

Current Status

Laparoscopic techniques are used to bypass the occlusive disease of the aorto-iliac segment and for exclusion of aneurysmal disease. Laparoscopic techniques have also been described as adjuncts to endovascular interventions [58, 59] such as ligation of vessels causing endoleak [60] and other techniques such as repair of thoracoabdominal aneurysm [61], aortic endarterectomy [62] and thoracofemoral bypass [63]. The enthusiasm in laparoscopic surgery was not well supported by advancements in instrumentation which perhaps led to lukewarm response later on. Perhaps due to the sharp learning curve related to the totally laparoscopic approach, some of the enthusiasts went on to develop hand-assisted technique [22, 24] or minilaparotomy techniques as an alternative while yet others developed robot-assisted techniques [27, 64].

The new generation of vascular trainees are busy gaining experience in endovascular skills in addition to the open surgical skills. Together with shortened exposure to general surgical training, this has led to further reduction of laparoscopic skills among the vascular surgeons. However, laparoscopic surgery does offer an alternative minimally invasive route for the vascular surgeons and is making a steady progress as stated above.

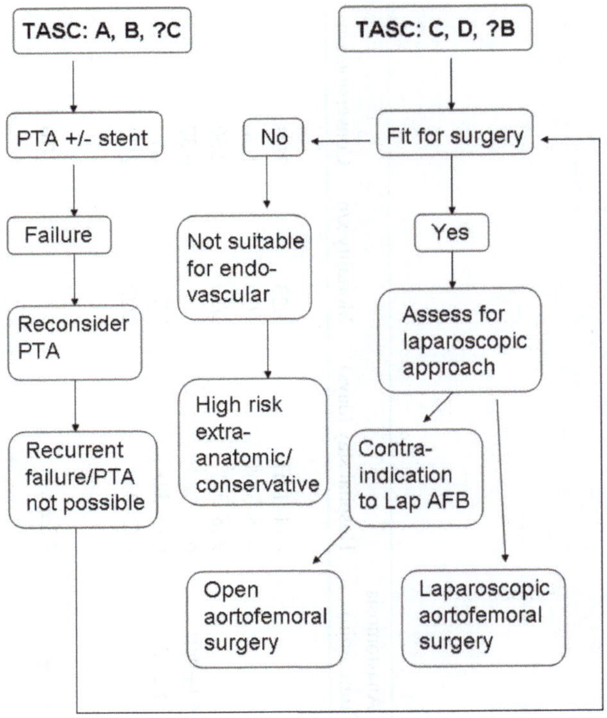

Fig. 27.1 Algorithm for managing aorto-iliac occlusive disease. TASC, Trans-Atlantic Inter-Society Consensus; PTA, percutaneous angioplasty; Lap AFB, Laparoscopic aortofemoral bypass

Indications

Trans-Atlantic Inter-Society Consensus (TASC II) document classified aorto-iliac disease into type A, B, C and D [2]. The basis for TASC recommendations in aorto-iliac segment disease comes from evidence obtained from expert committee reports or opinions and/or clinical experiences of respected authorities due to shortage of good quality studies in this area (grade C recommendation). According to the TASC recommendations, endovascular therapy is the treatment of choice for type A lesions and surgery is the treatment of choice for type D lesions. Endovascular treatment is the preferred treatment for type B lesions and surgery is the preferred treatment for good risk patients with type C lesions [2]. They recommended consideration of patient's co-morbidities, patient preference and the operator's long-term success rates when making decisions on type B and type C lesions. We believe laparoscopic aorto-iliac reconstruction should be considered in every case of occlusive disease needing open surgery and recommend the algorithm shown in Fig. 27.1 for treatment of aorto-iliac occlusive disease.

In young patients with abdominal aortic aneurysms where open surgery is the preferred option for durability of the procedure and in cases unsuitable for endovascular repair, laparoscopic approach should be considered as a feasible option in experienced centres. It could also be considered in bypass operations to the visceral arteries [65, 66] and as an adjunct to endovascular interventions in treating the endoleaks or for providing alternate access for deployment of the endovascular device [67].

Currently the contra-indications to the procedure include major alteration of anatomy from previous surgery or from congenital causes. It also includes major organ failures. Needless to say, the laparoscopic techniques should be performed by trained surgeons. Training courses are available to achieve the necessary basic skills and competency.

The Technique

Operative Technique

A summary of the technique performed by Dion et al. at St-Francois d'Assise Hospital in Quebec City follows. The technique has been extensively described previously [18, 19, 21]. All patients receive mechanical bowel preparation and prophylactic antibiotics and the surgery is performed under general anaesthesia with invasive monitoring. Patient is positioned at 45° right lateral oblique position using Gel supports or bean bag. This allows the chest and pelvis to be stabilised on the table while the table is tilted sidewise to achieve nearly 60° lateral position. The pelvis is relatively less obliquely placed in comparison to the chest wall to allow access to the femoral arteries. The left arm is positioned over the chest and secured with padding and bandages (Fig. 27.2).

The patient is positioned horizontally by tilting the table to the left. The femoral vessels are then exposed and slinged in standard fashion. The wounds are protected with saline swabs. An umbilical port and three more 10 mm ports are inserted as shown in Fig. 27.2. Laterally 12 mm ports are placed in the anterior axillary line with a little triangulation of the ports. The descending colon is mobilised with the main operator standing on the right side of the patient and the first assistant holding the camera on a 30° scope introduced through the umbilical port. The dissection starts in the left iliac fossa with the colon held in a bowel grasper passed through the supra-umbilical port and scissors through the sub-umbilical port. The assistant can use a grasper introduced through the epigastric port to give counter-traction on the parietal peritoneum. The gonadal vein is identified at the pelvic brim and dissection proceeds further to the splenic flexure of the colon taking care to avoid traction injury to the spleen. A progressive tilt of the table to the right up to about 70° will help developing the retroperitoneal plane anterior to the Gerota's fascia. The perirenal fat is identified from its distinctive yellow colour and the dissection is carried anterior to this. Tilting the table to maximum right lateral position will help further dissection along the gonadal vessels. Dion's technique of tracing the gonadal vein proximally will identify the left renal vein and the aorta medial to the left renal vein (Fig. 27.3).

The surgeon and the first assistant moves to the left side of the patient and dissection of the periaortic fascia is carried out starting from the left iliac artery

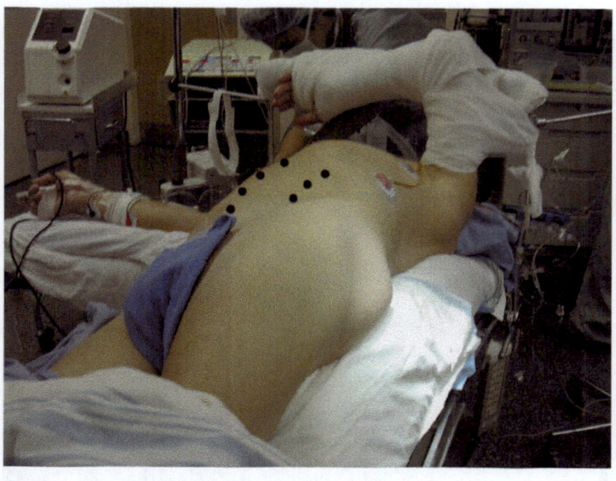

Fig. 27.2 Patient during positioning on the table. Note that the table can be rotated towards the *left* to allow femoral dissection when necessary. It can also be rotated to the *right* in cases where intraperitoneal organs would interfere with adequate visualisation of the operative field. *Black circles* represent the sites of trocar insertion for a totally laparoscopic procedure done on the aorto-iliac segment: four are located in the midline (one infra-umbilical site, one umbilical and two supra-umbilical) and three laterally on a line slightly medial to the anterosuperior iliac spine

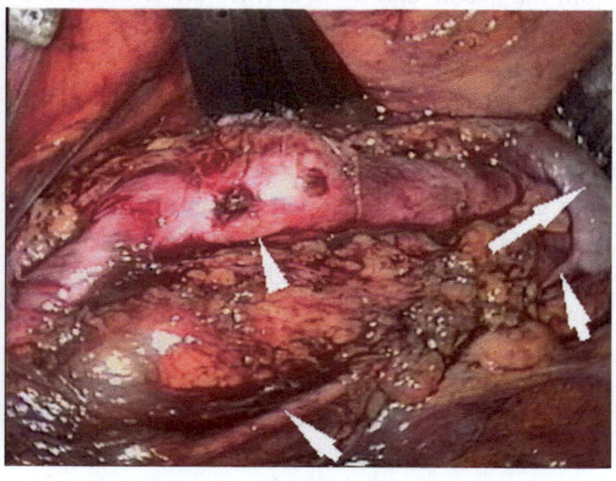

Fig. 27.3 Following totally laparoscopic transabdominal retrocolic dissection. The left mesocolon is seen in the background, retracted and held medially by a fan-shaped retractor. The left renal vein is seen to the *right* of the picture (*long arrow*) as well as the origin of the gonadal vein (*short arrow*) which can be followed up distally (*short arrow*). The infrarenal aorta (*arrowhead*) and the *left* common iliac arteries have been dissected. The *right* common iliac artery is next to be dissected in order to implant an aorto-bifemoral graft

moving proximally in occlusive disease and from the aortic neck moving downwards in aneurysm cases. The inferior mesenteric artery is doubly clipped and divided to facilitate further retraction of the descending colon and sigmoid. Two fan-shaped retractors are introduced through the median epigastric and umbilical ports to retract the colon to the right which is also helped by gravity. These retractors are held in position using table-fixed retractors (Omni-Lapo Tract by Omni-Tract surgical). At this point, the left ureter has long been identified because of its proximity to the left gonadal vein. The lumbar veins are seen and preserved. The left lumbar arteries are doubly clipped and divided to allow gentle lift on the aorta which will facilitate control of the remaining branches. The second assistant's contribution becomes important in progressively proceeding to the medial rotation of the aorta by retraction or counter-traction using a grabber or a suction device inserted through the sub-umbilical port. Care should be exercised in introducing instruments particularly through this port for fear of injury to the bowel. A short length of right common iliac artery is exposed by lifting the peritoneum with the grabbers, preferably to the level of the right ureter to create the tunnel behind it. The right and left iliac bifurcations can be reached if necessary.

The 3-0 Prolene sutures are divided at 24 cm from the needle and these stitches are terminated by 3 × 5 mm pledgets made out of the graft material. The bifurcated graft is introduced through the lateral 12 mm port after shortening the main body. It is pushed upwards into the abdominal cavity and then using a laparoscopic tunneller (or Crawford clamp) from the right groin first (with the peritoneum of right side of the pelvis lifted up with grabbers), the right limb of the graft is grasped and brought out to the right groin. The graft is pulled down to the desired position. A clamp placed on the limb of the graft in the right groin will prevent loss of pneumoperitoneum. Using a similar technique, the graft is tunnelled to the left groin. The left ureter is easily seen. On this side, care must be exerted not to open digitally the retroperitoneum from the groin since this would result in CO_2 leakage from the retroperitoneum. A specially designed 5 mm tunneller has been designed to minimize the potential for CO_2 leakage at the groin level. Intravenous heparin is given and the proximal aorta is clamped using a laparoscopic aortic clamp through the supra-umbilical port. When the bypass is performed for occlusive disease, an Endo GIA stapler is introduced, after removing its blade, through the left lateral 12 mm port. The distal aorta is cross-clamped with the stapler which leaves six rows of staples. The aorta is transected with laparoscopic aortic scissors while the first assistant uses the suction device through the sub-umbilical port to gently suck any oozing. The anastomosis is fashioned in two halves using the preformed stitches, starting at 9 O'clock position to finish at 3 O'clock position. Additional stitches are inserted as required on testing the suture line. The graft limbs are anastomosed to the femoral arteries and the circulation is re-established with standard technique. The peritoneal cavity is inspected again and haemostasis is ensured by specifically looking at the aortic stump. Bringing the colon back to the left side will enable the graft to be covered in its entirety. The ports are removed under direct vision and the wounds are closed after infiltration with local anaesthetic. The same technique is used for infrarenal aneurysms (Fig. 27.4). We do not advocate performance of three intracorporeal anastomoses (aortobi-iliac bypass) since this technique must be reserved for well-trained teams because of ischaemic time consideration. At the time of writing, at least three automated anastomotic techniques are being evaluated. They could significantly reduce clamping time and allow for routine bi-iliac anastomosis. Presently, we suggest that tube graft and aorto-bifemoral bypasses can be done when indicated for AAA treatment. When

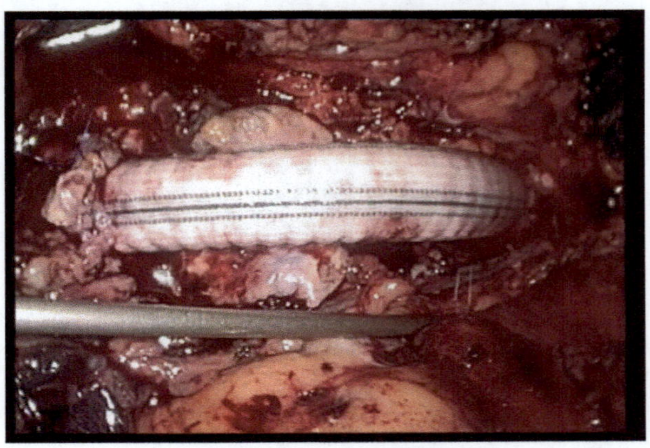

Fig. 27.4 A totally laparoscopic tube graft performed with a standard knitted Dacron graft and 3-0 polypropylene sutures. The proximal anastomosis is to the *right* of the picture and the distal anastomosis has been performed proximal to the aortic bifurcation

performing a tube graft, intracorporeal clamps (Karl Storz Endoscopy) are used to clamp the iliac arteries.

The naso-gastric tube is used only intraoperatively. The patient is started on oral fluid on the day after the operation to progress to diet as tolerated by the second postoperative day. This usually enables discharge by the third or fourth postoperative day.

Complications

The complications associated with laparoscopic aortic surgery are similar to those occurring after open surgery and are dealt with in a similar fashion. Large bowel injury is prevented by using graspers across the breadth of bowel wall and small bowel injury is prevented by careful retraction and by avoiding the bowels on change of instruments. Problems encountered during the operation include inadvertent dissection behind the kidney which could be prevented by careful dissection in front of the perirenal fat. The plane of dissection is obvious to the trained eye. Bleeding from injury to the gonadal vein or the spleen is easily avoided. Retroperitoneal venous bleed could be controlled with compression using laparoscopically adapted small raytex or with judicious use of diathermy or clips. Bleeding from the lumbar veins or from the communicating veins is prevented by identification and meticulous preservation; this is a rare occurrence and paradoxically, it can be more easily dealt with than at open surgery because a fair length of the vein can be seen with the laparoscope. In much calcified aorta difficulty could be encountered in firing the staples which could be helped by crushing the wall between the jaws of a clamp before re-applying the staples. Alternatively the aorta could be transected between clamps and the distal aortic stump can be sutured with running 3-0 polypropylene after laparoscopic endarterectomy. Suture line bleeding and back bleeding from the distal aortic stump are also controlled when they occur by appropriately placed stitches. Significant air embolism has not been encountered in our practice. Anticipation of a prolonged clamping time indicated conversion to an open procedure. If conversion is needed, relatively smaller incisions are placed at the most convenient location on the abdominal wall. Despite conversion to minilaparotomy, the patients benefit from the minimal invasiveness of the operation.

The Future

The cost-effectiveness of laparoscopic aortic surgery has not been formally studied. However, it is to be expected that future articles will make the case. Being a young addition to the vascular surgery world, laparoscopy is associated with research and development in instrument design and anastomotic devices. We believe it is a question of time before the laparoscopic anastomoses be done with automated devices rendering the procedure easier to the vascular surgeon. This advancement will also benefit the patient who will be submitted to shorter clamping times and operative procedures. It will also allow to address lesions of the thoracic aorta and of smaller arteries such as the renal arteries, IMA and SMA.

The generic skills in laparoscopic surgery acquired during training in general surgery are important but not entirely satisfactory to begin laparoscopic arterial surgery. Dedicated laparoscopic vascular surgical courses with hands-on training on animals are designed to help vascular surgeons to set up this practice. The steep learning curve could be mastered by starting with assisted procedures prior to progressing to the totally laparoscopic technique. Details of the courses offered in Quebec and membership to the International Endovascular and Laparoscopic Society can be found at www.vascularlaparoscopy.net.

Conclusion

Laparoscopic aorto-iliac reconstruction appears cost-effective and is a feasible way of treating occlusive and aneurysmal disease in the aorto-iliac arteries. It can also be used as an adjunct to endovascular interventions. Future modifications of devices are set to make laparoscopic vascular surgery more appealing.

References

1. Schneider JR: Extra-anatomic Bypass. In Rutherford RB, editor: *Vascular Surgery*, ed. 6, Philadelphia, 2005, Elsevier Saunders, pp. 1137–1153.
2. Norgren L, Hiatt WR, Dormandy JA et al.: Inter-society consensus for the management of peripheral arterial disease (TASC II), *J Vasc Surg* 45(1):S5–S67, 2007.

3. Dion YM, Katkhouda N, Rouleau C, Aucoin A: Laparoscopy-assisted aortobifemoral bypass, *Surg Laparosc Endosc* 3(5):425–429, 1993 October.
4. Berens ES, Herde JR: Laparoscopic vascular surgery: four case reports, *J Vasc Surg* 22:73–79, 1995.
5. Chen MH, Murphy EA, Halpern V, Faust GR, Cosgrove JM, Cohen JR: Laparoscopic-assisted abdominal aortic aneurysm repair, *Surg Endosc* 9(8):905–907, August 1995.
6. Chen MH, Murphy EA, Levison J, Cohen JR: Laparoscopic aortic replacement in the porcine model: a feasibility study in preparation for laparoscopically assisted abdominal aortic aneurysm repair in humans, *J Am Coll Surg* 183(2):126–132, August 1996.
7. Dion YM, Levesque C, Doillon CJ: Experimental carbon dioxide pulmonary embolization after vena cava laceration under pneumoperitoneum, *Surg Endosc* 9:1065–1069, 1995.
8. Dion YM, Chin AK, Thompson TA: Experimental laparoscopic aortobifemoral bypass, *Surg Endosc* 9:894–897, 1995.
9. Dion YM, Gracia CR: Experimental laparoscopic aneurysm resection and aortobifemoral bypass, *Surg Laparosc Endosc Percutan Tech* 6:184–190, 1996.
10. Dion YM, Gaillard F, Demalsy JC, Gracia CR: Experimental laparoscopic aortobifemoral bypass for occlusive aortoiliac disease, *Can J Surg* 39:451–455, 1996.
11. Ahn SS, Clem MF, Braithwaite BD, Concepcion B, Petrik PV, Moore WS: Laparoscopic aortofemoral bypass. Initial experience in an animal model, *Ann Surg* 222(5):677–683, November 1995.
12. Said S, Mall J, Peter F, Muller JM: Laparoscopic aortofemoral bypass grafting: human cadaveric and initial clinical experiences, *J Vasc Surg* 29(4):639–648, April 1999.
13. Chui PT, Gin T, Oh TE: Anaesthesia for laparoscopic general surgery, *Anaesth Intensive Care* 21:163–171, 1993.
14. McQuaide JR: Air embolism during peritoneoscopy, *S Afr Med J* 46:422–423, 1972.
15. De Plaizer RMH, Jones ISC: Non-fatal carbon dioxide embolism during laparoscopy, *Anaesth Intensive Care* 17:359–361, 1989.
16. Jones DB, Thompson RW, Soper NJ, Olin JM, Rubin BG: Development and comparison of transperitoneal and retroperitoneal approaches to laparoscopic-assisted aortofemoral bypass in a porcine model, *J Vasc Surg* 23(3):466–471, March 1996.
17. Schumaker HB: Midline extraperitoneal exposure of the abdominal aorta and the iliac arteries, *Surg Gynecol Obstet* 135:791–792, 1972.
18. Dion YM, Gracia CR: A new technique for laparoscopic aortobifemoral grafting in occlusive aortoiliac disease, *J Vasc Surg* 26(4):685–692, October 1997.
19. Dion YM, Gracia CR, Estakhri M et al.: Totally laparoscopic aortobifemoral bypass—a review of 10 patients, *Surg Laparosc Endosc Percutan Tech* 8:165–170, 1998.
20. Coggia M, Bourriez A, Javerliat I, Goeau-Brissonniere O: Totally laparoscopic aortobifemoral bypass: a new and simplified approach, *Eur J Vasc Endovasc Surg* 24(3):274–275, September 2002.
21. Dion YM, Thaveau F, Fearn SJ: Current modifications to totally laparoscopic "apron technique", *J Vasc Surg* 38(2):403–406, August 2003.
22. Alimi YS, Hartung O, Valerio N, Juhan C: Laparoscopic aortoiliac surgery for aneurysm and occlusive disease: when should a minilaparotomy be performed? *J Vasc Surg* 33(3):469–475, March 2001.
23. Kolvenbach R, Da SL, Deling O, Schwierz E: Video-assisted aortic surgery, *J Am Coll Surg* 190(4):451–457, April 2000.
24. Arous EJ, Nelson PR, Yood SM, Kelly JJ, Sandor A, Litwin DE: Hand-assisted laparoscopic aortobifemoral bypass grafting, *J Vasc Surg* 31(6):1142–1148, June 2000.
25. Da SL, Kolvenbach R, Pinter L: The feasibility of hand-assisted laparoscopic aortic bypass using a low transverse incision, *Surg Endosc* 16:173–176, 2002.
26. Jobe BA, Duncan W, Swanstrom LL: Totally laparoscopic abdominal aortic aneurysm repair, *Surg Endosc* 13(1): 77–79, January 1999.
27. Wisselink W, Cuesta MA, Gracia C, Rauwerda JA: Robot-assisted laparoscopic aortobifemoral bypass for aortoiliac occlusive disease: a report of two cases, *J Vasc Surg* 36(5):1079–1082, November 2002.
28. Kolvenbach R, Schwierz E, Wasilljew S, Miloud A, Puerschel A, Pinter L: Total laparoscopically and robotically assisted aortic aneurysm surgery: a critical evaluation, *J Vasc Surg* 39(4):771–776, April 2004.
29. Takagi H, Sugimoto M, Kato T, Matsuno Y, Umemoto T: Postoperative incision hernia in patients with abdominal aortic aneurysm and aortoiliac occlusive disease: a systematic review, *Eur J Vasc Endovasc Surg* 33(2):177–181, February 2007.
30. Raffetto JD, Cheung Y, Fisher JB et al.: Incision and abdominal wall hernias in patients with aneurysm or occlusive aortic disease, *J Vasc Surg* 37(6):1150–1154, June 2003.
31. Greenhalgh RM, Brown LC, Kwong GP, Powell JT, Thompson SG: Comparison of endovascular aneurysm repair with open repair in patients with abdominal aortic aneurysm (EVAR trial 1), 30-day operative mortality results: randomised controlled trial, *Lancet* 364(9437):843–848, September 4, 2004.
32. Endovascular aneurysm repair versus open repair in patients with abdominal aortic aneurysm (EVAR trial 1): randomised controlled trial, *Lancet* 365(9478):2179–2186, June 25, 2005.
33. Kolvenbach R, Ferrari M, Shifrin EG: Laparoscopic assisted aortic surgery. A review, *J Cardiovasc Surg (Torino)* 47(5):547–556, October 2006.
34. Coggia M, Javerliat I, Di Centa I et al.: Total laparoscopic versus conventional abdominal aortic aneurysm repair: a case-control study, *J Vasc Surg* 42(5):906–910, 2005 November.
35. de Vries SO, Hunink MG: Results of aortic bifurcation grafts for aortoiliac occlusive disease: a meta-analysis, *J Vasc Surg* 26(4):558–569, October 1997.
36. Ricco JB, Probst H: Long-term results of a multicenter randomized study on direct versus crossover bypass for unilateral iliac artery occlusive disease, *J Vasc Surg* 47(1):45–53, January 2008.

37. Nazzal MM, Hoballah JJ, Jacobovicz C et al.: A comparative evaluation of femorofemoral crossover bypass and iliofemoral bypass for unilateral iliac artery occlusive disease, *Angiology* 49(4):259–265, April 1998.
38. Maloney JD, Hoch JR, Carr SC, Acher CW, Turnipseed WD: Preliminary experience with minilaparotomy aortic surgery, *Ann Vasc Surg* 14(1):6–12, January 2000.
39. Turnipseed WD, Carr SC, Hoch JR, Cohen JR: Minimal incision aortic surgery (MIAS), *Ann Vasc Surg* 17(2): 180–184, March 2003.
40. Turnipseed WD: A less-invasive minilaparotomy technique for repair of aortic aneurysm and occlusive disease, *J Vasc Surg* 33(2):431–434, February 2001.
41. Alimi YS, De CG, Hartung O et al.: Laparoscopy-assisted reconstruction to treat severe aortoiliac occlusive disease: early and midterm results, *J Vasc Surg* 39(4):777–783, April 2004.
42. Olinde AJ, McNeil JW, Sam A, Hebert SA, Frusha JD: Totally laparoscopic aortobifemoral bypass: a review of 22 cases, *J Vasc Surg* 42(1):27–34, July 2005.
43. Kolvenbach R, Schwierz E, Wasilljew S, Miloud A, Puerschel A, Pinter L: Total laparoscopically and robotically assisted aortic aneurysm surgery: a critical evaluation, *J Vasc Surg* 39(4):771–776, April 2004.
44. Kalko Y, Ugurlucan M, Basaran M et al.: Standard open repair versus minilaparotomy approach for abdominal aortic aneurysms: what is the best approach in patients with ischemic heart disease? *Minerva Chir* 63(4):269–276, August 2008.
45. Dion YM, Griselli F, Douville Y, Langis P: Early and midterm results of totally laparoscopic surgery for aortoiliac disease: lessons learned, *Surg Laparosc Endosc Percutan Tech* 14(6):328–334, December 2004.
46. Coggia M, Javerliat I, Di Centa I et al.: Total laparoscopic bypass for aortoiliac occlusive lesions: 93-case experience, *J Vasc Surg* 40:899–906, 2004.
47. Velidedeoglu E, Williams N, Brayman KL et al.: Comparison of open, laparoscopic, and hand-assisted approaches to live-donor nephrectomy, *Transplantation* 74(2):169–172, July 27, 2002.
48. Shokeir AA: Open versus laparoscopic live donor nephrectomy: a focus on the safety of donors and the need for a donor registry, *J Urol* 178(5):1860–1866, November 2007.
49. Muzii L, Basile S, Zupi E et al.: Laparoscopic-assisted vaginal hysterectomy versus minilaparotomy hysterectomy: a prospective, randomized, multicenter study, *J Minim Invasive Gynecol* 14(5):610–615, 2007.
50. Song KY, Park CH, Kang HC et al.: Is totally laparoscopic gastrectomy less invasive than laparoscopy-assisted gastrectomy? Prospective, multicenter study, *J Gastrointest Surg* 12:1015–1021, 2008; PMID: 18256884.
51. Fourneau I, Sabbe T, Daenens K, Nevelsteen A: Hand-assisted laparoscopy versus conventional median laparotomy for aortobifemoral bypass for severe aorto-iliac occlusive disease: a prospective randomised study, *Eur J Vasc Endovasc Surg* 32(6):645–650, December 2006.
52. Kelly JJ, Kercher KW, Gallagher KA, Litwin DE, Arous EJ: Hand-assisted laparoscopic aortobifemoral bypass versus open bypass for occlusive disease, *J Laparoendosc Adv Surg Tech A* 12(5):339–343, 2002.
53. Fourneau I, Lerut P, Sabbe T, Houthoofd S, Daenens K, Nevelsteen A: The learning curve of totally laparoscopic aortobifemoral bypass for occlusive disease. How many cases and how safe? *Eur J Vasc Endovasc Surg* 35:723–729, February 20, 2008.
54. Waltman AC, Katzen BT, Ring EJ, Martin EC, Sos TA, Tegtmeyer CJ: Society of cardiovascular and interventional radiology: credentials criteria for peripheral, renal, and visceral percutaneous transluminal angioplasty, *Radiology* 167:452, 1988.
55. Subspecialty Training in Vascular Interventional Radiology. Bedford, 2008, British Society of Interventional Radiology.
56. Nio D, Diks J, Bemelman WA, Wisselink W, Legemate DA: Laparoscopic vascular surgery: a systematic review, *Eur J Vasc Endovasc Surg* 33(3):263–271, March 2007.
57. Cau J, Ricco JB, Marchand C et al.: Total laparoscopic aortic repair for occlusive and aneurysmal disease: first 95 cases, *Eur J Vasc Endovasc Surg* 31(6):567–574, June 2006.
58. Kolvenbach R, Pinter L, Raghunandan M, Cheshire N, Ramadan H, Dion YM: Laparoscopic remodeling of abdominal aortic aneurysms after endovascular exclusion: a technical description, *J Vasc Surg* 36(6):1267–1270, December 2002.
59. Wahlgren CM, Skelly C, Shalhav A, Bassiouny H: Hybrid laparorobotic debranching and endovascular repair of thoracoabdominal aortic aneurysm, *Ann Vasc Surg* 22(2): 285–289, March 2008.
60. Wisselink W, Cuesta MA, Berends FJ, van den Berg FG, Rauwerda JA: Retroperitoneal endoscopic ligation of lumbar and inferior mesenteric arteries as a treatment of persistent endoleak after endoluminal aortic aneurysm repair, *J Vasc Surg* 31:1240–1244, 2000.
61. Coggia M, Javerliat I, Di Centa I, Royer B, Kitzis M, Goeau-Brissonniere OA: Total videoscopic treatment of a type IV thoracoabdominal aneurysm, *J Vasc Surg* 41: 141–145, 2005.
62. Di C, Coggia I Javerliat I et al.: Total laparoscopic suprarenal aortic coral reef removal, *J Vasc Surg* 44(1): 194–197, July 2006.
63. Fukui S, Paraskevas N, Soury P, Gigou F, Petit MD, Laurian C: Totally videoendoscopic descending thoracic aorta to femoral artery bypass, *J Vasc Surg* 37(1):191–193, January 2003.
64. Diks J, Nio D, Jongkind V, Cuesta MA, Rauwerda JA, Wisselink W: Robot-assisted laparoscopic surgery of the infrarenal aorta: the early learning curve, *Surg Endosc* 21(10):1760–1763, October 2007.
65. Bakoyiannis C, Cagiannos C, Wasilljew S, Puerschel A, Pinter L, Kolvenbach R: Laparoscopic hybrid techniques for ectopic or accessory renal arteries debranching in complex endovascular aneurysm repair, *J Cardiovasc Surg (Torino)* 49(1):67–71, February 2008.
66. Bakoyiannis C, Cagiannos C, Wasilljew S, Pinter L, Kolvenbach R: Totally laparoscopic aortohepatic bypass for aortic debranching during endovascular thoracoabdominal aneurysm repair, *Eur J Vasc Endovasc Surg* 34(2):173–175, August 2007.
67. Kolvenbach R, Lin J: Combining laparoscopic and endovascular techniques to improve the outcome of aortic endografts. Hybrid techniques, *J Cardiovasc Surg (Torino)* 46(4):415–423, August 2005.

Endovenous Surgery

28

John J. Bergan and Nisha Bunke

Surgery of the veins was dominant in the early days of the modern era of vascular surgery up to about 1980. Now it has languished in performance and in progress. One of the many reasons for this is that arterial reconstruction is so spectacular and appealing to both patient and surgeon that performance of its procedures has crowded out teaching of venous disorders to students and surgical residents. Consequently, several generations of surgeons have learned little about venous pathophysiology and treatment. For them, endoluminal techniques of sclerotherapy and internal vein ablation have become an anathema. Therefore treatment of vein problems has lagged behind progress made on the other side of the circulation, in the arteries.

However, there is a sense of change in the surgical field. A new generation of surgeons is beginning to see the importance of venous treatment. They realize that diagnostic tools such as magnetic resonance phlebography and color duplex ultrasonography can unravel mysteries of venous pathophysiology. They see that minimally invasive interventions, so important to the patient's perception of success of operations, can be applied to veins. Therefore the future looks bright for endoluminal venous surgery. It is certainly appropriate to include a summary of its present status and future promise in this book.

At this time a variety of techniques have joined sclerotherapy and stripper introduction as endoluminal manipulations in the veins. Included in this armamentarium are angioscopy and several endoluminal endovenous ablative techniques including foam sclerotherapy. In addition, endoluminal, catheter-directed thrombolysis can be supplemented by percutaneous transluminal angioplasty (PTA) and stent placement. Also, subfascial video-endoscopy, although not truly endoluminal, must be considered in the same category because it provides outpatient, minimally invasive treatment to achieve the objectives of more traditional, older operations. This chapter considers the status of these advances in exploration of the venous system.

Current Status: Diagnosis

Progress in developing endoluminal venous surgery can proceed only after there is knowledge of the current status of venous interventions and the pathophysiology that they are designed to correct. Currently, in diagnosis, clinical examination provides a subjective categorization of venous dysfunction. This is then corroborated by instrumental objectivity. The hand-held, continuous-wave Doppler instrument lends such objectivity and has become an integral part of the venous examination [1]. It performs the same function as the Brodie–Trendelenburg test.

Commonly, the physical examination and hand-held Doppler examination are supplemented by a duplex examination. This is conducted in the supine patient when acute or chronic venous obstruction such as venous thrombosis is suspected and in the erect patient when reflux is assessed [2]. Additional imaging to search for venous obstruction can be achieved by CT scanning, magnetic resonance, or contrast phlebography [3]. Physiologic importance of chronic venous occlusions remains elusive to evaluate. Among

J.J. Bergan (✉)
Founder, Vein Institute of La Jolla, La Jolla, CA, USA

T.J. Fogarty, R.A. White (eds.), *Peripheral Endovascular Interventions*,
DOI 10.1007/978-1-4419-1387-6_28, © Springer Science+Business Media, LLC 1998, 2010

the methods that are being employed are impedance plethysmography (IPG), mercury strain gauge (MSG), and air plethysmography (APG). Duplex scans remain the most dominant of all methods of evaluation of venous function.

Global information about whole-limb reflux is obtained by venous pressure recovery time (VRT), photoplethysmography (PPG) recovery time, or LRR or APG examination. The venous pressure, PPG, and LRR recovery times are rendered imprecise by the vagaries of tourniquet application [1] but remain in common use. It is easily appreciated that precisely targeted therapy requires specific venous segment information regarding venous obstruction or reflux rather than the whole-limb data obtained by PPG, LRR, and APG. These may not even accurately assess grades of venous insufficiency.

After detection of venous reflux by continuous-wave Doppler sonography, duplex study identifies precisely the refluxing segment. This information is directly useful clinically. Duplex software can also give information about volume and velocity of reflux, as well as diameter and cross-sectional area of interrogated veins, but the utility of that information is questioned [4].

Accumulated information derived from imaging techniques and physiologic studies has led to better terminology in the diagnosis of venous disorders. For example, the term *postphlebitic state* has been replaced by *chronic venous insufficiency* (CVI). The former, easily traced to the pioneering observations of Homans [5], carried the connotation of an irreversible condition. CVI, in contrast, includes the entire cutaneous spectrum of findings of the postphlebitic state with the understanding that these may be caused by primary venous insufficiency. This can be treated for palliation and even cured [6]. This fact is of great importance to the development of endovenous surgery. Repair of venous valves, for example, can be done in primary venous dysfunction but not in the secondary, post-thrombotic state. The patient with the most advanced stigmata of CVI may profit from the manipulations of endovascular repair. The limb may not have to be relegated only to treatment with elastic support.

Despite the spate of new tools to measure venous physiology and pathophysiology, the ascending [7] and descending [8] phlebograms remain the standard against which all other imaging such as CT scanning and magnetic resonance phlebography are measured. Often in practice, these are left to be performed after an advanced surgical procedure is chosen.

Current practice holds that venous problems in their simplest form, the telangiectasias, and perhaps even reticular varicosities, need only physical examination and study by hand-held, continuous-wave Doppler. Varicose veins, the next step up the hierarchical ladder of severity, require physical examination supplemented by the hand-held, continuous-wave Doppler and, if any intervention is contemplated, corroboration by duplex scanning. Economic constraints of managed care limit the use of imaging and duplex scanning, although Duplex scans are held to be the gold standard in detection of reflux in superficial and deep veins. If duplex examination or clinical assessment suggests the presence of obstruction either in the iliofemoral segment or in the femoropopliteal segment, imaging techniques need to be performed, such as ascending phlebography or magnetic resonance phlebography. Low-frequency ultrasound studies (2–5 MHz) can image the iliocaval veins. If surgical reconstruction is thought to be necessary, or if subfascial perforator vein interruption is contemplated, ascending phlebography supplemented by descending phlebography for valve repair is usually done. Physiologic studies including APG are performed primarily as research tools rather than in selecting therapy.

Current Status: Treatment

Sclerotherapy and surgery are no longer considered to be competitive. Detection of axial reflux in the saphenous systems usually indicates surgical intervention rather than sclerotherapy but this fact is coming under question [9]. Size and location of varicosities also affect this judgment. Small varices, especially below the knee where compression therapy is most effective, may suggest treatment by sclerotherapy, especially, foam sclerotherapy, whereas large varices, especially those arising in the medial thigh, may dictate treatment by targeted intervention.

Reluctance to remove the saphenous vein led to a resurgence of interest in proximal saphenous vein ligation for correction of the gravitational reflux component of venous stasis after 1980. However, repeated comparisons of proximal ligation and stripping of the saphenous vein to the knee continue to show long-term superiority of the latter procedure when used in combination with varicectomy, perforator interruption, or sclerotherapy [9]. Saphenous ligation has the ability to return the operated patient back to work or military duty immediately but is inferior to other techniques in the long term. In situations where rapid return to normal activity is requisite, the lesser procedure may be justified.

Thus, after the various options have been explored, the one that produces the best long-term results has proven to be selective great saphenous vein stripping or Great Saphenous ablation to the knee combined with multiple stab avulsions of varices [10].

Because reflux is the dominant pathologic finding in nearly all cases of venous dysfunction, the first step in surgical treatment is usually directed toward correction of this abnormality. Superficial reflux, rather than deep insufficiency, has proven to be an important component of the total problem in well over 50% of legs with the most severe manifestations of CVI [11]. Therefore removal of the refluxing superficial veins by the endoluminal techniques to be described is a logical first step in surgical therapy. If this is inadequate treatment, surgical venous reconstruction should be considered.

Options in venous reconstruction, which are part of the current armamentarium, include bypass of physiologically important obstruction, repair or transplantation of venous valves, or redirection of the venous stream through competent proximal valves. All of these have acceptable late results [12] but are not endoluminal.

Endoluminal Venous Stripping

The actual technique of saphenous removal (stripping) became endoluminal after Van Der Stricht [13] revived the technique first proposed by Babcock at the turn of the century [14]. In brief, the method includes selection of patients by Doppler or duplex ultrasound to ensure that saphenofemoral reflux is present, introducing the disposable plastic stripper through an open venotomy in a distal direction after transecting the vein and ligating the stump proximally (Fig. 28.1). After the stripper is exposed distally at or just below the knee, a heavy ligature is tied around the vein and the stripper at its proximal end. The vein wall is grasped so that distal traction on the stripper will invert the vein into itself thus minimizing peri-venous trauma. Further traction allows it to exit through the lower incision. This technique minimizes tissue trauma because the relatively large stripper heads formerly used in saphenous stripping are not used. Thus the procedure accomplishes the objectives and needs of proximal saphenous vein removal and does so, incidentally, in an endovenous fashion [15].

Although saphenous vein removal has received criticism, it has been tested against the other vein-sparing techniques and remains convincingly the best method of preventing persistent distal reflux and recurrent varicosities. Proximal saphenofemoral junction ligation with or without excision of clusters of varicosities is another surgical option. Duplex scanning has determined the natural history of proximal saphenous vein ligation in treatment of greater saphenous reflux [16]. In 52 of 54 limbs in which actual proximal ligation was achieved, there were 24 in which reflux persisted. Similarly, Rutherford found that 70% of limbs undergoing proximal ligation for venous insufficiency showed persisting reflux [17], and others have documented a similar experience [18]. Even when proximal ligation is supplemented by distal sclerotherapy, phlebographically controlled perforator ligation, or even surgical stab avulsion, the results are not as satisfactory as when the same maneuvers are added to saphenous vein removal to knee level [9].

Endoluminal Sclerotherapy

Treatment of venous dysfunction by purely endoluminal sclerotherapy has a time-honored history that dates back to the invention of the syringe over 150 years ago. Modern studies relating to foam sclerotherapy have clarified indications for this form of venous ablation [19, 20]. Sclerotherapy is used for the treatment of telangiectasias, reticular varicosities, postoperative persistence of varicosities, or when treatment is requisite in the aged or infirm [21].

When patients are found with no saphenofemoral or saphenopopliteal reflux, sclerotherapy can be considered. Such sclerotherapy must be planned so as to deal with the source of venous hypertension and the distribution of the various varicose clusters. No universally accepted single sclerotherapy technique has emerged. However, foam sclerotherapy is gaining popularity. An important contribution of the French school

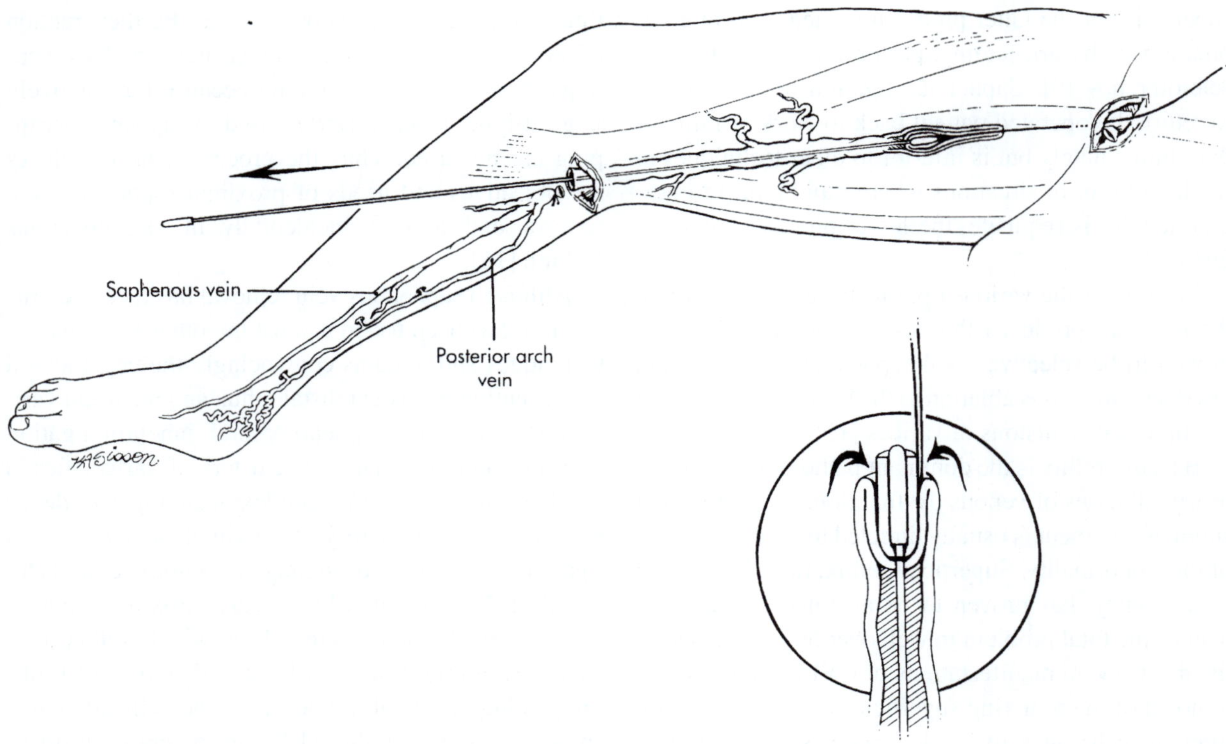

Fig. 28.1 Removal of the thigh portion of the saphenous vein is the mainstay in surgical treatment of primary venous insufficiency. The endoluminal device, commonly a disposable plastic stripper, can be introduced from above downward and the vein ligated around the stripper proximally. As distal traction is applied, the vein is inverted into itself and removed distally in the region of the knee. This minimizes tissue trauma but accomplishes the desired result of detaching the superficial venous system from perforating veins that are transmitting inter-compartmental pressure to unsupported subcutaneous venous networks

of sclerotherapy was emphasis on proximal-to-distal treatment [22]. A completely opposite point of view held that the largest diameter vessels must be treated first, since these are most likely to be transmitting pressure to smaller vessels. This is especially true when the source of venous hypertension is a perforating vein such as the anteromedial-calf-perforating vein named for Boyd. This method could result in distal-to-proximal treatment. Despite this and other controversies, some guiding principles remain in liquid and foam sclerotherapy: (1) empty veins should be treated rather than full veins; (2) the most dilute solution that will accomplish sclerosis should be used; (3) small amounts of sclerosant should be instilled at each injection site; (4) duration of compression will vary directly with the size of the vessel being treated: telangiectasias may need little or no compression or require only 12–24 h of compression, whereas large varicosities (4–6 mm in diameter) may require as much as 7–14 days of compression; and (5) ambulation is believed to cause rapid dilution of sclerosing solution, which prevents high concentrations of this solution from affecting deep veins.

Risks of deep venous thrombosis are lessened by adhering to the principle of injecting no more than 0.5–1.0 ml per injection site [23].

In foam sclerotherapy an upper limit of 15 ml/limb is usually adhered to. The greatest success is obtained when treating the smallest vessels. Subdermal reticular veins that are in intimate contact with telangiectasias are in this category. This technique requires 30-gauge needles, and the volume injected is 0.1–0.5 ml per reticular injection site. Treatment of the reticular veins before treatment of the telangiectasias greatly reduces the recurrence rate and minimizes side effects [24].

Endoluminal Endoscopy

Although venous thrombectomy is little used in the United States, the angioscope has been found to be invaluable in controlling completeness of thrombectomy in those situations where it has been chosen. Venous thrombectomy of the left iliofemoral system, in particular, lends itself to intravenous angioscopy. When this shows proximal thrombus clearance to be incomplete, the procedure can be terminated by further thrombectomy or a cross-femoral bypass from the common femoral vein to the contralateral external iliac vein with or without an arteriovenous fistula. Since venous thrombectomy is used only in situations of great need, having the option of intraoperatively monitoring clearance of thrombus is a valuable adjunct.

Miniaturization of endoscopic equipment allows exploration of the superficial venous system with visualization of the inside of the veins in situ and in vivo. Video recording of the morphology, dynamics, and kinetics of the valves is possible. Although this technique is currently in a stage of exploration, clearly the future holds hope for endovenous therapy, as is indicated below. Just as duplex ultrasound permits observation of the movements of valve leaflets, endoscopy provides a direct view of these valves. These are not seen in a physiologic state as the patient is supine and the valves are subject to irrigating fluid. However, many observations have been made that are of some value.

The classification of venous valves into three types has been made by Van Cleef [25]. Further, when passed from below, the angioscope with its internal illuminating system is able to transilluminate the veins from within, allowing very accurate location of the saphenofemoral junction and thus minimizing the external incision to control this point. This can be a very important adjunct when operations are done for varicose recurrence after proximal ligation. After failed proximal ligation of the saphenous vein, the angioscope passed from below minimizes the proximal dissection by identifying the exact point of ligature so that this can be exposed and dealt with properly.

Endoscopic evaluation of the saphenous vein has revealed it to have a preferential flattening that acts parallel to the surface of the skin. This gives a vein two walls, one internal and the other external, and two borders. The valves are inserted on each of the vein walls. The valve commissures are located on the borders; thus the free margins of the valves are parallel with the surface of the skin. Observation of valve function has revealed that transitory functional incompetence does occur in the valves (Fig. 28.2). This results from inertia of the valve leaflets and adherent flattening of the valve leaflet against the vein wall with resultant loss of coaptation.

The intercorunal or commissural space allows reflux along the margin of the valve. This important observation, made by Van Cleef, implies that external suture of the commissural space may restore competency to a refluxing valve. This observation supports the work of Kistner in performing external valve plasty. Finally, endoscopic observation has identified actual valve lesions such as stretching, splitting, and tearing that are de novo lesions clearly distinct from thickening, retraction, and adhesion of valves typically caused by previous phlebitis [26].

Angioscopy of the saphenous vein in particular has therapeutic implications. The frequent finding of long segments of apparently valveless greater saphenous veins suggests that total obliteration of the valve cusps has occurred [27]. Although chronic venous hypertension is a possibility in producing this type of valve destruction, a more likely possibility is leukocyte trapping, collagenase activation, and destruction of the supporting structure of the valve. Angioscopic observation of long, valveless segments of saphenous vein confirms the earlier work of Leonard Cotton. He

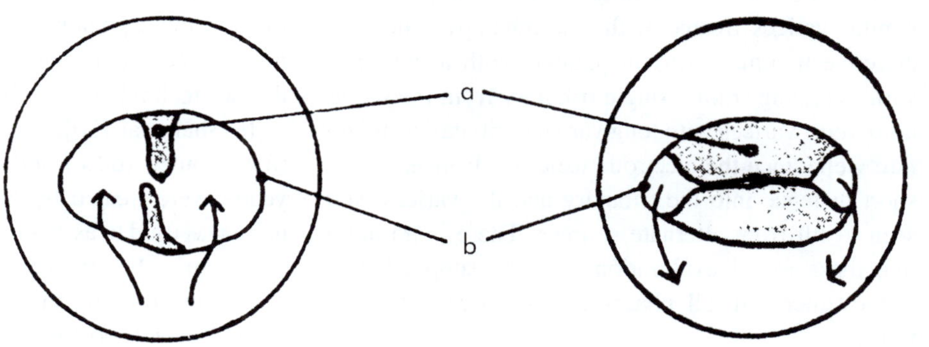

Fig. 28.2 Angioscopic observation of valve function has clarified origin of venous reflux. This occurs at the valve commissure **a**, and initiates reflux, which then proceeds along the margin of the valve, **b** (From Van Cleef et al. [26], with permission of Elsevier.)

reported long segments of avalvular greater saphenous vein in his dissections of veins removed from varicose vein patients [28].

Of further therapeutic importance are our observations that the greater saphenous vein is valveless or has no hemodynamically functional valves from the groin to the upper calf. The competent valves are frequently found near the anteromedial-calf-perforating vein (vein of Boyd). This observation confirms the advantage of greater saphenous stripping and ablative treatment only to the upper calf [10].

Since veins draining clusters of varicosities can readily be identified through the angioscope, it is logical to assume that endoscopically controlled obliteration of such veins might be of great therapeutic advantage in treating varicose clusters. Several groups have tried endovascular obliteration of tributary veins to the saphenous trunk in performance of in situ saphenous vein arterial bypass. Occlusion coils have been used. However, the technique is technically challenging, is sometimes ineffective, and causes intimal damage.

Endovenous Obliteration

More relevant to venous surgery, Gradman used venoscopically controlled endovascular obliteration of tributary veins in treatment of varicose clusters [29]. Monopolar electrocautery, available in most operating rooms, was used, and the electric current was delivered through a long, 0.4-mm steel alloy electrode insulated for most of its length with Teflon (Fig. 28.3). The 1-cm exposed electrode was directed into tributary veins where a 1-second burst was delivered with the energy system set for delivery of 10–15 W of power. Postoperatively, the appearance of varices thrombosed using endovascular coagulation was comparable to similar varices treated with sclerotherapy. The most effective treatment was in patients with a cluster of varices arising from a single tributary from the saphenous vein. Varices with long variceal tributaries did not fare well, since the electrode usually advanced only a short distance into the tributary and the varices were seen to fill from alternate sources. There is no doubt that these initial explorations will be supplanted by improvements in all phases of the procedure in the future.

Another endovenous approach to therapy has been explored by the VNUS Medical Technologies Company of Sunnyvale, California. Their two projects included endovenous occlusion and endovenous shrinking. The former was to obliterate grossly refluxing valve segments such as the saphenous vein, and the latter was to restore valve competence in axial veins when shrinkage could be applied (e.g., a refluxing but small-diameter saphenous vein). Their latter technique of vein shrinkage was abandoned long ago.

The VNUS system consists of a radiofrequency generator that displays power, impedance, temperature, and the time elapsed during which the pulse is delivered. There is a temperature control, and the system delivers the minimum power necessary to maintain a preset electrode temperature. Messages to the operator are supplied. The closure catheter consists of four collapsible electrodes surrounding a microthermacouple, which measures and delivers information about vein temperature. It is designed to be used in 2- to 6-mm veins through a 5F (1.7 mm) catheter. In practice, the closure catheter is inserted into the desired segment of vein; once in position, the electrodes are deployed, and a radiofrequency energy is initiated. The vein wall contracts owing to the increased temperature initiated by the electrodes, and the catheter is slowly withdrawn, closing vein segments as it moves.

The system in practice is designed to close segments of the greater saphenous vein or lesser saphenous vein. In theory, it can be inserted into major tributaries to the greater saphenous vein at the groin such as the anterolateral vein or the posteromedial vein with its connections to the vein of Giacomini. This variation in technique has been successfully explored. Whether the system could be used for recurrent varices depends on the potential accessibility of those varices and the ability to thread the catheter through them [29].

The endovenous laser has also become popular in treating the saphenous reflux of severe venous insufficiency. As foam sclerotherapy has become available, the two techniques have been compared.

In Shanghai [30], a consecutive series of patients (639 women [60%] and 421 men [40%] age 23–79 years) were treated by laser techniques. A questionnaire was used to assess preoperative and postoperative symptoms. The primary outcomes for assessing safety were mortality and morbidity, including laser-related adverse events, postoperative infection, and thrombotic

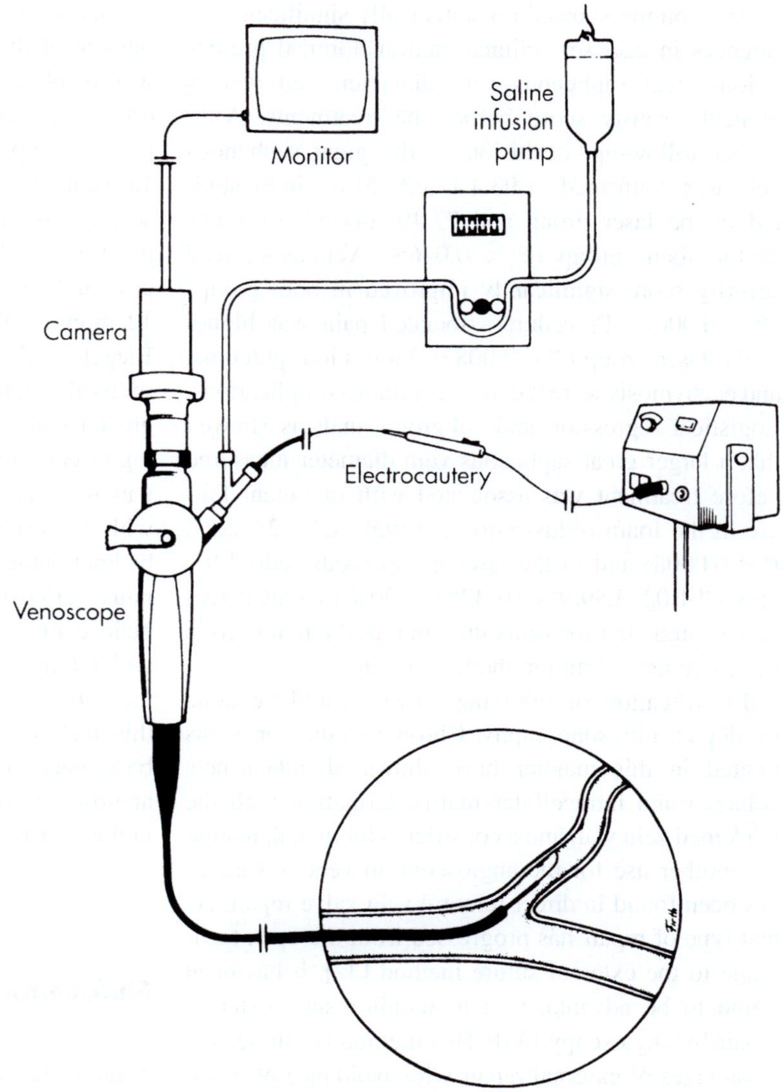

Fig. 28.3 Monopolar electrocautery delivered to the orifice of veins draining varicose clusters can obliterate those tributaries and the control points for the cluster itself (From Gradman et al. [55], with permission of Wiley.)

events. Effectiveness was assessed by the obliteration of the vein, disappearance of varicosities. All patients tolerated the procedure well, recovered uneventfully, and returned to daily activities and work 3–14 days after the operation. Treatment with laser plus ligation of the GSV resulted in occlusion in all cases at 2 weeks follow-up and in 1169 of 1186 (99%) patients at 6-month follow-up.

As foam sclerotherapy has emerged as a viable treatment option, it has been compared with alternate techniques [31]. A non-randomized prospective controlled study was designed (1) to test the hypothesis that endovenous laser treatment is more effective than foam sclerotherapy in the closure of the refluxing GSV and (2) to record the associated complications of echo-guided endovenous chemical ablation with foam and endovenous laser therapy for the treatment of great saphenous vein reflux and to identify risk factors associated with treatment failure. Patients seeking treatment of varicose veins were assessed for study. Inclusion criteria were (1) presence of great saphenous vein reflux and (2) C2-6, according to the CEAP classification. The selected patients consented to the study and were allowed to choose between foam (53 patients) and laser (45 patients) treatment. Duplex examinations were performed prior to treatment and at 7 and 14 days, 4 weeks, 6 months, and 1 year after treatment. Venous clinical severity score was assessed pre-treatment and at 1-year post-procedure.

The cohorts showed no statistically significant differences in age, sex, clinical and anatomical presentation, great saphenous vein diameter, and venous clinical severity score before the treatments. After 1-year follow-up, occlusion of the great saphenous vein was confirmed in 93.4% (42/45) of limbs studied in the laser group and 77.4% (41/53) of limbs in the foam group ($P < 0.0465$). Venous clinical severity score significantly improved in both groups ($P < 0.0001$). Procedure-associated pain was higher in the laser group ($P < 0.0082$). Induration, phlebitis, and ecchymosis were the most common complications. Logistical regression and subgroup analysis showed that a larger great saphenous vein diameter measured before treatment was associated with treatment failure in the foam (odds ratio 1.68, 95% CI 1.24–2.27, $P < 0.0008$) and in the laser group (odds ratio 1.91, 95% CI 1.02–3.59, $P < 0.0428$). A 90% treatment success is predicted for veins <6.5 mm in the foam group versus veins <12 mm in the laser group.

Identification of refluxing valves would be done by duplex ultrasonography. Chronic studies on veins treated in this manner have shown abundant new collagen and intracellular matrix formation with the thickened vein wall and a constricted luminal diameter.

Another use for the angioscope in venous surgery has been found in direct femoral vein valve repair. As that type of repair has progressed from the open technique to the external suture method [32], it has been found to be advantageous to monitor such external repair by angioscopy [33]. This method combines the advantages of external repair with avoidance of venotomy yet with accurate suture placement to ensure that the needle passes through the vein lumen and captures the edges of the elongated valve cusps. The angioscope allows discovery of hypoplastic or absent valve leaflets, which would preclude valve repair. Further, the angioscope allows final direct assessment of the repair so that valve competence is assured before surgical closure of the incision. With external vein plasty, multiple vein valves can be repaired at one operative sitting. Even greater saphenous vein valvular incompetence can be corrected if the angioscope is passed through one of the tributary veins near the saphenofemoral junction. A disadvantage of the technique is angioscope-induced trauma to venous intima or valve leaflets. Further, intraluminal pressures must be controlled very accurately to avoid disruption of the delicate valve repair.

Advocates of sclerotherapy would herald the development of the small-caliber angioscope as a possible way of obliterating greater saphenous reflux without open operation. Biegeleisen explored this possibility [34]. In 16 patients, attempts were made to obliterate 18 veins by angioscopic sclerotherapy. The angioscope was successfully passed to the saphenofemoral junction in 14 patients, and there was short-term success in 12 of them. In nine veins followed for up to 12 months, all nine recanalized in that time period. Biegeleisen's conclusion was that the magnitude of reflux through the saphenofemoral junction was much greater than had been imagined previously. This finding of complete recanalization was disparate from the patient's observations. Patients were generally satisfied with the results, but it was "evident, however, that we had not obtained durable obliteration of greater saphenous varicosities with this method." Because some believe that greater saphenous ablation can be done with purely endoluminal, sclerotherapeutic techniques, the subject is not closed [35]. The future holds that this technique may receive selective application or be replaced entirely by foam sclerotherapy. Clearly, angioscopy may find a place in direct venous surgery in the near future.

Endovenous Thrombolysis

Though thrombolytic therapy offers the potential of removing acute thrombus and preserving valvular integrity, concern for patient safety (based on bleeding complications associated with early trials of systemic infusions) has prevented its widespread use [36]. In addition to bleeding complications, systemic thrombolytic therapy is ineffective for treating lower extremity venous occlusion, as flow is shunted to collaterals and the superficial veins, away from the thrombosed segments.

The introduction of catheter-directed thrombolysis, unlike systemic thrombolysis, which has limited benefit in lower extremity deep venous thrombosis (DVT) due to preferential flow into collateral veins, offers an alternative method for treating DVT. Catheter-directed thrombolysis with urokinase has shown promise in treating both arterial and venous peripheral vascular diseases [37–40]. Evidence reveals that 75–79% of patients treated for DVT with this technique demonstrated complete or partial lysis of thrombus, improved vessel patency, and alleviation of symptoms [41, 42]. Although some investigators have stated that the estimated age of the thrombus is inversely correlated with technical success, we have shown clinical benefits from improved venous flow after treating chronic thrombosis as well [41, 43]. Urokinase has been recommended as the agent of choice for treating DVT because of its margin of safety and low complication rate [44, 45].

With its varying degrees of severity, DVT is a complex disease to treat. Experience suggests that thrombolysis offers advantages over anticoagulation alone, particularly for maintaining valvular competence. We have concluded that thrombolysis with urokinase is a safe, effective alternative to heparin anticoagulation for treating DVT. Furthermore, when comparing patients treated for a first known episode of DVT, urokinase patients experienced significantly less postthrombotic pain. This observation endured throughout the 10-year follow-up and suggests that removal of thrombus mitigates, if not prevents, valvular damage that leads to venous hypertension. Although most patients with chronic venous insufficiency have reflux without thrombosis, 10–15% of this population are afflicted by residual obstruction. This represents a large number of patients who suffer from apparently preventable postthrombotic sequelae.

Patient selection for thrombolysis remains a challenge and appears to include active patients with extensive, multisegmental obstructing thrombosis. Our unreported data suggest that thrombolysis versus standard therapy provides a clinical challenge to this group. This advantage could result in less venous disease over a lifetime and might represent a significant decrease in health-care costs to society.

Venous Stenting

Intravascular stents have been designed for use in arteries; experience with stents in the venous system is more limited but remains favorable. The longest reported clinical follow-up of arterial stenting is in the 5- to 10-year range. Therefore there is no conclusive evidence that long-term results will be satisfactory in the venous system. At present, venous stenting, a truly endoluminal technique, is restricted to a highly selected group of individuals who are poor surgical candidates but who have venoocclusive disease caused by thrombosis, prior surgery, and even angioplasty. Despite this, it has become increasingly apparent that percutaneous procedures are useful in opening venous conduits that are closed, compressed, or stenotic.

Endoluminal stents are fully described elsewhere in this book. Stents currently in use include stainless steel, tantalum, and nickel–titanium alloy. These have been fashioned into rigid tubes, flexible wire cylinders, woven meshes, and other designs that have been created to enhance desirable characteristics. The future holds that complex polysaccharide matrixes may be employed in an effort to obtain bioresorptive lattice works. The stents may be balloon expandable, such as the Palmaz stent, or self-expanding such as the Wallstent or the Gianturco Z stent. The latter are stainless steel, but their designs and methods of deployment are quite different.

The largest experience of venous stenting reported to date is that of the Stanford group [46]. Their experience includes treatment of the vena cava, the innominate, the subclavian, thoracic outlet venous compression, and iliofemoral veins (Figs. 28.4 and 28.5). Nearly half of their patients have had regional

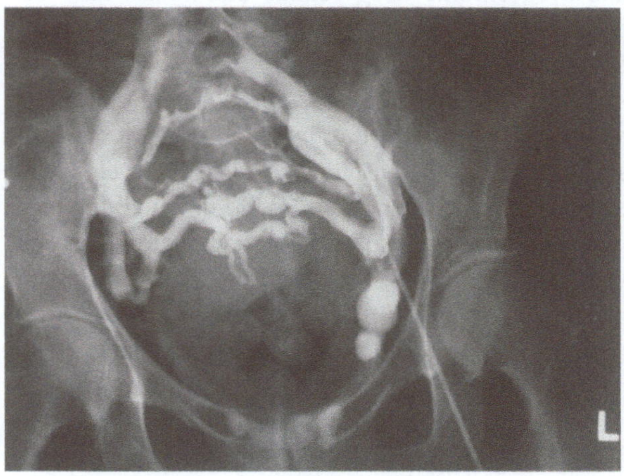

Fig. 28.4 This left iliac phlebogram shows the characteristic appearance of the May–Thurner syndrome with right iliac artery compression of the left common iliac vein. The patient is a 27-year-old woman with refractory venous stasis ulceration who demonstrated superficial reflux in the greater saphenous system distal to this lesion. Ablation of such reflux did not result in ulcer healing, and therefore the procedure of left iliac venous dilation and stenting was planned

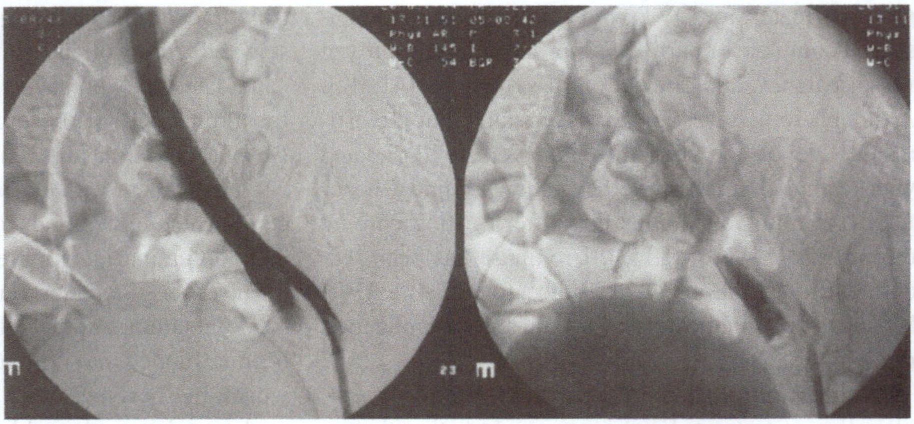

Fig. 28.5 These photographs taken during venous stenting in Fig. 28.4 demonstrate placement of the self-expanding Wallstent and the smooth venous channel that results after its insertion. Note the absence of crossover venous collateral vessels. This indicates that the physiologic obstruction present with the May–Thurner syndrome has been totally relieved

thrombolysis. In those without thrombus, a significant pressure gradient and/or residual stenosis was observed after percutaneous transluminal dilatation. They averaged placement of 2.8 stents per patient, with a resolution of venous obstructive symptoms in 97% of treated patients. Late follow-up revealed a 10% occlusion rate, but secondary patency was achieved in 95% of these. The Stanford group, with its vast experience, favors placement of stents in malignant obstructions. However, they have addressed the problem of failing hemodialysis access conduits in which the results are usually palliative but safe. In treating venous thrombosis, results with acute thromboses have been dramatic, and even chronic deep venous thrombosis has been benefited by treatment with catheter-directed thrombolysis and stent placement.

When lytic agents are used before stent placement, access can be gained through proximal arterial infusion or retrograde installation into foot veins with external compression. Ultrasound-directed popliteal puncture or even ipsilateral or contralateral femoral vein access is also a possibility. The transjugular placement of an infusion catheter directly into the thrombus has been found to be a favorable alternative because this provides easy access, prevention of further deep venous thrombosis from catheter placement, and sparing of the femoral vein from catheter-related trauma.

Advantages of the thrombolysis stent placement technique are obvious. No surgical procedure is required; no arteriovenous fistula is constructed [47]. However, as with any treatment modality, long-term careful observation is mandatory. These techniques may be only of short-term benefit.

Subfascial Endoscopy

Although technically not endovenous, subfascial operations using endoscopy should be included in this review because they fulfill the requirements of achieving therapeutic objectives in a minimally invasive fashion that allows outpatient, economically advantageous procedures to be accomplished. Perforator vein interruptions have been performed for decades in the treatment of severe chronic venous insufficiency. However, long hospitalization time required by slow secondary healing of long incisions from knee to ankle has discouraged wide application of these procedures.

Introduction of laparoscopic general surgery spurred investigation of minimally invasive approaches to venous surgery. Accumulating experience suggested that video-assisted techniques might be applicable to subfascial perforator interruption because 90% of incompetent perforating veins occur in the lower leg in the posterior arch vein distribution [48].

Clinically significant perforators include the gastrocnemius point, soleal point, and perforating veins identified at varying distances from the heel pad [49]. All of these are accessible by endoscopic coagulation or clipping. Such interruption occludes the perforating vein proximal to its branchings, and this approach allows transsection of all perforators that are thought to be clinically significant. An appealing aspect of the procedure is that it can be performed on an outpatient basis. Furthermore, the surgical incision is made proximal to affected skin even in patients with far-advanced changes of lipodermatosclerosis and healed ulceration.

We have chosen to modify the open technique of Reinhard Fischer of St. Gallen, Switzerland [50]. The incision is made on the anteromedial leg posterior to the tibia. The 3-cm skin and subcutaneous incision is retracted to expose the fascia that is incised. A subfascial space is created by inserting the endoscope and manipulating it anteriorly as far as is feasible and then posteriorly as far as needed. For us, foam sclerotherapy has totally replaced subfascial perforator interruption.

In subfascial exploration, it is relatively easy to distinguish a normal perforating vein that is competent from one that is incompetent. The normal perforator exhibits one or more veins with parallel walls that are not tortuous or dilated. The accompanying artery is often seen. In contrast, the incompetent perforating vein is often thick, passes transversely, is apparently white, and looks bloodless if a tourniquet is used and exsanguination of the limb has preceded the exploration. Without the tourniquet the incompetent perforating vein looks like any other varicose vein. Frequently the incompetent perforating vein is seen to branch into one or more tributaries before penetrating the fascia. Recognition of perforating veins is much more accurate by the subfascial approach than by phlebography or preoperative Doppler or duplex techniques.

On the other hand, significant incompetent perforating veins manifest themselves clinically in two ways. First, they are adjacent to or are involved in areas of severe hyperpigmentation and lipodermatosclerosis. Second, they may be identified close to ulcers that have not responded to standard techniques of foam sclerotherapy, varicose cluster removal, VNUS closure, or laser ablation of incompetent veins.

Limitations of subfascial video endoscopic perforator interruption are found in the most distal aspect of the leg. This is a dangerous area anatomically. Here there is reduced maneuverability of the instrumentation. The most serious distal consequences of the procedure include damage to the posterior tibial nerve. Complications may be avoided by keeping the scope strictly close to the fascia in every step throughout the endoscopy. Also, no structure should be divided unless one is absolutely sure it is a perforating vein. Before applying the cautery, extreme care must be taken that the structure being clamped, cauterized, or clipped is a perforating vein and not the accompanying artery or posterior tibial nerve [51].

Division of the crural fascia in patients with the most severe forms of chronic venous insufficiency has been advocated by many [52, 53]. The subfascial endoscopic perforator interruption technique lends itself to such fasciotomy. After division of the perforating veins and thorough exploration of the available space, the procedure is terminated by passing a fasciotomy knife through the scope and incising the fascia from above downward or from below upward (Fig. 28.6). The pathophysiologic indication for this is the severe fascia fibrosis and elevated compartment pressures found in the fascia in severe chronic venous insufficiency [54]. Thickening, induration, and elevated pressures are thought to limit transfascial blood flow. Transcutaneous partial pressure of oxygen ($TCPO_2$) levels has been measured in patients before and after fasciotomy. In all instances the measurements were made 2 cm proximal to the ulceration and 2, 5, and 10 days after surgical manipulations. An increase in $TCPO_2$ was observed immediately postoperatively, and by the 10th postoperative day all patients showed $TCPO_2$ levels that were at least 100% higher than before surgery. The impressive increase in $TCPO_2$ was confirmed at 8 weeks after the procedure [53].

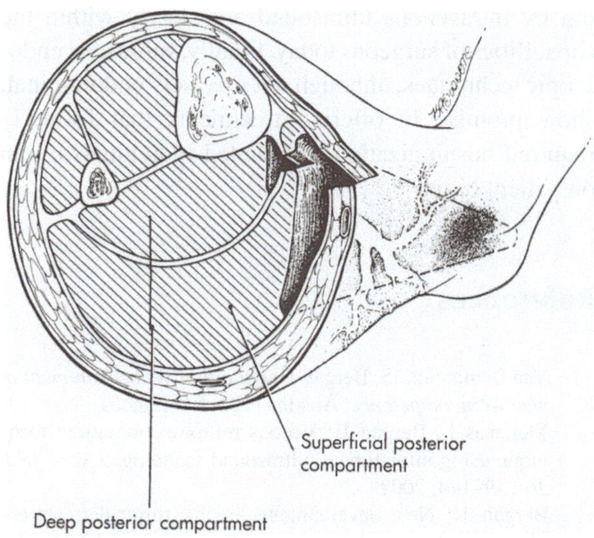

Fig. 28.6 Proximal incision and space that can be treated by subfascial endoscope. Perforator veins emanating from the superficial posterior compartment can be clipped and divided or electrocoagulated and divided using endoscope and video visualization. Paratibial perforating veins emanating from the deep posterior compartment can be identified after incision into fascia of the deep posterior compartment and exposure of those very important paratibial perforating veins

Von Langer measured compartment pressures in 12 patients with varicose veins, 18 with severe chronic venous insufficiency, and 6 with the postthrombotic syndrome [54]. Compartment pressures were lowest in those patients with primary venous insufficiency, intermediate in patients with severe chronic venous insufficiency, and highest in those with the postthrombotic syndrome. In all instances in these 36 patients a laser fasciotomy decreased the postoperative compartment pressures to one-half of the preoperative level. Since the broad fasciotomy split has been observed to remain open at least 6 months after the procedure, it appears that fasciotomy in situations of most severe chronic venous insufficiency is clearly an important addition to the minimally invasive armamentarium.

Conclusion

Endovenous surgery has passed through its infancy. Standard endoluminal techniques of saphenous ablation and sclerotherapy have now been joined by endoluminal thrombolysis and stenting in selected cases. Furthermore, explorations and angioscopy, electrodesiccation of selected venous tributaries, and monitoring by intravenous ultrasound are clearly within the capabilities of surgeons today. Finally, subfascial endoscopic techniques, although not precisely endoluminal, show promise in offering treatments that formerly required hospitalization to afflicted individuals on an outpatient basis.

References

1. Van Bemmelen JS, Bergan JJ: *Quantitative measurement of venous incompetence*, Austin, 1992, RG Landes.
2. Mekenas L, Bergan JJ: Venous reflux examination: technique using miniaturized ultrasound scanning, *J Vasc Tech* 26:139–144, 2002.
3. Bergan JJ: New developments in the surgical treatment of venous disease, *J Cardiovasc Surg (Torino)* 1:624–631, 1993.
4. Moulton S, Bergan JJ, Beeman S et al.: Gravitational reflux does not correlate with clinical status of venous stasis, *Phlebology* 8:2–6, 1993.
5. Homans J: Thrombophlebitis of the lower extremities, *Ann Surg* 87:641–651, 1928.
6. Walsh JC, Bergan JJ, Beeman S et al.: Femoral venous reflux is abolished by greater saphenous vein stripping, *Ann Vasc Surg* 8:566–570, 1994.
7. Lea Thomas M et al.: A simplified technique of phlebography for the localization of incompetent perforating veins of the legs, *Clin Radiol* 23:486, 1972.
8. Kamida CB, Kistner RL: Descending phlebography: the Straub technique. In Bergan JJ, Kistner RL, editors: *Atlas of venous surgery*, Philadelphia, 1992, WB Saunders.
9. Bunke N, Mekenas L, Bergan JJ: Non-saphenous treatment of venous insufficiency by foam sclerotherapy, *Ann Vasc Surg* (In Press).
10. Sarin S, Scurr JH, Coleridge-Smith PD: Assessment of stripping the long saphenous vein in the treatment of primary varicose veins, *Br J Surg* 79:889–893, 1992.
11. Shami SK, Sarin S, Cheatle TR et al.: Venous ulcers and the superficial venous system, *J Vasc Surg* 17:487, 1993.
12. Bergan JJ: Reconstruction of deep veins. In Negus D, editor: *Leg ulcers: a practical approach to management*, ed. 2, London, 1994, Butterworth-Heinemann.
13. Van Der Stricht J: La crossectomie. Quant et Pourquoi? *Extrait de Phlebologie* 39(1):47, 1986.
14. Babcock WW: A new operation for extirpation of varicose veins, *NY Med J* 86:1553, 1907.
15. Bergan JJ: Ambulatory surgery of varicose veins. In Bergan JJ, Goldman MP, editors: *Ambulatory treatment of venous disease: an illustrative guide*, St Louis, 1995, Mosby.
16. McMullin GM, Coleridge-Smith PD, Scurr JH: Objective assessment of high ligation without stripping the long saphenous vein, *Br J Surg* 78:1139–1142, 1991.
17. Rutherford RB, Sawyer JD, Jones DN: The fate of residual saphenous vein after partial removal or ligation, *J Vasc Surg* 12:422–428, 1990.
18. Friedell ML, Samson RH, Cohen MJ et al.: High ligation of the greater saphenous vein for treatment of lower extremity varicosities. The fate of the vein and therapeutic results, *Ann Vasc Surg* 6:5–8, 1992.
19. Hobbs JT: A random trial of the treatment of varicose veins by surgery and sclerotherapy. In Hobbs JT, editor: *The treatment of venous disorders*, Philadelphia, 1977, JB Lippincott.
20. Jakobsen BH: The value of different forms of treatment for varicose veins, *Br J Surg* 66:182–184, 1979.
21. Goldman MP, Weiss RA, Bergan JJ: Diagnosis and treatment of varicose veins: a review, *J Am Acad Dermatol* 3:393–414, 1994.
22. Tournay R, Caille JP, Chatard H et al.: *La sclerose des varices*, Paris, 1980, Expansion Scientifique.
23. Vanscheidt W, Heidrich H, Jünger M, Rabe E: Phlebology study group of the Austrian society of dermatology; German society of angiology; German society of phlebology; swiss society of phlebology. Guidelines for testing drugs for chronic venous insufficiency, *Vasa* 29(4): 274–278, November 2000.
24. Weiss RA, Weiss MA: Painful telangiectasias: diagnosis and treatment. In Bergan JJ, Goldman MP, editors: *Varicose veins and telangiectasias: diagnosis and treatment*, St Louis, 1993, Quality Medical Publishers.
25. Van Cleef JF, Desvaux P, Hugentobler JP et al.: Endoscopie Veneuse, *J Mal Vasc* 16:184–187, 1991.
26. Van Cleef JF, Hugentobler JP, Desvaux P et al.: Etude endoscopique des reflux valvulaires sapheniens, *J Mal Vasc* 17:113–116, 1992.

27. Gradman WS, Segalowitz J, Grundfest W: Venoscopy in varicose vein surgery: initial experience, *Phlebology* 8:145–150, 1993.
28. Cotton LT: Varicose veins: gross anatomy and development, *Br J Surg* 48:589–598, 1961.
29. Gradman WS: Venoscopic obliteration of variceal tributaries using monopolar electrocautery: preliminary report, *J Dermatol Surg Oncol* 20:482–485, 1994.
30. Lu X, Ye K, Li W, Lu M, Huang X: Endovenous ablation with laser for great saphenous vein insufficiency and tributary varices: a retrospective evaluation, *J Vasc Surg* 48(3):675–679, 2008.
31. Luebke T, Brunkwall J: Systematic review and meta-analysis of endovenous radiofrequency obliteration, endovenous laser therapy, and foam sclerotherapy for primary varicosis, *J Cardiovasc Surg* 49:213–233, 2008.
32. Kistner RL: Valve reconstruction for primary valve insufficiency. In Bergan JJ, Kistner RL, editors: *Atlas of venous surgery*, Philadelphia, 1992, WB Saunders.
33. Gloviczki P, Merrell SW, Bower TC: Femoral vein valve repair under direct vision without venotomy: a modified technique with use of angioscopy, *J Vasc Surg* 14:645–648, 1991.
34. Biegeleisen K: Failure of angioscopically guided sclerotherapy to permanently obliterate greater saphenous varicosity, *Phlebology* 9:21–24, 1994.
35. Raymond-Martimbeau P: Two different techniques for sclerosing the incompetent saphenofemoral junction: a comparative study, *J Dermatol Surg Oncol* 16:626–631, 1990.
36. Ricotta JJ, Dalsing MC, Ouriel K et al.: Research and clinical issues in chronic venous disease, *Cardiovasc Surg* 5:343–349, 1997.
37. Graor RA, Young JR, Rusius B, Ruschhaupt WF: Comparison of cost-effectiveness of streptokinase and urokinase in the treatment of deep venous thrombosis, *Ann Vasc Surg* 1:524–528, 1987.
38. Ouriel K, Shortell CK, DeWeese JA et al.: A comparison of thrombolytic therapy with operative revascularization in the initial treatment of acute peripheral arterial ischemia, *J Vasc Surg* 19:1021–1030, 1994.
39. Janosik JE, Bettmann MA, Kaul AF, Souney PF: Therapeutic alternatives for subacute peripheral arterial occlusion: comparison by outcome, length of stay, and hospital charges, *Invest Radiol* 26:921–925, 1991.
40. Van Breda A, Graor RA, Katzen BT et al.: Relative cost-effectiveness of urokinase versus streptokinase in the treatment of peripheral vascular disease, *J Vasc Interv Radiol* 2:77–87, 1991.
41. Bjarnason H, Kruse JR, Asinger DA et al.: Iliofemoral deep venous thrombosis: safety and efficacy outcome during five years of catheter-directed thrombolytic therapy, *J Vasc Interv Radiol* 8:405–418, 1997.
42. Comerota AJ, Katz ML, White JV: Thrombolytic therapy for acute deep venous thrombosis: how much is enough? *Cardiovasc Surg* 4:101–104, 1996.
43. Thorpe PE, Zhan XX, Sides SN: Endovascular therapy for chronic venous disease [abstract], *J Vasc Interv Radiol* 9:175, 1998.
44. Semba CP, Dake MD:: Venous thrombosis. In Ouriel K, editor: *Lower extremity vascular disease*, Philadelphia, 1995, Saunders, pp. 312–330.
45. Tomera JF, Kaul AF: Regional thrombolytic infusion for peripheral arterial occlusion and deep venous thrombosis: tried and true, *Am J Health Syst Pharm* 54:1988–1991, 1997.
46. Semba CP, Dake MD: Iliofemoral deep venous thrombosis: aggressive therapy with catheter-directed thrombolysis, *Radiology* 191:487–494, 1994.
47. Janssen HJ, Antonucci F, Stuckman G et al.: Behandlung von venenstenosen und verschlussen benigner Atiologie mit vaskularen endoprothesen: ein neues, nichtoperatives therapiekonzept, *Vasa* 23:66–73, 1994.
48. Jugenheimer M, Junginger T: Endoscopic subfascial sectioning of incompetent perforating veins in treatment of primary varicosis, *World J Surg* 16:971–975, 1992.
49. Sherman RS: Varicose veins: anatomy, reevaluation of Trendelenburg tests, and operating procedure, *Surg Clin North Am* 44:1369, 1964.
50. Fischer R: Erfahrungen mit der endoskopischen Perforantensanierung, *Phebologie* 21:224–229, 1992.
51. Fischer R, Sattler G, Vanderpuye R: Le traitement endoscopique des perforantes (TEP) situation actuelle, *Phlebologie* 46:701– 707, 1993.
52. Hauer G et al.: Endoskopische subfasziale diszision der perforansven. In Bruner H, editor: *Der unterschenkel. Aktuelle probleme in der angiologie*, Stuttgart, 1988, Huber.
53. Vanscheidt W, Peschen M, Kreitinger J et al.: Paratibial fasciotomy, *Phlebology* 23:45–48, 1994.
54. Von Langer C, Vorpahl U, Atamer C, Schack R: Die endoskopische laserfasciotomie. In Schatz R, Bruch H-P, Weiss H-D, editors: *Neue trends in diagnostik und therapie von venenleiden*, Labeck, 1993, Norddeutsche Angiologentage.
55. Gradman WS, Segalowitz J, Grundfest W: Venoscopy in varicose vein surgery: initial experience, *Br J Surg* 48: 589–598, 1961.

Thoracic Outlet Syndrome: Endoscopic Transaxillary First Rib Approach—23 Years Experience (1985–2008)

29

Bernardo D. Martinez and Angela M. Gerhardinger

Thoracic outlet syndrome is a condition related to compression of the subclavian axillary vein, artery, and brachial plexus due to significant congenital anomalies of the scalenus muscle's insertion at the first rib. In situations associated with trauma or occupational demand on the upper extremity, the functional relationship between these neurovascular structures, scalenus muscles, and the first rib appears to be altered.

Surgical Decisions

The surgical procedure elected depends on the patient's clinical manifestations. Most importantly, the decision for surgical intervention is based on worsening of the clinical symptoms of the patient, confirmation of the abnormal physical examination findings, the degree of disability, and failure of a conservative home exercise program to relieve neurogenic symptoms of compression. When symptoms of arterial and vein compression manifest, a thoracic outlet home exercise program is contraindicated.

Historical Remarks

The transaxillary approach for first rib resection was first described by Roos in 1966 [1], offering a lesser invasive alternative to the previously described anterior or supraclavicular approach [2], or the posterior approach [3]. The concept of adjunctive endoscopic video was adopted by us in 1983 because of the relative inaccessibility of the anatomic surgical area during the transaxillary approach [4]. This technique demonstrated the benefits of magnifying the anatomic surgical area, which ensures a greater measure of safety during the transaxillary approach [5, 6]. In 1982, the concerns for safety of transaxillary first rib resection was widely reported [7]. In addition, intraoperative endoscopic video during the transaxillary approach offers direct visualization of the congenital anomalies of the scalenus muscles and their compression of vital structures, greatly enhancing the likelihood of preserving functional integrity of the nerve, artery, and vein.

Congenital cervical band anomalies were first described by Roos in 1976 [8] and provided the concept that cervical bands are the key of the pathogenesis of thoracic outlet syndrome.

Most recently, we have adopted in the evolution of computer-enhanced instrumentation the application of robotic instrumentation during endoscopic transaxillary first rib resection [9]. Eighty-nine endoscopic transaxillary first rib resection procedures were completed with the first-generation robotic arm (Aesop/Hermes) with integrated voice control instrumentation. Forty-two surgical procedures were performed using the daVinci Surgical System.

It is our intention to report to you the current approach to endoscopic transaxillary first rib resection, having completed 115 transaxillary first rib resections using the daVinci Surgical System.

B.D. Martinez (✉)
Vascular Surgeon, Department of Vascular Surgery, The Toledo Hospital, Toledo, OH, USA

T.J. Fogarty, R.A. White (eds.), *Peripheral Endovascular Interventions*,
DOI 10.1007/978-1-4419-1387-6_29,

Anatomical Applications of the Cervical Bands and Scalenus Muscle into the First Rib During Endoscopic Transaxillary First Rib Resection

To understand the biomechanics of this surgical procedure, it is essentially important to review the basic anatomic landmarks of the first rib and its muscular insertions. Figure 29.1 shows the left first rib from a superior view, indicating that the most anterior muscular structure insertion is the subclavius muscle. This muscle orientation and hypertrophy are important in the development of venous compression in association with the costoclavicular ligament and the most anterior fibers of the scalenus anterior muscle, which inserts behind the vein. These three elements are key to the pathogenesis of extrinsic venous compression by a type 7 band [6, 8, 9], particularly in athletic muscular individuals. It is important to appreciate that the length of rib that lies underneath the clavicle remains anterior to the vein (Fig. 29.1), joining the sternum to create a relatively large surface area where the vein has to traverse the venous compartment of the thoracic outlet.

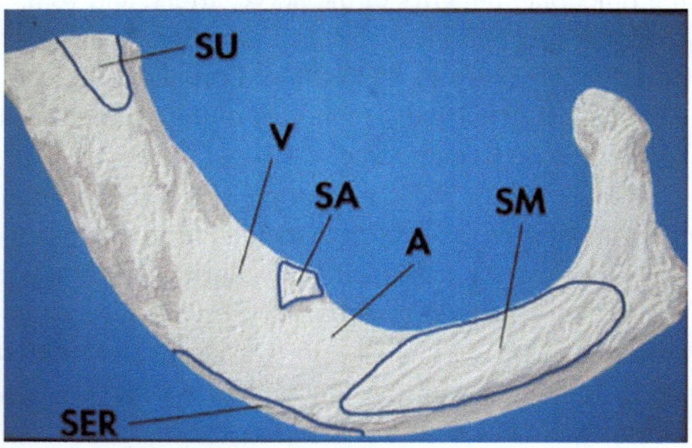

Fig. 29.1 The *left* first rib shows its muscular insertions. *SU*, subclavius; *V*, venous space; *SA*, scalenus anterior; *A*, arterial space; *SER*, serratus anterior; *SM*, scalenus medius

As a result of traversing the rib, venous and arterial rib notching is noted (Fig. 29.1) as well as the scalenus tubercle, the site of insertion of the scalenus anterior, that has significant anatomical variations. Obviously, a wide insertion of this muscle narrows the thoracic outlet space, producing neurovascular compression.

The scalenus medius is an important muscle and a key factor in neurogenic compression. Its broad insertion can produce the type 3 cervical band, which is a derivative of the most medial fibers of the scalenus medius in the inner border of the first rib and is the most common of all the congenital bands. Type 3 band is a critical factor in the compression of C8-T1 branches of the brachial plexus providing ulnar nerve distribution sensory clinical manifestations. Another important frequent band is the type 5, or scalenus minimus, which may have its lower insertion in the first rib or the Sibson fascia, called type 6, between the artery and the nerve (Fig. 29.2a–c).

Type 4 band is less frequent than the previous type 3 and type 5 bands; however, it is a very powerful band capable of severe compression of the nerve and the artery. This band, like a sling under the artery and the nerve, is composed of the most posterior fibers of the scalenus anterior and the most medial fibers of the scalenus medius (Fig. 29.3).

Severe neurovascular compression results from this type 4 cervical band that many times leaves practically no outlet to the nerve and the artery. This band could also be defined as an arcuate ligament that is around the nerve and the artery as a V shape rather than U shape, significantly compressing the neuro-arterial outlet space. Complete resection of the first rib and partial resection of the scalenus anterior and scalenus medius assure complete decompression of the neuro-arterial thoracic outlet space, therefore relieving the symptoms. Many times an area of indentation in the nerve is seen as the result of the previous compression by the type 4 cervical bands. The visualization of the articular surface of the transverse process of T1 vertebrae is a clear demonstration of complete excision of the first rib.

In our latest group of patients treated surgically with the daVinci Surgical System with 115 patients between February 2003 and August 2008, 15 patients or 13% had concomitant cervical ribs. Cervical ribs come in two forms. Type 1, which is the long cervical rib with the short tendinous portion connecting the cervical rib to the first rib at the scalenus tubercle (Fig. 29.4). Type 2 is the short cervical rib with a long tendinous portion of cervical band between the bony portion of the rib and the scalenus tubercle (Fig. 29.5). Old-fashioned cervical spine x-ray is the primary means of diagnosis of the cervical rib. These patients should be approached by a combined decompression of

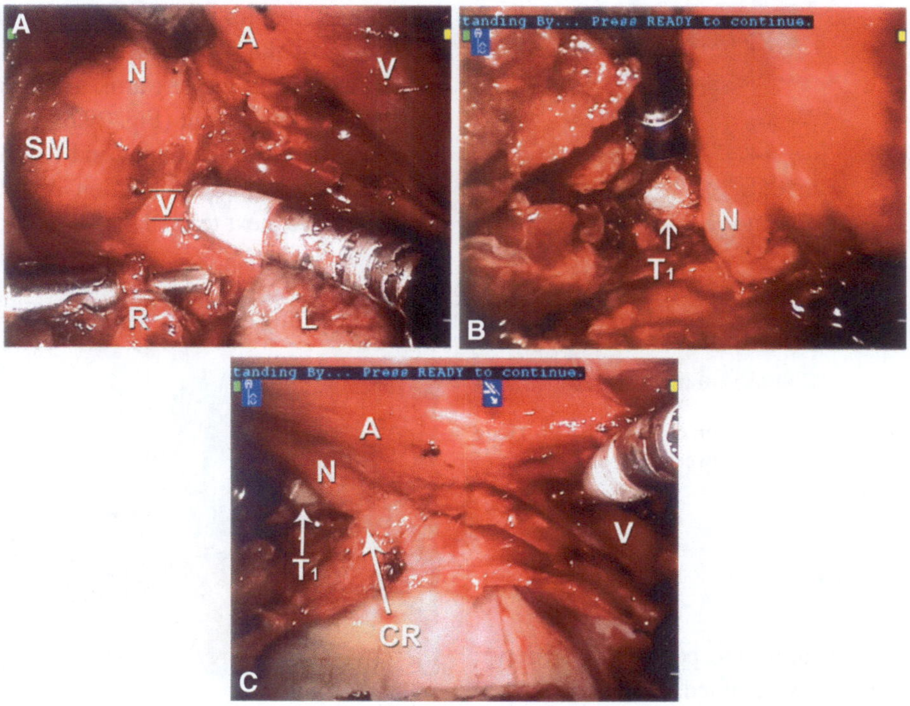

Fig. 29.2 **a–c**, The scalenus minimus may have its lower insertion in the first rib or the Sibson fascia, called type 6, between the artery and the nerve

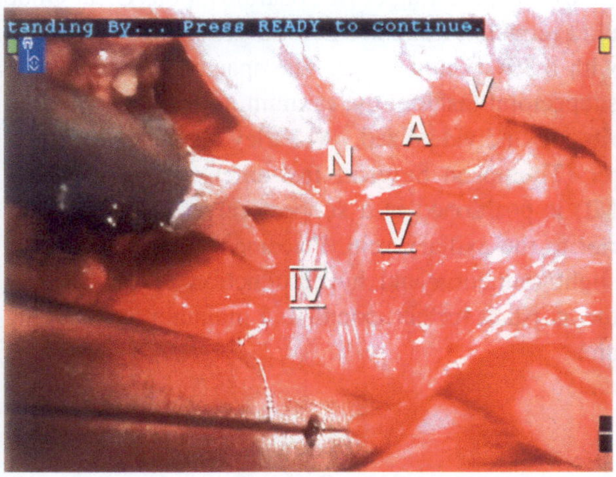

Fig. 29.3 The type 4 band is composed of the most posterior fibers of the scalenus anterior and the most medial fibers of the scalenus medius

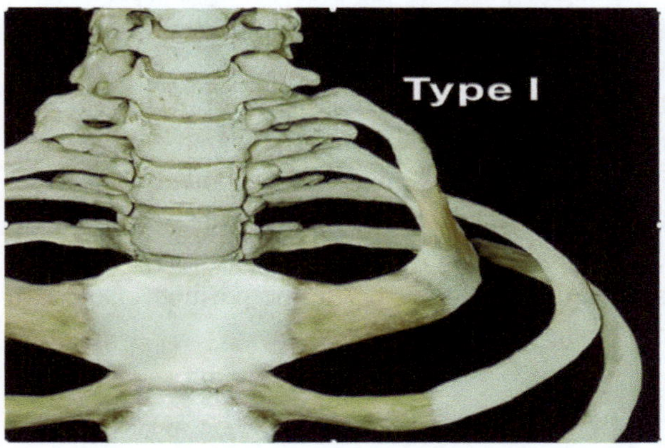

Fig. 29.4 Cervical rib type 1 is the long cervical rib with the short tendinous portion connecting the cervical rib to the first rib at the scalenus tubercle

supraclavicular excision of the cervical rib, disattachment of the cervical band, type 1 or type 2, and the transaxillary endoscopic approach to decompress the lower thoracic outlet area. Since our experience indicates that the combination of cervical bands, type 3, type 4, and type 5, with the cervical rib is clearly seen in three-fourths of our patients, our recommendation in cervical rib patients is to do a decompression supraclavicularly and transaxillarily for maximum benefit postoperatively.

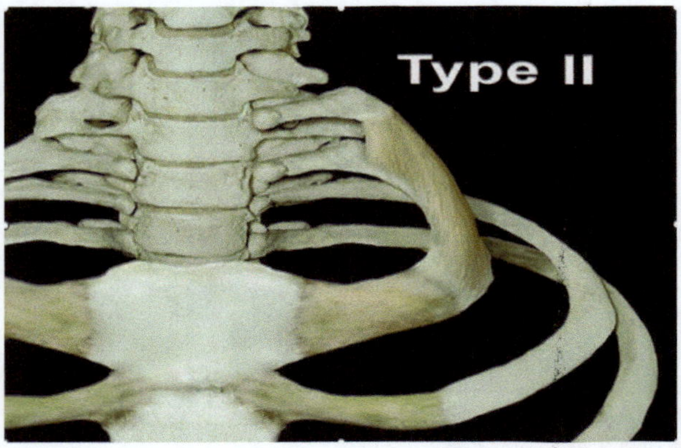

Fig. 29.5 Cervical rib type 2 is the short cervical rib with a long tendinous portion of cervical band between the bony portion of the rib and the scalenus tubercle

Surgical Procedure

Informed consent indicating the possibility of nerve, artery, or vein injury was obtained. A qualified anesthesiologist inserted a dual endotracheal tube-34F or 35F for females and 37F for males (Broncho-Cath with CPAP, Mallinckrodt Medical, Cormandy. Ireland). Standard anesthesia methods were used.

A supine position was used during a supraclavicular approach for a cervical rib resection or total anterior scalenectomy. A lateral position with 35° flexion of the leg was used for the transaxillary approach. The arm on the surgical side was fully prepared and wrapped in stockinette (Western Medical Limited, Camarillo, CA). Measures were taken to avoid unnecessary manual compression on the arm. A full-time assistant is always in place to supervise the position of the arm during the procedure.

Surgical Access

During the Aesop/Hermes procedures, a 30 mm mini-incision is performed transversely at the base of the axilla. A separate 10 mm port placement incision is made in the anterior axillary line, and a 512 Endopath SD trocar (Ethicon Endo-Surgery, Cincinnati, OH) is placed for the introduction of the endoscope.

In the daVinci subgroup, a 30 mm incision is made at the same level as in the first subgroup. Five centimeters distal from the working incision, three different ports are aligned for the right arm, the left arm, and the endoscope of the daVinci Surgical System. Between the right arm and the left arm, a base of 9–11 cm is used for port placement (Fig. 29.6). Port placement is between the pectoralis major and the latissimus dorsi musculature. Particular attention is paid to the long thoracic nerve, next to the latissimus dorsi.

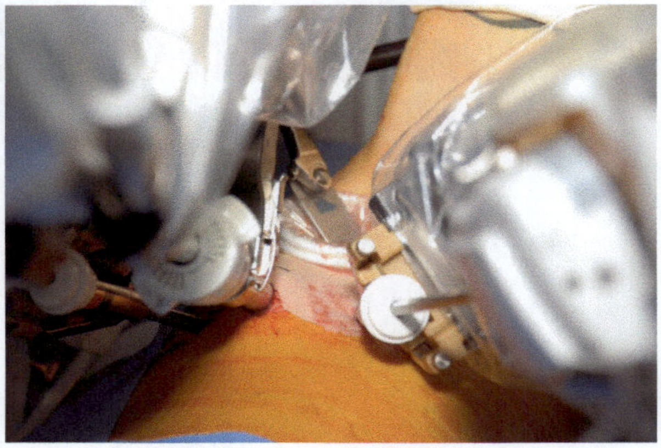

Fig. 29.6 Between the right arm and the left arm, a base of 9–11 cm is used for port placement

Creation of the space is initiated using a medium endovein harvesting device (Cardiovations Clear Glide ultra retractor, Ethicon Endo-Surgery, Cincinnati, OH) with a 30°, 5 mm scope. The space is dissected in a subpectoral fashion; the sternum, first rib, and second rib are individualized. A Farley Thompson retractor (Thompson Surgical Instruments, Traverse City, MI) is positioned in a subpectoral fashion just anterior to the axillary vein. Placement of this blade and slight retraction and hyperadduction of the arm by the assistant further extend and maintain the working area.

Engagement of the Robotics

In the Aesop/Hermes subgroup, the robotic arm is placed in front of the patient with a 20–30° pivotal rotation cephalad. The daVinci engagement is done at three levels: the endoscope-camera complex (8 mm), right-arm robotic instrumentation (5 mm), and left-arm instrumentation (5 mm). The robotic system approaches the patient head on, but slightly (15°) tilted posteriorly (Fig. 29.7a, b).

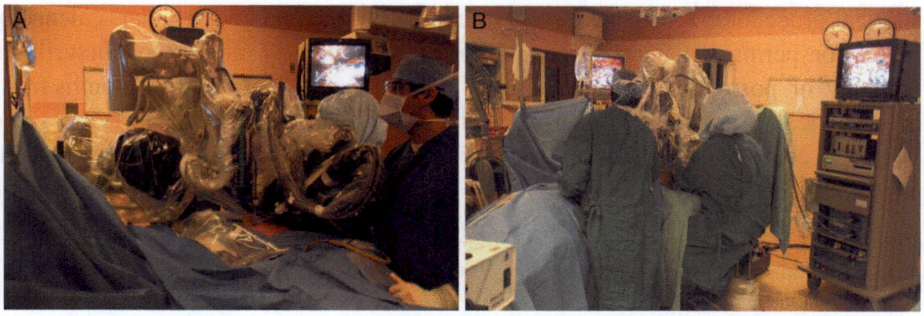

Fig. 29.7 **a** and **b**, The robotic system approaches the patient head on, but slightly (15°) tilted posteriorly

Dissection of Soft Tissue, First Rib, and Space Invasion with Collapse of Lung

The intercostal muscles between the first and the second rib are excised, and the parietal pleura is visualized and purposely opened. The lung is collapsed using the dual endotracheal tube. Owing to the reduction of the lung field, there is now a noticeable increase in the endoscopic working space.

Disengagement of the First Rib and the Concept of Floater Rib

Careful attention is made to protect the vein as the first rib is disconnected anteriorly from the sternal cartilage (Fig. 29.8). As the first rib is freed anteriorly, the rib can be mobilized superiorly and inferiorly—thus, the concept of a floater rib. The attachments of the scalenus muscle fibers (anterior and medius) are easily individualized as we create the floating rib. Cervical bands become stretched, making them easier to identify and safely excise, thus relieving pressure on the neurovascular structures. The dissection is carried posteriorly all the way to the transverse process of the T I vertebra. The various cervical bands are resected as they are encountered. The rib is resected in small pieces by rongeurs and is considered completely resected when the soft white cartilage is visualized at the transverse process (see Fig. 29.2b). This is the best indicator of complete resection of the rib posteriorly, as is the sternal cartilage the best indicator of complete excision anteriorly. The surgeon spends time at the console of the daVinci system to dissect the soft tissue area using DeBakey or Cadiere forceps on the left and electrocautery on the right. The surgeon comes to the standby position (next to the patient) to cut the rib. While the robot becomes an assistant, push the second rib down with one of the robotic arms.

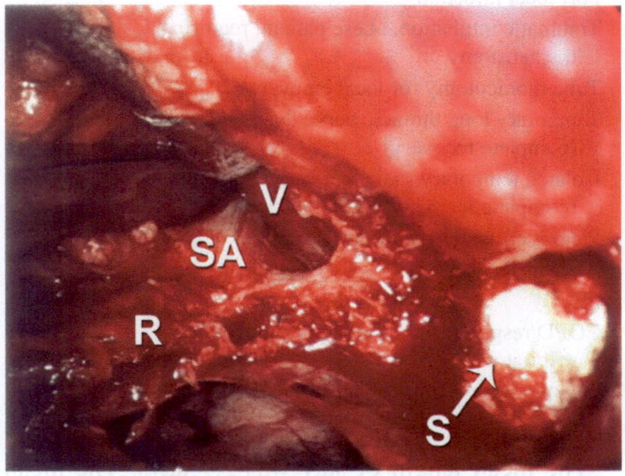

Fig. 29.8 Careful attention is made to protect the vein as the first rib is disconnected anteriorly from the sternal cartilage

Closure

Two red rubber catheters are left in the pleura cavity, and the lung is re-expanded. Subcuticular wound closure is completed using absorbable sutures. A chest radiograph is taken in the operating room.

Results

From November 1998 to August 2008, we have performed endoscopic transaxillary first rib resection using Aesop/Hermes in 89 patients and the daVinci Surgical System in 115 patients, for a total of 204 surgical procedures (Table 29.1). There were no mortalities or permanent neurovascular injuries intraoperatively or postoperatively. There was a 6.8% rate of complications, 14 out of 204 patients with postoperative complications. There was a 1% (2 of 204) conversion rate.

Table 29.1 Complications in endoscopic transaxillary first rib resection in 204 surgical procedures from November 1998 to August 2008

Complication	Number
Port local infection	1
Traumatic intubation, obese patient, requiring tracheostomy	1
Tube thoracotomy for local empyema	1
Temporary long thoracic nerve dysfunction (complete recovery)	2
Isolated temporary radial nerve dysfunction (complete recovery)	1
Pleural effusion/thoracentesis	2
Atelectasis	2
PE	1
COPD/respiratory failure requiring 48 h respirator	1
Pneumothorax requiring tube thoracotomy	2

The mean length of stay was 2.9 days. The mean follow-up for 90% of patients was 2 years. Complete or partial ablation of symptoms occurred in 85% of patients. Persistent myofibrositis of the parascapular muscles, usually of traumatic nature, occurred in about 1/3 of the patients and may persist as an individual clinical entity in the postoperative period. Staged supraclavicular scalenectomy was required in 18% (16 of 89 patients) in the group of Aesop/Hermes and 3% (4 out of 115 patients) in the daVinci group. Staged supraclavicular scalenectomy was performed at a mean 47 months post first rib resection in the Aesop/Hermes group and 16 months from the time of the original procedure in the daVinci group. No patient required a redo procedure for the transaxillary approach due to scar tissue formation. One patient required a sacrectomy of the supraclavicular previous scalenectomy approach.

References

1. Roos DB: Transaxillary approach for first rib resection to relieve thoracic outlet syndrome, *Ann Surg* 163:354–355, 1966.
2. Falconer MA, Li FWP: Resection of first rib in costoclavicular compression of the brachial plexus, *Lancet* 1:59–63, 1962.
3. Clagctt OT: Presidential address: research and pro-search, *J Thorac Cardiovasc Surg* 44:153–166, 1962.
4. Martinez BD: *Thoracic outlet syndrome, intraoperative endoscopic video recording evaluation*, American College of Surgeons Library, October 1985. Catalog ACS–1397.
5. Martinez BD: Thoracic outlet syndrome. In Cameron J, editor: *Current surgical therapy*, ed. 4, St. Louis, 1992, Mosby, pp. 753–757.
6. Martinez BD: *Adjunctive endoscopic video technique in transaxillary first rib resection for thoracic outlet syndrome: ten years experience*, American College of Surgeons library, October 1996. Catalog ACS-2008:8.
7. Dale WA: Thoracic outlet compression syndrome critique in 1982, *Arch Surg* 7:1437–1445, 1982.
8. Roos DB: Congenital anomalies associated with thoracic outlet syndrome, anatomy, symptoms, diagnosis and treatment, *Am J Surg* 132:771–778, 1976.
9. Martinez BD et al.: Computer-assisted instrumentation during endoscopic transaxillary first rib resection for thoracic outlet syndrome: a safe alternate approach, *Vascular* 13(6):327–335, 2005.

Prevention of Lesion Recurrence in Endovascular Devices

30

Adrienne L. Rochier and Bauer E. Sumpio

Although the use of autogenous bypass grafts is generally considered the optimal technique of augmenting perfusion to poorly perfused limbs, many patients do not have adequate conduit or are not at suitable risk for invasive surgery. One of the innovations over the last few decades has been the development of techniques to restore flow through endovascular methods such as angioplasty and vascular stents. Intra-arterial stent placement to treat atherosclerotic obstruction was proposed by Dotter and Judkins in 1964. The first use of percutaneously implanted stents in human arteries was the placement of the Wallstent in coronary, iliac, and femoral arteries in 1987 [1]. Shortly thereafter, favorable results in a multicenter trial with the Palmaz stent in iliac arteries were reported [2]. Stents were approved by the US Food and Drug Administration for use in iliac arteries in the United States in 1991. Although initially introduced as a method to salvage failed balloon angioplasty, stents and stent grafts have allowed the indications for percutaneous interventions to be extended to include treatment of lesions that previously were not considered suitable for balloon angioplasty, and these devices are now accepted as a primary therapy [3].

Recent studies have claimed that the long-term patency of arteries treated with stents may be comparable to that resulting from bypass surgery [4]. However, vessels after angioplasty and those containing stents may not respond to normal physiological activities and intravascular pressures in the same way as intact vessels. Angioplasty causes inflammation leading to a different healing process in atherosclerotic vessels compared with normal vessels. Stents fail to achieve a full endothelial lining, do not undergo the same vasomotor responses as native vessels, and can cause a reparative response that can lead to restenosis. This chapter focuses on the mechanisms underlying the development of intimal hyperplasia after angioplasty and stent placement and the potential strategies to prevent the occurrence of this common physiological response.

Mechanisms of Lesion Recurrence

Types of Lesions

Patency is widely used to assess the efficacy of revascularization and is an outcome measurement of success of the treatment. For instance, restenosis complicates 11–42% of renal artery angioplasties and 12–23% of renal artery stent procedures [5, 6]. Iliac angioplasty has been reported to have a 5-year patency rate of about 60%, while iliac stents have been reported to have a 5-year patency rate of 72% [7].

Many of the initial clinical reports on restenosis after stent placement or angioplasty derive from observations of human coronary vessels. Much of the mechanistic information we have about vessel response following endovascular procedures arise from investigations using animal models to mimic endovascular intervention, such as balloon injury of rat carotid artery. Data from these basic and clinical studies are extrapolated to predict the performance of peripheral endovascular interventions and guide the direction of future human trials.

A.L. Rochier (✉)
Postdoctoral Associate, Department of Vascular Surgery, Yale University School of Medicine, New Haven, CT, USA

T.J. Fogarty, R.A. White (eds.), *Peripheral Endovascular Interventions*,
DOI 10.1007/978-1-4419-1387-6_30, © Springer Science+Business Media, LLC 1998, 2010

Intimal Hyperplasia—Reparative Response to Vessel Injury

Intimal hyperplasia is the predominant cause for restenosis after angioplasty and stenting [8, 9]. Intimal hyperplasia is found in 30–60% of coronary arteries within 1 year of post-angioplasty [10]. Although stents decrease the risk of restenosis in selected lesions, peripheral arterial in-stent restenosis is still a frequent and often intractable clinical problem (Fig. 30.1). Intimal hyperplasia is a normal proliferative response to disruption of the endothelium or mural injury that occurs as a response to balloon dilatation of the arterial wall or stent implantation. The pathogenesis of intimal hyperplasia involves a number of factors including hemodynamic factors, vasoactive and thrombotic factors as well as cytokines and growth factors. It involves a complex interaction between endothelial cells, macrophages, smooth muscle cells, platelets, and various cytokines activated during the normal response to injury. The degree of injury during the intervention is usually correlated with the hyperplastic response [11].

Inflammatory cells play a key role in post-injury intimal hyperplasia. Days after balloon angioplasty or stenting, monocytes are recruited to the injury site, where they become activated. The magnitude of macrophage infiltration in stented lesions has been correlated to subsequent intimal growth [12]. There are two main theories that underlie the genesis of intimal hyperplasia. These include the mechanical and biologic mechanisms.

Mechanical: Alterations in hemodynamic forces. Alterations in hemodynamic forces have been postulated to play an important role in the development of intimal hyperplasia. Areas of flow separation, recirculation, and stasis occur as a result of altered laminar flow following vascular intervention. According to this mechanical theory, differential patterns of flow are the stimulus for activation of this intimal hyperplastic response. Histologically, intimal hyperplasia occurs most commonly at areas of low wall shear stress. This development of intimal hyperplasia due to altered patterns of flow and hemodynamic forces maybe analogous to the development of atherosclerotic lesion at arterial bifurcation and proximal branch points [13].

After peripheral bypass surgery, intimal hyperplasia occurs commonly at various portions of distal anastamoses correlating with low wall shear stress and altered hemodynamic forces [14, 15]. Low wall shear stress is found at the floor of the arterial wall, where the blood flow divides proximally and distally (stagnation point), and at the heel of the anastomosis, and it is in these two areas that intimal hyperplasia is most likely to develop. Various hemodynamic factors and physical forces created as a result of the geometry of the anastomosis may cause chronic forms of injury and modulate vascular structure by altering the local cellular expression of biochemical factors secreted by cells in the vessel walls [15]. Cellular response may be

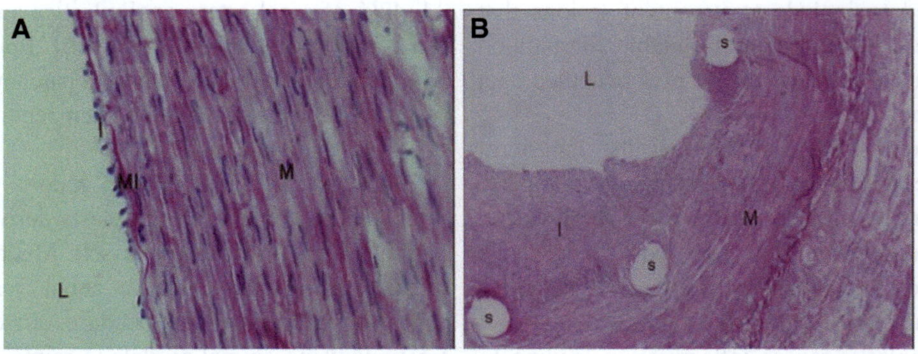

Fig. 30.1 Stent implantation injures the arterial wall, which results in the initiation of injury and thrombosis on the arterial wall. Growth factors and cytokines that are released stimulate smooth muscle cells that migrate causing intimal hyperplasia, resulting in restenosis in some patients. **a**, Normal uninjured left common carotid artery of a pig. HE staining. (L, lumen; I, intimal layer; M, medial layer; MI, medial–intimal interface.) **b**, Right common carotid artery of a pig 4 weeks after stent placement demonstrating intimal hyperplasia. HE staining (L, lumen; I, intimal layer; M, medial layer; S, stent fragment sites.) (Adapted from Pasa et al. [76], with permission.)

enhanced further due to compliance mismatch with the native vessel.

Biologic: Response to Endothelial cell disruption. Intimal hyperplasia is also the result of a triggered cellular response in the injured artery to certain cellular and noncellular components in the circulation. During injury of a rat carotid artery by a balloon catheter, the endothelial layer is denuded and platelets attach to the exposed media [16]. In this situation, fibrin does not accumulate, although it does in other types of injury, such as deep injury of the media, atherosclerotic plaque disruption, and repeat injury of established intima. Endothelial cell disruption following endovascular intervention leads to platelet aggregation and thrombosis. This process then continues with platelet activation and degranulation which in turn causes vasoactive and thrombotic factors to be released along with cytokines and growth factors. The most important of these are platelet-derived growth factor (PDGF) and basic fibroblast growth factor. Macrophages are thought to be important modulators in this injury response [17].

Medial injury is also incurred during ballooning of the vessel. Up to 30% of the smooth muscle cells can be damaged. The amount of damage to the media is important because it correlates with the subsequent wall thickening response (Fig. 30.2). This response has been demonstrated in human arteries as well [18, 19].

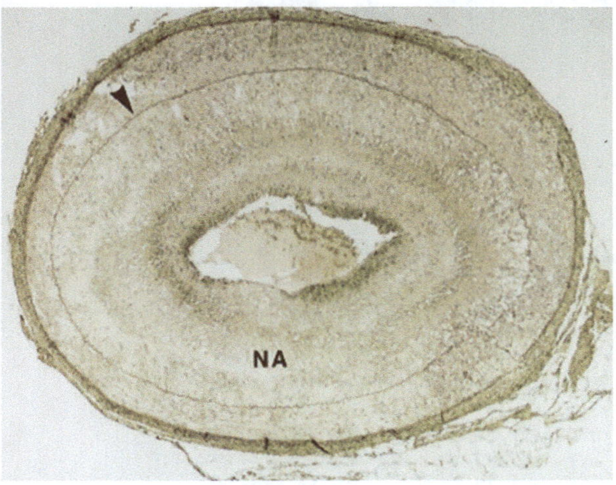

Fig. 30.2 Photomicrograph of rabbit common iliac artery 10 weeks after balloon denudation and 6 weeks after balloon dilation with markedly expanded neointimal area (NA). *Arrow* is pointing to the intact internal elastic lamina (Elastica van Gieson stain; original magnification, 40×.) (Adapted from Kalinowski et al. [77], with permission.)

Deeper injury causes cell proliferation in the media and the adventitia.

Prior to initiation of the reparative process, genes critical to cells leaving the resting state are induced in smooth muscle cells (Fig. 30.3). Within the first 24 h following injury, smooth muscle cells from the media start synthesizing DNA. The first few cycles allow repletion of damaged cells in the media [20]. This medial smooth muscle cell proliferation can be completely accounted for by the release of basic fibroblast growth factor (bFGF) from dying smooth muscle cells [21, 22]. By day 4, cells begin to move from the media to the intima, and smooth muscle cell division continues for 4 weeks and then stops spontaneously regardless of the degree of endothelial resurfacing, or earlier if endothelial coverage has been completed. Intimal thickening continues with deposition of large amounts of matrix, producing significant intimal thickening and luminal narrowing. In chronic situations, the intima is almost 80% matrix. The injury response described above has been shown to be immediate and short-lived in both animals and humans [11]. Changes that occur later are likely to have other sources such as progression of atherosclerotic disease rather than intimal hyperplasia.

There are various mechanisms by which injured vessels can be covered with endothelium, which is a primary response following injury unless inhibited by some process. Regeneration of the denuded endothelial layer is from nontraumatized cells adjacent to the injury zone. Experimentally, the maximum distance of migration and endothelial ingrowth is approximately 3 cm [16]. In the rat carotid artery, the endothelial layer is re-established at the ends but not the central denuded section. The smooth muscle cells in that region can adapt by forming a pseudoendothelium as a substitute if the areas of source endothelium are too far apart for the repair to go to completion. In interventions that delaminate the vessel wall, the transected vasa vasorum can serve as new sources of endothelium, as can invading microvessels from surrounding granulation tissue. It has also been suggested that endothelial cells can embolize from remote sites and form islands of endothelium with no obvious source.

Although many of these studies have been done in rat carotid arteries, the results have been extended to predict the response in human vessels. Studies of normal vessel response to injury are critical in our

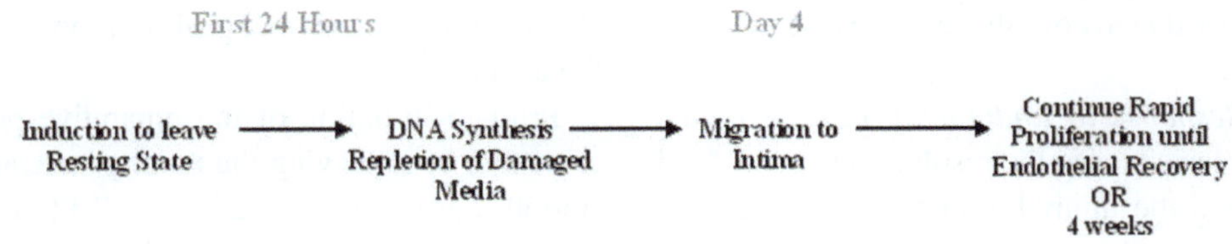

Fig. 30.3 Timeline of medial smooth muscle cell response to injury. Within the first 24 h, smooth muscle cells from the media start synthesizing DNA. The first few cycles allow repletion of damaged cells in the media. This medial smooth muscle cell proliferation can be completely accounted for by the release of basic fibroblast growth factor from dying smooth muscle cells. By day 4, cells begin to move from the media to the intima, and smooth muscle cell division continues for 4 weeks and then stops spontaneously regardless of the degree of endothelial resurfacing, or earlier if endothelial coverage has been completed

understanding of the healing response to injury in a diseased or atherosclerotic vessel.

Vascular Remodeling—Recoil and Chronic Vasospasm

Vascular remodeling describes the changes in luminal and external diameters in response to chronic changes in flow and pressure by the induction of various constricting or dilating pathways [23]. The initial response of the elastic fibers of the arterial wall to overstretching by balloon catheter is elastic recoil (Fig. 30.4). Elastic recoil characterizes the early phase of restenosis and is responsible for the loss of gain obtained during balloon inflation [24]. Vessel spasm following injury to the vessel may promote thrombus formation at the site of injury enhancing wall thickening and contributing to luminal narrowing [16].

Lafonte et al. observed that a chronic constriction occurred 3–4 weeks after balloon dilation of rabbit femoral artery and appeared to be an important correlate of restenosis [25]. This finding has important basic and clinical implications, since it suggests that restenosis is not solely related to neointimal–medial growth. This study also suggests that constriction at the site of angioplasty may be affected by multiple structural changes, including rearrangement of not just

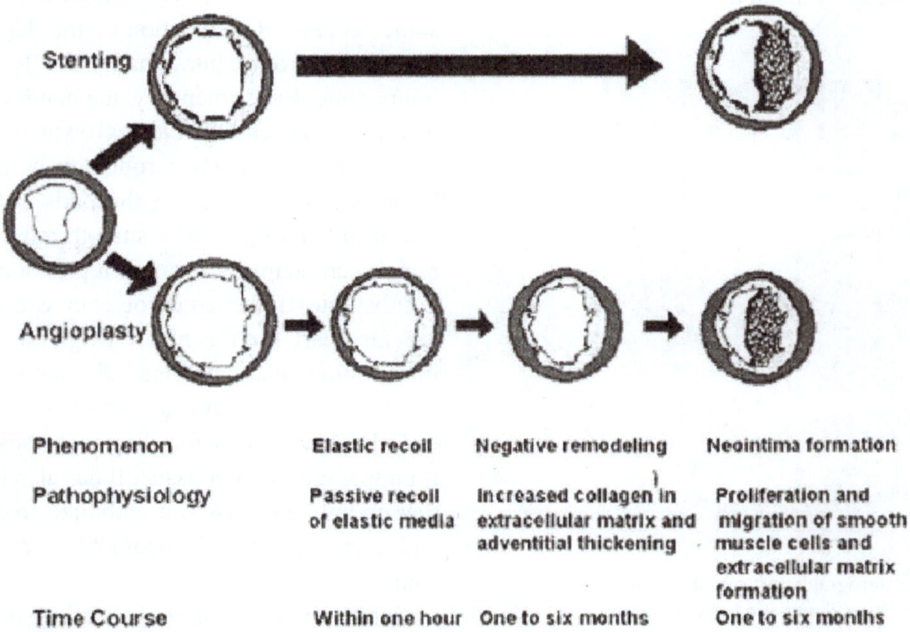

Fig. 30.4 Vascular remodeling and mechanisms contributing to restenosis. Elastic recoil and negative remodeling (*lower*) are two contributors to restenosis. Stenting effectively controls these processes (*upper*) but does cause neointimal proliferation (Adapted from Dobesh et al. [78], with permission.)

the intima and the media but also the adventitia. The changes in the adventitia are unlikely related to procedures used to form the initial lesion, since control lesions treated identically but without angioplasty did not exhibit constriction or such adventitial changes. In their study, a chronic constriction, perceived at the level of the external elastic lamina, correlated more closely with luminal narrowing after angioplasty than did neointimal–medial growth.

Constrictive remodeling has been identified as a major contributor to restenosis following angioplasty. An increase in wall shear stress can lead to luminal enlargement until normalization of the shear stress; an increase in the tension on the artery wall may induce a proliferative response [25]. Angioplasty-related healing may involve an analogous series of changes that may lead in some instances to chronic constriction. What is thought to be a variable constrictive response may result instead from a variable absence of relaxing influences. The degree of endothelial injury and regrowth may thereby influence vascular tone in the repairing vessel wall.

Recently, Ryan and colleagues looked at transforming growth factor-β (beta)(TGF-β)-mediated cellular events in the adventitia and their contribution to vascular remodeling [26]. They used a balloon catheter to denude rat carotid artery. Rats were treated with either vehicle or a TGF-β inhibitor, a soluble TGF-β receptor type II (TGF-βR:Fc). They observed that adventitial cell proliferation peaked 4 days after injury and was characterized by the de novo formation of several cell layers surrounding the outer adventitia. These neoadventitial cells expressed an abundance of collagen type I and a fetal isoform of fibronectin, and the expression of both proteins was suppressed in the presence of TGF-βR:Fc. Lumenal narrowing was apparent 14 days after injury, but inhibition of TGF-β signaling was found to promote vessel enlargement. As a result, lumen size did not change despite neointimal formation. Adventitial fibrosis with abundant collagen matrix deposition but not adventitial cell proliferation was dependent upon endogenous TGF-β activity. Furthermore, inhibition of TGF-β signaling prevented injury-induced reduction in lumen area by promoting vessel enlargement. These results suggest that TGF-β may be a worthwhile target in preventing restenosis by inhibition of TGF-β-dependent vascular remodeling.

Inward arterial remodeling may be another major cause for the delayed failure of angioplasty procedures [27]. Although the contribution of the different layers of the vessel wall is apparent, the role of the adventitia has traditionally been underappreciated. Many studies have demonstrated that the adventitia plays an active role in the vessel's response to injury, and may serve as a source of both cells and mediators to recruit additional cell types. In addition, the adventitia may be an optimal site to apply therapeutic agents, compared to application within the lumen, in the prevention of restenosis due to injury related processes.

Restenosis Due to Progression of Atherosclerotic Disease

Lesion recurrence may also occur as part of an ongoing process that initiated development of the atherosclerotic lesion. Atherosclerosis is a disease process that involves formation of multiple focal lesions in the internal and medial layers of vessel walls resulting in decreased elasticity and a narrowed lumen. The atherosclerotic process is the result of a long-lasting physiological response to factors having a harmful influence on the vessel wall leading to a chronic, proliferative inflammatory process. Atherosclerosis has a progressive character that continues through the aging process unless somehow inhibited. It is influenced by cardiovascular risk factors and individual profile. Observed trends include an earlier onset and faster progression of the process in males as well as an increase after menopause in women [28]. Endovascular intervention, per se, does nothing to address this process, which contributes to restenosis after angioplasty or stent placement unless some intervention is done to slow or stop the process. Two main strategies to prevent lesion recurrence are to target at the local vessel level and by systemic modification of risk factors.

Mechanisms of Prevention of Lesion Recurrence at the Local Level

There are a number of strategies to prevent intimal hyperplasia at the site of angioplasty and/or stenting (Table 30.1).

Table 30.1 Prevention of lesion recurrence strategies

Local prevention of intimal hyperplasia
⇒Optimizing stent material
⇒Local drug delivery
o Actinomycin D
o Paclitaxel
o Sirolimus
⇒Brachytherapy
⇒Gene therapy
o VEGF
o Nitric oxide synthase
o E2F decoy
o MCP-1
Systemic prevention of progression of atherosclerotic disease
⇒Statins
⇒Anticoagulation/antiplatelet therapy
⇒Risk factor modification

Optimization to Decrease Injury to Vessel Wall

Arteries exhibit a nonlinear degree of stretch and deformation in relation to increasing intraluminal pressure and are therefore termed anisotropic. The initial vessel dilatation causes the elastin fibers to stretch, but later as the pressure continues to increase, the less elastic collagen fibers are deformed.

Stents and stent grafts demonstrate less compliance and considerable stiffness at varying pressure ranges because they cannot contract or dilate in response to normal stimuli. Mismatch in the elastic or compliance properties of the stent with the native artery at the transition point has been implicated in the origin of intimal hyperplasia [11]. This variance is thought to activate smooth muscle cells exposed to cyclic strain forces and mitogens released from platelets activated by turbulent flow. The endothelial and smooth muscle cells that form a new endothelial covering are derived from the artery adjacent to the stent or transmural microvessels. The devices become embedded into the vessel wall as cell migration and new growth occur through the interstices and cover the stents. The synthetic material can also induce a chronic inflammatory response and is thrombogenic until the endothelial covering is formed. Newer stent materials and stent designs are being tested to reduce the contributions to the hyperplastic response and are addressed in other sections of this book.

Local Drug Delivery

Another method to decrease lesion recurrence involves the use of adjunctive drug treatments or conduit coating. The intent is for pharmacologic modulation of the local vasculature without imparting systemic toxicity. Different drug delivery methods or stent coating allow for variable release of the pharmacologic agent in specific target areas where lesion recurrence is most prevalent. This is currently a very popular strategy and clinical trials studying different types of stent coating, antiproliferative agents, immunosuppressants, and collagen inhibitors are all currently underway. In 2001, the first human study was published showing a nearly complete abolition of restenosis by using a sirolimus-eluting stent at 8 months clinical follow-up [24]. Since then, a few other agents have been found to show potential in this area and are currently under investigation to assess their efficacy in the prevention of lesion recurrence.

Actinomycin D

Actinomycin D is an antibiotic previously used in the treatment of certain malignancies, including Wilms tumor and soft tissue sarcomas, because it forms a stable complex with double-stranded DNA and inhibits DNA-primed RNA synthesis (Fig. 30.5a). Actinomycin D is a more potent and cytotoxic antiproliferative agent than the other two drugs discussed below, sirolimus and paclitaxel [29]. The ACTION trial looked at safety and performance of an actinomycin D-coated stent in the treatment of patients with single de novo native coronary lesions. Their results showed that while in-hospital and 1-month outcomes were similar in each group, by 6 months there was increased restenosis, late lumen loss, and target vessel revascularization in the treated stent arm. The trial demonstrated that not all antiproliferative drugs are effective in the prevention of restenosis and that promise in early preclinical studies (30 days) does not necessarily translate into clinical effectiveness at 6 months or long term [30]. Actinomycin D is currently still in clinical trials to assess the antiproliferative properties and efficacy when used in conjunction with endovascular devices.

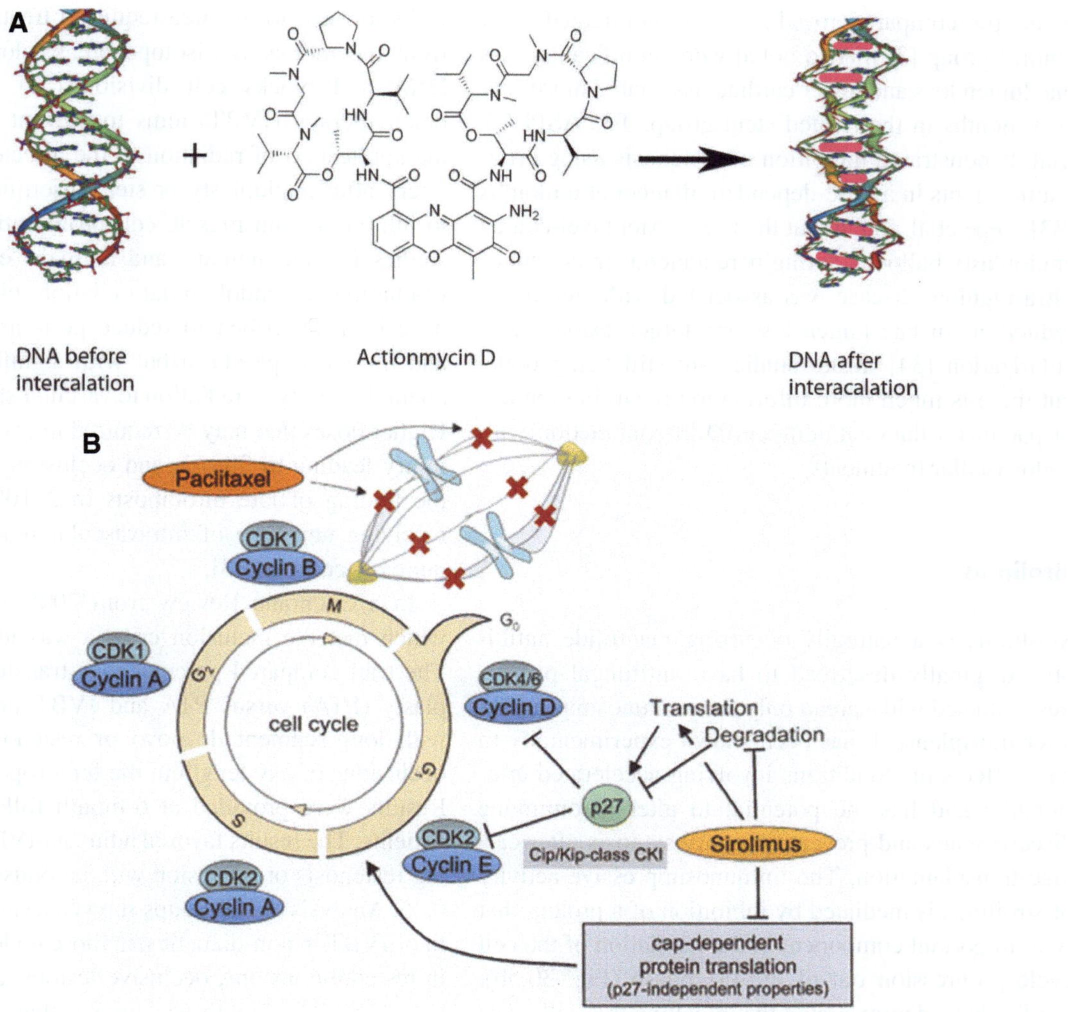

Fig. 30.5 **a**, Actinomycin D, an intercalating agent composed of aromatic macrocycles, can be inserted between the stacked base pairs of DNA. The bases are forced apart to accommodate these so-called intercalating agents, causing an unwinding of the helix to a more ladder-like structure. (From Garrett and Grisham [79], with permission.) **b**, Schematic illustration of the cell cycle and its regulatory mechanisms are relevant for the inhibitory effect imposed by sirolimus and paclitaxel. Critical cell cycle regulators in smooth muscle cells are involved. Subsequent to binding its intracellular receptor, sirolimus inhibits the activity of mammalian target of rapamycin (mTOR). mTOR is a pivotal protein kinase that mediates mitogen-induced cell proliferation. Sirolimus blocks cell cycle progression (G1 to S), thereby blocking T-cell and smooth muscle cell proliferation and migration. Paclitaxel impacts predominantly during cell division in the mitosis (M) phase of the cell cycle through centrosomal impairment, induction of abnormal spindles, and suppression of spindle microtubule dynamics. Paclitaxel interferes with microtubule formation and inhibits mitosis. Together, they block restenosis at multiple levels (From Wessely et al. [80], with permission from Elsevier.)

Paclitaxel

Paclitaxel is an antineoplastic agent that is commonly used to treat breast and ovarian cancer. It acts on the microtubule assembly process (Fig. 30.5b), in which the formation of stable components is followed by the inhibition of proliferation and migration, and then signal transduction. Paclitaxel impacts cell division in the mitosis (M) phase of the cell cycle through centrosomal impairment, induction of abnormal spindles, and suppression of spindle microtubule dynamics.

In clinical trials, paclitaxel has been shown to inhibit smooth muscle cell proliferation, but this action is dose dependent [31]. In the TAXUS I trial, a randomized controlled trial using paclitaxel-treated stents, the patients with treated stents showed 0% restenosis at

6 months compared to 11% in the nontreated stent control group [32]. Also noted were significantly less late lumen loss and lower cardiac-associated morbidity at 3 months in the treated stent group. The ASPECT trial demonstrated inhibition of restenosis using drug-eluting stents in a dose-dependent manner at 6 months [33]. Tepe et al. found that the use of paclitaxel-coated angioplasty balloons during percutaneous treatment of infra-inguinal disease was associated with significant reductions in late lumen loss and target-lesion revascularization [34]. More studies are still being done, but there is much more information regarding the use of paclitaxel than actinomycin D in conjunction with endovascular treatments.

Sirolimus

Sirolimus is a naturally occurring macrolide antibiotic, originally described to have antifungal properties, but used widespread only for immunosuppression after transplants. It has been shown experimentally to have effects on conditions involving accelerated arteriopathy and has the potential to alter autoimmune disease states and prevent coronary stenosis after cardiac transplantation. The immunosuppressive activity of sirolimus is mediated by inhibition of a protein that is an important component in the regulation of the cell cycle progression out of the G1 phase (Fig. 30.5b). Studies have demonstrated that blocking this cell cycle progression in smooth muscle cells decreases T-cell proliferation [35].

Sirolimus-coated stents showed no significant intra-stent or edge restenosis at 4, 6, and 12 months in nonrandomized studies. The RAVEL trial, a randomized controlled trial, demonstrated 0% restenosis using sirolimus-coated stents compared with 26% restenosis in the noncoated stent group at 6 months [36]. Many other trials involving stents coated with these and other pharmacologic treatments are underway, but long-term follow-up reports are just not yet available.

Brachytherapy

Radiation has been used in the treatment of many types of proliferative lesions. Brachytherapy is a form of radiotherapy in which a radioactive source is placed inside or next to the area requiring treatment. Energy from the radioactive isotope breaks double-stranded DNA and blocks cell division [37]. Intravascular brachytherapy (IVBT) aims to prevent restenosis by the application of radiation to the affected part of the artery after angioplasty or stent insertion in an effort to inhibit smooth muscle cell proliferation. In recent studies in both humans and animals, external beam irradiation and endoluminal radiation following injury have been described to reduce peri-vascular fibrosis and intimal hyperplasia but with significant concern about the safety of radiation to vascular structures [11]. Higher doses that may be required may cause vascular injury leading to fibrosis and occlusion. Furthermore, the finding of late thrombosis in 3–10% of patients receiving any type of intravascular brachytherapy is quite concerning [38].

In a Cochrane Review from 2005, only one trial which met the inclusion criteria was identified [39]. The trial compared percutaneous transluminal angioplasty (PTA) versus PTA and IVBT in 117 patients with long-segment de novo or restenotic lesions or occlusions of any length in the femoropopliteal artery. Results were provided at 6-month follow-up in 107 patients. The results favored adjuvant IVBT in preventing restenosis or occlusion with an odds ratio (OR) of 0.35. Analysis of subgroups showed a significant benefit of IVBT in non-diabetics, in those undergoing IVBT in restenotic lesions, occlusive lesions, and lesions in which the PTA length was greater than 10 cm. These results suggest that IVBT is effective at improving the patency of femoropopliteal arteries undergoing PTA in the short term, particularly in non-diabetics with long occlusions (>10 cm). In another study published in 2006 with a 5-year follow-up, Wolfram and colleagues found that radiation as prophylaxis following angioplasty in infra-inguinal vessels significantly delayed the onset of restenosis [38].

Although the results are intriguing, more research is needed, especially regarding the long-term effects and complications of this treatment. One unique characteristic of brachytherapy to blood vessels is the development of restenosis beyond the stent edge or the radiation delivery area, thought to be due to a drop-off effect of the radiation. The first reports of edge restenosis following brachytherapy occurred 4–6 months after implantation of ^{32}P-radioactive stents, located at or near the margins of the stent [40]. This effect came to be known as a "candy-wrapper"

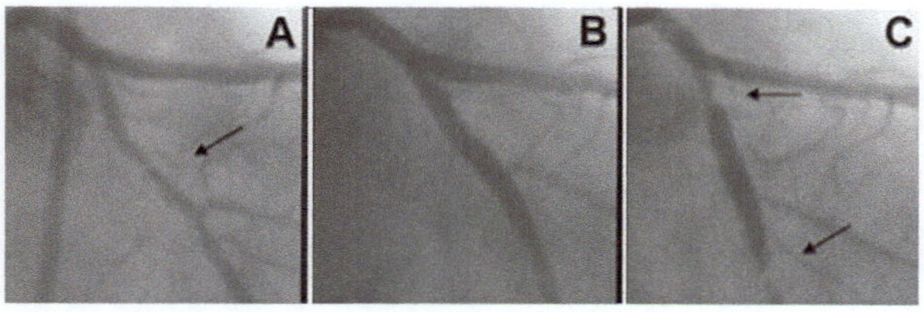

Fig. 30.6 "Candy-wrapper" (edge) stenosis after brachytherapy (From Albiero and Colombo [81], with permission.)

effect due to its radiographic appearance (Fig. 30.6). The incidence of edge restenosis after initial stent implantation without radiation has been reported to be between 5 and 10%. Although the mechanism of edge restenosis remains unclear, Kim et al. observed that it occurred in 21% of edges in their study in which the radioactive source did not adequately cover the entire segment of artery injured during the primary catheter-based treatment of stenosis [41]. This inadequate coverage, or anything less than the radiation protocol-mandated source coverage of at least 5 mm proximal and distal to the end of each lesion, is known as geographical miss. In the ^{32}P-emitting stent, the candy-wrapper effect is mostly a result of neointimal proliferation. After ^{32}P beta irradiation plus nonradioactive stent implantation, edge restenosis is caused by neointimal proliferation in lesions without geographical miss and negative remodeling in lesions with geographical miss.

Edge restenosis can be explained as a fall in dose to the point where it is inadequate to inhibit the restenosis process. Edge restenosis following gamma irradiation treatment of in-stent restenosis is related to a mismatch between the segment of artery injured during the primary catheter-based intervention and the length of the radiation source. This suggests that careful attention to the distribution of the treatment, confining it to the stenosed segment with maximal coverage of the treated segment with radiation sources, should be taken in order to avoid edge restenosis.

Radioactive stents are among the newer methods of radiotherapy. A recent study by Albeiro and colleagues described a beta-emitting Isostent with varying doses of radiation [42]. In this study, in-stent intimal hyperplasia was significantly decreased in those with higher doses of radiation. However, others have suggested that low doses in fact stimulate neointimal formation at segments subjected to trauma. Thus, significant concerns still remain in the field of brachytherapy and more clinical trials defining the benefits of radiotherapy and safety will be necessary before widespread clinical application can ensue.

Gene Therapy

Techniques of intervention to prevent lesion recurrence at the gene expression level are now available due to increased understanding and studies of cellular signaling involved in cell proliferation. One use of gene therapy is an attempt to correct underlying diseases or conditions by introducing normal genes into somatic cells to induce or inhibit the synthesis of certain gene products in vivo. Gene augmentation, or the introduction of normal foreign gene sequences for the defective gene, is one of the most commonly used techniques in vascular disease therapy [43].

Certain RNA sequences known as antisense oligonucleotides bind to specific mRNA sequences to inhibit translation. Other RNA sequences known as ribozymes cleave mRNA at target sites. Double-stranded DNA, which is more stable, has been used to alter gene expression by forming "decoy" sequences that have high affinity for specific target sites [44]. Studies done most recently have concentrated on gene transfer and expression using vascular endothelial growth factor (VEGF), nitric oxide synthase (NOS), the antisense oligodeoxynucleotide E2F decoy, and a mutant chemokine of MCP-1.

VEGF

It has been hypothesized that endothelial cells, during their rapid regeneration after injury, may modulate vascular growth through endothelial-derived antiproliferative cytokines in the development of intimal hyperplasia. Recent experiments have shown that VEGF is the crucial mediator of downstream events that ultimately lead to enhanced endothelial cell survival and increased vascular density (Fig. 30.7). Therapeutic angiogenesis using VEGF gene transfer was initially studied in a clinical trial in 1994 by Isner and colleagues. They noted improvements in the circulation of a group of patients shown on angiography, such as increased collateral circulation, after injecting VEGF

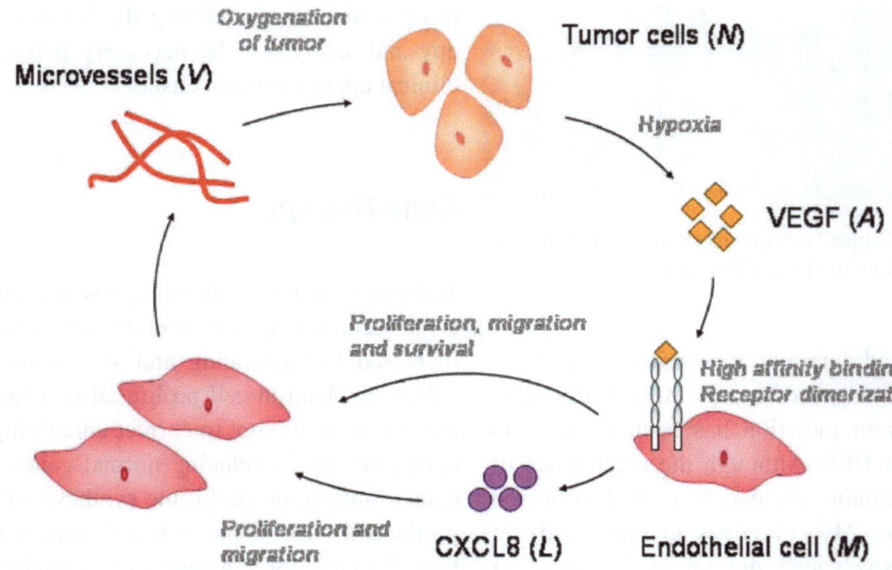

Fig. 30.7 Recent experiments show that vascular endothelial growth factor (VEGF) is the crucial mediator of downstream events that ultimately lead to enhanced endothelial cell survival and increased vascular density. The newly discovered pathway involves upregulation of the anti-apoptotic protein Bcl-2, which in turn leads to increased production of interleukin-8 (CXCL8) causing increase in proliferation and migration of vascular smooth muscle cells (From Jain et al. [82], with kind permission from Springer Science + Business Media.)

plasmids into the muscle of patients with critical limb ischemia [45]. Other studies using VEGF have shown significant inhibition of neointimal formation, increase in myocardial blood flow, and subjective improvement in overall functional status. In 2007, Leong-Poi et al. used a plasmid gene delivery system to study ischemic muscle in rats and found that it was possible to increase blood flow to ischemic areas after introducing VEGF [46]. These clinical trials have had a wide range of clinical outcomes but one unifying theme; there is great potential for the use of VEGF gene therapy in the future angiogenic treatment of patients with coronary and peripheral arterial disease in addition to or in patients not amenable to other vascular interventions.

Nitric Oxide Synthase

Nitric oxide is a molecule that has dual functions depending on the type of cell. In activated immune cells, it functions as a killer molecule, but in nerve and endothelial cells, it functions as a signaling molecule. Nitric oxide (NO) affects vascular cells by inhibiting vascular smooth muscle cell migration and proliferation, mediating vasorelaxation, and reducing platelet activation and vascular inflammation. Decreasing the smooth muscle cell migration and proliferation has been a central theme in strategies to decrease intimal hyperplasia. The production and catabolism of NO can be affected by disease states such as diabetes, hypertension, and atherosclerosis, to cause a decrease in NO bioactivity. Impaired NO activity in the vessel wall is thought to lead to dysregulation of cell growth, migration, and matrix deposition leading to pathologic vascular remodeling.

Recent studies have demonstrated that NO inhibits smooth muscle cell proliferation. Von der Layen demonstrated inhibition of stent-induced lesions using gene transfer of nitric oxide synthase (NOS) [47]. Urano et al. found that increasing NO production promotes both angiogenesis (de novo capillary vessel formation) and arteriogenesis (collateral vessel formation) [48]. Other studies have shown that increased NO production promotes increased vascularization as well as more mature vascular structure leading to decreased lesion recurrence [49]. More studies continue to be designed using NOS alone or in conjunction with other factors to improve prevention of restenosis.

Transcription Factor Decoy

In understanding restenosis after endovascular intervention, smooth muscle cell proliferation is at the center of intimal hyperplasia. Proliferation depends on the activation of cell cycle regulatory genes, and formation of the E2F/Cyclin A/CDK1 complex is a critical process of the cycle progression. E2F must be released from a regulatory complex which involves the hyperphosphorylation of the retinoblastoma gene product during late G1 phase. The E2F transcription factor upregulates the expression of many genes involved in DNA synthesis and cell cycle progression which results in cellular proliferation.

In clinical studies, an E2F decoy has been used to bind free E2F which does not allow activation of the cell cycle regulatory genes and stops cycle progression. Morishita et al. was able to successfully transfect an E2F decoy into rat vascular smooth muscle cells which proceeded to bind dissociated E2F and inhibit smooth muscle cell proliferation and intimal hyperplasia [50]. These studies demonstrated the safety of E2F decoy and feasibility in treatment after vascular intervention. However, the inhibition of intimal hyperplasia by E2F decoy has not been equivalent in all peripheral vascular procedures. Conte et al. demonstrated that an E2F decoy was no more effective than placebo in preventing restenosis causing peripheral bypass graft failure in the phase III of the PREVENT trial, underscoring the fact that success in animal studies does not necessarily correlate with success in human disease [51].

Mutant MCP-1

Monocyte chemoattractant protein-1 (MCP-1) is another target for clinical studies. MCP-1 is a specific monocyte chemokine that attracts inflammatory mediators to areas of vascular interventions causing neointimal formation. A mutant form of MCP-1, with key amino acids deleted, called 7ND was transfected into cells to try to prevent monocyte chemotaxis-related inflammation and neointimal formation. Tatewaki and colleagues showed that blockade of MCP-1 by adenoviral gene transfer of 7ND limits neointimal formation in dogs [52]. Ohtani et al. demonstrated that transfection of the mutant MCP-1 gene (*7ND*) suppressed monocyte infiltration and activation in the stented arterial wall and markedly reduced the development of neointimal hyperplasia in rabbits (Fig. 30.8). The mechanism of action of 7ND involved suppression of local expression of MCP-1 and inflammatory cytokines [53]. Therefore, inhibition of MCP-1-mediated inflammation was shown to be effective in reducing in-stent restenosis. This study highlights the potential therapeutic benefit of local anti-MCP-1 therapy for prevention of neointimal formation associated with endovascular therapy failure in humans, but more studies will be needed to determine in vivo application.

Systemic Prevention of Progression of Atherosclerotic Disease

In addition to the above local strategies for limiting restenosis after angioplasty and stenting, there are some systemic therapies which may enhance long-term patency (Table 30.1).

Statin Therapy

The use of HMG-CoA reductase inhibitors, also known as statins, has been shown to slow progression of atherosclerosis. The use of statins results in stabilization of atherosclerotic plaque by reducing the number of macrophages, collagen production, and smooth muscle cells. Many clinical trials have confirmed the role of statins and their multiple potential effects to slow progression of atherosclerosis [54]. Statin therapy has also been associated with regression of atherosclerosis when LDL is substantially reduced and HDL is increased by more than 7.5% [55]. Recently, it has been reported that statins exert many pleiotropic effects on the vascular wall, including improving endothelial function, inhibiting vascular smooth muscle cell proliferation, inhibiting platelet aggregation, reducing vascular inflammation, and averting antioxidative action. These so-called pleiotropic effects of statins have been the subject of considerable research over

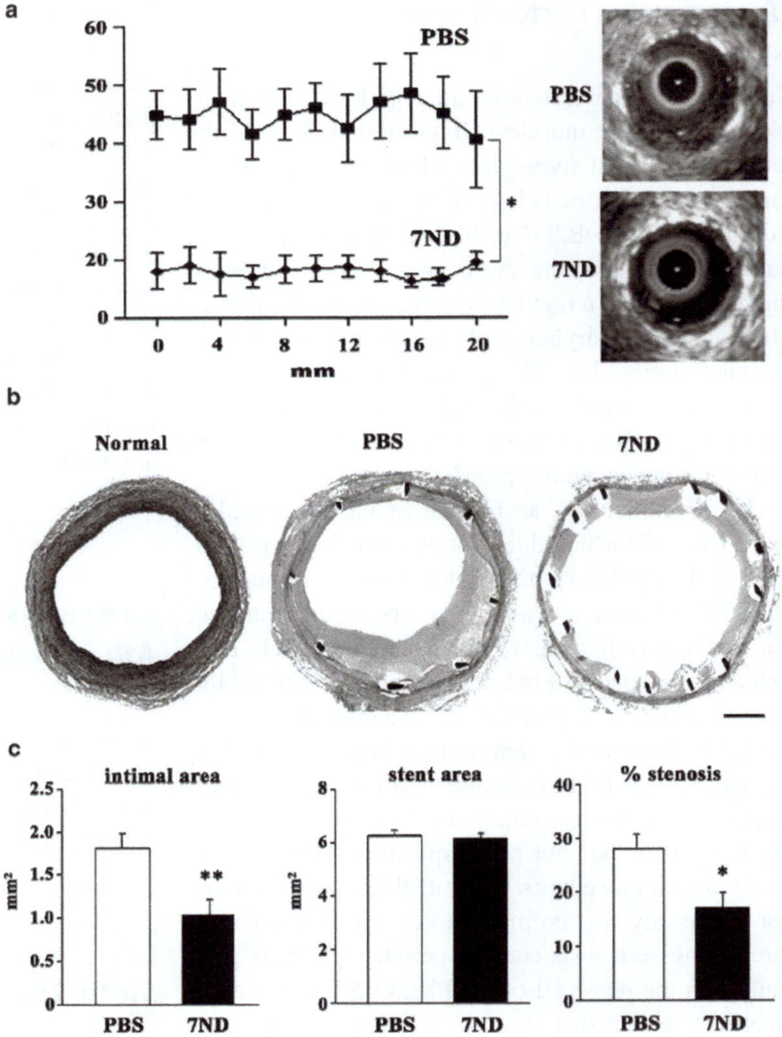

Fig. 30.8 Effects of *7ND* (mutant MCP-1) gene transfer on in-stent neointimal hyperplasia in rabbits. **a**, *Left*: mean percent area stenosis within stent in the PBS-treated and 7ND-transfected rabbits as assessed by intravascular ultrasound. *X*-axis: distance from the distal to the proximal stent end; *Y*-axis: percentage cross-sectional stenosis. The *upper right panel* shows an intravascular ultrasound cross-sectional image in PBS-treated animal with large neointimal hyperplasia. The *lower right panel* displays an intravascular ultrasound cross-sectional image in 7ND-transfected animal with small neointimal hyperplasia. **b**, Noninjured control artery section (*left panel*) and artery sections from the PBS-treated group (*middle*) and 7ND-transfected group (*right*) 28 days after stenting stained with elastic van-Gieson in rabbits. **c**, Effect of *7ND* gene transfer on intimal area, stented area, and percentage stenosis 28 days after stenting in rabbits versus PBS (From Ohtani et al. [53], with permission.)

recent years. Some effects are attributable to the inhibition of cholesterol biosynthesis, because substrates downstream from mevalonate in the synthesis cascade supply a number of different metabolic pathways [56]. One such substrate is geranylgeranyl pyrophosphate, which serves as a lipid attachment to Rho. This guanosine triphosphate-binding protein coordinates a number of specific cellular responses by interacting with downstream targets, and it is involved in stress fiber formation, monocyte adhesion, and monocyte transmigration through the endothelium.

Lovastatin and simvastatin have been shown to induce eNOS gene transcription in human endothelial cells. Interestingly, pravastatin improved endothelial function in monkeys at doses that do not decrease plasma LDL concentrations [57]. In this study, cynomolgus monkeys were fed an atherogenic diet for 2 years, followed by a 2-year treatment phase in which they were fed a lipid-decreasing diet containing or not containing pravastatin. Coronary arteries of those monkeys treated with pravastatin dilated, whereas those of control monkeys constricted in response to acetylcholine. Pravastatin has also been shown to increase the bioavailability of nitric oxide in atherosclerotic arterial walls, and it activates eNOS independently of its cholesterol-decreasing features [58].

Bandoh and colleagues investigated treatment of rabbits with fluvastatin at doses that did not cause a significant change in serum lipids [59]. After the femoral artery was injured surgically by balloon catheter, the rabbits demonstrated morphological deterioration of the intima and were noted to have intimal thickening. Excess proliferation of vascular smooth muscle cells which were identified in the intima was suppressed in rabbits on chronic treatment of fluvastatin. They concluded that fluvastatin at low doses insufficient to lower lipids in serum still attenuated the progression of intimal thickening following balloon catheterization. The effect of statins may be independent of their lipid-lowering effects and depend mainly on the pleiotropic effects on the vascular wall [60]. The beneficial effects of statins may contribute to reduction of neointimal hyperplasia and restenosis after stenting.

Anticoagulation/Antiplatelet Therapy

Anticoagulant and antiplatelet agents have been used to enhance vessel patency for many years. Aspirin is an antiplatelet agent that acts on platelets to prevent aggregation by irreversibly inactivating the cyclooxygenase activity of prostaglandin synthase, and this has been noted to decrease peri-operative thrombosis but not vessel restenosis. In one study, aspirin combined with clopidogrel showed an increased inhibition of platelet aggregation ex vivo as compared to aspirin alone, or aspirin with ticlopidine [61]. A Cochrane review of the literature in 2005 found aspirin (50–330 mg) alone or in combination with dipyridamole to reduce the incidence of reocclusion at 6–12 months after peripheral angioplasty, when compared to placebo or vitamin K antagonists [62]. The previous use of these drugs has been to prevent early thrombosis and platelet aggregation leading to occlusion which is now thought to possibly contribute to intimal hyperplasia at a later date. However, since platelet aggregation is not the sole cause for intimal hyperplasia, platelet inhibitors alone may not have a significant effect on reduction of intimal hyperplasia.

Abciximab belongs to a class of drugs that inhibit the glycoprotein IIb/IIIa receptor (GPIIb-–IIa), which is involved in the final common pathway of platelet activation, and has been shown to decrease the incidence of major cardiac adverse events. One other postulated theory is that glycoprotein IIb/IIIa inhibitors may also inhibit smooth muscle cell proliferation but also this has yet to be proven in clinical trials.

Clopidogrel and ticlopidine belong to the class of drugs known as thienopyridines. This class of drugs is known to block platelet activation by their inhibition of ADP-related platelet aggregation providing a complementary function to that of aspirin, but clopidogrel is more effective at inhibiting platelet function. High doses of clopidogrel inhibit not only platelet activation due to ADP stimulation but also the expression of GPIIb–IIIa. A meta-analysis in 2001 found that clopidogrel had less adverse side effects and decreased the rate of major adverse cardiac events compared to ticlopidine and recommended aspirin plus clopidogrel as the standard post-stent treatment [63]. Current clinical studies have not shown promising results for thienopyridine monotherapy.

Cilostazol is a quinolinone derivative that inhibits phosphodiesterase III and is used in the treatment of intermittent claudication. Min et al. investigated the efficacy of aspirin plus clopidogrel or ticlopidine with or without the addition of cilostazol on the prevention of in-stent neointimal hyperplasia [64]. IVUS were performed and repeated at 6 months to assess luminal diameter and in-stent neointimal hyperplasia volume. At 6-month follow-up, in-stent narrowing was significantly less in the triple therapy group. Volumetric IVUS at 6 months demonstrated that in-stent intimal hyperplasia volume was significantly greater in the double therapy group. Their findings suggest that triple antiplatelet therapy including cilostazol may be more effective than a dual antiplatelet regimen at preventing in-stent neointimal hyperplasia.

Warfarin is a traditional anticoagulant that inhibits vitamin K-dependent coagulation factors. Traditional anticoagulation includes heparin started immediately and continued until the patient is therapeutic on warfarin. This therapy, however, caused higher bleeding risks and adverse events without efficacy in preventing reocclusion. STARS was a major randomized, multicenter trial that looked at aspirin and ticlopidine compared with aspirin alone or aspirin with warfarin [65]. The results were unequivocal: the rate of stent occlusion was significantly lower with aspirin and ticlopidine than with conventional anticoagulation or aspirin alone. More recently, Bertrand et al. demonstrated that the use of antiplatelet therapy alone after stent implantation was associated with a reduction in the overall rate of bleeding complications and in the rate of subacute stent occlusion without significantly changing the rate of overall mortality and nonfatal MI between patients treated with antiplatelet therapy alone and those treated with conventional anticoagulant therapy [66]. After studies failed to show any benefit either as monotherapy or in conjunction with another agent, warfarin has not been generally recommended as post-endovascular therapy to prevent restenosis.

One other anticoagulant that binds thrombin and blocks the activation of platelets is from the European leech and is known as hirudin. Hirudin is a small peptide that penetrates thrombi and inhibits thrombin bound to fibrin [67]. Hirudin reduces fibrin deposition in areas of deep arterial injury and can eliminate mural thrombosis and almost eliminate platelet deposition in high doses [68]. However, this is effective in reducing only the early revascularization failures due to thrombosis but has no effect on intimal hyperplasia. As a result, it may be useful as an interventional anticoagulant but not as post-intervention treatment.

Risk Factor Modification

The most effective way patients can impact their risk of lesion recurrence is by decreasing their risk factors for atherosclerosis. Prospective epidemiologic studies have identified several risk factors for atherosclerosis, and most can be a target intervention. The most widely recognized risk factors for atherosclerotic disease include age, gender, cigarette smoking, sedentary lifestyle, elevated LDL, reduced HDL, hypertension, and diabetes. The consistency of associations between these factors and progression of atherosclerotic disease across populations is substantial [69].

It has been shown that smoking cessation increases the overall survival rate [70]. Faulkner et al. reported that patients with symptomatic peripheral arterial disease who quit smoking had almost twice the 5-year survival rate compared to those who continued to smoke [71].

Regular aerobic exercise not only improves the quality of life and functional capacity but also can be as beneficial in these areas as bypass surgery or more beneficial than angioplasty [72]. A meta-analysis of 10 randomized trials demonstrated an increase in maximal walking time of 150%, which exceeded that of angioplasty and was not significantly different from that of surgical revascularization [73]. Although exercise training is not associated with substantial changes in blood flow to the legs, exercise does improve endothelial vasodilator function, skeletal muscle metabolism, blood viscosity, and inflammatory responses. In older patients, exercise also lowers serum cholesterol and decreases systolic blood pressure, which are risk factors for progression of atherosclerosis [74]. While exercise is a negative predictive factor, Krause et al. found that high-energy expenditures at work are associated with an accelerated progression of atherosclerosis even after control for virtually all known cardiovascular risk factors, especially among older workers and workers with preexisting ischemic heart disease or carotid artery stenosis [75].

Conclusion

Vascular occlusive disease is prevalent in our society and commonly requires intervention. Although endovascular techniques to restore blood flow continue to improve, lesion recurrence still remains a concern. Restenosis occurs in up to 30% of all forms of revascularization. Failure of stenting and angioplasty is due to the progression of underlying disease states and proliferative lesions formed in the reparative process, most notably intimal hyperplasia. Ongoing studies on intimal hyperplasia are elucidating new treatment modalities including systemic or local pharmacologic therapy and gene therapy.

References

1. Sigwart U, Puel J, Mirkovitch V, Joffre F, Kappenberger L: Intravascular stents to prevent occlusion and restenosis after transluminal angioplasty, *N Engl J Med* 316:701–706, 1987.
2. Palmaz JC, Richter GM, Noeldge G et al.: Intraluminal stents in atherosclerotic iliac artery stenosis: preliminary report of a multicenter study, *Radiology* 168:727–731, 1988.
3. Pentecost MJ, Criqui MH, Dorros G et al.: Guidelines for peripheral percutaneous transluminal angioplasty of the abdominal aorta and lower extremity vessels: a statement for health professionals from a special writing group of the councils on cardiovascular radiology, arteriosclerosis, cardio-thoracic and vascular surgery, clinical cardiology, and epidemiology and prevention, the American heart association, *Circ J* 89:511–531, 1994.
4. Murphy TP, Ariaratnam NS, Carney WI, Marcaccio EJ, Slaiby JM, Soares GM, Kim HM: Aortoiliac insufficiency: long-term experience with stent placement for treatment, *Radiology* 231:243–249, 2004.
5. Ivanovic V, McKusick MA, Johnson CM 3rd, Sabater EA, Andrews JC, Breen JF, Bjarnason H, Misra S, Stanson

AW: Renal artery stent placement: complications at a single tertiary care center, *J Vasc Intervent Radiol* 14(2 Pt 1): 217–225, 2003.
6. Henry M, Amor M, Henry I, Ethevenot G, Tzvetanov K, Courvoisier A, Mentre B, Chati Z: Stents in the treatment of renal artery stenosis: long-term follow-up, *J Endovasc Surg* 6(1):42–51, 1999.
7. Cunningham LD, Conte MS: Lower-extremity arterial disease, *Perspect Vasc Surg Endovasc Ther.* 17(4):351–361, 2005.
8. Trabattoni D, Bartorelli AL: Late occlusive in-stent restenosis of a bare-metal stent presenting with ST-elevation anterior MI: is restenosis better than a late stent thrombosis? *Int J Cardiol* 34:186–94, 2008.
9. Farb A, Sangiorgi G, Carter AJ, Walley VM, Edwards WD, Schwartz RS, Virmani R: Pathology of acute and chronic coronary stenting in humans, *Circ J* 99:44–52, 1999.
10. Geary RL, Williams JK, Golden D, Brown DG, Benjamin ME, Adams MR: Time course of cellular proliferation, intimal hyperplasia, and remodeling following angioplasty in monkeys with established atherosclerosis, *Arterioscler Thromb Vasc Biol* 16:34–43, 1996.
11. Borromeo JR, Sumpio BE: Strategies in preventing intimal hyperplasia. In Whittemore A, Bandyk D, Cronenwett J, Herrtzer N, White R, editors: *Advances in vascular surgery*, St. Louis, MO, 2002, Mosby, pp. 201–218.
12. Feldman LJ, Aguirre L, Ziol M, Bridou JP, Nevo N, Michel JB, Steg PG: Interleukin-10 inhibits intimal hyperplasia after angioplasty or stent implantation in hypercholesterolemic rabbits, *Circ J* 101:908–916, 2000.
13. Frangos S, Gahtan V, Sumpio BE: Localization of atherosclerosis: role of hemodynamics, *Arch Surg* 134:1142–1149, 1999.
14. Kohler TR, Kirkman TR, Kraiss LW, Zierler BK, Clowes AW: Increased blood flow inhibits neointimal hyperplasia in endothelialized vascular grafts, *Circ Res* 69:1557–1565, 1991.
15. Steinthorsson G, Sumpio BE: Clinical and biological relevance of vein cuff anastomosis, *Acta Chir Belg.* 99: 282–288, 1999.
16. Kohler TR, Clowes AW: Prevention of lesion recurrence in endovascular devices. In White RA, Fogarty, TJ, editors.: Peripheral Endovascular Interventions, ed. 2, New York, 1999, Springer-Verlag New York, Inc, 539–553.
17. Sumpio BE: Atherosclerosis: biological and surgical considerations, In Ascher E, Hollier L, Strandness DE, editors: *Haimovici's vascular surgery*, ed. 5, Malden, MA, 2004, Blackwell Science, Inc, pp. 137–163.
18. Pasterkamp G, de Kleijn DP, Borst C: Arterial remodeling in atherosclerosis, restenosis and after alteration of blood flow: potential mechanisms and clinical implications, *Cardiovasc Res* 45(4):843–852, 2000.
19. Haruguchi H, Teraoka S: Intimal hyperplasia and hemodynamic factors in arterial bypass and arteriovenous grafts: a review, *J Artif Organs.* 6(4):227–235, 2003.
20. Schwartz SM, de Blois D, O'Brien ER: The intima. Soil for atherosclerosis and restenosis, *Circ Res* 77(3):445–465, 1995.
21. Lindner V, Reidy MA: Proliferation of smooth muscle cells after vascular injury is inhibited by an antibody against basic fibroblast growth factor. *Proc Natl Acad Sci USA*, 88:3739–3743, 1991.
22. 22.Olson NE, Chao S, Lindner V, Reidy MA: Intimal smooth muscle cell proliferation after balloon catheter injury: the role of basic fibroblast growth factor, *Am J Pathol* 140:1017–1023, 1992.
23. Langille BL: Remodeling of developing and mature arteries: endothelium, smooth muscle, and matrix, *J Cardiovasc Pharmacol* 21(suppl 1):S11–S17, 1993.
24. Fattori R, Piva T: Drug-eluting stents in vascular intervention, *The Lancet* 361(9353):247–249, 2003.
25. Lafont A, Guzman LA, Whitlow PL, Goormastic M, Cornhill JF, Chisolm GM: Restenosis after experimental angioplasty. Intimal, medial, and adventitial changes associated with constrictive remodeling, *Circ Res* 76(6): 996–1002, 1995.
26. Ryan ST, Koteliansky VE, Gotwals PJ, Lindner V: Transforming growth factor-beta-dependent events in vascular remodeling following arterial injury, *J Vasc Res* 40(1):37–46, 2003.
27. Paszkowiak JJ, Maloney SP, Kudo FA, Muto A, Teso D, Rutland RC, Westvik TS, Pimiento JM, Tellides G, Sessa WC, Dardik A: Evidence supporting changes in Nogo-B levels as a marker of neointimal expansion but not adaptive arterial remodeling, *Vascul Pharmacol* 46(4):293–301, 2007.
28. Assmus B, Walter DH, Lehmann R, Honold J, Martin H, Dimmeler S, Zeiher AM, Schächinger V: Intracoronary infusion of progenitor cells is not associated with aggravated restenosis development or atherosclerotic disease progression in patients with acute myocardial infarction, *Eur Heart J* 27(24):2989–2995, 2006.
29. Hiatt BL, Ikeno F, Yeung AC, Carter AJ: Drug-eluting stents for the prevention of restenosis: in quest for the Holy Grail, *Catheter Cardiovasc Interv* 55(3):409–417, 2002.
30. Serruys PW, Ormiston JA, Sianos G, Sousa JE, Grube E, den Heijer P, de Feyter P, Buszman P, Schömig A, Marco J, Polonski L, Thuesen L, Zeiher AM, Bett JH, Suttorp MJ, Glogar HD, Pitney M, Wilkins GT, Whitbourn R, Veldhof S, Miquel K, Johnson R, Coleman L, Virmani R: ACTION investigators. Actinomycin-eluting stent for coronary revascularization: a randomized feasibility and safety study: the ACTION trial, *J Am Coll Cardiol* 44(7):1363–1367, 2004.
31. Siablis D, Karnabatidis D, Katsanos K, Diamantopoulos A, Christeas N, Kagadis GC: Infrapopliteal application of paclitaxel-eluting stents for critical limb ischemia: midterm angiographic and clinical results, *J Vasc Interv Radiol* 18(11):1351–1361, 2007.
32. Grube E, Siber MS, Hauptmann KE: Prospective, randomized, double-blind comparison of NIRx stents coated with paclitaxel in a polymer carrier in de-novo coronary lesions compared with uncoated controls, *Circ J* 104(suppl):II-463, 2001.
33. Hong MK, Mintz GS, Lee CW, Song JM, Han KH, Kang DH, Song JK, Kim JJ, Weissman NJ, Fearnot NE, Park SW, Park SJ: Paclitaxel coating reduces in-stent intimal hyperplasia in human coronary arteries a serial volumetric intravascular ultrasound analysis from the ASian Paclitaxel-Eluting Stent Clinical Trial (ASPECT), *Circ J* 107:517–520, 2003.

34. Tepe G, Zeller T, Albrecht T, Heller S, Schwarzwälder U, Beregi JP, Claussen CD, Oldenburg A, Scheller B, Speck U: Local delivery of paclitaxel to inhibit restenosis during angioplasty of the leg, *N Engl J Med* 358(7):689–699, 2008.
35. Sousa JE, Costa MA, Abizaid A, Abizaid AS, Feres F, Pinto IM, Seixas AC, Staico R, Mattos LA, Sousa AG, Falotico R, Jaeger J, Popma JJ, Serruys PW: Lack of neointimal proliferation after implantation of sirolimus-coated stents in human coronary arteries: a quantitative coronary angiography and three-dimensional intravascular ultrasound study, *Circ J* 103:192–195, 2001.
36. Morice MC, Serruys PW, Sousa JE, Fajadet J, Ban Hayashi E, Perin M, Colombo A, Schuler G, Barragan P, Guagliumi G, Molnàr F, Falotico R: A randomized comparison of a sirolimus-eluting stent with a standard stent for coronary revascularization, *N Engl J Med* 346(23):1773–1780, 2002.
37. Teirstein PS, Kuntz RE: New frontiers in interventional cardiology. *Circ J* 104:2620–2626, 2001.
38. Wolfram RM, Budinsky AC, Pokrajac B, Potter R, Minar E: Endovascular brachytherapy for prophylaxis of restenosis after femoropopliteal angioplasty: five-year follow-up–prospective randomized study, *Radiology* 240(3):878–884, 2006.
39. Hansrani M, Overbeck K, Smout J, Stansby G: Intravascular brachytherapy for peripheral vascular disease, *Cochrane Database Syst Rev* 4:CD003504, 2002.
40. Albiero R, Nishida T, Adamian M, Amato A, Vaghetti M, Corvaja N, Di Mario C, Colombo A: Edge restenosis after implantation of high activity ^{32}P radioactive beta-emitting stents, *Circ J* 101:2454–2457, 2000.
41. Kim HS, Waksman R, Cottin Y, Kollum M, Bhargava B, Mehran R, Chan RC, Mintz GS: Edge stenosis and geographical miss following intracoronary gamma radiation therapy for in-stent restenosis, *J Am Coll Cardiol* 37:1026–1030, 2001.
42. Albiero R, Adamian M, Kobayashi N: Short- and intermediate-term results of ^{32}P radioactive (beta) β-emitting stent implantation in patients with coronary artery disease. The Milan dose-response study, *Circ J* 101:18–24, 2000.
43. Feldman LJ, Tahlil O, Steg G: Perspectives of arterial gene therapy for the prevention of restenosis, *Cardiovasc Res* 32(2):194–207, 1996.
44. Nikol S, Huehns TY: Preclinical and clinical experience in vascular gene therapy: advantages over conservative/standard therapy, *J Invasive Cardiol* 13(4):333–338, 2001.
45. Brogi E, Wu T, Namiki A, Isner JM: Indirect angiogenic cytokines upregulate VEGF and bFGF gene expression in vascular smooth muscle cells, whereas hypoxia upregulates VEGF expression only, *Circ J* 90:649–652, 1994.
46. Leong-Poi H, Kuliszewski MA, Lekas M, Sibbald M, Teichert-Kuliszewska K, Klibanov AL, Stewart DJ, Lindner JR: Therapeutic arteriogenesis by ultrasound-mediated VEGF165 plasmid gene delivery to chronically ischemic skeletal muscle. 2007 American Heart Association, Inc, *Circ Res* 101(3):295–303, 2007.
47. Von der Leyen HE, Dzau VJ: Therapeutic potential of nitric oxide synthase gene manipulation, *Circ J* 103:2760–2765, 2001.
48. Urano T, Ito Y, Akao M, Sawa T, Miyata K, Tabata M, Morisada T, Hato T, Yano M, Kadomatsu T, Yasunaga K, Shibata R, Murohara T, Akaike T, Tanihara H, Suda T, Oike Y: Angiopoietin-related growth factor enhances blood flow via activation of the ERK1/2-eNOS-NO pathway in a mouse hind-limb ischemia model, *Arterioscler Thromb Vasc Biol* 28(5):827–834, 2008.
49. Benest AV, Stone OA, Miller WH, Glover CP, Uney JB, Baker AH, Harper SJ, Bates DO: Arteriolar genesis and angiogenesis induced by endothelial nitric oxide synthase overexpression results in a mature vasculature, *Arterioscler Thromb Vasc Biol* 28(8):1462–1468, Published online May 22, 2008.
50. Morishita R, Tomita N, Kaneda Y, Ogihara T: Molecular therapy to inhibit NFkappaB activation by transcription factor decoy oligonucleotides, *Curr Opin Pharmacol* 4(2):139–146, 2004.
51. Conte MS, Bandyk DF, Clowes AW et al.: Results of PREVENT III: a multicenter, randomized trial of edifoligide for the prevention of vein graft failure in lower extremity bypass surgery, *J Vasc Surg* 43(4):742–751, 2006.
52. Tatewaki H, Egashira K, Kimura S, Nishida T, Morita S, Tominaga R: Blockade of monocyte chemoattractant protein-1 by adenoviral gene transfer inhibits experimental vein graft neointimal formation, *J Vasc Surg* 45(6): 1236–1243, 2007.
53. Ohtani K, Usui M, Nakano K, Kohjimoto Y, Kitajima S, Hirouchi Y, Li XH, Kitamoto S, Takeshita A, Egashira K: Antimonocyte chemoattractant protein-1 gene therapy reduces experimental in-stent restenosis in hypercholesterolemic rabbits and monkeys, *Gene Ther* 11:1273–1282, 2004.
54. Morka J, Krzemińska-Pakuła M, Drożdż J, Morka A: Factors affecting the progression of atherosclerosis in the coronary arteries, *Kardiol Pol* 65:1307–1311, 2007.
55. Nicholls SJ, Tuzcu EM, Sipahi I, Grasso AW, Schoenhagen P, Hu T, Wolski K, Crowe T, Desai MY, Hazen SL, Kapadia SR, Nissen SE: Statins, high-density lipoprotein cholesterol, and regression of coronary atherosclerosis, *JAMA* 297(20):2197, 2007.
56. 56.Von Haehling S: Treatment options for endothelial dysfunction, *Heart and Metab* 22:22–28, 2004.
57. Williams JK, Sukhova GK, Herrington DM, Libby P: Pravastatin has cholesterol lowering effects on the artery wall of atherosclerotic monkeys, *J Am Coll Cardiol* 31(3):684–691, 1998.
58. Kaesemeyer WH, Caldwell RB, Huang J, Caldwell RW: Pravastatin sodium activates endothelial nitric oxide synthase independent of its cholesterol-lowering actions, *J Am Coll Cardiol* 33(1):234–241, 1999.
59. Bandoh T, Mitani H, Niihashi M, Kusumi Y, Ishikawa J, Kimura M, Totsuka T, Sakurai I, Hayashi S: Inhibitory effect of fluvastatin at doses insufficient to lower serum lipids on the catheter-induced thickening of intima in rabbit femoral artery, *Eur J Pharmacol* 315(1):37–42, 1996.
60. Kamishirado H, Inoue T, Sakuma M, Tsuda T, Hayashi T, Takayanagi K, Node K: Effects of statins on restenosis after coronary stent implantation, *Angiology* 58(1):55–60, 2007.

61. Chaer RA, Graham JA, Mureebe L: Platelet function and pharmacologic inhibition, *Vasc Endovascular Surg* 40(4):261–267, 2006.
62. Dorffler-Melly J, Koopman MMW, Prins MH, Buller HR: Antiplatelet and anticoagulant drugs for prevention of restenosis/reocclusion following peripheral endovascular treatment, *Cochrane Database Syst Rev* 1:CD002071, 2005.
63. Bhatt DL, Bertrand ME, Berger PB, L'Allier PL, Moussa I, Moses JW, Dangas G, Taniuchi M, Lasala JM, Holmes DR, Ellis SG, Topol EJ: Meta-analysis of randomized and registry comparisons of ticlopidine with clopidogrel after stenting, *J Am Coll Cardiol* 39(1):9–14, 2002.
64. Min PK, Jung JH, Ko YG, Choi D, Jang Y, Shim WH: Effect of cilostazol on in-stent neointimal hyperplasia after coronary artery stenting: a quantitative coronary angiography and volumetric intravascular ultrasound study, *Circ J* 71(11):1685–1690, 2007.
65. Leon MB, Baim DS, Gordon P, Giambotolomei A, Williams D, Diver DD, Senerchia C, Fitzpatrick M, Popma J, Kuntz RE: Clinical and angiographic results from the Stent Anticoagulation Regimen Study (STARS), *Circ J* 94(suppl I):I-685, 1996.
66. Bertrand ME, Legrand V, Boland J, Fleck E, Bonnier J, Emmanuelson H, Vrolix M, Missault L, Chierchia S, Casaccia M, Niccoli L, Oto A, White C, Webb-Peploe M, Van Belle E, McFadden EP: Randomized multicenter comparison of conventional anticoagulation versus antiplatelet therapy in unplanned and elective coronary stenting, *Circ J* 98:1597–1603, 1998.
67. Greinacher A, Warkentin TE: The direct thrombin inhibitor hirudin, *Thromb Haemost* 99(5):819–829, 2008.
68. Chesebro JH, Webster MW, Zoldhelyi P, Roche PC, Badimon L, Badimon JJ: Antithrombotic therapy and progression of coronary artery disease: antiplatelet versus antithrombins, *Circ J* 86(suppl III):100–110, 1992.
69. Budoff M: Aged garlic extract retards progression of coronary artery calcification, *J Nutr* 136(3):741S–744S, 2006.
70. Faulkner KW, House AK, Castleden WM: The effect of cessation of smoking on the accumulative survival rates of patients with symptomatic peripheral vascular disease, *Med J Aust* 1:217–219, 1983.
71. Willigendael EM, Teijink JA, Bartelink ML, Peters RJ, Buller HR, Prins MH: Smoking and the patency of lower extremity bypass grafts: a meta-analysis, *J Vasc Surg* 42:67–74, 2005.
72. Regensteiner JG, Steiner JF, Hiatt WR: Exercise training improves functional status in patients with peripheral arterial disease, *J Vasc Surg* 23:104–115, 1996.
73. Leng GC, Fowler B, Ernst E: Exercise for intermittent claudication, *Cochrane Database Syst Rev* 2:CD000990, 2000.
74. Izquierdo-Porrera AM, Gardner AW, Powell CC, Katzel LI: Effects of exercise rehabilitation on cardiovascular risk factors in older patients with peripheral arterial occlusive disease, *J Vasc Surg* 31:670–677, 2000.
75. Krause N, Brand RJ, Kaplan GA, Kauhanen J, Malla S, Tuomainen TP, Salonen JT: Occupational physical activity, energy expenditure and 11-year progression of carotid atherosclerosis, *Scand J Work Environ Health* 33(6): 405–424, 2007.
76. Pasa MB, Pereira AH, Júnior CC: Morphometric analysis of intimal thickening secondary to stent placement in pig carotid arteries, *Acta Cir Bras* 23(2):165–172, 2008.
77. Kalinowski M, Alfke H, Bergen S et al.: Comparative trial of local pharmacotherapy with L-arginine, r-hirudin, and molsidomine to reduce restenosis after balloon angioplasty of stenotic rabbit iliac arteries, *Radiology* 219:716–723, 2001.
78. Dobesh PP, Stacy ZA, Ansara AJ, Enders JM: Drug-eluting stents: a mechanical and pharmacologic approach to coronary artery disease, *Pharmacotherapy* 24(11):1554–1577, 2004.
79. Garrett RH, Grisham CM: Structure of Nucleic Acids. In *Biochemistry*, ed. 2, Fort Worth, TX, 1999, Saunders College Publishing, pp. 356–394.
80. Wessely R, Schömig A, Kastrati A: Sirolimus and paclitaxel on polymer-based drug-eluting stents, *J Am Coll Cardiol* 47:708–714, 2006.
81. Albiero R, Colombo A: European high-activity (32)P radioactive stent experience, *J Invasive Cardiol* 12(8): 416–421, 2000.
82. Jain HV, Nör JE, Jackson TL: Modeling the VEGF-Bcl-2-CXCL8 pathway in intratumoral angiogenesis, *Bull Math Biol* 70:89–117, 2008.

Management of the Percutaneous Puncture Site

31

Melissa E. Hogg, Ashley K. Vavra, and Melina R. Kibbe

Over the past quarter century there has been rapid growth of percutaneous endovascular procedures. The estimated total amount of open and endovascular cardiac and vascular surgery procedures is close to 7 million per year [1]. According to the American Heart Association's Heart Disease and Stroke Statistics, approximately 1,285,000 angioplasty procedures were performed in 2004 [1]. The number of stents placed annually is now well over 1 million per year with 615,000 coronary stents, 400,000 peripheral stents, and 40,000 stents for renal artery stenosis, in addition to stents at other sites [1, 2, 3]. Endovascular procedures are performed in venues ranging from operating rooms to catheterization laboratories and are performed by a wide array of specialists including interventional radiologists, neurosurgeons, cardiologists, cardiothoracic surgeons, and vascular surgeons. Furthermore, these procedures are commonly performed all over the body: cerebral, carotid, subclavian, coronary, mesenteric, renal, and peripheral arteries. The common gradient in all these procedures is the percutaneous puncture site.

Knowledge, familiarity, and comfort in management of the percutaneous access site should not be taken lightly. Every specialist performing these interventions should have knowledge of access options and limitations, and be able to troubleshoot problems and manage complications. This chapter will outline the main percutaneous access sites, paying attention to indications for their use, techniques in gaining access, options for closing the arteriotomy, and complications that can arise.

Overview of Access Locations

Various locations can be used for percutaneous arterial access. It is important to understand the different advantages, disadvantages, and complications associated with each site (Table 31.1). This includes a working knowledge of anatomy, arterial size, and vessel tortuosity as it relates to target lesion site.

Femoral

The common femoral artery is the most often used access site for percutaneous endovascular procedures. There are two approaches to the common femoral artery access: retrograde and antegrade. Retrograde punctures allow access to the iliac arteries, the aorta and its branches, and the entire contralateral limb, while antegrade punctures allow only for procedures of the ipsilateral superficial femoral artery and its distal branches. Virtually every procedure can be accomplished from common femoral artery access and most of the industry's product inventions and developments have been designed with the femoral approach in mind [4]. Benefits of femoral access include palpable pulse, compressible artery, simple puncture technique, safe, well tolerated, and allows access to almost all arterial territories [5]. Furthermore, the common femoral artery is centrally located, large, can easily accommodate sheaths up to 24 French (F), and has an ergonomic

M.E. Hogg (✉)
Resident, Department of Surgery, Northwestern University Feinberg School of Medicine, Chicago, IL, USA

T.J. Fogarty, R.A. White (eds.), *Peripheral Endovascular Interventions*,
DOI 10.1007/978-1-4419-1387-6_31, © Springer Science+Business Media, LLC 1998, 2010

Table 31.1 Comparison of arterial puncture locations

Artery	Advantages	Disadvantages	Possible complications
Femoral	Easy, ergonomic access	Delayed ambulation	Bleeding/hematoma
	Patient comfort	Atherosclerotic disease	Pseudoaneurysm
	Can access entire arterial system	Obesity	Thrombosis
	Compress against femoral head	Long working distance for remote sites	Embolus
	Large arterial diameter		Dissection
	Immobile target		
	Can easily access both sides		
Brachial	Usually atherosclerotic free	Mobile target	Same as femoral artery
	Relatively large arterial diameter	Spasm	Spasm and thrombosis more pronounced
	No delay in ambulation time	Left side preferable	Nerve injury secondary to hematoma
	Patient comfort	Long working distance	
		Tortuous catheter routes	
Radial	Easy access	Spasm	Bleeding
	Easily compressible	Small arterial diameter	Thrombosis
	Minimal complications	Left side preferable	Spasm
	No delay in ambulation	Long working distance	Hand ischemia
	Less personnel required for hemostasis	Must assess Allen's test	Nerve injury
	Possible early discharge		Radial artery cannot be used as a conduit
	Patient preference		
Axillary	Large arterial diameter	Technically challenging	Same as femoral artery
	Close proximity to arch vessels	Mobile target	Axillary sheath hematoma
		Patient discomfort	Nerve injury
		Hemostasis more difficult to achieve	Arteriovenous fistula
Popliteal	Good for proximal SFA disease	Technically challenging	Same as femoral artery
	Good for CFA disease	Patient discomfort	Arteriovenous fistula
		Obesity	
Cervical	Good for proximal CCA disease	Technically challenging	Same as femoral artery
		Patient discomfort	Stroke associated with any emboli

SFA: Superficial femoral artery; CFA: common femoral artery; CCA: common carotid artery.

space with respect to fluoroscopy [4]. Also, both sides are accessible and puncture complications can usually be managed easily [6]. There are drawbacks to this site which include increased bleeding risk and delayed ambulation [4]. Also, vessel tortuosity and atherosclerotic disease can make procedures technically difficult or impossible and remote targets have a long pathway for catheter manipulations. Obstacles for attaining access include obesity and absent or diminished pulses. Additional obstacles exist for antegrade punctures: the anterior abdominal wall and the inguinal ligament make vessel puncture difficult and there is an increased risk of superficial femoral artery puncture with this approach which has greater reported complications [5].

Brachial

The brachial artery is the second most frequent site for percutaneous access [5]. One advantage to using the brachial artery is that it is usually patent and disease free [6]. The left side is preferred to the right to avoid crossing the carotid and vertebral arteries which could precipitate cerebral complications. Sheath sizes 5–7 F are well tolerated and, given the size of the brachial artery, a Micropuncture Kit (Cook, Bloomington, IN) should be used for entry [5]. Brachial artery access is not typically used to perform procedures below the knee due to the length of the catheters required to reach the target vessels. Indications for left brachial artery access include left subclavian artery stenosis, renal artery stenosis (especially if the vessel takes a sharp downward angle), celiac and mesenteric procedures, cases of aortic occlusion or bilateral iliac artery stenosis or occlusion preventing femoral access, groin scars making femoral access difficult, absence of femoral pulses, and failure of femoral access or a common femoral artery aneurysm [7]. Indications for right-sided access include left subclavian artery stenosis, innominate stenosis, and failure of left brachial access [7]. That being said, brachial access is best for angiography and simple interventions. However, some reports have also touted the brachial artery as a potentially useful adjunct or even first line for procedures. Criado et al. reported the use of a second access via the brachial artery to facilitate endovascular aortic aneurysm repair (EVAR) in 103 patients [8]. This group found the brachial access specifically useful to overcome tortuous aortoiliac anatomy, which allowed the surgeon to stabilize the transfemoral wire and facilitate tracking and advancement of the delivery sheath to the desired location. Advantages of the use of an upper extremity access point are decreased time-to-patient ambulation and improved patient comfort. However, despite these potential advantages, more tortuous catheter routes and a higher perceived complication rate have limited the use of the brachial artery as a preferred access site [9]. Unlike the common femoral artery, the brachial artery has a limited sheath size and increased risk of ischemic complications. Upper extremity vessels are prone to spasm and can thrombose in response to instrumentation; thus there is a need for aggressive administration of vasodilators and heparin through the sheath when using this access [4].

Radial

Radial access used to be a novelty but has recently gained more acceptance as an alternative access site, especially with cardiac procedures. This access site has now been studied extensively as an alternative access site for coronary-based procedures but has also been described for use in cerebral angiography and in peripheral procedures such as carotid stenting [10, 11]. Relative indications for the radial access are similar to brachial access and include obesity, inguinal scarring, severe peripheral vascular disease (PVD), aortic or iliac occlusion, and coagulopathy [12]. Advantages are that the artery is easily compressible and frequently does not require personnel for compression. The patient is able to ambulate early and possibly discharge early with the radial approach, which can lead to decreased hospital costs [13]. Also, morbidity can be lower. Gilchrist et al. compared radial and femoral access sites and, in their cohort, they had 12 patients with femoral access site complications (arteriovenous fistulas, pseudoaneurysms, and hematomas) compared with no access site complications in the radial arm [14]. Additionally, a quality-of-life study revealed that patients actually preferred radial artery puncture to common femoral artery puncture [14]. Disadvantages of this site include risk of spasm, thrombosis, hand ischemia, and potential nerve damage. Another consideration is that access of the radial artery can make it ineligible as a conduit for a bypass graft in the future [6]. Exclusion criteria for this site include absence of radial or ulnar pulse, digital ischemia upon performance of the Allen's test, and lesions necessitating large sheaths [12]. Typically, sheath sizes up to 6 F can be accommodated by the radial artery, but this depends mainly on the diameter of the individual radial artery. We advocate assessing the size of the radial artery with duplex ultrasonography before accessing the radial artery to confirm the appropriateness of the radial artery for a given sheath size. In addition, newer hydrophilic-coated sheaths have the potential to minimize access-related complications for the radial artery.

Axillary

Axillary artery access has many of the same uses and indications as the previously discussed upper extremity access sites, but it is currently rarely used and often not recommended [7]. In some reports, referenced use of the axillary artery simply refers to use of a proximal brachial artery puncture. Benefits of using the axillary or proximal brachial artery include a larger vessel diameter and close proximity to the carotid and splanchnic vessels, making it an advantageous approach for procedures involving these sites [15]. Also, a 7–8-F sheath can easily be accommodated at this access site. The type of complications associated with axillary access is also similar to those seen with the brachial artery and include hematoma, pseudoaneurysm formation, thrombosis, arteriovenous fistula, and distal embolus. However, proximity of the axillary artery to the brachial plexus places patients at increased risk for nerve injury in the setting of bleeding complications. Because axillary access has an increased risk of insecure hemostasis, bleeding can cause an intra-sheath hematoma which can lead to a compressive neuropathy of the brachial plexus, necessitating urgent operative decompression [5]. Additionally, the puncture can be tricky and arm positioning is uncomfortable to the patient.

Popliteal

Like the common femoral artery access site, the popliteal artery can be punctured in an antegrade or a retrograde fashion. Access via the popliteal artery is usually performed via a retrograde approach, although antegrade approaches can be performed. The popliteal artery can easily accommodate 5–7-F sheaths and can accommodate larger sheaths if the diameter is >6 mm [5, 16]. Popliteal access is indicated when femoral access is contraindicated or not technically feasible and when use of the brachial artery is contraindicated. This access choice, however, is also based on the location of the lesions: superficial femoral artery (ostial, proximal, or diffuse) or common femoral artery. Contraindications exist when the patient is unable to lay prone, is obese, has respiratory insufficiency, has femoropopliteal obstruction near the puncture site, or if the patient has the inability to hyperextend the knee [16]. The retrograde approach is frequently used for iliofemoral lesions close to a potential common femoral artery puncture site [5]. This access, particularly the antegrade puncture, is technically challenging and requires experience. No large antegrade popliteal puncture experiences exist, only isolated reports in the literature [17, 18, 19].

Cervical

Cervical access is mainly considered for supra-aortic trunk lesion interventions and can be performed in an antegrade or a retrograde fashion [20]. It can be performed via a percutaneous puncture, cutdown, or a hybrid operation performed simultaneously with a carotid intervention. Indications for this access site include arch calcification, arch elongation, proximal common carotid artery disease, carotid tortuosity, redo operations (scarring and increased risk of cranial nerve injury), and mobile arch atheroma where embolism is a hazard for gaining access to the aorta [20]. Another time to consider this technique is with a bovine arch, which occurs in about 15% of patients [21]. A bovine arch can make access to the internal carotid artery difficult, given the acute angulations involved, thus necessitating an alternative access approach [21]. While cervical access has very specific indications, it is a technically challenging approach, and one that is associated with a significant risk of stroke from an embolus of air or particulate debris. Thus, this approach should be utilized with great caution.

Percutaneous Access Techniques

Regardless of access site location or procedure, there are a few basic principles of obtaining access: the needle puncture, Seldinger technique, and the use of introducer sheaths. Methods of arterial puncture are the single-wall entry and the through-and-through technique [6]. With a single-walled entry, only the anterior wall is traversed. For this procedure the bevel should remain up. This technique has a potential to dissect the vessel upon advancing the wire because blood may return, but the needle may only be partially within the arterial lumen. Clues of subintimal dissection include lack of smooth intraluminal wire passage and curling of guidewire in a short distance on fluoroscopy [5]. For the through-and-through technique, access is achieved to the vessel when pulling back. The same needle employed for single-walled entry can be used, but often a multipart needle is used [6]. The Seldinger over-the-wire technique involves passing a wire through the needle to maintain the path from the skin into the artery. For virtually all procedures, an introducer sheath is used in order to maintain access. The sheath secures access and allows for safe and rapid exchanges of wires, balloons, stents, and other devices needed to successfully complete the endovascular intervention. Furthermore, sheaths allow for administration of pharmacologic agents and contrast injections, and can transduce an arterial waveform. Additionally, adjunct techniques can be employed to access the artery if palpation is not effective: hand-held Doppler, ultrasound probes, and a SMART needle (Cardiovascular Dynamics, Irvine, CA). SMART needles have an ultrasound probe built into the tip so that when the artery is approached, an auditory signal is heard.

Femoral

The patient is placed on the angiography table in the supine position. The femoral head is imaged using fluoroscopy to mark the transverse midpoint as the site of puncture (Fig. 31.1). Several have addressed the anatomical consideration of the common femoral artery with respect to the femoral head [4, 5, 22, 23]. Rupp et al. indicates that the femoral artery is 1 cm lateral to the most medial cortex of the femoral head [23]. Criado et al. use the medial third of the femoral head as a reference point [24]. Additionally, obtaining access fluoroscopically has been shown to decrease the incidence of pseudoaneurysm fourfold [25]. Fewer arterial injuries have been observed when practitioners use fluoroscopy compared to no fluoroscopy. Once the landmarks are identified, a horizontal stab incision is made approximately 2–3 cm below the midpoint of the femoral head depending on the girth of the patient. Using an 18-gauge needle, arterial access is gained through the anterior wall of the common femoral artery directly overlying the midpoint of the femoral head. A technical consideration at this point is to keep the angle between the needle and the artery 30–45°. Otherwise, it can be hard to pass a guidewire if too steep, while if too parallel, the puncture may be too proximal and not enter the artery in an infrainguinal location [5]. Use of the above described technique will place the needle entry site directly in the common femoral artery away from the superficial femoral artery and profunda femoral artery bifurcation, and will allow for direct compression of the common femoral artery against the femoral head in the event that manual compression is planned or required. After arterial entry, a J wire is advanced into the aorta and the access site is secured with an introducer. Our group performs an angiogram of the common femoral artery for every percutaneous puncture in order to assess the puncture site and determine appropriateness for closure devices. This "Fem-Shot" is obtained by using an ipsilateral 25° oblique view of the femoral head, while digital subtraction images are taken during contrast injection.

Antegrade femoral puncture has the same setup and anatomical landmarks as a retrograde femoral puncture. The needle stick should also be done in a 30–45° needle to artery angle [5]. The anterior abdominal wall and the inguinal ligament make vessel puncture difficult, especially in an obese patient where keeping

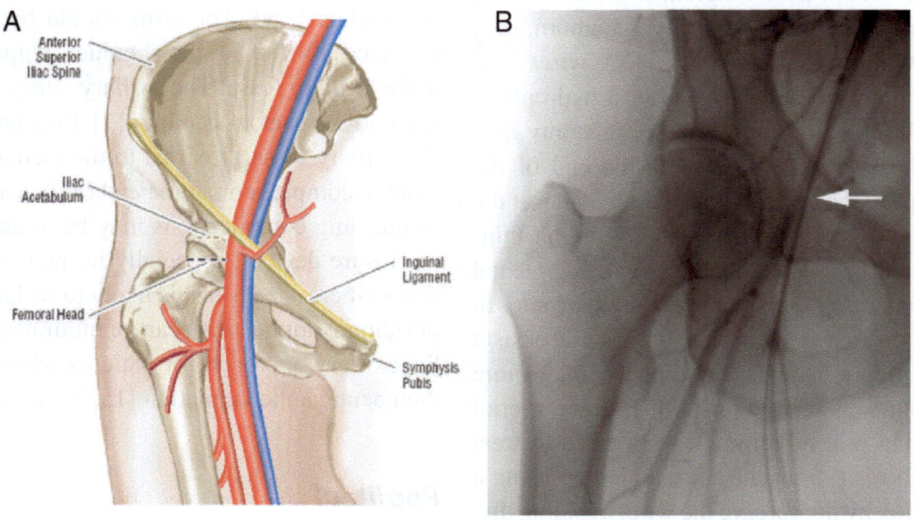

Fig. 31.1 **a**, Illustration of the common femoral artery and its relationship to the femoral head; **b**, Angiogram of the common femoral artery depicting its relationship to the femoral head. Reproduced from with permission from Hogg and Kibbe [47], copyright owned by BC Decker, Inc

the entry angle from being too steep can be difficult. Standing to the left of the patient often makes this puncture technically easier for a right-handed surgeon. Given the risk of puncturing the superficial femoral artery, we will frequently use a Micropuncture Kit to obtain access until common femoral artery confirmation is obtained.

Brachial

Brachial artery access is also achieved with the patient in a supine position. The arm should be supinated, extended, and in 30–90° abduction [7]. The brachial artery is fixed and superficial at or above the antecubital fossa. Thus, the arteriotomy should be achieved at this level. The practitioner should take care to immobilize the brachial artery between his/her second and third digits prior to arterial puncture, given that the brachial artery is less fixed within its facial plane (i.e., compared to the common femoral artery which is relatively fixed in its location). The puncture should be performed superficially and obliquely in a proximal and internal direction along the axis of brachial–radial artery using a Micropuncture needle. After wire access is obtained, an introducer sheath should be placed and constantly perfused with heparinized saline. The long and tortuous path to the site of intervention may be difficult and wire choice is critical. Ledesma et al. prefer Bentson (Cook, Bloomington, IN, USA), Storq (Cordis, Johnson & Johnson company, Langhorn, PA), or Wholey (Guidant, Indianapolis, IN) wires [5]. Gengler et al. prefer a Teflon-coated or a hydrophilic wire, especially for tortuous arterial anatomy [7]. Removal of the sheath is required at the end of the case, and compression of the brachial artery against the humerus should be performed for 15–20 min at minimum. The main pitfall of this technique is brachial spasm. This may necessitate using an alternate site. In Barnett et al.'s series of 438 patients, arterial spasm caused failure in four patients. This appears to be more common in smokers and women [7]. Intra-arterial nitroglycerin and oral nifedipine can be used to treat spasm. Thrombosis can usually be avoided by using a one-piece needle, by not forcing the wire, avoiding dissection, heparinized saline administration, and using a maximum of 6-F sheath for brachial access or 8-F sheaths for axillary access [7].

Radial

Accessing the radial artery on the right is easier if the surgeon is right-handed. The patient should be placed in the supine position with the arm supinated and the wrist extended or hyperextended [12]. Palpate the styloid process. Entry into the artery should occur approximately 1 cm proximally to the styloid process. An 18–22-gauge needle should be used to gain access. Advance the needle at a 30–45° angle relative to the artery. Once access is obtained, use a short (7 cm), a standard (13 cm), or a long (23 cm) sheath. Each has its advantages and disadvantages. Long sheaths have less spasm and easier movement, but they are harder to withdraw. For all radial artery access procedures, administration of anti-spasm and anti-thrombosis medication is critical. Fast-acting nitrates and prolonged acting verapamil should be given followed by heparin [12]. Upon completion of the intervention, remove the sheath immediately. Compress the radial artery while placing a tourniquet to hold pressure on the artery for 30–45 min. Following this a non-circumferential compressive bandage should be placed for 6 h.

Axillary

Axillary artery access is technically difficult and positioning is usually uncomfortable for the patient [7]. Place the patient in a supine position with his or her hand under head. The arms should be supinated and extended 90–180° at the shoulder. Palpate for a pulse in the axillary fossa. The axillary artery is located posterior to the pectoralis minor [7]. Puncture the artery in the axillary fossa proximal to the median nerve. Hold manual compression at the end of the case. Prevention of bleeding complications may be assisted by the use of closure devices, especially in interventional procedures where sheath size is likely to be larger. However, bleeding complications can be minimized by reserving the axillary approach for patients who do not require therapeutic anticoagulation [15, 26, 27].

Popliteal

There have been multiple techniques reported to access the popliteal artery. Positioning of the patient is critical and varies per technique. For retrograde punctures, the needle puncture is accomplished in a prone position. The artery can be visualized using adjunct technologies, such as ultrasound, an EchoDoppler, or a SMART needle [16]. Regardless of the method utilized to localize the artery, it should be accessed just proximal to the joint [16]. Careful attention should be paid toward veering medially or laterally, given that the popliteal artery runs with the tibial nerve and the popliteal vein (Fig. 31.2). CT (computed tomography) imaging of the popliteal fossa in a study by Trigaux et al. demonstrated that the popliteal artery and the vein lie in close proximity within a common sheath with the artery anterior or anteromedial to the vein in the majority of cases [28]. If the vein is inadvertently punctured in an attempt to access the popliteal artery or if the needle traverses the artery, patients are at significantly increased risk for arteriovenous fistula development. The introducer should be withdrawn at the end of the procedure. Manual compression can be applied or a closure device can be utilized [16].

Antegrade popliteal artery access has seldom been reported. It is a technique best left in the hands of skilled interventionalists. The patient can be placed in a left lateral position. This provides a straight route to the tibioperoneal trunk. Ultrasound guidance will help with arterial puncture. A maximum of a 6–7-F sheath is recommended. Although, some have described the use of no sheath for interventions requiring only angioplasty [18].

Cervical

Cervical access can be performed in a retrograde or an antegrade fashion. Feldtman et al. describe an antegrade cervical approach by utilizing a small, low cervical incision [21]. The incision is made 2 cm above the sternal head. Then, a 4-mm transverse counter incision is made approximately 1 cm inferior to the vertically placed cervical incision. The common carotid artery is visualized for direct puncture. The puncture should be kept well below the bifurcation. The vagus nerve, which commonly lies posterior to the artery, must be identified and protected. The sheath is advanced 1 cm into the common carotid artery and secured over the patient using an Ioban (3 M, St. Paul, MN). After the removal of the sheath, a stitch can be used to close the arteriotomy in the common carotid artery.

Diethrich et al. describe another technique for direct antegrade cervical access [29]. General anesthesia is recommended due to difficult positioning and patient comfort. The neck should be hyperextended and rotated laterally. The ipsilateral shoulder should

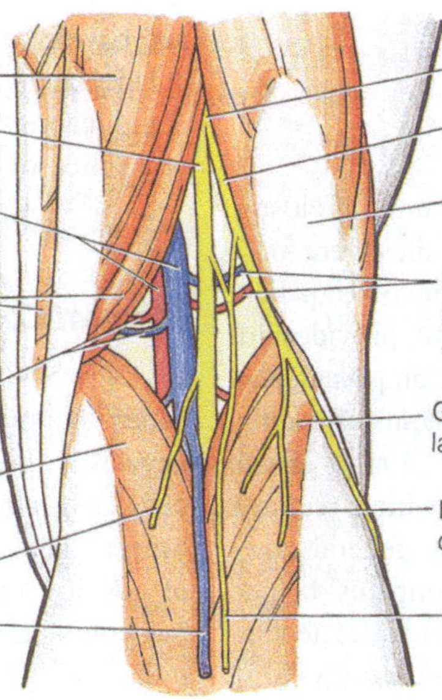

Fig. 31.2 Illustration of the popliteal artery with the posterior–lateral location of the popliteal vein with respect to the popliteal artery. Also, note the close proximity of the tibial nerve to the vascular structures. Reproduced with permission from Moore and Agur [102], copyright owned by Lippincott, Williams and Wilkins

be elevated and the carotid palpated as proximal to the aorta as possible. The needle entry should be 2 cm above the clavicle, just medial to the sternocleidomastoid muscle. An 18-gauge, single-wall entry needle should be advanced until a flash of blood indicates the artery has been accessed. A small contrast bolus can be used to confirm position, and a guidewire can be passed into the external carotid artery. A dilator should be passed prior to the placement of a short sheath. Care should be taken to minimize thrombosis with the use of heparinized saline and systemic heparin. All injections should be meticulously checked for air as possible sources of embolization. Injection should be gentle, given direct access to the cerebral circulation. Lastly, we use half-strength contrast injections to minimize the risk for contrast-induced seizure. After the procedure, an activated clotting time (ACT) should be checked prior to sheath removal.

The technique for a direct cervical retrograde puncture is frequently performed as a hybrid procedure, but it is also possible via a puncture or cutdown approach [30]. It utilizes the same anatomy and equipment. Needle entry should be at the upper third of the cervical carotid [29]. The patient should be systemically heparinized and a sheath is then inserted [20, 30]. After the procedure, the sheath is removed. For a puncture, pressure can be held, and for a cutdown, vascular stitches can be placed for hemostasis.

Closure of the Arteriotomy

Prior to the inception of percutaneous arterial closure devices, small sheath arterial puncture sites were managed with manual compression, which involved patient discomfort and required a health-care provider for compression or the application of a C-clamp, sand bag, or the FemStop (RADI Medical Systems, Reading, MA) until hemostasis was achieved. Large sheath sizes were managed with cutdowns which required a surgeon, an operating room, usually general anesthesia, and scarring [31, 32]. The impetus behind the development of closure devices includes technical requirements, patient comfort, and safety [33]. Closure devices reduce or eliminate the time needed for manual compression and allow earlier ambulation, both of which increase patient satisfaction. In addition, percutaneous devices were also developed to increase efficiency and turnover in response to the growing volume of cardiac catheterizations in the 1990s.

Closure devices were originally developed for the retrograde femoral access site and initially designed to close arteriotomies made by sheath sizes 10 F or smaller. Early devices included the use of procoagulant glues and bioabsorbable sponges, small suture-mediated closure devices, and clip-based systems. Modified techniques, though, have allowed the use of these devices to close sheaths twice that size and have extended their use to include arteries other than the common femoral artery. Devices may be classified according to the mechanism of hemostasis or according to intravascular versus extravascular delivery of closure. Many different closure devices currently exist on the market (Table 31.2). Some of the more popular devices include the Angio-Seal (Kensey-Nash, Exton, PA), the VasoSeal (Datascope, Montvale, NJ), the Duett (Vascular Solutions, Minneapolis, MN), the Closer (Abbott Vascular Devices, Redwood City, CA), the ProGlide (Abbott Vascular Devices, Redwood City, CA), the Prostar XL, the SuperStitch (Sutura, Fountain Valley, CA), the Techstar (Petclose Inc., Redwood City, CA), the StarClose (Abbott Vascular Devices, Redwood City, CA), and the EVS Vascular Closure System (Angiolink Corporation, Taunton, MA). Most investigators have reported experiencing a significant learning curve with the initial use of these devices and have continued to caution that even though a percutaneous approach is utilized, prompt recognition of complications is critical for immediate treatment and prevention of adverse sequelae.

Manual Compression

When comparing manual compression to closure devices, two main factors have been evaluated: efficacy and outcome. Efficacy measurements include time to hemostasis, time to ambulation, and length of hospital stay. In almost all series comparing manual compression to any number of closure devices, it has been found that devices have a shorter time to hemostasis, a quicker time to ambulation, and a shorter hospital stay compared to those undergoing manual compression [34, 35]. Even though devices cost money, there is potentially decreased total cost

Table 31.2 Closure devices and FDA arteriotomy size approval

Device (Manufacturer)	FDA approved size
Seal devices	
Angio-Seal (Kensey-Nash, Exton, PA)	6-8 F
VasoSeal (Datascope, Montvale, NJ)	6-8 F
Duett (Vascular Solutions, Minneapolis, MN)	5-9 F
Matrix Vascular Sealing Gel (Access Closure, Mountain View, CA)	5-7 F
Suture-mediated devices	
Prostar XL (Abbott Vascular Devices, Redwood City, CA)	6-10 F
SuperStitch (Sutura, Fountain Valley, CA)	6-8 F, 12 F in development but not approved
ProGlide (Abbott Vascular Devices, Redwood City, CA)	5-8 F
Clip-based devices	
StarClose (Abbott Vascular Devices, Redwood City, CA)	5-6 F
EVS Closure System (Angiolink Corporation, Taunton, MA)	6-8 F

F: French; FDA: Food and Drug Administration.

when these efficacy endpoints are considered. Less personnel time is required for the closure devices and earlier discharge offers savings to the patient. However, data from the cardiac literature remains variable in regard to outcomes of manual compression compared to closure devices. Gerckens et al. reported decreased vascular complications and reduced time to hemostasis and ambulation with the use of either the Prostar or the Techstar [36]. With the use of these suturing devices, when compared to manual compression, the incidence of vascular complication was 5.7% vs. 11.3%. Applegate et al. showed that, in patients receiving IIb/IIIa inhibitors, no increased risk of major complications (death, surgery, occlusion, bleed, loss of pulse) was observed with Angio-Seal or Perclose compared to manual compression [37]. However, these reports have been contradicted by additional studies. Kahn reported higher minor and major complications using the Prostar Plus device compared to manual compression [38]. These complications included pseudoaneurysm 2.7%, hematoma 9.8%, and need for surgical intervention 0.67%. Two large meta-analyses have been published and reported that the use of closure devices, including Angio-Seal, VasoSeal, and Prostar Plus, may not improve outcome [34, 36]. One consisted of 4,000 patients from 30 randomized, controlled trials and concluded that closure devices were only marginally effective and may have increased hematoma and pseudoaneurysm rates [34]. A larger meta-analysis that included a review of a total of 37,066 patients revealed no difference in risk of access site-related complications between manual and device groups, but in general favored manual compression [39]. Most of the studies included demonstrated reduced time to hemostasis and ambulation with the use of closure devices, but there was a wide range of failure rates amongst the device groups (up to 20%). Regardless, closure devices are currently used in approximately 50% of cardiac catheterization procedures performed annually, not to mention their use in many other endovascular interventions, and they have generally shown efficacy rates greater than 90% [34]. Therefore, it is important to be familiar with these devices, their limitations, and complications because even though many different specialists deploy these devices during procedures, complications can be severe and require further interventions.

With respect to manual compression, there have been no randomized controlled trials delineating exactly how large an arteriotomy can successfully achieve hemostasis by manual compression alone. Quinn et al. hypothesized that manual compression is feasible and safe for arteriotomies 12 F or less in non-obese patients with a normal coagulation profile [40]. Shawl et al. reported using manual compression for 107 patients undergoing percutaneous cardiopulmonary bypass using 20 F and 18 F sheath sizes [41]. Of the first 41 patients who received a 20-F sheath, the sheath was removed immediately following the procedure, regardless of the ACT, and manual compression was performed followed by the application of an external clamp for 13 h. The complication rate was 9.8%, and 34% of the patients required postoperative blood transfusions. In the second group of patients ($n = 66$) that underwent placement of an 18-F sheath, the sheath was removed once the ACT was less than 240 s followed by manual compression and clamp application. In this group, the complication rate was only 1.5%, and 9% of these patients required transfusions. While these results suggest that manual compression is possible with larger sheath sizes, it is clear that one must be diligent with respect to the technique and the anticoagulation status of the patient.

Seal and Plug Devices

Utilization of the coagulation cascade is the main mechanistic strategy behind these biologic seals and plugs. The most popular devices on the market include Angio-Seal, VasoSeal, and Duett. Others include Matrix Vascular Sealing Gel (Access Closure, Mountain View, CA), DISC-Close-Sure (Biointerventional Corp., Pleasanton, CA), DISC-Close-Sure+ (Biointerventional Corp., Pleasanton, CA), and Scio Clo-Sur PAD (Scion Cardio-Vascular, Miami, FL) [33]. The Matrix Vascular Sealing Gel uses collagen to promote rapid formation of a thrombotic plug. The DISC-Close-Sure deploys an intraluminal impermeable disk to occlude the puncture. The next generation, the DISC-Close-Sure+, adds the delivery of hemostatic agent to the puncture site as well. The Scio Clo-Sur PAD incorporates a naturally occurring biopolymer polyproleate acetate and this chain of positive charges yields pro-coagulant properties [33]. Below are pros, cons, sheath sizes, technical considerations, and potential complications of the Angio-Seal, VasoSeal, and Duett seal systems. In a meta-analysis by Koreny et al., no difference in subgroup analysis was found between Angio-Seal, VasoSeal, Duett, and Perclose in terms of safety and efficacy [34].

The Angio-Seal uses collagen to promote rapid formation of a thrombotic plug (Fig. 31.3a). It is a true mechanical plug with three components: a footplate, a collagen plug, and a suture [33]. It is an intravascular device that uses an intraluminal anchor. Advantages to this device include the need for only one operator, ease of deployment, no need for manual compression, and a secure plug-based system [33]. A major drawback to this system is the inability to re-puncture this site for several weeks. Other disadvantages include a 3-h ambulation delay and enlargement of puncture hole with deployment [33]. Intraluminal anchors can be problematic due to complications of

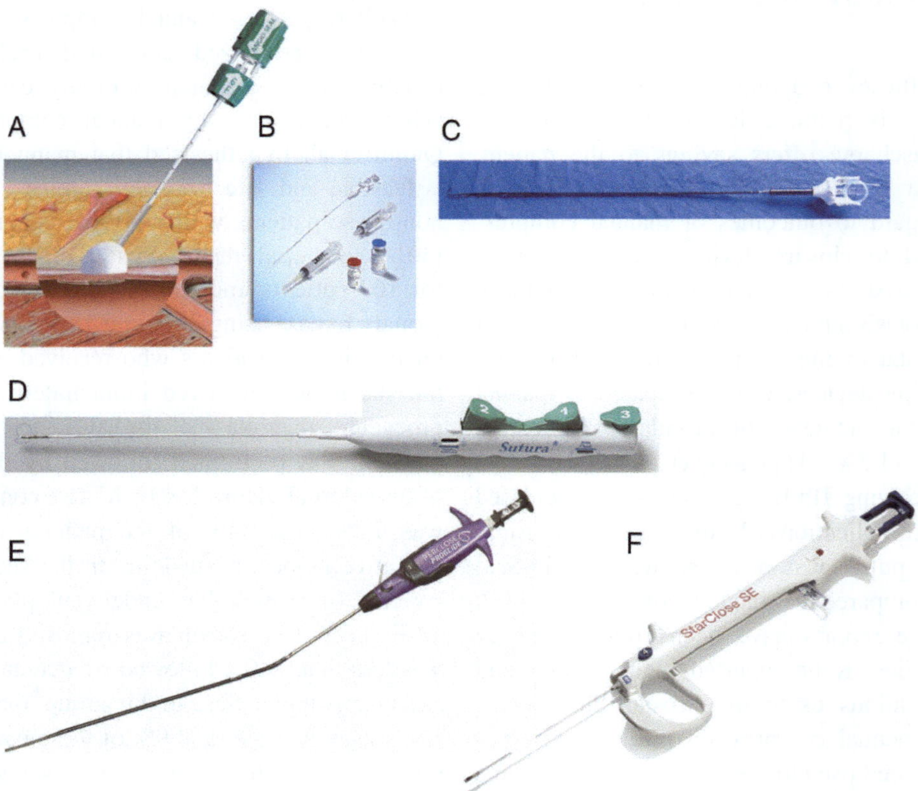

Fig. 31.3 **a**, Angio-Seal, seal device; **b**, Duett, seal device; **c**, Prostar XL, suture-mediated device; **d**, SuperStitch, suture-mediated device; **e**, Proglide, suture-mediated device; and **f**, StarClose, clip-based device. Reproduced with permissions from St. Jude Medical Inc, Vascular Solutions Inc., Abbott Vascular Inc. (© 2008 Abbott Laboratories. All rights reserved) and Sutura, Inc

dissection, thrombosis, and embolization. Major complications are rare (<1%) but can be catastrophic. They consist of the need for vascular surgery, major bleeding with transfusions, retroperitoneal hematoma, thrombosis or loss of pulses, groin infections, groin hematoma, and death [42]. Kussmaul et al. conducted a randomized controlled trial and showed that Angio-Seal had a decreased time to hemostasis and successful deployment 96% of the time [43]. No difference in pseudoaneurysm formation was noted when compared to manual compression. Heparin was associated with a higher complication rate in the manual compression arm but had no effect on the device group [43]. Several other reports exist in the literature with cohorts between 20 and almost 2,000. Deployment success ranged from 88 to 100% and total complications ranged from 0.49 to 23% [33]. Eggebrecht et al. reported on 1,317 patients closed with the Angio-Seal [42]. They found that predictors of access complications include female gender, even though females received less heparin than did males [42]. Also, giving IIb/IIIa inhibitors increased time to hemostasis. In their report, five patients required surgery for complications. Most sheath sizes were 8 F but some utilized 9–11-F sheaths. In these patients, deployment success was 83% compared to 96.3% when an 8-F sheath was used. They suggested that the learning curve consists of a specialist's first 50 cases and that it is also a predictor of deployment failure [42].

VasoSeal also uses collagen to promote rapid formation of a thrombotic plug. The device inserts a bovine collagen sponge into the soft tissue tract over the puncture. The VasoSeal is easy to learn, can seal diseased and calcified arteries, allows for early re-puncture, and is easy to convert to manual compression [33]. It is an extravascular delivery system even though deployed through a sheath. This prevents complications like dissection and embolization, but the VasoSeal upsizes the subcutaneous track to 11.5 F. Further disadvantages include high failure rates in obese patients and 1–3 h ambulation delays. Also, to properly deploy the device, inflow occlusion is needed and can be accomplished by proximal arterial compression at the time of deployment [33]. This requires two people. Bos et al. performed a meta-analysis to assess the efficacy and cost of the VasoSeal compared to manual compression [44]. They found a decrease in patient complications requiring treatment with the use of the VasoSeal: 16:1,000 patients compared to 31:1,000 in the manual compression group. In terms of cost of the procedure, the VasoSeal was more expensive than manual compression: $177 versus $42. However, use of the device is cost-effective if complications are averted at a cost of $9,000 per puncture site or if such a device truly reduces hospital stay by at least 1 day [44].

The Duett closure device uses collagen to promote rapid formation of a thrombotic plug (Fig. 31.3b). It does not enlarge the arteriotomy and requires only one operator, but temporary balloon occlusion of the artery is necessary. This requires an intravascular component, the balloon, as well as the extravascular injection of collagen/thrombin through a side port of the sheath. Like the VasoSeal, the Duett allows for simple conversion to manual compression and immediate re-puncture, but it should not be used in diseased vessels. A European multicenter registry was established to evaluate the safety and procedural success of the Duett sealing device in a broad range of patients undergoing diagnostic or interventional endovascular procedures [45]. Standard sheath size was 5–9 F, patients were required to have an ACT $\leq$400 s, and the use of glycoprotein IIb/IIIa platelet receptor antagonist was permitted. Deployment success was achieved in 96.2% of patients with complete hemostasis within 2–5 min in over 95% of the patients. The complication-free rate was 96.4%. Complications included arterial occlusions (4 patients), pseudoaneurysm (34 patients), and major complications were 2.6% (41 of 1,587 patients). These results demonstrate that the Duett sealing device can be used with a high procedural success following diagnostic and interventional endovascular procedures.

Suture-Mediated Devices

On the market, the main suture-mediated devices include Prostar XL, Proglide, and SuperStitch. These devices are designed for sheaths between 5 and 10 F but have been used off-label to close larger arteriotomies. The technical applications of these devices can be difficult and can require a long learning curve. The original sheath has to be exchanged for the closure device, which can enlarge the subcutaneous track up to 21 F depending on the device used. Patients in a study by Carere et al. reported less pain during suture closure compared with mechanical compression using a

C-clamp based on surveys and questionnaires [46]. One benefit of suture-mediated devices is their potential use in procedures which require a larger sheath size. Of the different mechanisms of action of the arterial closure devices, including the bioabsorbable sponges, collagen plugs, fibrin and thrombin glues, clip closure, and suture-mediated devices, only the suture-mediated devices can be used off-label safely and effectively in conjunction with larger sheath sizes [47].

The Prostar XL is a suture-mediated device deploying two sutures and is available for up to 10-F sheath applications (Fig. 31.3c). This device does not need compression and allows for immediate ambulation, but a steep learning curve exists, along with an increased technical failure compared to the biomaterial seals. The device consists of a hydrophilic J-shaped sheath which contains two pairs of sutured needles, a needle guide which precisely controls the needles around the puncture site, a rotating barrel, and a marker lumen. The marker lumen exits from the hub of the device proximally and allows a pathway for pulsatile back bleeding from the femoral artery that ensures proper device positioning within the artery. The needle delivery system's handle is connected to two sets of needles attached to braided sutures.

The Preclose technique using the Prostar XL for closing large arteriotomies has previously been described in detail by our group [47]. The technique is largely the same with some variations between institutions. Our group utilized one 10-F Prostar device with the Knot Pusher but without the use of the Arterial Tamper. Other institutions routinely use two Prostar XL devices, an 8-F and a 10-F or two 10-F devices, in order to deploy four sutures instead of two [40, 48–52]. For example, Quinn et al. reports using two devices for all sheath sizes greater than 12 F but only one device for sheath sizes 12 F or smaller [40]. The second device is rotated to varying degrees (25–90°) to allow for altering locations of suture positioning. Complication rates in the single device group range from 0 to 6.7% with success rates of 93–100% [31, 53–56]. The ranges are larger in the two-device group with complications occurring in 0–12.7% and success rates of 66–100% [40, 48–52, 57]. Potential problems exist when using two devices. The needles of the second device can pierce the sutures of the first causing deflection, suture breakage, or inability to capture in the barrel. Too many threads can cause entanglement with other sutures and disrupt the vessel wall [40]. These devices are also costly and increase the price of the procedure [24].

Starnes et al. performed a literature review on the Prostar XL closure for EVAR procedures [54]. This included 483 patients, 728 total sites, and sheath sizes from 12 to 25 F. The review revealed an overall technical success rate ranging from 66 to 100%, with a mean of 90%. Complication rates varied from 0 to 12.7%, and conversion rates varied from 0 to 35%. The wide range in success, complication, and conversion rates appears to be related in part to the experience of the user. Proper instrument deployment is often influenced by operator error as well as patient selection. During each step of the Preclose technique, there is a possibility of failure or complication. Recognition of this is imperative to successful deployment.

In trials evaluating closure devices during cardiac catheterizations, patients with peripheral vascular disease were first excluded. There have since been studies looking at this patient population. Mackrell et al. reported the use of Prostar and Closer devices in 500 patients with peripheral vascular disease (ankle-brachial index <0.8) undergoing either diagnostic angiography or intervention [58]. Overall success of the closure device was 95% with a 1.4% complication rate. Complications included bleeding, limb ischemia, and pseudoaneurysm formation. Overall, this study demonstrated that closure devices for small sheath sizes can be safely used in this patient population.

SuperStitch is a suture-mediated device that is indicated for 6–8-F sheaths, but has a 12-F device currently in development (Fig. 31.3d). It is safe and effective allowing for immediate closure and initial results show that it is quick, easy to use, and can be deployed through the existing femoral puncture. It applies one non-absorbable surgical suture. The device also contains two suture-carrying arms, a plunger handle, and two needles. The proper deployment of this device has previously been described in detail [59]. It is placed at the end of the procedure without wire guidance through the sheath. The first report of the device's clinical feasibility was by Eggebrecht et al. [59]. Their cohort exclusion criteria were the following: <18 years old, pre-existing hematoma, multiple puncture attempts on the artery, and PVD [59]. They reported a 92% deployment success. The SuperStitch application took 91±33 s and achieved 77% immediate hemostasis

[59]. Manual pressure was held if immediate hemostasis was not achieved and 92% of patients achieved hemostasis at 2 min and 97.5% at 10 min [59]. In this study, 150 patients underwent deployment of the device. There was one fatality from rapid hemorrhagic shock despite emergency vascular surgery. Other complications included groin pain during the procedure (12%), late bleed (4.7%), and groin hematoma (4%). Also, infection was observed in between 0.3 and 1.1% of patients, which can potentially cause extensive morbidity [59].

The Perclose Proglide is another suture-mediated closure device which was designed for 5–8-F sheath closures (Fig. 31.3e). It deploys a single 3-0 polypropylene suture using a pair of nitinol needles. It is commonly used for a variety of peripheral and coronary interventions. A randomized controlled trial was conducted by Martin et al. comparing the Proglide, the Angio-Seal, and manual compression following coronary interventions (CAP Trial) [60]. There were no differences in vascular complications between these three groups. Time to hemostasis and ambulation was longest in the manual compression group. The Proglide group had more deployment failures, a longer time to ambulation, and a longer time to hemostasis compared to the Angio-Seal group [60].

The Preclose technique has also been described utilizing deployment of two 6-F Proglide devices angled 90° to one another prior to the insertion of larger sheaths for aortic procedures [61]. Lee et al. report a technical success of 91.4% for sheath sizes 18–24 F and 99.0% for sheath sizes 12–16 F, for an overall success of 94.3% [61]. Failures were mainly attributable to obesity, device malfunction, severe calcific disease, and faulty arterial punctures. Short-term complications (not counting device deployment failures) included bleeding, dissection, and pseudoaneurysm formation. All of these complications required intervention to avoid sequelae of hemorrhage and limb threat. This original series had two cases of severe retroperitoneal bleed requiring emergent deployment of a covered stent. One infectious complication of a mycotic pseudoaneurysm on post-operative day 27 was reported and necessitated replacement of the common femoral artery with autologous vein. No access-related mortality was observed. Lee et al. also report their midterm results with the Proglide Preclose technique on 100 patients totaling 156 femoral arteries [62]. Using CT angiograms they identified three (1.92%) late complications in three patients: one asymptomatic femoral dissection and two femoral artery pseudoaneurysms [62]. The former patient had no symptoms and stable scans, thus no intervention was necessary. The latter patients required surgical repair. One of these pseudoaneurysms was precipitated by a draining sinus from the wound, subsequent wound infection, and femoral artery thrombosis. Another group has reported a small series using the same technique [63]. They report an 81% primary success rate but had only 17 patients in their series.

Clip-Based Devices

Clip-based hemostatic devices offer another method for closing arteriotomies after vascular procedures. The clip-based system should have minimal risk of post-closure luminal obstruction, and since delivery is extravascular, it avoids risk of dissection, thrombosis, and embolization. The main device on the market is the StarClose. Another system is the EVS Vascular Closure System. This is a purse-string staple closure utilizing a staple made from titanium alloy. While it is FDA approved for 6–8 F sheath sizes, its use has been reported for larger sheath sizes up to 20 F [33].

The StarClose device provides circumferential, extravascular closure of the femoral puncture site by delivering a small and flexible nitinol clip (Fig. 31.3f). It is approved for sheath sizes ranging from 5 to 6 F [64]. Exclusion criteria proposed for this device are artery diameter <5 mm, punctures at or distal to the bifurcation of superficial and profunda femoral arteries, and punctures created in areas of calcified plaque [64]. Some studies list obesity and calcification as exclusion criteria for closure devices, but these patients are included in some StarClose patient series [64]. Imam et al., however, did report difficulty in extracting the clip applier in four cases of severely calcified arteries [64]. An extra sheath exchange step is still necessary before deployment of the StarClose permanent external clip; therefore, the same risk of infection and scarring exists with the current closure device [64]. Manual compression can be used if deployment of the device is unsuccessful. The device has been successfully deployed with good outcomes in the face of anticoagulation with aspirin, Plavix, and IIb/IIIa inhibitors [65]. No data exists regarding re-puncture after product deployment [64]. One study performed a sub-group analysis on patients undergoing closure, StarClose, after an artery had been previously accessed the week before; however, none of the initial access had been closed by deploying the StarClose [65]. In this cohort, 24% of patients were undergoing repeat punctures, and no difference in this sub-group analysis was observed compared to patients who were having the artery accessed for the first time. They did, however, require 12 h bed rest because this use was new [65].

The Closure in Percutaneous Procedures (CLIP) study indicates that the StarClose device is similar to manual compression in regard to the primary safety endpoint for both diagnostic and therapeutic interventions, but the median time to hemostasis was 16.8 s versus 15 min with manual compression [65, 66]. There has been a prospective, non-randomized trial comparing the StarClose with the Angio-Seal. Ratnam et al. showed an increased need for manual compression after initial success in achieving hemostasis by StarClose device compared to Angio-Seal [67]. They also showed an increased risk of major puncture site complications in women with PVD. In one review, device success was reported between 86.8 and 94.1%, and major complications ranged from 0 to 1.9% [65]. Major complications include large hematoma, hemorrhage requiring transfusion, surgery, pseudoaneurysm, arteriovenous fistula, distal embolization, groin infection, and death [64]. Fantoni et al. reported on 30 patients undergoing StarClose deployment for antegrade femoral puncture [68]. They experienced 100% delivery success. The device had an approximate delivery time of 1 min, a hemostasis time of 21 ± 19 s, and an ACT of 226 ± 37 s [68]. They immobilized patients for 6 h and had no major vascular complication immediately or within 30 days [68]. A group of interventional radiologists reported a 96% successful deployment rate, an average of 48 s deployments, and no major complications with the use of the StarClose [64]. Minor complications included 8% small hematoma, 3% mild oozing, 8% groin ache [64]. There has been a report of device misplacement with subsequent vascular stenosis and need for surgical removal and plastic reconstruction [69]. These cases are rare, and, from the reports published, the StarClose has high technical success and good clinical efficacy [64]. No long-term complications after the use of the StarClose have been reported, but Tay et al. advocate close observation because of the potential for recurrent bleeding, especially in patients with partial device success [65].

Complications

Access site complications are essentially the same regardless of puncture site. They include bleeding, hematomas, pseudoaneurysm, arteriovenous fistula, arterial dissection, arterial thrombosis, plaque embolization, and infection. However, each of these complications can have different effects on morbidity and mortality depending on the access site and the size of the arteriotomy. Also, if closure devices have been utilized, some have unique sets of complications specific to the delivery mechanism of the device. The key is that practitioners maintain a high index of suspicion to look for potential complications when the patient has symptoms. Also, prompt action on troubleshooting these complications is mandatory, especially if it requires emergent surgery to correct potentially fatal hemorrhage.

Femoral

The common femoral artery is the most common access site and it is the most common site of device deployment. General principles introduced here apply to each of the other access sites as well. Complications have well-described risk factors and can be classified as early or late. Subsequently, early and late vascular access site complications will be delineated. Also, device-specific complications exist. Some of these have been described in the previous section, and others will be outlined below. Additionally, complications of the common femoral artery access site, and all other access sites, can be due to location alone.

Several risk factors have been delineated for predicting access site complications (Table 31.3). In a single-center experience of access site complications, Applegate et al. showed that female gender was the strongest independent predictor of any vascular complication after cardiac catheterization or coronary intervention [70]. They also observed that the incidence of vascular complications in women decreased

Table 31.3 Risk factors for femoral access site complications

Female gender
Overweight
Underweight
Older age
Uncontrolled hypertension
Previous access at same site
Peripheral vascular disease
High level of anticoagulation
Larger sheaths
Renal failure
Device failure
Concomitant venous sheath
Prolonged sheath duration
Location of arteriotomy

over the course of the study, likely attributable to use of smaller sheaths and fewer closure devices over the course of the study [70]. It is likely that the increased trend toward vascular complications may be from intrinsic biologic factors in addition to a relative increase in the distribution of adverse covariates.

In general, complications include bleeding, acute arterial thrombosis, arterial embolization, arterial dissection, aneurysm, arteriovenous fistula, pseudoaneurysm, and injury to local structures [71]. Of these complications, the most commonly encountered early complication is bleeding, which can range from a minor hematoma to a large retroperitoneal hemorrhage resulting in death. Two deaths from cardiac arrests secondary to hypovolemic shock have been reported with the Prostar XL and one previously mentioned with the SuperStitch [49, 54, 59]. Vascular injuries ranging from arterial dissection, thrombosis, and embolization of either pre-existing plaque or peri-sheath thrombus have been observed and can be limb threatening. As long as these early bleeding and vascular injury complications are recognized at the time of the procedure or immediately thereafter, and repair is initiated promptly, overall outcome can be good. Minor and often self-limited complications of nerve entrapment or irritation causing persistent pain at the arteriotomy site or nervus ilioinguinalis, or paresthesias and numbness in the groin area, have also been described [36, 72].

Late complications include arterial stenosis, wound infection, suture infection, and pseudoaneurysm formation. Of the late complications, in the suture-mediated group, infection of the sutures can lead to a devastating outcome if not recognized early and treated. A variety of infectious complications have been reported, including cellulitis, abscess formation, necrotizing fasciitis, infectious arteritis, mycotic pseudoaneurysm, septic emboli, and *methicillin-resistant Staphylococcus aureus* sepsis resulting in death [73, 74]. These can result from pre-existing infectious sources, secondary infection of a foreign body (i.e., suture), or from improper sterile technique at the time of deployment. However, a study specifically performed to look at infectious complications after the use of suture-mediated devices failed to note any relationship between infection and diabetes, obesity, or anticoagulation [74].

In determining whether an artery is suitable for use with a percutaneous arterial closure device, several factors are important. Potential pre-procedural patient exclusion categories include obesity, small arteries, prior groin surgery, prior use of a closure device, the presence of significant arterial calcifications, a common femoral artery aneurysm, arterial tortuosity, and arterial occlusive disease [31, 49, 50, 54, 75]. These risk factors have been hypothesized to exhibit an increased risk of complications and in some studies have been shown to have decreased success rates [49, 50, 54]. The concerns of using a device in these patients are due to (1) increased resistance and inadequate final positioning of the deployed sutures secondary to scar tissue; (2) embolization of calcifications; (3) arterial dissection from manipulating the device in a tortuous vessel; (4) device needle deflection secondary to calcifications; (5) arterial narrowing following closure in small arteries; and (6) increased overall device failure in the face of obesity and aneurysmal tissue [31, 49, 50, 54, 55, 75]. Applegate et al. reported on over 21,000 patients undergoing common femoral artery closure using manual compression, Angio-Seal, VasoSeal, Quikseal, Duett, and Perclose devices [76]. Reported complications across the groups were low: major 0.76% and minor 0.86–1.07%.

Specific to the common femoral artery, location of the needle entry and thus arteriotomy is critical for subsequent complications. A high puncture does not allow for effective compression due to inguinal ligament interference. This leads to retroperitoneal bleeding and pseudoaneurysm formation. A low puncture may have higher complication rates from dissection, thrombosis, and embolization due to the puncture of the superficial femoral artery, the profunda femoral artery, or at the bifurcation [5]. Sherev et al. looked at angiographic consideration of femoral access site complications [71]. They broke up the anatomy into four zones: (1) distal to superficial and femoral artery bifurcation, (2) common femoral artery proximal to bifurcation but below lower most part of inferior epigastric artery, (3) from lower most curve of epigastric artery to ostium of inferior epigastric artery, and (4) external iliac artery [71]. They found that most complications occurred in zones 1, 3, and 4 and that all retroperitoneal hemorrhages occurred in zones 3 and 4. Complications in group 2, the desired location for access, were exclusively hematomas [71].

Brachial

Overall complication rates for diagnostic or therapeutic angiographic procedures utilizing the brachial artery for access range between 1 and 25% [9, 77–79]. The risk of complication is increased with the use of anticoagulation or larger sheath size and includes failed access in addition to both minor and major complications of the procedure. Success rates for brachial artery canalization range from 90 to 100% of attempts [9, 80–83]. Reasons for failure include multiple prior punctures in the antecubital fossa, spasm of the brachial artery resulting in temporary loss of pulse, as well as small artery size. In most cases, however, the use of the opposite brachial artery after failure to canalize resulted in success leading to an ultimate failure rate of between 0.5 and 1.5% [80, 82]. Additional complications reported include brachial artery thrombosis, brachial artery pseudoaneurysm formation, bleeding complications resulting in ecchymoses and/or hematoma, and finally neurologic complications ranging from local pain or paresthesia to transient ischemic attack.

Complications which potentially require subsequent surgical intervention are classified as major and include brachial artery thrombosis and pseudoaneurysm formation. The incidence of brachial artery thrombosis ranges between 0.5 and 6% of brachial artery punctures [77–79, 84, 85]. The incidence may vary with the type of procedure and with artery size. In a series with patients undergoing both diagnostic and therapeutic procedures for peripheral arterial interventions, the incidence of brachial artery thrombosis was reported to be 0.5–1.2% [9, 80, 82]. Armstrong et al. also found an increased risk of thrombosis in women [9]. In a series of 1,326 angiograms via brachial access in peripheral vascular disease patients, women had a significantly higher incidence of brachial artery thrombosis and failed access ($p < 0.001$). The authors felt this increased risk may be related to the smaller average brachial artery size found in women and pointed to similar findings by Rath et al. in a smaller series of patients. In this series, two patients developed thrombosis of the brachial artery. Both of these patients were women and duplex scans demonstrated that the arterial size of both patients was in the lowest 10th percentile of the series [85]. The authors recommended considering routine imaging of the brachial artery to determine appropriate candidates for brachial access. In general, most patients who presented with brachial artery thrombosis present early in the post-operative course and were treated successfully with surgical thrombectomy. There were no instances of tissue loss or amputation in these series [9, 77–80, 82, 84, 85].

Brachial artery pseudoaneurysm is another complication which frequently requires surgical intervention for repair. Although relatively uncommon, pseudoaneurysm of the brachial artery still occurs with more frequency when compared to pseudoaneurysm development following femoral artery puncture (0.3–2.7% vs. 0.05–0.5%) [9, 82, 86–88]. Most patients require surgical intervention but additional treatment options included ultrasound-guided compression or injection of thrombin [9, 82]. Although there have been reports of success with these alternative treatments, the latter is associated with a higher risk of subsequent thrombosis as seen in a series by Kang et al. in which one out of the five patients with brachial artery pseudoaneurysm treated with thrombin injection developed thrombosis [89]. However, the thrombosis did resolve spontaneously and overall they had excellent results with a low recurrence.

Although some minor complications do occasionally require further intervention, most resolve with observation and without significant sequelae. These minor complications consisted of minor bleeding such as hematoma and ecchymoses and neurologic symptoms like paresthesias and pain. Although there are instances in which larger hematomas resulting in compression of the brachial artery or the median nerve require intervention, surgical drainage is not necessary in most cases. In a series by Gritter et al.,

9.5% of patients developed a hematoma but only 0.15% of these required surgical drainage [80]. Other series report between 2 and 16.7% incidence of hematoma, none of which required drainage [83, 86, 87]. Ecchymoses were not always reported as complications in every series but when mentioned, they appeared to be common (between 13 and 50% of patients) but minor in severity [80, 82]. Most neurologic sequelae reported consist of pain or paresthesias in up to 8% of patients, all of which resolved spontaneously. More importantly, using the brachial artery for access potentially poses a higher risk for stroke or transient ischemic attack (TIA), secondary thromboembolic events via the carotid (depending on the side) or the vertebral artery. Armstrong et al. reported an incidence of TIA of 0.075% in 1,326 angiograms. A TIA also occurred in one out of 37 interventions by Ernst et al. when trying to negotiate the proximal anastomosis of a prior bypass graft [9, 86]. No reports of stroke were noted in these series.

Radial

The radial approach is associated with decreased complication rates when compared to access via the femoral artery. In a meta-analysis by Agostoni et al. comparing coronary procedures using either radial or femoral access, entry site complications were significantly lower in the radial group (0.3% vs. 2.8%, $p < 0.0001$) [13]. The lower complication rate associated with radial access is in part due to the anatomy of the radial artery which has excellent collateralization in most patients and is not in close proximity to any major nerves or veins. As a result, when complications occur, they are not often associated with significant sequelae. Bleeding complications including hematoma and pseudoaneurysm formation are rare and thrombosis of the radial artery is not considered a major event. In two series by Kiemeneij et al. and Goldberg et al., the incidence of radial artery thrombosis was between 5 and 7% and none of the patients had associated ischemic complications [87, 90]. There are limitations of this approach, however, which include a steep learning curve for obtaining access to the radial artery and the smaller caliber of the artery which limits sheath size and makes the vessel prone to spasm. As a result, despite the wide range of success and limited complications, approximately 1 in 14 patients will still require conversion to another approach due to these technical challenges [13].

Axillary

Overall complication rates for the use of the axillary artery have been reported as high as 27% in a series by AbuRhama et al., with the incidence of nervous system and brachial plexus injury at 11 and 13%, respectively, although rates in several other series were significantly lower, between 0.6 and 2.8% [91–94]. Complications at the axillary access site are principally caused by bleeding. Holding compression after a procedure is particularly difficult at this site due to the anatomy of the axilla. Hematomas in this area can lead to brachial nerve compression. Injury to the brachial plexus occurs after hematoma or pseudoaneurysm formation within the medial brachial fascial compartment, resulting in the compression of the adjacent nerves of the brachial plexus, most commonly the median nerve [26, 95]. This medial brachial fascial syndrome has been described in the literature and may be under-diagnosed since both motor and sensory symptoms may be delayed [92, 94, 95]. In addition, the hematoma after axillary puncture may not be obvious on clinical examination since symptoms can occur with relatively small hematomas. In a series by Chitwood et al., of 842 transaxillary procedures, only 71% of the patients with nerve injury had readily identifiable hematomas on exam [26]. Patients who were treated with urgent exploration on the basis of symptoms were more than eight times more likely to have resolution of deficit when compared to patients treated with delayed exploration [26]. Thus, a high index of suspicion for complications is necessary when performing these procedures.

Popliteal

At the popliteal access site, the average complication rates for these procedures vary between 4 and 7.5% [19, 96–98]. Although complications such as hematoma, thrombosis, and pseudoaneurysm are reported [19, 96–98], the most serious and specific complication of the use of the popliteal artery is development of arteriovenous fistula with an incidence rate between 6 and 14% [96, 99–101]. Methods to prevent the development of arteriovenous fistula involve various imaging techniques to guide needle placement such as fluoroscopy, ultrasound, and Doppler. Although fluoroscopy provides accurate localization of the artery, it requires a second access site for an angiogram and then requires subsequent repositioning of the patient for popliteal access. Yilmaz et al. performed retrograde popliteal artery catheterization on 174 patients using ultrasound guidance without development of arteriovenous fistula [19]. The authors noted that ultrasound is readily available at many institutions, provides real-time guidance for puncture, and does not necessitate a second puncture site for angiogram. Kluge et al. also demonstrated improved incidence of arteriovenous fistula with the use of the Doppler-equipped SMART needle [96]. They reported a 1.7% incidence of arteriovenous fistula, which is significantly decreased from the previously reported range of 6–14%. However, 3.4% of their initially planned transpopliteal interventions had to be aborted because the arterial and venous signals could not be differentiated. An additional limitation of the retrograde popliteal approach is the inability to treat distal embolic events at the time of the procedure [19]. In addition, the use of the popliteal artery may worsen ischemia by compromising collaterals or through occlusion of the popliteal segment distal to collateralization. However, it should be considered as an option since many of the patients reported in these series were not candidates for alternate access or open bypass and, therefore, would have required amputation as an alternative to the transpopliteal procedure performed.

Cervical

There is a paucity of information addressing complications of cervical access. Complications through this access site can be related to the access site itself in addition to the procedure. The same types of complications can occur: hematoma, dissection, thrombosis, embolization, pseudoaneurysm, and arteriovenous fistulas. Given the proximity of the cerebral circulation, these complications can be devastating since they can manifest as a stroke. Hematoma is the most common complication seen. Given close proximity to the trachea and the risk of airway obstruction, this could potentially be fatal.

Conclusion

As technology progresses, more types of procedures are being performed endovascularly. Many factors should be considered when developing a technical strategy for these procedures. The decision of where and how to access the artery is as important as determining what stent to use or where to land a device. Factors to consider include location of the access, anatomic considerations relating to the patient's arterial anatomy and body habitus, techniques on puncturing the artery to avoid undue trauma or complications, and decisions on how to achieve hemostasis at the end of the procedure. Sheath sizes and proficiency of deploying arterial closure devices play a critical role in determining the method of hemostasis. Although, in general, these procedures have relatively low complication rates, most of the complications occur at the site of access. These complications can be as mild as pain at the puncture site or as severe as death from retroperitoneal hemorrhage. Diligence in monitoring the patient post-procedure and knowledge of the signs and symptoms of common complications per access site or device used are essential for any endovascular specialist, regardless of their specialty or the actual procedure being performed.

References

1. Rosamond W, Flegal K, Friday G et al.: Heart disease and stroke statistics—2007 update: a report from the American heart association statistics committee and stroke statistics subcommittee, *Circulation* 115(5): e69–e171, February 6, 2007.
2. Myles O, Thomas WJ, Daniels JT, Aronson N: Infected endovascular stents managed with medical therapy alone, *Catheter Cardiovasc Interv* 51(4):471–476, December 2000.
3. Dworkin LD, Jamerson KA: Case against angioplasty and stenting of atherosclerotic renal artery stenosis, *Circulation* 115(2):271–276, January 16, 2007.
4. Dauterman K, Casserly IP, Bajzer CJ, General A, Interventional P: In Casserly I, Sachar R, Yadav J, editors: *Manual of peripheral vascular interventions*,

Philadelphia, 2005, Lippincott Williams and Wilkens, pp. 39–45.
5. Ledesma DF, Domer GS, Criado Frank J: Techniques of arterial access for endovascular intervention. In Heuser RR, Henry M, editors: *Textbook of peripheral vascular interventions*, New York, 2004, MD Martin Dunitz Taylor and Francis Group, pp. 79–85.
6. Andros G, Arterial A In Moore WS, Ahn SS, editors: *Endovascular Surgery*, ed. 3, Philadelphia, 2001, W.B. Saunders Company, pp. 37–47.
7. Gengler L, Rodde A: Transbrachial and transaxillary approach: indications, techniques, pitfalls, and complications. In Heuser RR, Henry M, editors: *Textbook of peripheral vascular interventions*, New York, 2004, MD Martin Dunitz Taylor and Francis Group, pp. 87–91.
8. Criado FJ, Wilson EP Abul-Khoudoud O, Barker C, Carpenter J, Fairman R: Brachial artery catheterization to facilitate endovascular grafting of abdominal aortic aneurysm: safety and rationale, *J Vasc Surg* 32(6): 1137–1141, December 2000.
9. Armstrong PJ, Han DC, Baxter JA, Elmore JR, Franklin DP: Complication rates of percutaneous brachial artery access in peripheral vascular angiography, *Ann Vasc Surg* 17(1):107–110, January 2003.
10. Folmar J, Sachar R, Mann T: Transradial approach for carotid artery stenting: a feasibility study, *Catheter Cardiovasc Interv* 69(3):355–361, February 15, 2007.
11. Yamashita T, Imai S, Tamada T et al.: Transradial approach for noncoronary angiography and interventions, *Catheter Cardiovasc Interv* 70(2):303–308, August 1, 2007.
12. Henry I, Henry M, Transradial A In Heuser R, Henry M, editors: *Textbook of Peripheral Vascular Interventions*, New York, 2004, MD Martin Dunitz Taylor and Francis Group, pp. 93–5.
13. Agostoni P, Biondi-Zoccai GG, De Benedictis ML et al.: Radial versus femoral approach for percutaneous coronary diagnostic and interventional procedures; systematic overview and meta-analysis of randomized trials, *J Am Coll Cardiol* 44(2):349–356, July 21, 2004.
14. Gilchrist IC, Moyer CD, Gascho JA: Transradial right and left heart catheterizations: a comparison to traditional femoral approach, *Catheter Cardiovasc Interv* 67(4): 585–588, April 2006.
15. Inglese L, Lupattelli T, Carbone GL et al.: Axillary artery access for interventional procedures, *J Endovasc Ther* 11(4):414–418, August 2004.
16. Henry M: Popliteal access site. In Hauser RR, Henry M, editors: *Textbook of peripheral vascular interventions*, New York, 2004, MD Martin Dunitz Taylor and Francis Group, pp. 95–100.
17. Wholey MH, Solomon N, Jarmolowski CR: Antegrade popliteal puncture: technical note, *Cardiovasc Intervent Radiol* 15(2):123–125, March 1992.
18. Glasby MJ, Bolia A: Subintimal angioplasty of a crural vessel via an antegrade popliteal artery puncture, *Eur J Vasc Endovasc Surg* 34(3):347–349, September 2007.
19. Yilmaz S, Sindel T, Luleci E: Ultrasound-guided retrograde popliteal artery catheterization: experience in 174 consecutive patients, *J Endovasc Ther* 12(6):714–722, December 2005.
20. Monge M, Eskandari M: Hybrid procedure for Supra-aortic trunk lesions. In Pearce WH, Matsumura JS, Yao JS, editors: *Vascular surgery in the endovascular era*, Evanston, 2008, Greenwood Academic, pp. 353–61.
21. Feldtman RW, Buckley CJ, Bohannon WT: How I do it: cervical access for carotid artery stenting, *Am J Surg* 192(6):779–80, December 2006.
22. Criado FJ, Twena M, Halsted M, Abul-Khoudoud O. Percutaneous femoral puncture for endovascular treatment of occlusive arterial lesions, *Am J Surg* 176(2):119–121, August 1998.
23. Rupp SB, Vogelzang RL, Nemcek AA Jr, Yungbluth MM: Relationship of the inguinal ligament to pelvic radiographic landmarks: anatomic correlation and its role in femoral arteriography, *J Vasc Interv Radiol* 4(3):409–413, May 1993.
24. Criado FJ: Percutaneous arterial puncture and endoluminal access techniques for peripheral intervention, *J Invasive Cardiol* 11(7):450–456, July 1999.
25. Fitts J, Ver LP, Hofmaster P, Malenka D: Fluoroscopy-guided femoral artery puncture reduces the risk of PCI-related vascular complications, *J Interv Cardiol* 21(3):273–278, June 2008.
26. Chitwood RW, Shepard AD, Shetty PC et al.: Surgical complications of transaxillary arteriography: a case-control study, *J Vasc Surg* 23(5):844–849, May 1996.
27. Mulligan B, Espinosa GA, Mafee M: Prevention of brachial plexus injury during transaxillary artery catheterization, *Mil Med* 148(6):518–520, June 1983.
28. Trigaux JP, Van BB, De Wispelaere JF: Anatomic relationship between the popliteal artery and vein: a guide to accurate angiographic puncture, *AJR Am J Roentgenol* 157(6):1259–1262, December 1991.
29. Diethrich EB, Marx P, Wrasper R, Reid DB: Percutaneous techniques for endoluminal carotid interventions, *J Endovasc Surg* 3(2):182–202, May 1996.
30. Criado FJ, Twena M: Techniques for endovascular recanalization of supra-aortic trunks, *J Endovasc Surg* 3(4):405–413, November 1996.
31. Morasch MD, Kibbe MR, Evans ME et al.: Percutaneous repair of abdominal aortic aneurysm, *J Vasc Surg* 40(1):12–16, July 2004.
32. Morasch MD: Percutaneous thoracic and abdominal aortic aneurysm repair, *Ann Vasc Surg* 19(4):585–589, July 2005.
33. Criado FJ, Abul-Khoudoud O, Martin JA, Wilson EP. Current developments in percutaneous arterial closure devices, *Ann Vasc Surg* 14(6):683–687, November 2000.
34. Koreny M, Riedmuller E, Nikfardjam M, Siostrzonek P, Mullner M: Arterial puncture closing devices compared with standard manual compression after cardiac catheterization: systematic review and meta-analysis, *JAMA* 291(3):350–357, January 21, 2004.
35. Sanborn TA, Gibbs HH, Brinker JA, Knopf WD, Kosinksi EJ, Roubin GS: A multicenter randomized trial comparing a percutaneous collagen hemostasis device with conventional manual compression after diagnostic angiography and angioplasty, *J Invasive Cardiol* 11(suppl B):6B–13B, September 1999.
36. Gerckens U, Cattelaens N, Lampe EG, Grube E: Management of arterial puncture site after catheterization

procedures: evaluating a suture-mediated closure device, *Am J Cardiol* 83(12):1658–1663, June 15, 1999.

37. Applegate RJ, Grabarczyk MA, Little WC et al.: Vascular closure devices in patients treated with anticoagulation and IIb/IIIa receptor inhibitors during percutaneous revascularization, *J Am Coll Cardiol* 40(1):78–83, July 3, 2002.
38. Kahn ZM, Kumar M, Hollander G, Frankel R: Safety and efficacy of the Perclose suture-mediated closure device after diagnostic and interventional catheterizations in a large consecutive population, *Catheter Cardiovasc Interv* 55(1):8–13, January, 2002.
39. Nikolsky E, Mehran R, Halkin A et al.: Vascular complications associated with arteriotomy closure devices in patients undergoing percutaneous coronary procedures: a meta-analysis, *J Am Coll Cardiol* 44(6):1200–1209, September 15, 2004.
40. Quinn SF, Kim J: Percutaneous femoral closure following stent-graft placement: use of the Perclose device, *Cardiovasc Intervent Radiol* 27(3):231–236, May 2004.
41. Shawl FA, Quyyumi AA, Bajaj S, Hoff SB, Dougherty KG: Percutaneous cardiopulmonary bypass-supported coronary angioplasty in patients with unstable angina pectoris or myocardial infarction and a left ventricular ejection fraction < or = 25%, *Am J Cardiol* 77(1):14–19, January 1, 1996.
42. Eggebrecht H, Haude M, Woertgen U et al.: Systematic use of a collagen-based vascular closure device immediately after cardiac catheterization procedures in 1,317 consecutive patients, *Catheter Cardiovasc Interv* 57(4): 486–495, December 2002.
43. Kussmaul WG III, Buchbinder M, Whitlow PL et al.: Rapid arterial hemostasis and decreased access site complications after cardiac catheterization and angioplasty: results of a randomized trial of a novel hemostatic device, *J Am Coll Cardiol* 25(7):1685–1692, June 1995.
44. Bos JJ, Hunink MG, Mali WP: Use of a collagen hemostatic closure device to achieve hemostasis after arterial puncture: a cost-effectiveness analysis, *J Vasc Interv Radiol* 7(4):479–486, July 1996.
45. Silber S, Tofte AJ, Kjellevand TO, Grube E, Gershony G: Final report of the European multi-center registry using the Duett vascular sealing device, *Herz* 24(8):620–623, December 1999.
46. Carere RG, Webb JG, Buller CE et al.: Suture closure of femoral arterial puncture sites after coronary angioplasty followed by same-day discharge, *Am Heart J* 139(1 Pt 1):52–58, January 2000.
47. Hogg ME, Kibbe MR: Percutaneous thoracic and abdominal aortic aneurysm repair: techniques and outcomes, *Vascular* 14(5):270–281, September 2006.
48. Haas PC, Krajcer Z, Diethrich EB: Closure of large percutaneous access sites using the prostar XL percutaneous vascular surgery DEVICE, *J Endovasc Surg* 6(2): 168–170, May 1999.
49. Teh LG, Sieunarine K, Van SG et al.: Use of the percutaneous vascular surgery device for closure of femoral access sites during endovascular aneurysm repair: lessons from our experience, *Eur J Vasc Endovasc Surg* 22(5):418–423, November 2001.
50. Traul DK, Clair DG, Gray B, O'Hara PJ, Ouriel K: Percutaneous endovascular repair of infrarenal abdominal aortic aneurysms: a feasibility study, *J Vasc Surg* 32(4):770–776, October 2000.
51. Howell M, Doughtery K, Strickman N, Krajcer Z: Percutaneous repair of abdominal aortic aneurysms using the AneuRx stent graft and the percutaneous vascular surgery device, *Catheter Cardiovasc Interv* 55(3): 281–287, March 2002.
52. Rachel ES, Bergamini TM, Kinney EV, Jung MT, Kaebnick HW, Mitchell RA: Percutaneous endovascular abdominal aortic aneurysm repair, *Ann Vasc Surg* 16(1):43–49, January 2002.
53. Peterson BG, Matsumura JS, Morasch MD, West MA, Eskandari MK: Percutaneous endovascular repair of blunt thoracic aortic transection, *J Trauma* 59(5):1062–1065, November 2005.
54. Starnes BW, Andersen CA, Ronsivalle JA, Stockmaster NR, Mullenix PS, Statler JD: Totally percutaneous aortic aneurysm repair: experience and prudence, *J Vasc Surg* 43(2):270–276, February 2006.
55. Torsello GB, Kasprzak B, Klenk E, Tessarek J, Osada N, Torsello GF: Endovascular suture versus cutdown for endovascular aneurysm repair: a prospective randomized pilot study, *J Vasc Surg* 38(1):78–82, July 2003.
56. Howell M, Villareal R, Krajcer Z: Percutaneous access and closure of femoral artery access sites associated with endoluminal repair of abdominal aortic aneurysms, *J Endovasc Ther* 8(1):68–74, February 2001.
57. Quinn SF, Duke DJ, Baldwin SS et al.: Percutaneous placement of a low-profile stent-graft device for aortic dissections, *J Vasc Interv Radiol* 13(8):791–798, August 2002.
58. Mackrell PJ, Kalbaugh CA, Langan EM III et al.: Can the Perclose suture-mediated closure system be used safely in patients undergoing diagnostic and therapeutic angiography to treat chronic lower extremity ischemia? *J Vasc Surg* 38(6):1305–1308, December 2003.
59. Eggebrecht H, Naber C, Woertgen U et al.: Percutaneous suture-mediated closure of femoral access sites deployed through the procedure sheath: initial clinical experience with a novel vascular closure device, *Catheter Cardiovasc Interv* 58(3):313–321, March 2003.
60. Martin JL, Pratsos A, Magargee E et al.: A randomized trial comparing compression, Perclose Proglide and Angio-Seal VIP for arterial closure following percutaneous coronary intervention: the CAP trial, *Catheter Cardiovasc Interv* 71(1):1–5, January 1, 2008.
61. Lee WA, Brown MP, Nelson PR, Huber TS: Total percutaneous access for endovascular aortic aneurysm repair ("Preclose" technique), *J Vasc Surg* 45(6):1095–1101, June 2007.
62. Lee WA, Brown MP, Nelson PR, Huber TS, Seeger JM: Midterm outcomes of femoral arteries after percutaneous endovascular aortic repair using the preclose technique, *J Vasc Surg* 47(5):919–923, May 2008.
63. Dosluoglu HH, Cherr GS, Harris LM, Dryjski ML: Total percutaneous endovascular repair of abdominal aortic aneurysms using Perclose ProGlide closure devices, *J Endovasc Ther* 14(2):184–188, April 2007.

64. Imam A, Carter RM, Phillips-Hughes J, Boardman P, Uberoi R: StarClose vascular closure device: prospective study on 222 deployments in an interventional radiology practice, *Cardiovasc Intervent Radiol* 30(4):738–742, July 2007.
65. Tay EL, Co M, Tai BC et al.: Clinical experience of StarClose vascular closure device in patients with first and recurrent femoral punctures, *J Interv Cardiol* 21(1): 67–73, February 2008.
66. Hermiller JB, Simonton C, Hinohara T et al.: The StarClose vascular closure system: interventional results from the CLIP study, *Catheter Cardiovasc Interv* 68(5):677–683, November 2006.
67. Ratnam LA, Raja J, Munneke GJ, Morgan RA, Belli AM: Prospective nonrandomized trial of manual compression and Angio-Seal and Starclose arterial closure devices in common femoral punctures, *Cardiovasc Intervent Radiol* 30(2):182–188, March 2007.
68. Fantoni C, Medda M, Mollichelli N et al.: Clip-based arterial haemostasis after antegrade common femoral artery puncture. *Int J Cardiol* April 5, 2008.
69. Stock U, Flach P, Gross M, Meyhofer J, Albes J, Butter C: Intravascular misplacement of an extravascular closure system: StarClose, *J Interv Cardiol* 19(2):170–172, April 2006.
70. Applegate RJ, Sacrinty MT, Kutcher MA et al.: Vascular complications in women after catheterization and percutaneous coronary intervention 1998–2005, *J Invasive Cardiol* 19(9):369–374, September 2007.
71. Sherev DA, Shaw RE, Brent BN: Angiographic predictors of femoral access site complications: implication for planned percutaneous coronary intervention, *Catheter Cardiovasc Interv* 65(2):196–202, June 2005.
72. Wagner SC, Gonsalves CF, Eschelman DJ, Sullivan KL, Bonn J: Complications of a percutaneous suture-mediated closure device versus manual compression for arteriotomy closure: a case-controlled study, *J Vasc Interv Radiol* 14(6):735–741, June 2003.
73. Smith TP, Cruz CP, Moursi MM, Eidt JF: Infectious complications resulting from use of hemostatic puncture closure devices, *Am J Surg* 182(6):658–662, December 2001.
74. Boston US, Panneton JM, Hofer JM et al.: Infectious and ischemic complications from percutaneous closure devices used after vascular access, *Ann Vasc Surg* 17(1):66–71, January 2003.
75. Brown DB, Crawford ST, Norton PL, Hovsepian DM: Angiographic follow-up after suture-mediated femoral artery closure, *J Vasc Interv Radiol* 13(7):677–680, July 2002.
76. Applegate RJ, Sacrinty MT, Kutcher MA et al.: Propensity score analysis of vascular complications after diagnostic cardiac catheterization and percutaneous coronary intervention 1998–2003, *Catheter Cardiovasc Interv* 67(4):556–562, April 2006.
77. Grollman JH Jr, Marcus R: Transbrachial arteriography: techniques and complications, *Cardiovasc Intervent Radiol* 11(1):32–35, 1988.
78. Watkinson AF, Hartnell GG: Complications of direct brachial artery puncture for arteriography: a comparison of techniques, *Clin Radiol* 44(3):189–191, September 1991.
79. Heenan SD, Grubnic S, Buckenham TM, Belli AM: Transbrachial arteriography: indications and complications, *Clin Radiol* 51(3):205–209, March 1996.
80. Gritter KJ, Laidlaw WW, Peterson NT: Complications of outpatient transbrachial intraarterial digital subtraction angiography. Work in progress, *Radiology* 162(1 Pt 1):125–127, January 1987.
81. Uchino A: Selective catheterization of the brachiocephalic arteries via the right brachial artery, *Neuroradiology* 30(6):524–527, 1988.
82. Chatziioannou A, Ladopoulos C, Mourikis D, Katsenis K, Spanomihos G, Vlachos L: Complications of lower-extremity outpatient arteriography via low brachial artery, *Cardiovasc Intervent Radiol* 27(1):31–34, January 2004.
83. Bilecen D, Bongartz G, Ostheim-Dzerowycz W: Off-label use of Angio-Seal vascular closure device for brachial artery puncture closure-deployment modification and initial results after transbrachial PTA, *Eur J Vasc Endovasc Surg* 31(4):431–433, April 2006.
84. Cohen M, Rentrop KP, Cohen BM: Safety and efficacy of percutaneous entry of the brachial artery versus cutdown and arteriotomy for left-sided cardiac catheterization, *Am J Cardiol* 57(8):682–684, March 1, 1986.
85. Rath J, Ganschow US, Kelm M et al.: [Duplex ultrasound risk stratification of percutaneous puncture of the brachial artery for diagnostic and interventional coronary angiography], *Z Kardiol* 87(4):249–257, April 1998.
86. Ernst S, Fischbach R, Brochhagen HG, Heindel W, Landwehr P: Transbrachial thrombolysis, PTA and stenting in the lower extremities, *Cardiovasc Intervent Radiol* 26(6):516–521, November 2003.
87. Kiemeneij F, Laarman GJ, Odekerken D, Slagboom T: van der WR: A randomized comparison of percutaneous transluminal coronary angioplasty by the radial, brachial and femoral approaches: the access study, *J Am Coll Cardiol* 29(6):1269–1275, May 1997.
88. Kresowik TF, Khoury MD, Miller BV et al.: A prospective study of the incidence and natural history of femoral vascular complications after percutaneous transluminal coronary angioplasty, *J Vasc Surg* 13(2):328–333, February 1991.
89. Kang SS, Labropoulos N, Mansour MA et al.: Expanded indications for ultrasound-guided thrombin injection of pseudoaneurysms, *J Vasc Surg* 31(2):289–298, February 2000.
90. Goldberg SL, Renslo R, Sinow R, French WJ: Learning curve in the use of the radial artery as vascular access in the performance of percutaneous transluminal coronary angioplasty, *Cathet Cardiovasc Diagn* 44(2):147–152, June 1998.
91. Aburahma AF, Robinson PA, Boland JP et al.: Complications of arteriography in a recent series of 707 cases: factors affecting outcome, *Ann Vasc Surg* 7(2):122–129, March 1993.
92. Molnar W, Paul DJ: Complications of axillary arteriotomies. An analysis of 1,762 consecutive studies, *Radiology* 104(2):269–276, August 1972.
93. Westcott JL, Taylor PT: Transaxillary selective four-vessel arteriography, *Radiology* 104(2):277–281, August 1972.

94. Smith DC, Mitchell DA, Peterson GW, Will AD, Mera SS, Smith LL: Medial brachial fascial compartment syndrome: anatomic basis of neuropathy after transaxillary arteriography, *Radiology* 173(1):149–154, October 1989.
95. Tsao BE, Wilbourn AJ: The medial brachial fascial compartment syndrome following axillary arteriography, *Neurology* 61(8):1037–1041, October 28, 2003.
96. Kluge A, Rauber K, Breithecker A, Rau WS, Bachmann G: Puncture of the popliteal artery using a Doppler-equipped (SMART) needle in transpopliteal interventions, *Eur Radiol* 13(8):1972–1978, August 2003.
97. Saha S, Gibson M, Magee TR, Galland RB, Torrie EP: Early results of retrograde transpopliteal angioplasty of iliofemoral lesions, *Cardiovasc Intervent Radiol* 24(6):378–382, November 2001.
98. Tonnesen KH, Sager P, Karle A, Henriksen L, Jorgensen B: Percutaneous transluminal angioplasty of the superficial femoral artery by retrograde catheterization via the popliteal artery, *Cardiovasc Intervent Radiol* 11(3): 127–131, June 1988.
99. Henry M, Amicabile C, Amor M, Beron R, Henry I, Mentre B: [Peripheral arterial angioplasty: value of the popliteal approach. Apropos of 30 cases], *Arch Mal Coeur Vaiss* 86(4):463–469, April 1993.
100. McCullough KM: Retrograde transpopliteal salvage of the failed antegrade transfemoral angioplasty, *Australas Radiol* 37(4):329–331, November 1993.
101. MacIntyre PA, Samra G, Hatch DJ: Preliminary experience with the Doppler ultrasound guided vascular access needle in paediatric patients, *Paediatr Anaesth* 10(4): 361–365, 2000.
102. Moore KL, Agur AMR: *Essential clinical anatomy*, ed. 3, Baltimore, 2007, Lippincott Williams & Williams, p. 354.

Endovascular Practice in Asia-Pacific

32

Stephen W.K. Cheng

The Asia-Pacific consists of countries with wide diversities in population, ethnicity, language, and clinical practice. With improvement in health care, many developed economies in the region have an aging population. The incidence and detection rates of occlusive and aneurysmal diseases are on the rise, although not yet approaching that in the United States.

The development of vascular surgery in Asia is slow, and most countries have only a small group of dedicated vascular surgeons. Peripheral vascular surgery is often practiced within the domain of general or cardiac surgery. With the rapid evolution of endovascular procedures, there is an increasing awareness to develop these technologies in Asia, but the task is made more difficult by the lack of a cohesive force, stern competition from other disciplines, and the difficulty in obtaining devices and training.

The growth of endovascular surgery, particularly endovascular stent grafts, is met with distinct variations in practice, device availability, regulations, and reimbursement among Asian countries. In those with matured economies and established funding structures such as Japan, government regulations and conservatism have hindered the introduction of industrial devices. On the other hand, developing worlds such as China have no strict regulation for devices, but the absence of reimbursement mechanism has restricted availability to only the more affluent. In others, the endovascular treatment option is simply not possible due to economic constraints. Culturally many patients are less receptive to pay for medical devices and consumables for conditions that they do not perceive as immediately life threatening—such as peripheral arterial disease and aneurysms. These factors are the main obstacles in the advancement of endovascular surgery in Asia.

To deliver an up-to-date and accurate summary of endovascular surgery in Asia is a grand task. I would attempt to describe the evolution and current practice of endovascular aortic aneurysm repair (EVAR) as representative of current developments in key countries including China, India, Japan, and Korea and the South East Asian states of Hong Kong, Singapore, Malaysia, Taiwan, Thailand, and to a lesser extent, Malaysia, Philippines, Indonesia, and Vietnam. For this purpose the Caucasian population of Oceania is not included. With a tremendous economic growth in the region, we expect that endovascular practice will evolve at an equally rapid pace, and information presented in this chapter may soon become obsolete.

Diversity

Maturity of Vascular Surgery as a Specialty

With modernization and changing dietary habits, we are witnessing an increase in the incidence of arterial pathologies, but peripheral vascular disease in Asia is still less prevalent than in the West. As a result vascular surgery as a specialty is not well developed in Asia. There is a proliferation of different practices based on patient access, equipment, and referral patterns. Many cardiologists and interventional

S.W.K. Cheng (✉)
Professor, Department of Surgery, Chief, Division of Vascular Surgery, Queen Mary Hospital, The University of Hong Kong, Hong Kong, China

T.J. Fogarty, R.A. White (eds.), *Peripheral Endovascular Interventions*,
DOI 10.1007/978-1-4419-1387-6_32, © Springer Science+Business Media, LLC 1998, 2010

radiologists participated in peripheral vascular work, particularly lower limb angioplasty and stenting.

Currently in many countries vascular surgery is practiced predominantly by general surgeons. In China, there is an increasing trend of specialization in major cities, and the Chinese Vascular Society comprise both dedicated vascular surgeons and general surgeons. Japan, Korea, and India have well-formed regional vascular surgery societies. Nevertheless many aortic aneurysm repairs are done by cardiovascular surgeons in these countries, while lower limb reconstructions are seldom performed. Primary amputation is still widely practiced. Most vascular surgeons work inside university practices, and vascular surgery in its current form as in the United States does not exist.

Training and certification requirements are also different. Local training institutions and facilities are very limited, and many vascular surgeons have sought additional overseas experience in reputed centers in the United States, Australia, or Europe as fellowships or short-term attachments. These surgeons form the backbone of the modern generation vascular surgeons in Asia and are often the pioneers in endovascular intervention.

Health Statistics

Due to the relative underdevelopment of vascular surgery, it is a universal phenomenon in Asia that there is no organized national database or health registry of peripheral vascular disease. Information is often gathered from local institution-based research data, and the overall disease prevalence is not known.

Economy and Health-Care Structure

Asia is also diversified in terms of wealth. There are regions that are considered developed, with health-care systems on par with the West, such as Japan, Hong Kong, and Taiwan. In other, less developed countries endovascular surgery is still very much in its infancy due to the non-availability of infrastructure and resources. In some countries, expensive devices such as aortic endograft are realistically out of the general population's financial means. Most countries also have no universal health insurance, and the costs of devices have to be borne by the patients, which generally limits the accessibility of devices to the more affluent population.

Language

Each of the Asian countries speaks its own language, sometimes several languages and dialects, and English is not widely spoken even by physicians except perhaps in India, Hong Kong, and Singapore. When it comes to advanced endovascular procedures, international academic exchange, training, and proctorship, language barrier is an important concern. Very often the promulgation of a technology is left to a few English-speaking pioneers in the country.

Device Market

There are additional difficulties of making all devices available in Asia, particularly in the smaller countries. Most device companies regard Japan and China as their chief targets, the former due to its wealth and pricing structure, and the latter due to its economic growth and vast population. The degree of technical and product support in many countries in Asia is sadly at best haphazard and at worst non-existent. The uncertainties of government regulations, import restrictions, lack of good local training infrastructure, and domestic distribution issues have made many companies hesitant in moving into Asia. There are the additional legal concerns of patents and property rights and competition from domestic-manufactured devices. For the aortic endografts, only three industrial companies are currently having a real presence in Asia, namely Cook Medical (Bloomington IN), Gore (Flagstaff, AZ), and Medtronic (Santa Rosa, CA). In the smaller countries, access to new devices is often very limited due to the lack of company representation, knowledgeable sales personnel, and good technical support.

Government Regulations

Japan and Taiwan have FDA-type strict government regulations on the import and use of new medical devices. Endografts have to undergo a rigorous clinical trial stage before approval can be granted. This has also resulted in a setback of several years before current generation devices are made available for use outside clinical trials. In many South East Asian countries, on the other hand, government regulations are less stringent, and any new devices are accepted as long as they have been marketed in a Western country and possess either a CE mark or FDA approval rating. Many branched and fenestrated devices are therefore made available also in Asia, notably Hong Kong and Singapore. With strict FDA regulations in the United States, some companies are already conducting their trials of new innovative devices in Asia.

Anatomy

Asians are generally smaller in stature and have smaller vessels. Superficial femoral artery diameters of 5–6 mm are common among women, and this has a negative impact on the results of angioplasty and stenting. The use of covered stents in the lower limbs is also not met with great success due to the inherent bulk of the graft. Likewise small access vessels have limited the application of endovascular aortic stent grafts. In our own experience half of the thoracic endografts implanted in women require the construction of an iliac conduit. Percutaneous stent graft insertion is seldom feasible, and this has also limited the adoption of endovascular aortic stent graft by interventional cardiologists in Asia.

The common iliac artery in Asians is often shorter and wider than their Western counterparts [1]. The average length of the common iliac artery is in the region of 25–30 mm, with diameters of 16–20 mm. Short and wide common iliacs result in two main issues: length of the main body and a lack of adequate distal seal. As a result planning for EVAR has to be more demanding and execution more accurate in Asians. Many abdominal stent grafts, originally designed according to Caucasian anatomy, were too long for Asians. Placement of the distal components had to be as close to the iliac bifurcation as possible to maximize seal. A three-component system such as the Zenith endograft (Cook Medical, Bloomington, IN) is popular. The main body can be introduced first without concern of the length of the ipsilateral leg, and the iliac components added at a second stage to achieve an accurate landing as close to the iliac bifurcation as possible. The Zenith graft also has a wide choice of body lengths and large diameter iliac extensions up to 24 mm to accommodate variations in Asian anatomy.

Preservation of the internal iliac arteries also is a challenge. Even with large diameter iliac extensions, more than 40% of our patients would need sacrifice of one internal iliac artery. The newer generation iliac bifurcation grafts have also found a good testing ground in this part of the world.

China

China has a population of 1.3 billion. There is, however, no national training body for vascular and endovascular surgery. Vascular surgery is not a popular specialty, but there are large individual hospitals and units in major cities dedicated to cardiovascular and peripheral vascular work. Over the last decade, there has been a tremendous development of health care in China, although most remain regional based. New hospitals with modern equipment, including state-of-the art CT scanners and interventional theaters, are being built at a fast pace.

Endovascular intervention is shared by many specialists who have access to patients and equipment. Peripheral and carotid angioplasty and stenting had proliferated but unregulated and is practiced by cardiologists, neurologists, radiologists, and vascular surgeons alike.

EVAR is largely carried out by surgeons in operating theatres. Currently more than 2,000 cases are performed annually in about 200 regional centers. Prominent leading centers in endovascular surgery are located mainly in Shanghai, Beijing, and Guangzhou. The Chinese have embraced the thoracic endovascular stent graft technology to treat aortic dissections, and several centers have accumulated experiences in excess of 200 implants, among the most experienced in the world. At the Department of Vascular Surgery at Fudan University in Shanghai, some 110 thoracic endovascular repairs (TEVAR) were performed for dissection in 2006, compared to 20 in 2000. Treating acute Type B dissection by TEVAR has become the standard first choice procedure in China. There is a disproportionally large percentage of thoracic endograft implants compared with its abdominal counterpart – it is estimated that at least 60–75% of endografts in China are done for thoracic dissections. Although hypertension and smoking may be more prevalent in China, the high number of aortic dissections being treated in China may not actually reflect a high incidence of the disease, but a higher detection rate from emergency departments. EVAR comprises about half of TEVAR numbers in China, but with the rapid modernization of health-care systems and improved detection of abdominal aortic aneurysms (AAA), endovascular repair of AAA has been growing fast.

There is no strict license for devices, and a variety of foreign-manufactured stent grafts are available. The Medtronic Talent and Valiant grafts currently dominate the stent graft market, with the Cook Zenith coming second. These devices are often sold for prices in the region of US $20,000, and there is no national reimbursement system or medical insurance. Except in the military and some private companies, the patients are expected to pay for the device out of their own resources.

There are a number of domestically manufactured stent grafts which comprise about half of the total market. The Microport Hercules device (Microport Medical, Shanghai, China) is a thoracic stent graft made of polyester fabric sutured on nitinol stents, similar to the Talent design. It is available in diameters up to 44 mm and lengths from 40 to 160 cm and delivered through a 16–24 Fr sheath. The company also offers an abdominal bifurcated AEGIS graft (Microport Medical, Shanghai), consisting of an e-PTFE fabric supported by a cobalt–chromium–nickel–molybdenum–iron alloy (Conichrome) with suprarenal stents, similar to the Powerlink (Endologix Inc, Irving, CA) design, and comes in diameters from 20 to 38 mm. The Ankura (Lifetech Scientific Inc, Shenzhen, China) device consisted of an e-PTFE embedded non-suture stent graft with a suprarenal stent cone. These domestic devices are available for about two-thirds of the costs of a "Western" device and are attractive alternatives to patients. There is also a large market for domestically developed medical cardiovascular products, from balloons to peripheral, carotid, and intracranial stents, drug-eluting coronary stents, IVC filters, occluders, to endovascular stent grafts. There are plans for a central tendering system from the Beijing government, but at the time of writing the choice and pricing of devices are largely hospital administered.

A lot of innovative work has been done in China to adopt endografts in unconventional situations, such as Type A aortic dissections, and homemade branched devices for the aortic arch have also been developed [2]. The main issue about endovascular surgery in China is the adequacy of follow-up. Many patients who seek treatment in reputed centers are from rural areas and without means of further surveillance or communication. This alone poses a significant barrier to promulgating the many novel procedures currently done in China.

Vascular surgeons in China are currently doing more than 90% of EVAR, and it is expected that their role will continue to dominate in future.

Japan

Vascular surgery is also not well recognized and underdeveloped as a specialty in Japan. The entire country has only four professors of vascular surgery among 80 medical schools. Open surgery is largely done by cardiac surgeons, while carotid disease is managed by neurosurgeons. Few procedures such as carotid endarterectomy or distal bypasses were performed. Lower limb and renal angioplasty are less commonly done and largely in the hands of cardiologists. Although the Japanese Society for Vascular Surgery has almost 2,000 members, the majority are cardiothoracic surgeons who perform aneurysm repairs and lower limb procedures. Nevertheless it is estimated that 10,000 AAA repairs were done annually in Japan. Over 80% of EVAR currently is being performed by cardiovascular surgeons and the remaining by interventional radiologists and cardiologists.

The Minister of Health, Labor, and Welfare has a very strict process of licensing stent grafts, which has led to a delay of their commercial availability. In the last decade Japan has developed, by domestic manufacturers, a number of homemade thoracic endografts, with proprietary branch and fenestration arrangements. The Najuta stent graft was developed by the Tokyo Medical University, with custom-made Z stents covered with PTFE and containing fenestrations and sutured only at proximal and distal ends to allow for the aortic curvature [3]. Other designs include the

Matsui–Kitamura graft consisting of a nitinol stent spiral skeleton covered with Dacron and also curved to match the arch anatomy [4] and the branched abdominal and thoracic versions of the Inoue graft [5]. A few hundred of these devices have been implanted in Japan under research permits in several centers, but they are not widely available.

Japan has always been regarded as one of the largest market for cardiovascular devices in the world, second only to the United States, due to its health-care system and high pricing. There is no universal insurance, but once a device is registered, it is reimbursable by a health insurance company based on a fixed price controlled by the government and only if the patients are deemed at high risk unsuitable for open surgery. Currently an EVAR device costs about US $15,000 in Japan.

Three industry-made abdominal aortic stent grafts have been approved by the Minister of Health, Labor, and Welfare: the Zenith (Cook Medical, Bloomington, IN) in July 2006, Excluder (Gore & Associates, Flagstaff, AZ) in January 2007, and Powerlink (Endologix Inc, Irving, CA) in April 2008, 7 years behind the United States. The training requirements mandate the first two cases to be done in the presence of a proctor and the first ten under strict scrutiny. About 1,500 EVARs have since been performed in the first 2 years of launch, compared to only 100 in 2006. In early 2008 the Gore TAG device had been approved, and in the first 4 months some 300 TEVARs had been performed. It is anticipated that after the initial adoptive phase, there will be an explosive growth in the use of these devices in the next 1–2 years. The total number of endografts done to date in Japan approximates 2,000.

As of the time of writing the largest endovascular surgery unit had been established at the Jikei University in Tokyo, where approximately 300 aortic stent grafts were performed yearly. In the last 2 years, more than 360 EVARs were performed in this university, of which about 60% were Zenith and 40% Excluder implants. Current workload has increased to about 30 EVARs a month, and some 30 branched graft cases have been performed [6].

The Angioguard/Precise carotid stent was approved in 2007. Four Japanese centers have recently been recruited into the Cook Zilver PTX drug-eluting stent's trial. The situation is promising, and with better device access in future, it is foreseeable that there will be an endovascular revolution in Japan.

Korea

Similar to Japan, there are no large numbers of vascular surgeons in Korea, and interventional radiologists have traditionally dominated peripheral endovascular work. Surgeons and cardiologists are, however, showing an interest in endografts. Currently about 300 EVARs and 100 TEVARs have been performed in the country.

Reimbursement of the device is government controlled with a diagnosis-related group-based payment and the prices are generally lower. Registrations of foreign devices are relatively slow. Three industry-made endografts are currently approved in Korea – the Zenith (Cook Medical, Bloomington, IN), AneuRx (Medtronic, Santa Rosa, CA), and Excluder (Gore, Flagstaff, AZ).

Korea has developed a domestic thoracic endograft which had originated in 1997 with S&G Biotech, currently named SEAL. The graft is based on a percutaneous 12 Fr design with an outer Dacron fabric supported at both ends with nitniol stents and reinforced by a second stage inner lattice of bare nitinol stents [7]. The graft has been approved by the Korean FDA in March 2008 and is marketed mainly in Korea and also in Indonesia.

India

Despite its large population of more than 1.1 billion, vascular surgery is still in its developing phase in India. In 2008 it was estimated that there were only 70 full-time vascular surgeons in the country. Only 10 out of 24 medical schools in India have a vascular surgery unit, and only seven centers have a training program for 12 vascular trainees annually. There are about 5,000 arterial reconstructions per year, and most of the work is done by cardiac and general surgeons. There is no medical insurance, and patients with the financial means will have to pay for the consumables. Endovascular surgery has not been widely available to the general population, mainly due to the prohibitive costs of the devices, and the general public often prefers the less expensive open option. Availability of interventional facilities is another factor, as most are controlled by cardiologists and radiologists. As far as endografting is concerned at this time India remained a small market of 100–200 devices per year, and the work is largely done by vascular surgeons and cardiologists working in private hospitals. Endovascular training is generally obtained overseas, but a company has established a training facility in New Delhi. Progress at present remains slow.

Hong Kong

Vascular surgery practice is mainly confined to two university hospitals, and the rest are performed by general surgeons. Following largely a British system, the territory provides affordable health care for all citizens, but expensive devices were not included and patients have to pay for endografts and stents. Insurance is picking up but still not popular among the aged.

There is an increasing interest of vascular surgeons to practice endovascular surgery, and many have obtained training overseas in United States and Australia. Nevertheless they face keen competition from cardiologists and some interventional radiologists for peripheral vascular work. Carotid angioplasty and stenting are not commonly done, and around 80 are done yearly in the region. In general, peripheral endovascular surgery is still not popular due to reluctance of the patients to undergo intervention and to pay for expensive devices. Endovascular stent graft remained at this time largely in the hands of surgeons, working in operating room setting either individually or in cooperation with radiologists.

Regulation of devices is not stringent, and any device with CE or FDA approval can be used in Hong Kong. The first EVAR was performed as early as 1997, and to date about 150–200 have been performed yearly, largely in three public hospitals. Currently at the largest vascular center at Queen Mary Hospital, the University of Hong Kong, approximately 60 aortic endografts are performed annually, accounting for 60–70% of all its aneurysm repairs.

The biggest obstacle to the endovascular program in Hong Kong is reimbursement. The Hospital Authority, which controls all funding to public hospitals, does not restrict the use of EVAR, but also does not provide financial support. After more than 10 years of regular usage, EVAR is still regarded as a new technology and remains unfunded. Most patients would have to be self-financed, with a small proportion of disadvantaged patients supported by meager charity grants.

Due to issues of representation and difficulty of technical support, only a few devices are currently available. The first endograft was the AneuRx (Medtronic, Santa Rosa, CA), which was later replaced by the Talent. The Zenith (Cook Inc, Bloomington, IN) graft became the market leader since its introduction in 2003, taking about 80% of share because of its range of diameters suited for Asian anatomy. There have been sporadic Excluder (Gore, Flagstaff, AZ) implants. In the thoracic market, the Zenith TX2 and Medtronics Valiant are the popular grafts.

Hong Kong has benefitted from a relative freedom in importing devices and has always enjoyed the latest grafts on the market (such as the Zenith FLEX and TX2 with Flexor sheaths, fenestrated grafts, and branched devices and the newer Medtronic Endurant). Due to the unique common iliac anatomy, we have come to the need to sacrifice one internal iliac artery in almost half of the patients with EVAR. This has prompted the introduction of a proprietary iliac bifurcated branched graft and later a bifurcated main body version in the territory.

With a relatively small population of 7 million, the endograft market has matured in Hong Kong, and the number will stay stable. The funding system has found a balance, and there is no apparent incentive in the health-care administration to advance this arrangement.

Singapore

Similar to Hong Kong, Singapore is a mature but smaller market. With a population of about 4.5 million, less than 100 endografts are performed in the country yearly, largely in cardiac laboratories or radiology suites in two public institutions. The work is shared between vascular surgeons, cardiologists, and radiologists. Singapore has a more mature specialty structure, and vascular surgery is better recognized in the region. There is a small government fund to support a small number of grafts, but most patients have to pay for the devices.

Taiwan

Vascular surgery only gained recognition as a specialty in the mid-2000s, when the Taiwan Society for Vascular Surgery was established. Prior to this endovascular work was largely in the hands of cardiologists. There has been a significant volume of carotid and vertebral angioplasty and stenting done by the Division of Cardiology at the National University of Taiwan Hospital. EVAR development was late in Taiwan due to government regulations mandating a FDA-type trial before any devices can be registered for use. EVAR was formally approved only in July 2005 after a series of slow trials, and currently only the AneuRx (Medtronic, Santa Rosa, CA), Zenith TriFab (Cook Medical, Bloomington, IN), and Excluder (Gore, Flagstaff, AZ) endografts are on the market. EVAR is being performed largely by cardiovascular surgeons, with some 150 AAA and 100 TAAs and dissections per year. This is also a growing market, although most patients have to pay for the devices and no universal insurance coverage is in place.

Thoracic endografting was officially approved in November 2006 with the registration of the Zenith TX2 device. The current leading center in Taiwan is the Veterans General Hospital, where annually about 60 TEVAR and 50 EVARs are performed in the cardiothoracic department, many in combination with extracorporeal circulation or hybrid procedures. There has been a steady growth in endovascular stent grafts in other centers over the territory.

Thailand

Endovascular surgery has also proliferated significantly in Thailand in the last few years. Initially supported and reimbursed by the government, covering 80% of device costs, there has been a rapid growth of endovascular stent grafts, but at significant expenses to the government. Currently EVARs are mainly done by cardiothoracic surgeons in Bangkok.

Malaysia

EVAR and other endovascular surgery is limited to a very few private vascular surgeons who have the facilities and the patients to afford the devices. Currently this remains a very small market.

Philippines and Indonesia

These countries do not have a well-differentiated vascular surgery program and are also limited by device costs. There is really only a token number of cases performed each year, and the market is not looking at expanding in the near future.

In conclusion, endovascular surgery practice is very varied in Asia, but shows good promise in at least several countries. There is a universal phenomenon of under-recognition of vascular surgery, and limitation in facilities and reimbursement became the major obstacles for vascular surgeons. It is anticipated, however, that with increasing disease numbers and awareness we will see a continuing bloom of endovascular surgery in this part of the world.

References

1. Cheng SWK, Ting ACW, Ho P, Poon JTP: Aortic aneurysm morphology in Asians: features affecting endovascular stent graft application and design, *J Endovasc Ther* 11:605–612, 2004.
2. Wang ZG, Li C: Single-branch endograft for treating Stanford type B aortic dissections with entry tears in proximity to the left subclavian artery, *J Endovasc Ther* 12: 588–593, 2005.
3. Ishimaru S, Kawaguchi S, Yokoi Y: Fenestrated options for aortic arch applications, *Endovasc Today* 6:86–87, 2007.
4. Sanada J, Matsui O, Terayama N, Kobayashi S, Minami T, Kurozumi M, Ohtake H, Urayama H, Endo M: Clinical application of a curved nitinol stent-graft for thoracic aortic aneurysms, *J Endovasc Ther* 10:20–28, 2003.
5. Saito N, Kimura T, Odashiro K, Toma M, Nobuyoshi M, Ueno K, Kita T, Inoue K: Feasibility of the Inoue single-branched stent-graft implantation for thoracic aortic aneurysm or dissection involving the left subclavian artery: short- to medium-term results in 17 patients, *J Vasc Surg* 41:206–212, 2005.
6. Ohki T: The dawn of AAA stenting in Japan, *Endovasc Today* 6(3):47–52, 2007.
7. Kang SG, Lee DY, Maeda M, Kim ES, Choi D, Kim BO, Yoon HK, Sung KB, Song HY: Aortic dissection: percutaneous management with a separating stent-graft – preliminary results, *Radiology* 220:533–539, 2001.

Future Imaging and Guidance for Endovascular Procedures

33

Jean Bismuth, Christof Karmonik, Neal Kleiman, Miguel Valderrábano, and Alan B. Lumsden

The considerations which are fundamental when assessing the value of an imaging modality in the endovascular arena are that (1) the equipment must have adequate *definition* and thereby be able to characterize tissues and define boundaries between anatomic structures; (2) the system must be *interactive* and *intuitive*; (3) *three-dimensional* capabilities are necessary when navigating vascular anatomy; and (4) finally, the *fourth dimension*, namely, the ability to evaluate *motion*. The vascular bed is a dynamic one and therefore not including motion could allow for misinterpretation during both preoperative planning and postoperative evaluation. By this we mean that motion affects operative planning for proper stent sizing as well as movement during function (i.e., superficial femoral artery stents during knee movement).

Patients and clinicians alike are demanding better endovascular results and a minimization of device-related complications, while continuing to expand its use to a larger proportion of patients. The element which has and continues to plague endovascular therapies is a reported higher incidence of post-procedural device-related complications, as well as re-intervention rates that greatly supersede open vascular surgery.

Preoperative and intraoperative imaging plays a crucial role in determining the feasibility and success of such therapies. We have long ignored motion in our imaging modalities, but much of the developments seen in multiple imaging techniques indicate that motion is a critical feature. Understanding motion by magnetic resonance imaging, computed tomography, intravascular ultrasound, transesophageal ultrasound, and contrast ultrasound has been shown to display disease not previously appreciated and the potential to avoid endovascular errors and catastrophes. Blood vessels are an integral part of the structures which surround them, often subject to a variety of external forces. The advantages of each modality are listed in Table 33.1.

Table 33.1 Features of various imaging modalities

Study	Lumen	Anatomy	Motion	Plaque characteristics
Arteriography	+	–	–	–
CT[a] scan	+	+++	+++	–
MRI/MRA[b]	+	++	+++	++
IVUS[c]	+	–	++	+++
DynaCT	+	++	–	–

[a]Computed tomography.
[b]Magnetic resonance.
[c]Intravascular ultrasound.

There are essentially three phases where a variety of imaging modalities play a fundamental role in appropriate application of endovascular therapeutics: (1) procedural planning, (2) operative intervention, and (3) follow-up. We will herein discuss a number of imaging methods and how we believe they apply to these three phases of endovascular therapy (Table 33.2).

Imaging

Magnetic Resonance Imaging

In contrast to any other clinical medical image modality, MRI has unique capabilities. These originate in

J. Bismuth (✉)
Assistant Professor, Cardiovascular Surgery Associates, The Methodist Hospital, Houston, TX, USA

T.J. Fogarty, R.A. White (eds.), *Peripheral Endovascular Interventions*,
DOI 10.1007/978-1-4419-1387-6_33, © Springer Science+Business Media, LLC 1998, 2010

Table 33.2 Proposed points of use of imaging/therapeutics during the three stages of endovascular therapy

Procedural planning	Operative intervention	Follow-up
Dynamic CT[a]/MR[b]	DynaCT	Dynamic CT/MR
Contrast ultrasound/ echo[c]	TEE	Contrast ultrasound
3D Echo	IVUS[d]	Robotics
Virtual reality simulator	Robotics	
	TCD[e]	

[a] Computed tomography.
[b] Magnetic resonance.
[c] Echocardiography.
[d] Intravascular ultrasound.
[e] Transcranial Doppler.

part from the dependence of the signal on its molecular environment, leading to intrinsic tissue contrast that can be utilized to characterize tissue composition, and in part from the procedure utilized for image formation, which relies on the sampling of a signal echo (gradient echo or spin echo) created from an original excitation of protons at a given location. The intrinsic time dependence of the MRI signal in the acquisition process allows the quantification of physiological flow processes directly in blood vessels or indirectly in tissue.

Another advantage of MRI is its widespread use. In the last decades, MRI has advanced to one of the major clinical imaging modalities and almost every hospital possesses at least one MRI scanner. Despite its higher operation costs and its (on average) longer image acquisition duration than computed tomography, the popularity of MRI may be at least in part founded in the fact that it has been proven to be very safe. It does not expose the patient or the operator to harmful radiation and therefore can be applied without concern in pediatric imaging.

Since the early days of MRI, applications for imaging the human vasculature have been developed [1]. With cardiovascular disease being the leading cause of death in the United States and the developing world, the capabilities of MRI for quantifying and characterizing atherosclerotic disease have been explored. Already 20 years ago, MRI had been shown to be able to discriminate between normal, smooth muscle wall, fatty plaque, complex, fibrous plaque, and calcified plaque [2]. With improvements in scanning and computing hardware and software, a virtual histology technique has been developed based on multi-contrast MRI [3]. This is validated with conventional histological procedures for quantifying atherosclerotic plaque composition in the carotid bifurcation [4] and for tracking the progression or the regression of carotid atherosclerotic plaque volume [5, 6]. The recent push in molecular imaging techniques has led to new developments of MRI contrast agents with the aim to selectively visualize tissues of different chemical composition in atherosclerotic plaque [7]. Within this development, ultra-small superparamagnetic particles of iron oxide (USPIO), for example, were found to be able to detect infiltration of macrophages in human atherosclerotic carotid plaque [8, 9]. Arterial wall and atherosclerotic lesion composition may be of great importance for the planning of endovascular treatments of various vascular beds and could potentially alter existing treatment paradigms.

Of equal or even greater importance is an accurate assessment of the geometry of the diseased arterial section, which may, for example, be an aneurysm, a stenosis, or a dissection. MRI time-of-flight (TOF) techniques are capable of easily visualizing the arterial lumen, provided that there is sufficient blood flow present. This is achieved by exploiting the difference in the MRI signal from moving protons compared to stationary protons (i.e., tissue) [10]. As slow or recirculating flow may lead to signal void, another approach of visualizing blood by optimizing its contrast to stationary tissue is achieved through administering an exogenous contrast agent intravenously. Contrast-enhanced MRI allows for a very good delineation of all arteries ranging from the aorta over the carotid artery to peripheral vessels of small diameter. Still, image accuracy is limited by the spatial resolution of MRI, which in many cases is not as good as the one achieved with computed tomographic angiography (CTA). However, as the sensitivity of MRI to detect effects caused by contrast agents is higher than that of X-rays, doses about 100–1,000 times lower can be given [11].

Besides visualization of static anatomical features, of far higher importance is the capability of MRI to provide time-resolved information. The presence of pulsatility in a dynamic environment such as in vascular structures almost necessitates our attention as this likely has a crucial role in future stent design and durability.

Improvements in real-time magnetic resonance (rtMRI) pulse sequences in recent years now enable the acquisition of images in tens of milliseconds [12]. At this rate, cardiac and respiratory motion does not create image artifacts, as known from conventional MRI. Instead, both types of motion can actually be visualized and quantified in almost real time. In addition to depict motion, physiological flow effects can also be characterized using phase contrast MRI (pcMRI). Using this method we exploit the fact that the phase of the MRI signal (in contrast to the magnitude, which is mainly used in conventional MRI) is dependent on the motion (velocity, acceleration) of the protons when flow-encoding gradients are implemented in the MRI pulse sequence. In particular, 2D pcMRI, where the MRI sequence is optimized for flow through the scanning plane, can be used to quantify the blood volumetric flow rate in arteries [10, 13, 14].

To map the phase difference to a velocity, the operator has to prescribe an additional parameter, commonly called VENC (for velocity encoding). If the VENC is too small, flow aliasing results may make the images unsuitable for flow analysis and if the VENC is too large, sensitivity is too poor, resulting in poor contrast-to-noise ratio and large errors in the flow analysis. For normal blood circulation, the maximum velocities in the major cerebral vessels are tabulated and these values can then be used to adjust the VENC. In pathologies such as stenoses, aneurysms, and arteriovascular malformations (AVM), maximum velocities can be increased several fold, which makes it more difficult to select an optimum VENC value.

Compared to the straight vessels of the peripheral vasculature, the placement of the MRI slice in the cerebral vessels is complicated by the tortuous nature of these vessels. The QMRA technique (VasSol, Inc., www.vassolinc.com) [13] has been developed to overcome this obstacle: based on a 3D surface reconstruction of the cerebral vasculature derived from a time-of-flight localizer, QMRA calculates the orientation of the MRI slice at a location on the vessel chosen by the operator. This orientation can then be entered on the MRI scanner console and the 2-D pcMRI images are acquired. After acquisition, the images are transferred to the QMRA computer and a computer-assisted analysis is performed yielding the average flow wave form for one cardiac cycle, the volumetric flow rate time-averaged over one cardiac cycle, and the blood velocities interpolated from the measurement data for the single time points (typically 20) during one cardiac cycle. Recent implementation of a 3D version of the pcMRI technique also allows the visualization of blood flow patterns [15].

Hemodynamic parameters are known to influence the artery wall, for instance, wall shear stress (WSS) has been shown to influence the organization of endothelial cells and to influence endothelial cell gene expression [16]. As there is still no reliable method to measure WSS in vivo, computational techniques, in particular computational fluid dynamics (CFD), has been extensively used to model the hemodynamics in a variety of vascular pathologies, such as stented and unstented abdominal aortic aneurysms (AAA), [17–25] the carotid bifurcation, [26–28] and for cerebral aneurysms [29–32]. CFD simulations need accurate geometries and inflow boundary conditions. Magnetic resonance angiography, either realized through TOF methods or contrast-enhanced techniques, has been demonstrated to provide this information [30, 31, 33, 34]. This concept is further illustrated in Fig. 33.1.

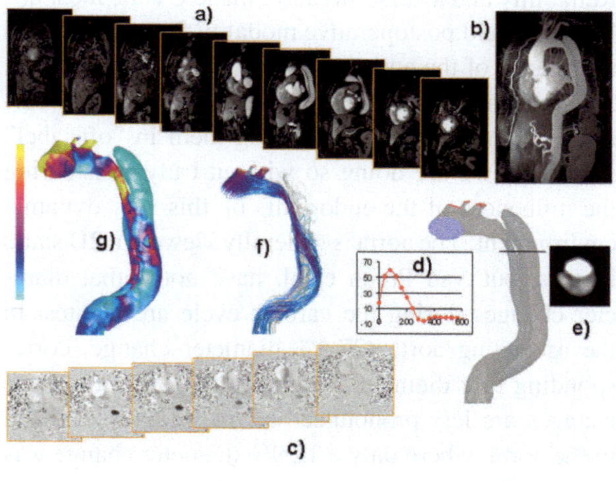

Fig. 33.1 Dynamic magnetic resonance imaging with computational fluid dynamics of Type B aortic dissection

With the advances in MRI described previously, it is clear that this imaging modality plays an essential role in the planning of an endovascular procedure by providing information about the composition of the vessel well, its geometry, the extent of motion in the vessel wall as well as hemodynamic parameters, in particular if combined with computational methods. An MRI may be even more important when considering device design and development.

In addition to this, extensive efforts also went into exploring the role of MRI in the operative invention itself. These efforts are driven primarily by enabling access of the interventionalist to the superior information MRI provides during the operation. Other considerations are reduced exposure of the patient and medical personnel to ionizing radiation. Such hybrid magnetic resonance/X-ray (XMR) suites have been successfully used for real-time guidance during cardiovascular catheterization [35] and drug delivery with MR guidance may soon be feasible in such a suite [36]. Combining MR with flexible robotics (see robotics section) is seen as another way of improving therapeutic goals during endovascular interventions. Current robotic catheters can easily be modified to be primarily nitinol based rather than metal, thereby making them MR friendly. This has the potential of pairing the best imaging modality with the most versatile catheter guidance technology.

Dynamic Computed Tomography

Reliability and availability have made CT the most utilized pre- and postoperative modality for evaluation of aneurysms of the aorta to support endovascular repair. As we continue to challenge the engineering of the current endografts, oftentimes using them in "off-label" situations, we are doing so without truly considering the influences of the endografts on this very dynamic environment. The aorta is generally viewed in 2D static images, but Van Prehn et al. have noted that diameter changes during the cardiac cycle are greatest in the ascending aorta (27.5% diameter change, corresponding to a diameter difference of 7.5 mm). These changes are less pronounced as one progresses distal in the aorta, where only a 12.9% diameter change was noted [37]. A stent graft placed within a structure with such profound movement must take into account how it affects the aortic motion, including side branches. As endovascular devices are being placed more frequently in the thoracic aorta, we find treating the arch or at times even the ascending aorta extremely appealing. Yet, grafts placed in these locations are actually indicated only for the descending aorta. It is important to understand and appreciate that the forces in the ascending aorta are very different from other locations.

When using static images, there is also a very real potential for undersizing with risk for migration or intermittent endoleaks. Therefore, sizing endografts during systole may better represent the percent oversizing actually required for the individual patient. Similarly, stent graft fatigue and fracture may also be a consequence of arterial pulsatility. As many factors are likely to play a role in the motion of the aorta, including but not limited to branches, calcification, tortuosity, and thrombus, it would seem fundamental that each patient be evaluated by dynamic imaging such as CT.

Muhs et al. [38] noted, for example, that placement of a transrenal or an infrarenal aortic device had no effect on renal artery motion but that fenestrated endografts with stents into the renal arteries decreased motion at both the proximal and the distal segment of these vessels. Their interest in looking at renal artery motion was based on their observation that stented renal arteries tended to result in renal complications far more commonly than did the non-stented fenestrations. Evidence has shown that patients who receive fenestrated endografts have a 16% incidence of renal insufficiency when they have a normal preoperative renal function, while patients with preoperative renal insufficiency have a 39% risk of an adverse renal event [39]. Lack of motion may be a critical factor in the clarification of this phenomenon and could potentially lead to changes in practice or endograft design. In the case of branched endografts, Sun et al. used CT virtual intravascular endoscopy (VIE) to investigate the intraluminal appearance of stents in fenestrated vessels [40]. This is based on multislice CT scans measuring 0.625–1 cm in thickness which are formatted on a workstation equipped with Analyze software (version 7.0; AnalyzeDirect, Inc., Lenexa, KS, USA), where the 3D VIE images are generated. This technique could potentially allow the interventionalist to appreciate stent deformities that are likely to give a poor long-term outcome.

Stented branches could also be evaluated by three-dimensional volumetric analysis with, for example, pcMRI and CFD, which could give you the opportunity to evaluate not only the relationships of flow in the renal arteries in relationship to the aorta but also dynamic flow patterns with information such as shear stress, pressure, and stent deformation during the phases of the cardiac cycle.

DynaCT (Digital Subtraction Angiography CT)

Several manufacturers have developed new combined angiography/CT suites, which use flat-panel detector

(FD) technology for improved resolution angiography that is also able to produce improved cone-beam volume CT images. The system permits 3D rotational digital subtraction angiography (DSA) or cone-beam volume CT interchangeably with the same c-arm so that patients do not have to be transferred to a separate unit in order to obtain both imaging modalities. Real-time feedback of endovascular procedures is possible for both DSA and CT. One of the most striking features of this technology is its simplicity, which allows for efficient and fluid endovascular procedures.

When comparing DynaCT to a 16-slice multidetector CT scanner (SOMATOM Sensation 16; Siemens Medical Solution, Erlangen, Germany), Irie et al. found that DynaCT was able to scan a wider area in a shorter period of time, while delivering superior quality coronal and sagittal reconstruction images [41]. DynaCT allows a contrast resolution of 10 HU as well as a slice thickness and in-plane resolution of <1 mm [42]. It is also ideal if the system is able to boast better coverage, which can be a clear advantage when treating an obese patient, but can also serve to decrease exposure times.

One of the concerns with this cone-beam technology is the amount of radiation exposure to the surgeon/interventionalist and the patient. It was found that the total radiation dose is 236 mGy for FD-based DynaCT, while the dose for 3D DSA using the same system is about 50 mGy [41]. Other authors revealed that the dose of radiation for a conventional head CT was similar to that of DynaCT, namely 60 mGy [43]. Numbers quoted by Seimens are 20–60 mGy for a typical CT of the head. Another significant limitation of DynaCT relative to conventional CT is that reconstructions can be quite time consuming, taking up to 5–10 min, although the updated *syngo* DynaCT from Seimens promises processing times of less than a minute and acquisition times of approximately 10 s.

One of the areas where DynaCT has the potential to garner the most advantage is as a navigational tool. As devices become more refined and are able to challenge more complex anatomy, DynaCT will be able to assist obtaining the indispensable 3D imaging necessary to situate and guide the instrument to its target. This can be a particularly attractive feature when one starts discussing potential applications for flexible robotics.

Although not of the quality of images acquired using traditional 64-slice CT scanners, the fluoro CT can be used to import and overlay previously acquired 64-slice images. This registration process allows interventionalists to intervene real time using a previously acquired high-resolution image. For the first time, surgeons will have the ability to rapidly acquire a CT image during the performance of a procedure and to evaluate the adequacy of an intervention. This CT capability is likely to dramatically affect how many procedures are performed, allowing point of service adjustment of an operative plan. A recent comparison of DynaCT with multidetector CT during endovascular repair of abdominal aortic aneurysms (EVARs) found that although multidetector CT had a higher visibility score than did DynaCT, the images obtained during fluoro CT were more than adequate to give measurements and relationships necessary to safely complete EVAR [44]. This realization has potentially important implications for the treatment of acute aortic syndromes, where patients can be taken directly to the operative hybrid suite, be rapidly imaged, while also permitting expedited endovascular or open repair.

It is the combination of this imaging technology with catheter robotics (Fig. 33.2) which potentially revolutionizes our ability to navigate catheters in three dimensions, remotely or semiautomatically over predetermined *glide paths*. The ability to perform real-time fluoro CT also fundamentally alters our ability to localize and biopsy lung or other intrathoracic lesions: CT-guided biopsy can immediately progress to thoracoscopic biopsy to immediate lesion resection. Many other combined or hybrid procedures will develop using open and endoluminal approaches.

The concepts that should remain fundamental today and in the future are that all technological advances in the fields of imaging and robotics should have a common goal. Improved safety and outcome is what one ultimately should measure these advances on. This should happen irrespective of the procedure, whether placing an endograft for Type B aortic dissection, performing a complex venous procedure, challenging a complex aortic arch to stent a carotid, or performing a peripheral intervention.

Intravascular Ultrasound

Intravascular ultrasound (IVUS) creates high-quality cross-sectional views of the vascular system. It therefore has the ability to interrogate vessels and give feedback about the quality of the vessel, its size, and now

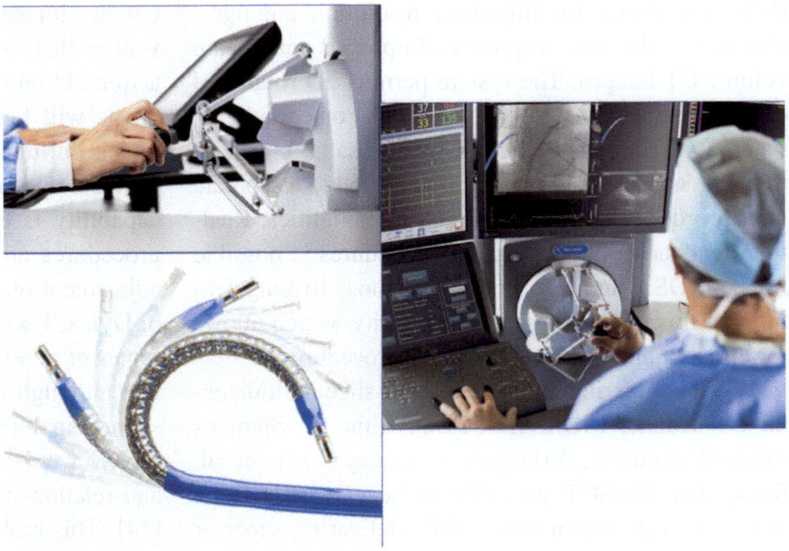

Fig. 33.2 This imaging technology combined with catheter robotics potentially revolutionizes our ability to navigate catheters in three dimensions, remotely or semiautomatically over predetermined *glide paths* (Courtesy of Hansen Medical, Mountain View, CA)

also the potential for virtual histology. Sizing a vessel becomes important in appraising the size of a device required for treatment as well as its proper placement post-deployment. Like any ultrasound image, IVUS is capable of discerning calcifications, thrombus, and stenoses.

Ex vivo validation of the approach has demonstrated accuracies at the highest level of confidence to be 97% for necrotic tissue, 98% for lipidic tissue, 95% for fibrotic tissue, and 98% for calcified tissue [45–47]. In addition, the test results obtained in vivo from a swine animal model showed a good agreement with histology. The ability to do this has not only clinical implications but also academic interests. Vulnerable plaques are more likely to embolize, and obtaining a better understanding of these plaques may guide our future interventions. The IVUS "map" has the ability to assist the interventionalist in understanding more fully how the target lesion will behave, whether it will be resistant to complete stent deployment or be predisposed to embolization. The implications are that the interventionalist may alter the approach and/or choice of device. IVUS provides a clearer appreciation of the interface between the vessel wall and the blood stream, the lumen size, and the success of treatment. Color flow IVUS creates real-time images that have the same appearance as color flow Doppler ultrasound. Therefore, it has improved the ability of the interventionalist to understand the arterial disease they are treating and to assess the completion of treatment [45]. Furthermore, today a larger proportion of our patients have renal insufficiency, and since IVUS has the ability to evaluate the treatment performed, one has the opportunity to decrease the contrast load to the patient and reduce the risk of contrast nephropathy.

IVUS catheters also have the advantage of measuring lengths, which CT scans often underestimate. IVUS is also helpful in the identification of the exact location of an aneurysm when intraluminal thrombus may create a normal angiographic arterial lumen at either landing zone. IVUS may be critical in the identification of a saccular aneurysm or arterial ulcerations filled by thrombus, and atheromatous sources of arterial emboli may at times be identified only by IVUS. However, there are two distinct concerns with IVUS measurements. The first is off-center measurements that confound the image and may misguide the surgeon. The second is tangential measurements on a curve, which would not reflect a true centerline diameter. These can be offset by the use of DynaCT.

It has been shown by Arko and colleagues that the magnitude of cyclic change in aortic diameter can be as high as 11% [48] and this is where the *fourth dimension*, namely movement, comes into play. Murphy et al. also showed the advantages of dynamic IVUS imaging in the low-pressure venous system, where the vena cava was, in the supine position, noted to be elliptical and deform anisotropically during the normal respiratory cycle. A marked displacement (36%) was observed in the short axis during a Valsalva maneuver [49]. This ability of IVUS to reliably define vessel wall excursion can also be a valuable perspective to have in cases such as endovascular exclusion of a Type B dissection.

In a direct comparison of 48 stent-graft implantations in 42 patients, Koschyk et al. were able to show that ultrasound techniques provide additional information superior to that of DSA, such as true and false lumen identification, detection of slow flow in the false lumen in a Type B aortic dissection after stent-graft implantation, and documentation of endoleaks or incomplete stent-graft apposition [50]. IVUS has the ability to help navigate guidewires and catheters in the true lumen of an aortic dissection. The advantages including safety and reliability are clearly reported, resulting in improved procedural outcomes. These advantages can be transmitted to many procedures outside the aorta such as peripheral interventions and carotid stenting.

Thoracic Echocardiography

Since the highly publicized death of the actor John Ritter, who succumbed to a misdiagnosed aortic dissection, there has been much focus on this disease. There is no place where that is more apparent than in the realm of endovascular surgery. Although, the mainstay of stable Type B aortic dissection remains medical therapy, the long-term results are poor with up to 50% mortality at 5 years. Early results with endografts have been promising, so early and definitive diagnosis becomes imperative in expediting care in a timely fashion. Three-dimensional transthoracic echocardiography (3DTTE) has an advantage over two-dimensional transthoracic echocardiography (2DTTE), namely that it can differentiate reverberations and linear artifact from a dissection flap [51]. The Philips iE33 system (Bothell, WA) and a 4× matrix transducer can easily depict not only the flap of the aortic dissection in the descending thoracic aorta, but also the entry tear [52]. The ability to have the resources for evaluating a patient in the emergency room with symptoms consistent with a dissection facilitates expedited care, which could include going to the hybrid suite with a diagnosis and plan in hand.

In the operating room, transesophageal echocardiography (TEE) then becomes important when treating aortic dissections. Koschyk et al. found that during endovascular treatment of aortic dissection, TEE was slightly less suited than IVUS to detect the false/true lumen, the slow flow in the false lumen, the incomplete stent apposition, and entry tears. On the other hand, TEE was much better than angiography. TEE was also better than all modalities at identifying endoleaks [50]. A combination of modalities such as IVUS, TEE, and angiography appears to improve identification of the necessary elements for safe endovascular management of aortic dissection.

Transcranial Doppler Monitoring Endovascular Interventions

Among the more than 150,000 carotid interventions (CIs) performed each year, stroke is the most dreaded complication. Strokes related to CIs are usually due to perioperative hypoperfusion, hyperperfusion, or, most commonly, thromboembolism. Published stroke rates range between 2 and 10%. In addition to symptomatic thromboembolic events, silent subclinical cerebroembolism occurs at an even higher rate. Monitoring for such events is critical to prevent, diagnose, and treat procedure-related embolism.

TCD is the only examination able to monitor intracranial blood flow in real time, thus detecting both asymptomatic and symptomatic cerebrovascular events as they actually happen. TCD shows the blood flow direction and velocity in the intra-cerebral vessels, adding physiologic information to the anatomical images obtained with other imaging modalities. TCD can also detect potential collateral flow signals in the ophthalmic, anterior communicating, and posterior communicating arteries caused by hemodynamically significant carotid stenosis. Understanding the collateral flow patterns can affect the intervention, carotid artery stenting (CAS), particularly when considering which embolic protection device (EPD) to use during CAS, based on the patient's intra-cerebral flow patterns.

One of the limitations of TCD remains its operator/interpretation dependence as well as the occasional suboptimal temporal bone windows, reportedly an issue in approximately 16% of cases [53]. Differentiating gas from particulate matter with a high level of sensitivity has been reported and would help determine the embolic source. The minimum detectable diameter of gaseous emboli has been reported at 10 μm, while particulate emboli can be detected from 40 μm [54]. The pore size of EPD becomes vital to cerebral protection as pore size determines which emboli have the ability to travel to MCA from the working areas. The major limitation of filter pore size is that decreasing the pore size also decreases flow.

Although, there is inconsistency in the actual effects of microemboli, showers of microemboli at post-dilation are strongly associated with adverse cerebral outcome [53]. Both distal filter and protection with carotid flow reversal have been shown to produce a remarkably low incidence of intra-procedural cerebral embolization [55, 56]. Despite this fact, several studies have shown that new intracranial lesions are detected by magnetic resonance (MR) diffusion-weighted imaging (DWI) [57–59]. Hammer et al. found that post-procedural DWI detected new focal ischemic lesions in 40% of patients [60].

During thoracic endograft (TAG) placement, it has been shown that risk factors for developing a stroke are obesity, blood loss, and vascular embolization. Manipulation of the aortic arch during cardiac catheterization has likewise been identified as a source of cerebral embolization. The influences of endograft placement on cerebral embolization and flow are not well described. We have used TCD to quantify the number of microembolic signals (MES,) velocities (VEL), as well as pulsatility index (PI) during different stages of the endograft placement. Our practice is to record middle cerebral artery (MCA) velocities, pulsatility index (PI), and embolic count. What we have noted during these procedures is that embolic counts are generally equal bilaterally, with emboli being most frequent during pigtail catheter use in the diagnostic stage. In the post-dilation stage the velocities and the pulsatility index increase significantly relative to baseline bilaterally. This has potential consequences, particularly in patients with altered extra- and intra-cerebral flow patterns. In this setting, TCD can also play an important role in the planning stages by allowing for preoperative mapping of the intra-cerebral circulation.

Robotics

Flexible Robotics

Hansen Medical is the global leader in flexible robotics and the developer of robotic technology for accurate three-dimensional control of catheter movement (Fig. 33.2). This technology is currently being applied in cardiology, more specifically in electrophysiology, for cardiac ablation therapy in the treatment of aberrant cardiac rhythms. That is because this is the only application for which it is FDA approved. More recently, surgeons have used the Hansen robot to assist in the placement of endovascular grafts for exclusion of an abdominal aortic aneurysm. Although these endografts are placed routinely without such advanced technology, surgeons are often presented with complex anatomy. This recent success speaks not only for its feasibility but also for its safety.

Fenestrated branched grafts for exclusion of thoracoabdominal aneurysms have been shown to have satisfactory results, [61, 62] but these grafts remain available only in select centers in the United States. Elsewhere, factors such as the inherent delay in manufacturing of fenestrated branched grafts, the high degree of planning, and the cost limit its widespread use. Riga et al. circumvented this limitation by performing robot-assisted antegrade in situ-fenestrated stent grafting using the Hansen Robotic system. The versatility of the Sensei robotic system, its accurate positional orientation, minimum instrumentation of the vessel wall, and the ability to reproducibly and precisely return to locations of interest during the procedure were found to be fundamental for success [63]. Potentially, DynaCT could further improve the benefits of such technology by allowing intraoperative 3D imaging. Likewise, guidance by IVUS could also be beneficial, potentially even mounting the IVUS directly on the Artisan Control Catheter.

The advantage of a catheter, which can be guided with a high degree of safety and precision, opens the door for a multitude of applications in vascular surgery. One immediately thinks of procedures which are today particularly challenging as current catheters surrender a tremendous amount of "pushability" and direction. Surgeons are often in the situation where a multitude of catheters are necessary to get to the site of the intended intervention. This is because diagnostic and interventional catheters are currently limited by the ability to simply rotate around one axis. Therefore, one depends on a variety of preformed catheters to fit the existing anatomy. As vascular anatomy is not uniform, catheters are often less than adequate and therefore present a veritable challenge. This can potentially place a patient at risk, particularly in the arterial tree with degenerative atherosclerotic disease. Having a catheter with which the surgeon can control movement in multiple planes would allow him/her to proceed through the arterial anatomy with greater precision, confidence, and safety. As endograft and stent technology improves, so must our ability to deploy these devices be. It is our opinion that flexible robotics will allow us to do just that. Robot-assisted surgery enables the surgeon to make fine, precise, and consistent movements. This ultimately increases procedural speed and reliability.

Surgical Robotics

In 1995, Intuitive Surgical, Inc. created the computer-enhanced robotic system known today as the *da Vinci* Surgical System. The goal of this device was to create familiar hand movements from open surgery while performing operations via a minimally invasive approach. This could effectively remove the difficulties that many surgeons experience using the laparoscopic technique. The advent of robotics in vascular surgery could suddenly make a technically challenging procedure practicable. This rationale is further supported by the development of Intuitive Surgical's *EndoWrist*, a form of telemanipulation that facilitates eye–hand coordination similar to the human brain and provides dual-channel (three-dimensional) vision necessary for the more dexterous maneuvers required to create vascular anastomoses [64]. In 1999, Mohr and colleagues were already successful in performing five coronary artery bypasses and four mitral valve repairs using the *da Vinci* Surgical System [65]. Animal studies confirmed the benefits of robotics, more specifically the *da Vinci* Surgical System, which was shown to reduce the time required to perform an anastomosis, reduce clamp time, and reduce total operative times [66, 67]. Refinements to the *da Vinci* Surgical System include the ability to ceiling mount the unit and again incorporate endoscopic imaging with high-definition flat-panel screens, which are already an integral part of the imaging system.

For thoracoabdominal aneurysms the fundamental question remains whether hybrid repairs are superior, worse, or equivalent to an open surgical repair or simply medical treatment alone. These procedures have been billed as "minimally invasive," but mortality and morbidity rates for these procedures remain high [68]. Robotics has the potential to rapidly advance hybrid procedures for thoracoabdominal aneurysms into a truly minimally invasive realm. Laparoscopic aorto-renal and aorto-mesenteric bypasses have already been performed successfully [69, 70]. Wahlgren et al. reported a successful laparorobotic debranching and endografting [71]. Refinements in technique and robotics should permit these operations to be done with greater ease and safety. Performing such operations in well-equipped hybrid operating rooms with 3D capability (DynaCT) also allows for precise robotic port placement, as well as identification of the target vessel.

Secondary interventions remain a trying issue in endovascular aortic repairs. The majority of these re-interventions remain transfemoral (60%), but at a rate of 6% over the first year and 14% at 4 years, it remains a significant problem. In the Eurostar report, Type II endoleaks are the cause for intervention in 23% [72]. This is another area where surgical robotics could potentially facilitate endovascular surgery. Endovascular exclusion of a Type II endoleak is not always feasible and can lead to surgical conversion if the aneurysm sac continues to expand. The ease of surgical exposure of the aorta and its branches permits interruption of the culprit branches, which are contributing to these endoleaks. This has the potential of preventing multiple endovascular interventions and/or surgical conversion of the aortic repair.

Simulation

Virtual Procedure Rehearsal

As surgeons and devices become better at challenging complex anatomy, a significant amount of time and money can be lost if the access strategy is not sound. Furthermore, there is a substantial risk of exposing the patient to large volumes of contrast and extending fluoroscopy time, with ensuing complications. Virtual procedure rehearsal has the potential of affording the interventionalist the opportunity to perform the procedure before the patient is on the table in order to work out the kinks. Virtually every aspect of endovascular surgery could benefit from such preparation, from a tortuous Type III aortic arch, complex carotid lesion morphology to a difficult hypogastric artery embolization. A recent abstract presented at the New England Society for Vascular Surgery by Hislop et al., but not yet published, used the *Simbionix* simulator to validate the process of rehearsing a case prior to performing the procedure. They found that indeed CTA-derived data could with a high degree of fidelity be converted to an endovascular simulator. In this case it held true for both the aortic arch and carotids.

There are a multitude of virtual simulators available on the market, including SimSuite (Medical Simulation Corporation, Denver, CO), Procedius Vascular Intervention System Training (VIST) Simulator (Mentice AB, Göteborg, Sweden), and the ANGIO Mentor (Simbionix, Cleveland, OH). Irrespective of which system one uses, it is imperative that simulator can with a great degree of reliability mimic actual live cases. Simulators have been used to afford trainees in all aspects of surgery the opportunity to improve their skills prior to "practicing" on patients. This becomes particularly important in our current training paradigms, where work hours are so closely monitored and limited. Furthermore, the wider acceptance of endovascular procedures for carotids, aorta, and lower extremity revascularizations emphasizes the importance of instituting appropriate endovascular training into the curriculum, thereby assuring competent delivery of care [73]. Simulators provide structured learning, meaning different levels of difficulty can be installed [74]. The most flexible units are able to not only provide training for the less experienced but also provide an established clinician to rehearse a case preoperatively.

In order for a simulator to accomplish this task, it must be easy to upload a patient's CT/MR-based films into the system, it must accurately be able to replicate reality, that is, produce reliable imaging and haptics, and must have a wide spectrum of catheters and devices available in its database to accommodate the variable approaches by interventionalists.

Lessons from the Cardiac Catheterization Lab

As in the operating room, the search for increased precision in the cardiac catheterization lab has accelerated as the case mix has increased in complexity and as the ability has appeared to deliver a permanent solution for cardiac problems. A variety of rudimentary robotic approaches have been developed to increase the precision with which intracardiac devices are placed. The first of these devices was the Stereotaxis (Stereotaxis, St. Louis, MO) Niobe system. This system consists of two permanent magnets that reside in close proximity to the patient's thorax, a computer software to control the orientation of their combined magnetic vector in three dimensions, and a magnet-tipped guidewire. By altering the magnetic vector created by the magnets, the operator is able to change the deflection on the guidewire tip and therefore allow it to be steered into the target coronary artery. The advantage is that as a guidewire is advanced around multiple bends, torque control at the wire tip is not lost, since the direction in which the tip is aimed is accomplished by the magnets rather than by manual rotation of the wire. This approach has thus far proved most useful in extremely tortuous vessels and vessels with sharply angled ostia. Research is currently directed at developing applications that will be useful to cross total occlusions.

The Carto System, used in cardiac electrophysiology (EP), was described in 1997 by Ben-Haim's group [75, 76]. The system is composed of a miniature passive magnetic field sensor, an external ultralow magnetic field emitter (location pad), and a processing unit (CARTO, Biosense). The mapped catheter, which is inserted into the body, typically contains conventional electrodes for recording of electrophysiological signals in the heart. Embedded in its tip is the location sensor. The location pad is mounted on a tray positioned underneath the patient's chest. This pad contains three magnetic coils that generate ultralow magnetic fields (5×10^{-6} to 5×10^{-5} T), which decay as a function of distance from that coil. The distance from each coil to the sensor in the catheter can be measured. The location is then determined from the intersection of the theoretical spheres whose radii are the distances measured by the sensor. The system can locate not only the three-dimensional coordinates of the catheter tip (its sensor in *x, y, z*), but also the yaw, the pitch, and the roll. Additionally, the electrodes record the extracellular field signals from the heart tissue in their proximity. When the location information is combined with the local electrical signal, the local activation time of that location, relative to a given reference (e.g., the QRS of the electrogram or that of a fixed intracardiac electrode, such as one in the coronary sinus), the system allows for the creation of three-dimensional activation maps of cardiac arrhythmias. Such three-dimensional maps can be enhanced by merging the geometry with that of previously acquired CT or MRI scans. Another system utilized in EP is the NavX–EnSite system (St Jude Medical). The system uses three pairs of electrode patches arranged along three orthogonal axes. Patches are conventionally placed in these locations: (1) sternum, (2) interscapular region, (3) anterior right neck, (4) left groin, (5) right lateral chest, (6) left lateral chest. With this distribution, three orthogonal electric fields are created using 5.7-kHz current sources driving the three pairs of opposing patches. The currents are sourced sequentially, allowing the potential at an intracardiac electrode to be sensed for each axis in turn. The potentials sensed are proportional to the distance from the patches, which allows determination of the location in three dimensions. A reference electrode in the heart (usually the coronary sinus) forms the origin of the coordinate system. Once the location of the catheter is known, roving the catheter around the cavity of interest allows for the creation of a three-dimensional shell of such chamber. Activation times can be simultaneously recorded. The system is particularly quick at generating chamber geometry, given the fact that multiple electrode catheters can be used and that signals are recorded from each electrode. Medical positioning devices have also come into use in the catheterization laboratory. The Mediguide system (Mediguide, Haifa, IL) uses a GPS-like detector that is mounted on the flat-panel detector and a probe that is miniaturized and placed on a catheter tip. Once an image is registered on the system, the medical positioning system can alert the operator when the intracardiac catheter reaches its target. Precision is approximately 1 mm. This operation can potentially be performed without fluoroscopy. A second application allows the lumen of the target vessel to be mapped with intravascular ultrasound (IVUS). A balloon or a stent can then be advanced through the vessel, and the course overlaid on a virtual image that is obtained from a three-dimensional reconstruction of the IVUS image. Since the IVUS reconstruction is able to provide more detail than does a coronary angiogram, this approach theoretically allows more precise placement of an intracardiac stent and may prove useful in placing ostial stents and avoiding side branches.

Conclusion

Appreciating how advances in imaging technologies can improve endovascular decisions and outcomes means that one is willing to embrace a variety of modalities. The reality is that there is not a single imaging apparatus, which by itself excludes all others. In order to be an accomplished interventionalist, one needs to be well aware of the different modalities including their advantages and pitfalls. As such we believe that it is fundamental that if you are evaluating a structure, which is in constant motion, you should include this dimension in your evaluation and planning. One should not view a stent as a structure placed within a static tube but rather seek to understand how delivering a device in a vessel will modify the motion of that vessel and how the vessel in turn will affect the structure of the device. This is most important when we consider that probably at last a third of the devices implanted in the vascular system are off-label interventions.

References

1. Fishman MC, Naidich JB, Stein HL: Vascular magnetic resonance imaging, *Radiol Clin North Am* 24(3):485–501, September 1986.
2. Merickel MB, Carman CS, Brookeman JR, Mugler JP 3rd, Brown MF, Ayers CR: Identification and 3-D quantification of atherosclerosis using magnetic resonance imaging, *Comput Biol Med* 18(2):89–102, 1988.
3. Saam T, Hatsukami TS, Takaya N et al.: The vulnerable, or high-risk, atherosclerotic plaque: noninvasive MR imaging for characterization and assessment, *Radiology* 244(1):64–77, July 2007.
4. Karmonik C, Basto P, Morrisett JD: Quantification of carotid atherosclerotic plaque components using feature space analysis and magnetic resonance imaging, *Conf Proc IEEE Eng Med Biol Soc* 1:3102–3105, 2006.
5. Martin K, Brownfield D, Karmonik C et al.: Short-term tracking of atherosclerosis in operated and unoperated human carotid arteries by high resolution magnetic resonance imaging, *World J Surg.* 31(4):723–732, April 2007.
6. Adams GJ, Greene J, Vick GW 3rd et al.: Tracking regression and progression of atherosclerosis in human carotid arteries using high-resolution magnetic resonance imaging, *Magn Reson Imaging* 22(9):1249–1258, November 2004.
7. Canet-Soulas E, Letourneur D: Biomarkers of atherosclerosis and the potential of MRI for the diagnosis of vulnerable plaque, *Magma* 20(3):129–142, June 2007.

8. Kawahara I, Nakamoto M, Kitagawa N et al.: Potential of magnetic resonance plaque imaging using superparamagnetic particles of iron oxide for the detection of carotid plaque, *Neurol Med Chir (Tokyo)* 48(4):157–161, April 2008; discussion 161–152.
9. Howarth S, Li ZY, Trivedi RA et al.: Correlation of macrophage location and plaque stress distribution using USPIO-enhanced MRI in a patient with symptomatic severe carotid stenosis: a new insight into risk stratification, *Br J Neurosurg* 21(4):396–398, August 2007.
10. Berstein MA, King KF, Zhou XJ: *Handbook of MRI pulse sequences*, New York, 2004, Elsevier, Academic Press.
11. Bogaert J, Dymarkowski S, Taylor AM: *Clinical Cardiac MRI*, Berlin Heidelberg New York, 2005, Springer.
12. Wintersperger BJ, Nikolaou K, Muhling O et al.: [Determining global heart function with real time TrueFISP in one respiratory cycle], *Radiologe* 44(2):152–157, February 2004.
13. Zhao M, Amin-Hanjani S, Ruland S, Curcio AP, Ostergren L, Charbel FT: Regional cerebral blood flow using quantitative MR angiography, *AJNR Am J Neuroradiol* 28(8):1470–1473, September 2007.
14. Zhao M, Charbel FT, Alperin N, Loth F, Clark ME: Improved phase-contrast flow quantification by three-dimensional vessel localization, *Magn Reson Imaging* 18(6):697–706, July 2000.
15. Meckel S, Stalder AF, Santini F et al.: In vivo visualization and analysis of 3-D hemodynamics in cerebral aneurysms with flow-sensitized 4-D MR imaging at 3 T, *Neuroradiology* 50:473–484, March 19, 2008.
16. Malek AM, Izumo S: Control of endothelial cell gene expression by flow, *J Biomech* 28(12):1515–1528, December 1995.
17. Kleinstreuer C, Li Z: Analysis and computer program for rupture-risk prediction of abdominal aortic aneurysms, *Biomed Eng Online* 5:19, 2006.
18. Kleinstreuer C, Li Z, Farber MA: Fluid-structure interaction analyses of stented abdominal aortic aneurysms, *Annu Rev Biomed Eng* 9:169–204, 2007.
19. Li Z, Kleinstreuer C: A new wall stress equation for aneurysm-rupture prediction, *Ann Biomed Eng* 33(2):209–213, February 2005.
20. Li Z, Kleinstreuer C: Blood flow and structure interactions in a stented abdominal aortic aneurysm model, *Med Eng Phys* 27(5):369–382, June 2005.
21. Li Z, Kleinstreuer C: Fluid-structure interaction effects on sac-blood pressure and wall stress in a stented aneurysm, *J Biomech Eng* 127(4):662–671, August 2005.
22. Li Z, Kleinstreuer C: Analysis of biomechanical factors affecting stent-graft migration in an abdominal aortic aneurysm model, *J Biomech* 39(12):2264–2273, 2006.
23. Li Z, Kleinstreuer C: Computational analysis of type II endoleaks in a stented abdominal aortic aneurysm model, *J Biomech* 39(14):2573–2582, 2006.
24. Li Z, Kleinstreuer C, Farber M: Computational analysis of biomechanical contributors to possible endovascular graft failure, *Biomech Model Mechanobiol* 4(4):221–234, December 2005.
25. Scotti CM, Shkolnik AD, Muluk SC, Finol EA: Fluid-structure interaction in abdominal aortic aneurysms: effects of asymmetry and wall thickness, *Biomed Eng Online* 4:64, 2005.
26. Lee SW, Antiga L, Spence JD, Steinman DA: Geometry of the carotid bifurcation predicts its exposure to disturbed flow, *Stroke* 39(8):2341–2347, August 2008.
27. Xue Y, Gao P, Lin Y, Dai C: Preliminary study of hemodynamics in human carotid bifurcation by computational fluid dynamics combined with magnetic resonance angiography, *Acta Radiol* 48(7):788–797, September 2007.
28. Xue YJ, Gao PY, Duan Q, Lin Y, Dai CB: Preliminary study of hemodynamic distribution in patient-specific stenotic carotid bifurcation by image-based computational fluid dynamics, *Acta Radiol* 49(5):558–565, June 2008.
29. Karmonik C, Benndorf G, Klucznik R, Haykal H, Strother CM: Wall shear stress variations in basilar tip aneurysms investigated with computational fluid dynamics, *Conf Proc IEEE Eng Med Biol Soc* 1:3214–3217, 2006.
30. Karmonik C, Klucznik R, Benndorf G: Comparison of velocity patterns in an AComA aneurysm measured with 2D phase contrast MRI and simulated with CFD, *Technol Health Care* 16(2):119–128, 2008.
31. Karmonik C, Klucznik R, Benndorf G: Blood flow in cerebral aneurysms: comparison of phase contrast magnetic resonance and computational fluid dynamics—preliminary experience, *Rofo* 180(3):209–215, March 2008.
32. Mantha A, Karmonik C, Benndorf G, Strother C, Metcalfe R: Hemodynamics in a cerebral artery before and after the formation of an aneurysm, *AJNR Am J Neuroradiol* 27(5):1113–1118, May 2006.
33. Kock SA, Nygaard JV, Eldrup N et al.: Mechanical stresses in carotid plaques using MRI-based fluid-structure interaction models, *J Biomech* 41(8):1651–1658, 2008.
34. Yoshida K, Nagao T, Okada K et al.: Development of a system for measuring wall shear stress in blood vessels using magnetic resonance imaging and computational fluid dynamics, *Igaku Butsuri* 27(3):136–149, 2008.
35. Rhode KS, Sermesant M, Brogan D et al.: A system for real-time XMR guided cardiovascular intervention, *IEEE Trans Med Imaging* 24(11):1428–1440, November 2005.
36. Arepally A: Targeted drug delivery under MRI guidance, *J Magn Reson Imaging* 27(2):292–298, February 2008.
37. van Prehn J, Vincken KL, Muhs BE et al.: Toward endografting of the ascending aorta: insight into dynamics using dynamic cine-CTA, *J Endovasc Ther* 14(4):551–560, August 2007.
38. Muhs BE, Vincken KL, Teutelink A et al.: Dynamic cine-computed tomography angiography imaging of standard and fenestrated endografts: differing effects on renal artery motion, *Vasc Endovascular Surg* 42(1):25–31, February–March 2008.
39. Haddad F, Greenberg RK, Walker E et al.: Fenestrated endovascular grafting: the renal side of the story, *J Vasc Surg* 41(2):181–190, February 2005.
40. Sun Z, Allen YB, Nadkarni S, Knight R, Hartley DE, Lawrence-Brown MM: CT virtual intravascular endoscopy in the visualization of fenestrated stent-grafts, *J Endovasc Ther* 15(1):42–51, February 2008.
41. Irie K, Murayama Y, Saguchi T et al.: Dynact soft-tissue visualization using an angiographic C-arm system: initial clinical experience in the operating room, *Neurosurgery* 62(3 Suppl 1):266–272, March 2008; discussion 272.

42. Meyer BC, Frericks BB, Albrecht T, Wolf KJ, Wacker FK: Contrast-enhanced abdominal angiographic CT for intra-abdominal tumor embolization: a new tool for vessel and soft tissue visualization, *Cardiovasc Intervent Radiol* 30(4):743–749, July–August 2007.
43. Heran NS, Song JK, Namba K, Smith W, Niimi Y, Berenstein A: The utility of DynaCT in neuroendovascular procedures, *AJNR Am J Neuroradiol* 27(2):330–332, February 2006.
44. Eide KR, Odegard A, Myhre HO, Lydersen S, Hatlinghus S, Haraldseth O: DynaCT during EVAR—a comparison with multidetector CT, *Eur J Vasc Endovasc Surg* 37(1):23–30, January 2009.
45. Diethrich EB, Irshad K, Reid DB: Virtual histology and color flow intravascular ultrasound in peripheral interventions, *Semin Vasc Surg* 19(3):155–162, September 2006.
46. Diethrich EB, Pauliina Margolis M, Reid DB et al.: Virtual histology intravascular ultrasound assessment of carotid artery disease: the Carotid Artery Plaque Virtual Histology Evaluation (CAPITAL) study, *J Endovasc Ther* 14(5):676–686, October 2007.
47. Irshad K, Millar S, Velu R, Reid AW, Diethrich EB, Reid DB: Virtual histology intravascular ultrasound in carotid interventions, *J Endovasc Ther* 14(2):198–207, April 2007.
48. Arko FR, Murphy EH, Davis CM 3rd, Johnson ED, Smith ST, Zarins CK: Dynamic geometry and wall thickness of the aortic neck of abdominal aortic aneurysms with intravascular ultrasonography, *J Vasc Surg* 46(5):891-896, November 2007; discussion 896–897.
49. Murphy EH, Johnson ED, Arko FR: Evaluation of wall motion and dynamic geometry of the inferior vena cava using intravascular ultrasound: implications for future device design, *J Endovasc Ther* 15(3):349–355, June 2008.
50. Koschyk DH, Nienaber CA, Knap M et al.: How to guide stent-graft implantation in type B aortic dissection? Comparison of angiography, transesophageal echocardiography, and intravascular ultrasound, *Circulation* 112(9 Suppl):I260–I264, August 30, 2005.
51. Htay T, Nanda NC, Agrawal G, Ravi BS, Dod HS, McGiffin D: Live three-dimensional transthoracic echocardiographic assessment of aortic dissection, *Echocardiography* 20(6):573–577, August 2003.
52. Yelamanchili P, Nanda NC, Patel V, Bogabathina H, Baysan O: Definitive diagnosis of descending thoracic aortic dissection by real time/live three-dimensional transthoracic echocardiography, *Echocardiography* 23(2):158–161, February 2006.
53. Ackerstaff RG, Suttorp MJ, van den Berg JC et al.: Prediction of early cerebral outcome by transcranial Doppler monitoring in carotid bifurcation angioplasty and stenting, *J Vasc Surg* 41(4):618–624, April 2005.
54. Georgiadis D, Uhlmann F, Astler M, Cencetti S, Zierz S: Automated identification of Doppler microembolic signals: comparison of two techniques, *Neurol Res* 22(7):738–740, October 2000.
55. Criado E, Fontcuberta J, Orgaz A, Flores A, Doblas M: Transcervical carotid stenting with carotid artery flow reversal: 3-year follow-up of 103 stents, *J Vasc Surg* 46(5):864–869, November 2007.
56. Ribo M, Molina CA, Alvarez B, Rubiera M, Alvarez-Sabin J, Matas M: Transcranial Doppler monitoring of transcervical carotid stenting with flow reversal protection: a novel carotid revascularization technique, *Stroke* 37(11):2846–2849, November 2006.
57. du Mesnil de Rochemont R, Schneider S, Yan B, Lehr A, Sitzer M, Berkefeld J: Diffusion-weighted MR imaging lesions after filter-protected stenting of high-grade symptomatic carotid artery stenoses, *AJNR Am J Neuroradiol* 27(6):1321–1325, June–July 2006.
58. Jaeger H, Mathias K, Drescher R et al.: Clinical results of cerebral protection with a filter device during stent implantation of the carotid artery, *Cardiovasc Intervent Radiol* 24(4):249–256, July–August 2001.
59. Palombo G, Faraglia V, Stella N, Giugni E, Bozzao A, Taurino M: Late evaluation of silent cerebral ischemia detected by diffusion-weighted MR imaging after filter-protected carotid artery stenting, *AJNR Am J Neuroradiol* 29(7):1340–1343, August 2008.
60. Hammer FD, Lacroix V, Duprez T et al.: Cerebral microembolization after protected carotid artery stenting in surgical high-risk patients: results of a 2-year prospective study, *J Vasc Surg* 42(5):847-853, November 2005; discussion 853.
61. Semmens JB, Lawrence-Brown MM, Hartley DE, Allen YB, Green R, Nadkarni S: Outcomes of fenestrated endografts in the treatment of abdominal aortic aneurysm in Western Australia (1997–2004), *J Endovasc Ther* 13(3):320–329, June 2006.
62. O'Neill S, Greenberg RK, Haddad F, Resch T, Sereika J, Katz E: A prospective analysis of fenestrated endovascular grafting: intermediate-term outcomes, *Eur J Vasc Endovasc Surg* 32(2):115–123, August 2006.
63. Riga CV, Bicknell CD, Wallace D, Hamady M, Cheshire N: Robot-assisted antegrade in-situ fenestrated stent grafting, *Cardiovasc Intervent Radiol* 23:220–26, 2008.
64. Martinez B: Robotics in vascular surgery, *Ann Vasc Surg* 18(5):619–620, September 2004.
65. Mohr FW, Falk V, Diegeler A et al.: Computer-enhanced "robotic" cardiac surgery: experience in 148 patients, *J Thorac Cardiovasc Surg* 121(5):842–853, May 2001.
66. Ruurda JP, Wisselink W, Cuesta MA, Verhagen HJ, Broeders IA: Robot-assisted versus standard videoscopic aortic replacement. A comparative study in pigs, *Eur J Vasc Endovasc Surg* 27(5):501–506, May 2004.
67. Malhotra SP, Le D, Thelitz S et al.: Robotic-assisted endoscopic thoracic aortic anastomosis in juvenile lambs, *Heart Surg Forum* 6(1):38–42, 2002.
68. Resch TA, Greenberg RK, Lyden SP et al.: Combined staged procedures for the treatment of thoracoabdominal aneurysms, *J Endovasc Ther* 13(4):481–489, August 2006.
69. Javerliat I, Coggia M, Bourriez A, Di Centa I, Cerceau P, Goeau-Brissonniere OA: Total laparoscopic aortomesenteric bypass, *Vascular* 12(2):126–129, March 2004.
70. Hsu TH, Gill IS, Sung GT, Meraney A, McMahon JT, Novick AC: Laparoscopic aortorenal bypass, *J Endourol* 14(2):123–131, March 2000.
71. Wahlgren CM, Skelly C, Shalhav A, Bassiouny H: Hybrid laparorobotic debranching and endovascular repair of thoracoabdominal aortic aneurysm, *Ann Vasc Surg* 22(2):285–289, March 2008.
72. Hobo R, Buth J: Secondary interventions following endovascular abdominal aortic aneurysm repair using current endografts. A EUROSTAR report, *J Vasc Surg* 43(5):896–902, May 2006.

73. Van Herzeele I, Aggarwal R, Neequaye S, Darzi A, Vermassen F, Cheshire NJ: Cognitive training improves clinically relevant outcomes during simulated endovascular procedures, *J Vasc Surg* 48(5):1223–1230, November 2008.
74. Tsang JS, Naughton PA, Leong S, Hill AD, Kelly CJ, Leahy AL: Virtual reality simulation in endovascular surgical training, *Surgeon* 6(4):214–220, August 2008.
75. Ben-Haim SA, Osadchy D, Schuster I, Gepstein L, Hayam G, Josephson ME: Nonfluoroscopic, in vivo navigation and mapping technology, *Nat Med* 2(12):1393–1395, December 1996.
76. Gepstein L, Hayam G, Ben-Haim SA: A novel method for nonfluoroscopic catheter-based electroanatomical mapping of the heart. In vitro and in vivo accuracy results, *Circulation* 95(6):1611–1622, March 18, 1997.

Index

T.J. Fogarty, R.A. White (eds.), *Peripheral Endovascular Interventions*,
DOI 10.1007/978-1-4419-1387-6, © Springer Science+Business Media, LLC 1998, 2010

U

MIX
Papier aus verantwortungsvollen Quellen
Paper from responsible sources
FSC® C105338
FSC
www.fsc.org

If you have any concerns about our products,
you can contact us on
ProductSafety@springernature.com

In case Publisher is established outside the EU,
the EU authorized representative is:
Springer Nature Customer Service Center GmbH
Europaplatz 3, 69115 Heidelberg, Germany

Printed by Libri Plureos GmbH
in Hamburg, Germany